PRIMARY HEMATOLOGY

PRIMARY HEMATOLOGY

Edited by

AYALEW TEFFERI, MD

*Consultant, Division of Hematology and Internal Medicine, Mayo Clinic
and Mayo Foundation; Associate Professor of Medicine, Mayo Medical School;
Rochester, Minnesota*

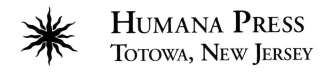

HUMANA PRESS
TOTOWA, NEW JERSEY

For additional copies, pricing for bulk purchases, and/or information about other Humana titles, contact Humana at 999 Riverview Drive, Suite 208, Totowa, NJ 07512 or at any of the following numbers: Tel: 973-256-1699; Fax: 973-256-8341; E-mail: humana@humanapr.com or visit our website at http://humanapress.com

As new scientific information becomes available through basic and clinical research, recommended treatments and drug therapies undergo changes. The authors and publisher have made all reasonable attempts to make this book accurate, up to date, and in accord with accepted standards at the time of publication. The authors, editor, and publisher are not responsible for errors or omissions or for consequences from application of the book, and make no warranty, expressed or implied, in regard to the contents of the book. Any practice described in this book should be applied by the reader in consultation with a physician and taking regard of the unique circumstances that may apply in each situation. The reader is advised always to check product information (package inserts) for changes and new information regarding dose and contraindications before administering any drug. Caution is especially urged when using new or infrequently ordered drugs. Nothing in this publication implies that Mayo Clinic endorses the products or equipment mentioned in this book.

All articles, comments, opinions, conclusions, or recommendations are those of the author(s) and do not necessarily reflect the views of the publisher or of Mayo Clinic.

Cover design by Patricia F. Cleary.
Cover illustration by Garry Post.

This publication is printed on acid-free paper. ⊚
ANSI Z39.48-1984 (American National Standards Institute)
Permanence of Paper for Printed Library Materials.

Photocopy Authorization Policy:
Authorization to photocopy items for internal or personal use, or the internal or personal use of specific clients, is granted by Humana Press Inc., provided that the base fee of US $10.00 per copy, plus US $00.25 per page, is paid directly to the Copyright Clearance Center at 222 Rosewood Drive, Danvers, MA 01923. For those organizations that have been granted a photocopy license from the CCC, a separate system of payment has been arranged and is acceptable to Humana Press Inc. The fee code for users of the Transactional Reporting Service is: [0-89603-664-2/01 $10.00 + $00.25].

Printed in the United States of America.   10 9 8 7 6 5 4 3 2 1

Library of Congress Cataloging-in-Publication Data

PREFACE

The discipline of hematology is enriched by tremendous diversity in pathology and its close identification with molecular biology. Routine clinical practice often involves the diagnosis and management of anemia, sickle cell disorders, hypercoagulable states, and monoclonal gammopathy of undetermined significance. Hematologic malignancies, including lymphoma and leukemia, are some of the most treatable cancers, and treatment outcome has been improved by the use of hematopoietic stem cell transplantation. Hematologists, oncologists, cardiologists, internists, and family practitioners are all equally interested in the problems of thrombosis and bleeding. Transfusion medicine, the use of hematopoietic growth factors, and cancer chemotherapy have all become integral components of hematology practice. A holistic approach to patient care requires some background information on ethics and statistics. This book was written with all of these considerations in mind.

I thank the authors of the chapters for their diligence in providing fine contributions. I am appreciative of the efforts of the Section of Scientific Publications at Mayo Clinic in the production of this book, especially Virginia A. Dunt, Mary L. Schwager, Mary K. Horsman, Roberta J. Schwartz, and LeAnn M. Stee.

Ayalew Tefferi, M.D.

To

Dr. Robert L. Phyliky

and

Dr. H. Clark Hoagland

decent human beings, master clinicians, and loyal friends

LIST OF COLOR PLATES

Color plates appear in an insert following p. 242.

CONTENTS

CONTRIBUTORS

ALEX A. ADJEI, MD, PHD • *Consultant, Division of Medical Oncology, Mayo Clinic and Mayo Foundation; Assistant Professor of Oncology, Mayo Medical School; Rochester, Minnesota*

JOSEPH H. BUTTERFIELD, MD • *Consultant, Division of Allergy and Outpatient Infectious Disease and Internal Medicine, Mayo Clinic and Mayo Foundation; Associate Professor of Medicine, Mayo Medical School; Rochester, Minnesota*

GERARDO COLON-OTERO, MD • *Consultant, Division of Hematology/Oncology, Mayo Clinic Jacksonville, Jacksonville, Florida; Assistant Professor of Medicine, Mayo Medical School; Rochester, Minnesota*

COSTAS L. CONSTANTINOU, MD • *Fellow in Hematology, Mayo Graduate School of Medicine, Rochester, Minnesota*

ANGELA DISPENZIERI, MD • *Senior Associate Consultant, Division of Hematology and Internal Medicine, Mayo Clinic and Mayo Foundation; Assistant Professor of Medicine, Mayo Medical School; Rochester, Minnesota*

VIRGIL F. FAIRBANKS, MD • *Consultant, Divisions of Hematology and Internal Medicine and Hematopathology, Mayo Clinic and Mayo Foundation; Professor of Medicine and of Laboratory Medicine, Mayo Medical School; Rochester, Minnesota*

RAFAEL FONSECA, MD • *Senior Associate Consultant, Division of Hematology and Internal Medicine, Mayo Clinic and Mayo Foundation; Assistant Professor of Medicine, Mayo Medical School; Rochester, Minnesota*

THOMAS M. HABERMANN, MD • *Consultant, Division of Hematology and Internal Medicine, Mayo Clinic and Mayo Foundation; Associate Professor of Medicine, Mayo Medical School; Rochester, Minnesota*

C. CHRISTOPHER HOOK, MD • *Consultant, Division of Hematology and Internal Medicine, Mayo Clinic and Mayo Foundation; Assistant Professor of Medicine, Mayo Medical School; Rochester, Minnesota*

ROBERT A. KYLE, MD • *Consultant, Division of Hematology and Internal Medicine, Mayo Clinic and Mayo Foundation; Professor of Medicine and of Laboratory Medicine, Mayo Medical School; Rochester, Minnesota*

MARK R. LITZOW, MD • *Head of a Section of Hematology and Internal Medicine, Mayo Clinic and Mayo Foundation; Assistant Professor of Medicine, Mayo Medical School; Rochester, Minnesota*

S. BREANNDAN MOORE, MD • *Chair, Division of Transfusion Medicine, Mayo Clinic and Mayo Foundation; Professor of Laboratory Medicine, Mayo Medical School; Rochester, Minnesota*

PIERRE NOËL, MD • *Chair, Division of Hematology/Oncology, Mayo Clinic Scottsdale, Scottsdale, Arizona; Assistant Professor of Medicine, Mayo Medical School; Rochester, Minnesota*

RAJIV K. PRUTHI, MD • *Consultant, Division of Hematology and Internal Medicine, Mayo Clinic and Mayo Foundation; Assistant Professor of Medicine, Mayo Medical School; Rochester, Minnesota*

GEORGENE SCHROEDER, MS • *Statistician, Cancer Center Statistics, Mayo Clinic and Mayo Foundation; Rochester, Minnesota*

LAWRENCE A. SOLBERG, JR., MD, PHD • *Chair, Division of Hematology/Oncology, Mayo Clinic Jacksonville, Jacksonville, Florida; Associate Professor of Medicir Mayo Medical School; Rochester, Minnesota*

AYALEW TEFFERI, MD • *Consultant, Division of Hematology and Internal Medicine Mayo Clinic and Mayo Foundation; Associate Professor of Medicine, Mayo Medical School; Rochester, Minnesota*

ZELALEM TEMESGEN, MD • *Consultant, Division of Infectious Diseases and Internal Medicine, Mayo Clinic and Mayo Foundation; Assistant Professor of Medicine, Mayo Medical School; Rochester, Minnesota*

I

ANEMIA AND OTHER CYTOPENIAS

1

A Practical Approach to the Diagnosis of Anemia

Ayalew Tefferi, MD

Contents

INTRODUCTION

Anemia can be defined as a persistent decline in either hemoglobin or hematocrit level from a previous baseline value. Because baseline values in individual patients are variable and often unavailable, the presence of anemia is implied from a statistically determined reference range that represents 95% of the "normal" population. As such, accurate interpretation of a particular hemoglobin level requires use of an appropriate age-, sex-, and race-adjusted reference range and realization that a value that is slightly below normal may be a statistical outlier rather than an indication of a disease state. In general, hemoglobin levels are 1 to 2 g lower in women and African-American men than in white males.

AN OVERVIEW OF THE CAUSES OF ANEMIA

Anemia occurs as a result of either decreased marrow output or excess peripheral blood loss (Fig. 1). In the former, the problem may either arise at the stem cell level (intrinsic or injury-associated stem cell defect) or affect the latter stages of effective red cell production. An intrinsic stem cell defect is often a clonal (neoplastic) process that usually results in either trilineage aplasia (aplastic anemia) or ineffective hematopoiesis (myelodysplastic process). The stem cell also may be injured by external causes (drugs, radiation exposure). Even when the stem cell compartment is relatively healthy and functional, effective red cell production may be impaired as a result of bone marrow infiltration (metastatic cancer, fibrosis), nutritional deficiency (iron, vitamin B_{12}, or folate), or erythroid hypoproliferation. Erythroid hypoproliferation may be mediated by

From: *Primary Hematology*
Edited by: A. Tefferi © Mayo Foundation for Medical Education and Research, Rochester, MN

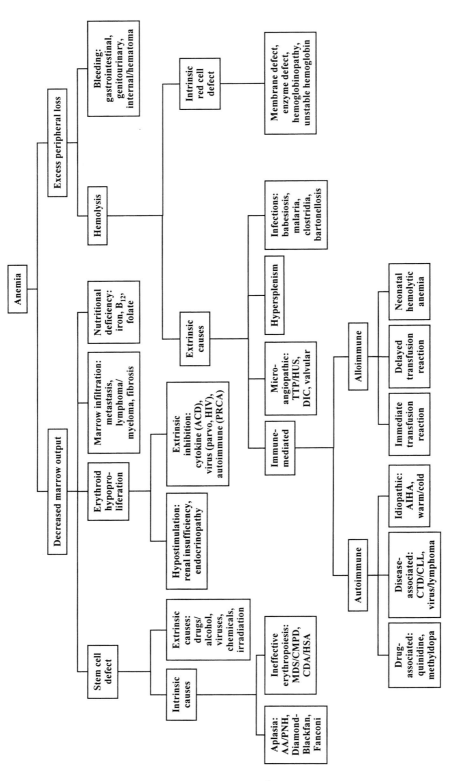

Fig. 1. Clinical classification of anemias. AA, aplastic anemia; ACD, anemia of chronic disease; AIHA, autoimmune hemolytic anemia; CDA, congenital dyserythropoietic anemia; CLL, chronic lymphocytic leukemia; CMPD, chronic myeloproliferative disease; CTD, connective tissue disease; DIC, disseminated intravascular coagulation and fibrinolysis syndrome; HIV, human immunodeficiency virus; HSA, hereditary sideroblastic anemia; HUS, hemolytic uremic syndrome; MDS, myelodysplastic syndrome; parvo, parvovirus; PNH, paroxysmal nocturnal hemoglobinuria; PRCA, pure red cell aplasia; TTP, thrombotic thrombocytopenic purpura.

cytokines (anemia of chronic disease), viruses (parvovirus infection), autoimmunity (pure red cell aplasia), or lack of growth factors or hormones (renal insufficiency, hypogonadism).

Peripheral blood loss may be caused by bleeding or hemolysis. Hemolysis occurs as a result of either an intrinsic red cell defect or an external cause (extrinsic). The red cell may be defective at the membrane (hereditary spherocytosis), hemoglobin (sickle cell anemia), or enzyme (glucose-6-phosphate dehydrogenase deficiency) level. Extrinsic hemolysis may either be immune-mediated or result from infections (malaria, *Clostridia*) or endothelial injury (microangiopathic hemolytic anemia) (Fig. 1). Drugs can cause hemolysis by either an immune (quinidine) or oxidative (dapsone) mechanism. In the latter instance, affected patients usually have an underlying red cell enzyme deficiency (glucose-6-phosphate dehydrogenase deficiency). Non–drug-associated immune hemolytic anemia may be either idiopathic or associated with viral infection, chronic lymphoproliferative disorders, or connective tissue disease. Finally, alloimmune mechanisms may also cause severe hemolysis (ABO mismatched transfusion, neonatal hemolytic anemia).

THE STEPWISE APPROACH TO DIAGNOSIS

History

The general symptoms of anemia are often nonspecific and indicate either decreased intravascular volume or the inadequacy of oxygen transport to tissues. Compensatory mechanisms include increased cardiac output and respiratory rate (palpitations, dyspnea on exertion, exercise intolerance). Symptoms of decreased oxygen delivery to the central nervous system include light-headedness, somnolence, headache, and lack of attention. Fatigue is a universal complaint but lacks specificity. In addition, anemia may precipitate angina or congestive heart failure in patients with underlying coronary artery disease or cardiomyopathy, respectively, and claudication in those with peripheral vascular disease. Alternatively, a gradual onset of anemia, regardless of severity, may be relatively asymptomatic because of physiologic adjustment by the body. Historical clues for a specific cause of anemia are outlined in Table 1.

Physical Examination

Anemia from acute blood loss or hemolysis is associated with signs of hypovolemia, including orthostatic hypotension, tachycardia, light-headedness, and exertional dyspnea. These signs are often not impressive in chronic anemia because of volume compensation. Mucocutaneous pallor signifies decreased hemoglobin and is appreciated best in the conjunctiva, nail beds, and roof of the mouth. Severe iron deficiency anemia may be associated with koilonychia (spooning of the nails), cheilitis (fissures in the corner of the mouth), glossitis (smooth and sore tongue), blue sclerae, and dysphagia from postcricoid esophageal web (Plummer-Vinson syndrome). Megaloblastic anemia (B_{12} deficiency) may be associated with a beefy and atrophic tongue, diarrhea, and neurologic signs (impaired gait, paresthesias, decreased vibration sense in distal extremities). The presence of lymphadenopathy or other signs of malignancy may require a bone marrow examination to exclude marrow invasion.

Jaundice accompanies severe hemolytic anemia that also may be associated with splenomegaly. The splenomegaly results from functional hypertrophy of the spleen. Clinical features of patients with major thalassemia include skeletal deformities (chip-

Table 1
Historical Clues for Specific Causes of Anemia

Type of anemia	Historical clue	Cause
Iron deficiency	Infants	Increased demand during growth, milk is poor in iron content
	Children	Increased demand during growth
	Young women	Loss of iron with menstruation
	Pregnancy	Diversion of iron to the fetus and placenta
	Chronic bleeding	Nose, lungs (IPH, GPS), gastrointestinal (ulcer, varices, hiatal hernia, colon cancer, polyps, angiodysplasia, AVM, IBD, Meckel's diverticulum, HHT), genitourinary (schistosomiasis, uterine fibroids, metro-menorrhagia), blood donation, NSAID use, intravascular hemolysis and loss in the urine (PNH, cardiac valve prostheses), factitious
	Pica	Craving for ice or other items
	Gastric surgery	Gastric acid is needed to reduce dietary Fe^{3+} to Fe^{2+}, which is better absorbed
	Intestinal surgery	Because iron is absorbed in the duodenum and proximal jejunum, reduced absorptive area and rapid transit time might affect absorption
	Intestinal parasites	Hookworm infestation in tropical countries
	Sprue	Decreased intestinal absorption
B_{12} deficiency	Gastric surgery or achlorhydria in elderly	Decreased availability of pepsin and gastric acid to release food-bound B_{12} and sometimes IF insufficiency
	Pancreatic insufficiency	Inability to release B_{12} from the R protein-B_{12} complex
	Intestinal parasites	*Diphyllobothrium latum* (fish tapeworm)
	Intestinal surgery	B_{12} is absorbed in the distal ileum
	Malabsorptive states	Celiac or tropical sprue, IBD (e.g., Crohn's disease)
	Strict vegetarian	Dietary B_{12} is found in animal products only. Animals get the vitamin from microorganism-infested plants. The B_{12} is synthesized by microorganisms
	NO exposure	Inhibition of methionine synthase
	Neurologic manifestations	Peripheral neuropathy, abnormal gait, impaired position sense, fatigue, poor memory, depression, psychosis
Folate deficiency	Malabsorption	Intestinal surgery, celiac or tropical sprue

Table 1 continued

Type of anemia	Historical clue	Cause
	Alcoholism	Poor dietary intake, impaired folate utilization
	Increased demand	Pregnancy, hemolysis, psoriasis (increased cell turnover)
	Drugs	Anticonvulsants (impaired intestinal absorption), sulfasalazine (impaired absorption and utilization)
Hemolysis	Drug history	Antimalarials, antiarrhythmics (quinidine, procainamide), sulfa drugs (dapsone), α-methyldopa
	Jaundice	Increased indirect bilirubin from hemoglobin catabolism
	Cholelithiasis	Pigmented (bilirubinate) stones
	Splenomegaly	Functional hypertrophy of spleen macrophages
	Neurologic signs	TTP
	Renal insufficiency	Hemolytic uremic syndrome, TTP
	Lymphoma, CLL, CTD	Immune hemolytic anemia
	Recent transfusion	Delayed transfusion reaction
	Recent travel	Malaria
Hemoglobinopathies	Ethnic origin	Ethnic groups from Africa, Asia, the Mediterranean basin
	Family history	Traits are dominant, disease usually recessive
	Leg ulcers	Sickle cell disease
Anemia of chronic disease	Chronic infections	AIDS, osteomyelitis, endocarditis
	Inflammatory state	Rheumatoid arthritis, temporal arteritis, SLE
	Chronic conditions	Diabetes
Marrow injury or disease	Chemotherapy	Stem cell toxicity
	Radiation therapy	Stem cell toxicity
	Benzene, lead	Stem cell toxicity
	Hematologic or nonhematologic malignancy	May be from ineffective erythropoiesis (MDS, AMM), autoimmune or viral suppression of RBC production (PRCA, AA), or marrow replacement (lymphoma, myeloma, metastatic cancer)
	Drugs	Chloramphenicol, chemotherapy, phenytoin (neutropenia), gold, antibiotics, NSAID
Hormone deficiency	Renal insufficiency	Relative hypoerythropoietinemia
	Orchiectomy	Hypoandrogenism
	Endocrine disorders	Hypogonadism, hypothyroidism

Abbreviations: AA, aplastic anemia; AIDS, acquired immunodeficiency syndrome; AMM, agnogenic myeloid metaplasia; AVM, arteriovenous malformation; CLL, chronic lymphocytic leukemia; CTD, connective tissue disease; GPS, Goodpasture's syndrome; HHT, hereditary hemorrhagic telangiectasia; IBD, inflammatory bowel disease; IF, intrinsic factor; IPH, idiopathic pulmonary hemosiderosis; MDS, myelodysplastic syndrome; NO, nitrous oxide; NSAID, nonsteroidal anti-inflammatory drug; PNH, paroxysmal nocturnal hemoglobinuria; PRCA, pure red cell aplasia; RBC, red blood cells; SLE, systemic lupus erythematosus; TTP, thrombotic thrombocytopenic purpura.

munk facies) from marrow expansion, splenomegaly, and features of hemochromatosis (bronze skin, hepatomegaly, cardiomyopathy, hypogonadism, arthritis, growth retardation). The hand-foot syndrome (acral dysesthesia accompanied by redness and swelling) may develop in children with sickle cell disease.

Telangiectasias around the mouth and tongue suggest hereditary hemorrhagic telangiectasia. Hemolytic anemia associated with Wilson's disease (hereditary defect in biliary copper excretion and toxic accumulation of copper in the liver and basal ganglia) may be accompanied by liver disease (cirrhosis), neurologic signs (dysarthria, incoordination), and Kayser-Fleischer ring (brown deposition of copper around the cornea that requires a slit-lamp examination for detection). A history of dark urine may indicate hemoglobinuria from intravascular hemolysis associated with either paroxysmal nocturnal hemoglobinuria or unstable hemoglobins. Finally, the presence of physical stigmata may suggest Fanconi's anemia (short stature, thumb hypoplasia, microcephaly, hypopigmentation) or dyskeratosis congenita (reticulated hyperpigmentation, dystrophic nails).

Complete Blood Cell Count

The initial laboratory approach in determining the cause of anemia is to use all available data from the complete blood cell count. This provides red cell indices (mean corpuscular volume, red blood cell count, and red blood cell distribution width) that are crucial in narrowing the diagnostic possibilities. One should start with classifying anemias according to red cell size; mean corpuscular volumes less than 80, 80 to 100, or more than 100 femtoliters (fL) define microcytic, normocytic, and macrocytic anemia, respectively. A differential diagnosis list can then be formulated for each of these three divisions (Table 2).

Within the context of a microcytic anemia, an increased red blood cell distribution width (a numerical quantification of anisocytosis) or increased platelet count suggests iron deficiency anemia. Iron deficiency anemia is one of the causes of reactive thrombocytosis. Alternatively, an increased red blood cell count suggests thalassemia minor, and the red blood cell distribution width in this instance is often, but not always, normal. In the presence of macrocytic anemia, a normal distribution width suggests round macrocytosis (e.g., alcohol), and an increased distribution width suggests oval macrocytosis (e.g., B_{12} or folate deficiency, myelodysplastic syndrome). Also, a mean corpuscular volume more than 110 fL is unusual in round macrocytosis and is consistent with vitamin B_{12} or folate deficiency, hydroxyurea therapy, or a hematologic malignancy (e.g., myelodysplastic syndrome, large granular lymphocytic leukemia, aplastic anemia).

Peripheral Blood Smear

After analysis of the complete blood cell count, the next step is to obtain a peripheral blood smear. In iron deficiency anemia, the smear usually shows anisocytosis (variation in size) and poikilocytosis (variation in shape), and in severe cases it may show cigar-shaped red blood cells and elliptocytes. Polychromasia (the Wright-Giemsa stain equivalent of reticulocytosis) and basophilic stippling are conspicuously absent. Target cells characterize thalassemia but also may be seen after splenectomy and in liver disease. The smear is unremarkable in anemia of chronic disease. Dimorphic red blood cells (two distinctly sized red cell populations) may be seen in myelodysplastic syndrome and in transfused patients. Macrocytes may further be classified as round (alcohol, tobacco, reticulocytosis) or oval (nutritional deficiency, myelodysplastic syndrome, drug-induced) (Table 2). In alcohol-related round macrocytosis, target cells are often appreciated.

Table 2
Classification of Anemia by Red Cell Size (Mean Corpuscular Volume, MCV)

Anemia		
Microcytic, MCV < 80 fL	*Normocytic, MCV 80-100 fL*	*Macrocytic, MCV > 100 fL*
Iron deficiency anemia	Anemia of chronic disease	Round macrocytosis
Thalassemia	Early iron deficiency anemia	Alcohol and tobacco abuse
Anemia of chronic disease	Anemia of renal insufficiency	Liver disease
Temporal arteritis	Hemolytic anemia	Hypothyroidism
Rheumatoid arthritis	Nonthalassemic	Acute hemolytic anemia
Chronic osteomyelitis	hemoglobinopathies	Oval macrocytosis
Miscellaneous	Aplastic anemia	Drug effect
Sideroblastic anemia	Pure red cell aplasia	Large granular lymphocyte
Mostly MDS (RARS)	Drug-induced BM suppression	disorder
Rarely hereditary	BM infiltrative process	Aplastic anemia
Rarely lead toxicity	Metastatic cancer	Vitamin B_{12} deficiency
Hodgkin's disease	Hematologic malignancy	Folic acid deficiency
Castleman's disease	Fibrosis	Myelodysplastic syndrome
Agnogenic myeloid		Hydroxyurea therapy
metaplasia		

Abbreviations: BM, bone marrow; MDS, myelodysplastic syndrome; RARS, refractory anemia with ringed sideroblasts.

Hypersegmented or hypolobulated (pseudo–Pelger-Huët anomaly) neutrophils accompany either B_{12} or folate deficiency or myelodysplastic syndrome, respectively.

The Peripheral Smear

The peripheral blood smear is the most practical diagnostic tool for the hematologist. A drop of blood is applied against a glass slide that is subsequently stained with polychrome stains (Wright-Giemsa) to permit identification of the various cell types. These stains are mixtures of basic dyes (methylene blue) that are blue and acidic dyes (eosin) that are red. As such, acid components of the cell (nucleus, cytoplasmic RNA, basophilic granules) stain blue or purple, and basic components of the cell (hemoglobin, eosinophilic granules) stain red or orange. In addition to the polychrome stains, monochrome stains are sometimes used to visualize young red cells (reticulocyte stain), denatured hemoglobin (Heinz body stain), or cellular iron (Prussian blue stain).

The peripheral blood smear examination also allows detection of red cell inclusion bodies. Howell-Jolly bodies (nuclear remnants) are present in both anatomical (surgical splenectomy) and functional (sickle cell disease, amyloidosis, celiac sprue) asplenia. Heinz bodies represent denatured hemoglobin and are present in drug-induced hemolytic anemias, thalassemias, unstable hemoglobinopathy, and glucose-6-phosphate dehydrogenase deficiency. A well-prepared smear may reveal intra-erythrocyte parasites, including malaria and babesiosis. Aggregates of ribosomes are sometimes visible and stain with the Wright-Giemsa stain as punctate basophilia and are seen as basophilic stippling. When such basophilic stippling is coarse rather than punctate, it implies lead poisoning or thalassemia.

The smear is also critical for revealing schistocytes (microangiopathic hemolytic anemia, including thrombotic thrombocytopenic purpura/hemolytic uremic syndrome and valvular hemolysis), sickle cells, tear-drop cells (associated with a bone marrow infiltrative process including metastatic cancer and bone marrow fibrosis), spherocytes (hereditary spherocytosis, autoimmune hemolytic anemia), acanthocytes (liver disease, abetalipoproteinemia, asplenia), and bite cells (drug-induced hemolysis, glucose-6-phosphate dehydrogenase deficiency, unstable hemoglobinopathies).

Specific Laboratory Tests

The final step requires, first, formulation of the most likely diagnostic possibilities (based on history, physical examination, complete blood cell count) and, second, the ordering of specific laboratory tests. The specific laboratory tests are discussed separately for each of the three major categories of anemia: microcytic, normocytic, and macrocytic.

MICROCYTIC ANEMIA

Figure 2 outlines an algorithm for the laboratory evaluation of microcytic anemia.

Step 1: Determination of Serum Ferritin

All patients with microcytic anemia should have determination of the serum ferritin value to exclude the presence of an iron-depleted state either by itself or in conjunction with another cause of microcytic anemia. The other serum iron studies (serum iron, total iron-binding capacity, transferrin saturation) lack specificity and therefore have limited value in the evaluation of iron deficiency anemia. If the serum ferritin value is low, it is diagnostic of an iron-depleted state. If it is more than 60 μg/L, iron deficiency anemia is unlikely. If the value is between 20 and 60 μg/L, then the possibility of an acute inflammatory state being responsible for the "inappropriately" normal serum ferritin is entertained (ferritin is an acute-phase reactant). However, we do not recommend a bone marrow biopsy (to evaluate marrow iron stores) for further clarification. Instead, an effort is made to make an alternative diagnosis or empirically treat the patient with iron supplements and reevaluate in 3 to 6 months.

Interpretation of Iron Studies

The amount of iron in the body is estimated by measuring iron and iron-associated proteins in the serum. Iron in the serum either is bound to a transporter protein called transferrin or is part of a soluble form of storage iron called ferritin (normal range, 20-300 μg/L). Serum iron bound to transferrin is measured as serum iron (normal range, 35-150 μg/dL). Free and iron-bound transferrin is measured as the total iron-binding capacity (normal range, 250-400 μg/dL). The serum iron value divided by the total iron-binding capacity and expressed in percentage is called the serum iron percentage saturation (normal range, 14%-50%). The most reliable test to assess iron deficiency anemia is measurement of serum ferritin. A low serum ferritin value is diagnostic of an iron-depleted state. A value more than 60 μg/L is unusual in iron deficiency anemia, and a value between 20 and 60 μg/L may occur in patients with liver disease and inflammatory diseases (rheumatoid arthritis) despite low body iron stores. We do not recommend determination of serum iron, total iron-binding capacity, or percentage saturation to evaluate iron deficiency anemia because values also may be low in anemia of chronic disease.

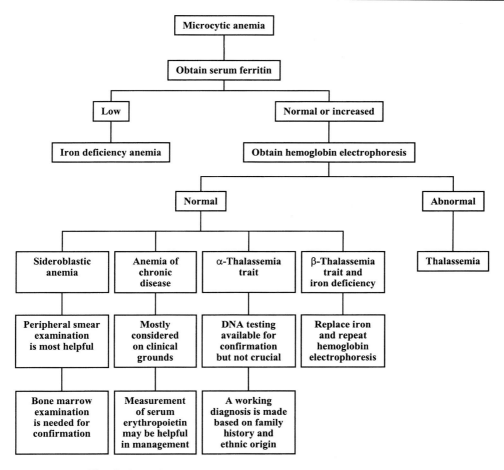

Fig. 2. Stepwise laboratory evaluation of microcytic anemia.

Step 2: Hemoglobin Electrophoresis

If the serum ferritin level is normal, the next step is to perform hemoglobin electrophoresis. This test is helpful for revealing the presence of some, but not all, thalassemic syndromes (hemoglobin disorders characterized by decreased globin-chain synthesis). Most thalassemia syndromes (α and β) do not involve structural variants of the hemoglobin molecule. As such, hemoglobin electrophoresis may not detect an abnormality. This is especially true for α-thalassemia. Like any other thalassemia syndrome, α-thalassemia may exist as either the trait (2 out of 4 allele deletion) or the disease (3 out of 4 allele deletion). In the former instance, the result of hemoglobin electrophoresis is normal. In the latter instance (hemoglobin H disease), the presence of β-chain tetramers (hemoglobin H) is revealed by hemoglobin electrophoresis (5%-30%).

β-Thalassemia also occurs as a trait (1 out of 2 allele mutation) or symptomatic disease (homozygous or double heterozygous allele defect). In β-thalassemia trait, the level of hemoglobin A_2 ($\alpha_2\delta_2$) may increase from the normal value of 2% to 3%-5%. However, if iron deficiency coexists, the hemoglobin A_2 level may be normal. Therefore, a normal hemoglobin A_2 level may not exclude the possibility of β-thalassemia trait unless a simultaneously measured normal serum ferritin level is documented. In β-thalassemia disease, the hemoglobin electrophoresis reveals mostly hemoglobin F ($\alpha_2\gamma_2$). Furthermore, severe microcytic anemia from any thalassemia disorder is associated with an increased serum level of lactic dehydrogenase because of the underlying ineffective hematopoiesis.

Finally, rare microcytic thalassemia disorders that result from structural hemoglobin variants are directly identified by hemoglobin electrophoresis. These include both β (hemoglobin Lepore) and α (hemoglobin Constant Spring) structural variants. Hemoglobin Lepore results from a nonhomologous crossover of β and δ gene sequences that creates a fusion β-chain variant (δβ), resulting in a disorder that is clinically similar to β-thalassemia. Similarly, hemoglobin Constant Spring is clinically similar to α-thalassemia and is a result of termination codon mutation that creates an elongated α chain. Finally, hemoglobin E (a structural hemoglobinopathy that is prevalent in Southeast Asia) is also characterized by microcytosis because of a decreased synthesis of the abnormal β chain. This results from an RNA splice site mutation associated with the production of an alternative mRNA that is not effectively translated.

Step 3: Microcytic Anemia Associated With Normal Serum Ferritin and Normal Hemoglobin Electrophoresis

As mentioned, the presence of a normal or increased serum ferritin value and a normal hemoglobin electrophoresis pattern does not rule out the possibility of α-thalassemia trait. Currently, there exists a molecular genetic test (polymerase chain reaction-based assay) that may detect the deletion defect in most patients with α-thalassemia. However, the test is expensive and suspected cases may be managed without laboratory confirmation. The information on ethnic origin and family history is often adequate to establish a working diagnosis and provide genetic counseling for affected patients.

Similarly, there is no positive blood test that confirms anemia of chronic disease or sideroblastic anemia. These are often considered on the basis of the clinical presentation, peripheral smear examination, and, if indicated, bone marrow examination. The microcytosis in sideroblastic anemia is accompanied by red cell dimorphism and coarse basophilic stippling, whereas the bone marrow reveals ringed sideroblasts. The peripheral smear in anemia of chronic disease is unremarkable. Moderate to severe microcytic anemia might accompany chronic infections (endocarditis), Hodgkin's disease, Castleman's disease (angiofollicular lymph node hyperplasia), temporal arteritis, rheumatoid arthritis, and other connective tissue diseases.

NORMOCYTIC ANEMIA

Step 1: Rule Out Readily Treatable Causes

The critical issue in the evaluation of any form of anemia is to recognize treatable causes early. In a patient with normocytic anemia, both iron and vitamin B_{12} deficiencies are possible causes despite their usual association with microcytic and macrocytic anemia, respectively. Other treatable causes of normocytic anemia include anemia of renal insufficiency, bleeding, and hemolysis. As such, the initial investigation of normocytic anemia should include determination of serum ferritin, B_{12}, or folate levels (to address nutritional causes) and the serum creatinine level (to address anemia of renal insufficiency). If the serum creatinine level is increased, determination of serum erythropoietin may be helpful for confirming relative hypoerythropoietinemia. If these initial tests are unrevealing and bleeding is not clinically suspected, then the possibility of hemolysis is considered (see below).

Step 2: The Hemolysis Workup

The hemolytic anemias can be broadly divided into extravascular hemolytic anemia occurring in the monocyte-macrophage system of the spleen and intravascular hemolytic anemia occurring by lysis inside the blood vessels. During both processes, laboratory evidence of increased cell destruction (increased lactic dehydrogenase), increased hemoglobin catabolism (increased levels of indirect bilirubin, carbon monoxide, and urinary urobilinogen), and bone marrow regenerative effort (reticulocytosis) may be appreciated. Therefore, when a hemolytic process is suspected, the initial tests should include measurement of lactic dehydrogenase, indirect bilirubin, and reticulocyte count. Because carbon monoxide and urinary urobilinogen also may be increased in smokers and patients with liver disease, respectively, and because the additional information is not critical, these tests are usually not used during the evaluation of hemolysis.

On the basis of the pathophysiologic discussions in the tip boxes on extravascular and intravascular hemolytic anemia (see below), serum haptoglobin is expected to be low in all intravascular cases and in moderate to severe extravascular cases because of hemoglobin spillage from macrophages during extravascular hemolysis. Therefore, determination of serum haptoglobin is more helpful in screening for the presence of hemolysis in general, rather than distinguishing intravascular from extravascular disease. Furthermore, serum haptoglobin also may be decreased in other disorders (Table 3). However, the demonstration of hemosiderinuria or free plasma and urine hemoglobin is relatively specific for intravascular hemolytic anemia. Of these tests, the determination of urinary hemosiderin is preferred because of better sensitivity, especially during intermittent (paroxysmal nocturnal hemoglobinuria) or low-grade (valvular) hemolysis.

Extravascular Hemolytic Anemia

In extravascular hemolytic anemia, the red cell is first phagocytosed (ingested) into the macrophage (mostly in the spleen), where the cell membrane is disrupted and the hemoglobin separates into heme and globin (via lysozymal enzymes). The globin disintegrates into its constituent amino acids and the heme is oxidized (heme oxygenase) by cleavage of the porphyrin ring into biliverdin, iron, and carbon monoxide. The biliverdin is reduced (biliverdin reductase) to bilirubin, which is released into the bloodstream, picked up by albumin, and carried to the liver (hepatocytes). This bilirubin is water insoluble and is called indirect bilirubin (unconjugated). In the hepatocytes, the indirect bilirubin is conjugated to glucuronic acid (bilirubin glucuronyl transferase), which makes it soluble, and then is secreted into the small intestine as direct bilirubin via the bile duct. Intestinal bilirubin is degraded by bacteria into urobilinogen, which may be reabsorbed and secreted in the urine.

Intravascular Hemolytic Anemia

In intravascular hemolytic anemia, free hemoglobin in the plasma readily dissociates into $\alpha\beta$ hemoglobin dimers. These are promptly picked up by haptoglobin (a plasma protein, α_2-globulin, which binds free hemoglobin) and are carried to the liver, where they undergo intrahepatocyte degradation in a similar fashion to that previously described for intramacrophage hemolysis. The leftover hemoglobin dimers (unbound to haptoglobin) in the plasma are filtered by the kidneys (32 kDa), or the iron in the dimers is oxidized into the ferric state (methemoglobin). The methemoglobin in the plasma splits into globin and ferriheme (non-enzymatic). Ferriheme is picked up by either albumin (methemalbumin) or hemopexin (another plasma protein that binds ferriheme) and carried to the liver (hepatocytes) for the usual heme degradation process. The hemoglobin dimers excreted by the kidneys are resorbed by the proximal tubular cells, where they are degraded into hemosiderin (a storage form of iron), bilirubin, and globin. The tubular cells are shed every 2 to 7 days and the cellular iron deposits can be demonstrated with a Prussian blue stain of spun urine sediment (hemosiderinuria). In severe intravascular hemolytic anemia, excess filtered hemoglobin appears in the urine (hemoglobinuria).

Table 3
Causes of Decreased Haptoglobin

Intravascular hemolysis
Moderate to severe extravascular hemolysis
Ineffective hematopoiesis (B_{12} deficiency, myelodysplastic syndrome)
Severe liver disease
Pregnancy or estrogen therapy
Rare cases of congenital haptoglobin deficiency

Step 3: Pinpointing the Specific Cause of Hemolysis

The aforementioned tests (reticulocyte count, lactic dehydrogenase, haptoglobin, indirect bilirubin) constitute the preliminary tests required in the evaluation of a general hemolytic state. In addition, if one suspects intravascular hemolytic anemia, determination of urinary hemosiderin is a useful additional test. Although plasma hemopexin, free plasma or urinary hemoglobin, and plasma methemalbumin can be measured, these tests are usually not ordered in clinical practice because of limited additional information. A stepwise algorithm for identifying the cause of intravascular hemolytic anemia is outlined in Figure 3.

Evaluation of extravascular hemolytic anemia requires a comprehensive examination of the history, peripheral smear, and additional specific laboratory tests. Ethnic origin from Southeast Asia, Africa, or the Mediterranean basin suggests the presence of a hemoglobinopathy or enzymopathy. Some of these abnormalities may be exacerbated by drug ingestion (dapsone, antimalarial agents, sulfa drugs, fava beans). The presence of spherocytes (densely pigmented small round red cells) in the peripheral blood smear suggests either hereditary spherocytosis or autoimmune hemolytic anemia. The two are distinguished by the presence of red cell-bound antibodies (Coombs test) in autoimmune hemolytic anemia but not in hereditary spherocytosis. Chronic extravascular hemolytic anemia is characterized by functional hypertrophy of the spleen (splenomegaly) and the occasional formation of pigment stones (bilirubinate stones). Other tests that may be useful in the evaluation of immune-mediated hemolytic anemia include cold agglutinin titer and the Donath-Landsteiner test. The aforementioned laboratory tests are done stepwise to investigate the cause of extravascular hemolytic anemia (Fig. 4).

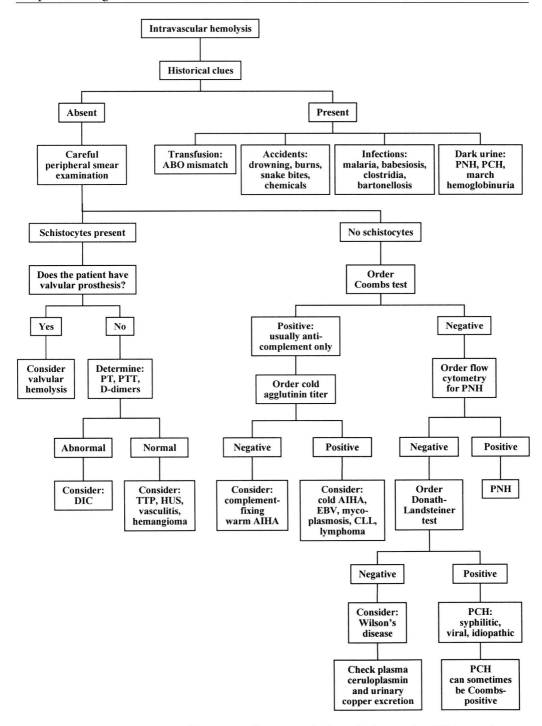

Fig. 3. Stepwise identification of the cause of intravascular hemolytic anemia. AIHA, autoimmune hemolytic anemia; CLL, chronic lymphocytic leukemia; DIC, disseminated intravascular coagulation; EBV, Epstein-Barr virus; HUS, hemolytic uremic syndrome; PCH, paroxysmal cold hemoglobinuria; PNH, paroxysmal nocturnal hemoglobinuria; PT, prothrombin time; PTT, partial thromboplastin time; TTP, thrombotic thrombocytopenic purpura.

The Coombs Test

The purpose of the Coombs test is to determine whether red cell-binding antibody (IgG) or complement (C3) is present on the red cell membrane (the direct Coombs test) or sera (the indirect Coombs test). In the direct test, the patient's red cells are incubated with polyspecific rabbit anti-human IgG and anti-complement. In the presence of red cell-bound antibodies or complement, red cell agglutination occurs (positive Coombs test). In the indirect test, red cells other than the patient's (heterologous red cells) are first incubated with the patient's serum (to allow circulating antibodies to bind to the red cells), and then a direct Coombs test is performed. Monospecific sera can be used to detect only IgG or complement on the red cell. However, the Coombs test does not detect IgM antibody and its presence is surmised by the detection of complement only on the red cells. A positive direct Coombs test suggests the presence of autoantibodies to red cells. A positive indirect Coombs with a negative direct test suggests the presence of alloantibodies to red cells. The indirect Coombs test is also helpful for determining red cell antigen specificity to antibody.

Cold Agglutinin Titer and the Donath-Landsteiner Test

The cold agglutinin titer test is used to detect and quantify cold-reacting immunoglobulins (mostly IgM). Red cells from affected patients are incubated at 4°C overnight in serially diluted autologous serum. The dilution factor that results in red cell agglutination is reported as the cold agglutinin titer. Clinically relevant hemolysis occurs at titers of more than 1:256. Most cold autoimmune hemolytic anemia is IgM-mediated, whereas paroxysmal cold hemoglobinuria is IgG-mediated. The laboratory diagnosis of paroxysmal cold hemoglobinuria involves the Donath-Landsteiner test. This test involves preincubation of a patient's red cells with autologous serum at 4°C followed by the addition of complement at 37°C. A positive test is characterized by visible hemolysis. Antigen specificity in cold autoimmune hemolytic anemia is "i" for infectious mononucleosis and "P" for paroxysmal cold hemoglobinuria.

Step 5: Normocytic Anemia Not Associated With Nutritional Deficiency, Renal Insufficiency, Bleeding, or Hemolysis

The primary consideration in this setting is either anemia of chronic disease or a primary bone marrow disorder. It is not always easy to differentiate the two. Obviously, the history is critical in this regard and also for excluding other causes of normocytic anemia, including drug effect, alcoholism, radiation therapy, chemical exposure, and recent trauma or surgery. The presence of comorbid conditions, increased erythrocyte sedimentation rate, and a peripheral smear study that is unremarkable support the diagnosis of anemia of chronic disease.

Alternatively, the peripheral smear examination may suggest a myelodysplastic syndrome (dimorphic red cell populations, pseudo-Pelger-Huët anomaly), a marrow infiltrative process such as metastatic cancer or bone marrow fibrosis (teardrop-shaped and nucleated red cells, immature myeloid precursors), multiple myeloma (red cell rouleaux formation), or lymphoma or leukemia (circulating neoplastic cells). In addition to anemia, a primary bone marrow disease also results in quantitative and qualitative abnormalities of white blood cells and platelets. A severe degree of unexplained anemia with a low reticulocyte count suggests either aplastic anemia or pure red cell aplasia.

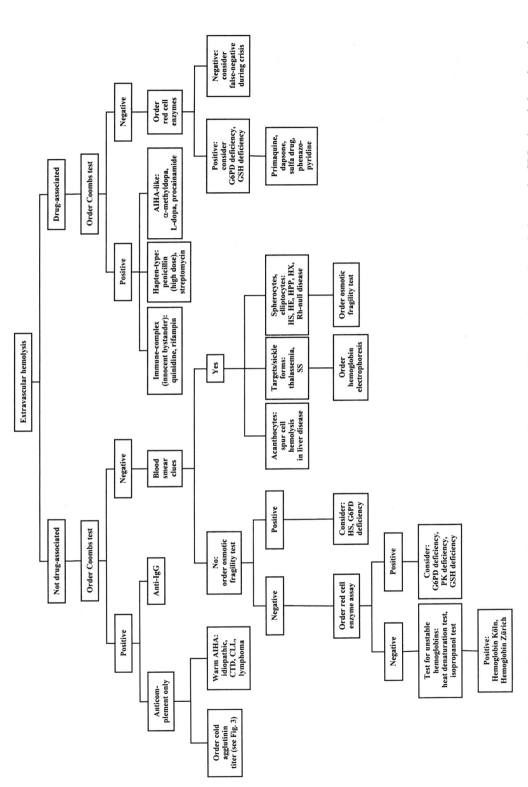

Fig. 4. Stepwise identification of the cause of extravascular hemolytic anemia. AIHA, autoimmune hemolytic anemia; CLL, chronic lymphocytic leukemia; CTD, connective tissue disease; G6PD, glucose-6-phosphate dehydrogenase; GSH, glutathione reductase; HE, hereditary elliptocytosis; HPP, hereditary pyropoikilocytosis; HS, hereditary spherocytosis; HX, hereditary xerocytosis; PK, pyruvate kinase deficiency; SS, sickle cell disease.

Laboratory results that are suggestive of specific diseases include increased total protein (multiple myeloma), hypercalcemia (multiple myeloma, metastatic cancer), and increased C-reactive protein (an inflammatory state). A definite diagnosis is often not possible even with additional information from bone marrow biopsy. Furthermore, the results from the bone marrow examination do not necessarily help modify management. Therefore, it is reasonable to formulate a working diagnosis based on history and peripheral smear data and to defer a more aggressive workup in case of clinical deterioration.

MACROCYTIC ANEMIA

Step 1: Rule Out the Presence of Drugs That Cause Macrocytosis

For evaluation of macrocytic anemia (Fig. 5), the first step is to exclude substance (alcohol, tobacco) or drug (hydroxyurea, methotrexate, trimethoprim, zidovudine [AZT], 5-fluorouracil) use that is associated with macrocytosis. Among the offenders, hydroxyurea is the most notorious and induces the largest increases in mean corpuscular volume (oval macrocytosis of > 110 fL). Lesser degrees of macrocytosis (100-110 fL) may result from the use of AZT (oval macrocytosis), chemotherapy (oval macrocytosis), or alcohol (round macrocytosis).

Step 2: Rule Out Nutritional Causes of Macrocytic Anemia

In any patient with macrocytosis, B_{12} or folate deficiency must be ruled out. In folate deficiency, serum folate levels are usually low. However, because recent dietary changes may affect the serum folate level, red blood cell folate levels are sometimes used to document chronic folate deficiency (red cells acquire folate at the time of birth and the cellular concentration does not change during their life span). Because red cell folate assays are not very accurate, the serum homocysteine level may be used, instead, to evaluate folate deficiency (the serum homocysteine level is increased during folate deficiency as a result of impaired folate-dependent conversion of homocysteine to methionine).

In B_{12} deficiency, serum B_{12} levels are usually low. However, B_{12} levels may be spuriously low during pregnancy, in elderly subjects, and in patients with low leukocyte counts. In these instances and in borderline-low B_{12} level, a more sensitive and highly specific test is measurement of the serum methylmalonic acid level (B_{12} cofactor activity is required to convert methylmalonyl coenzyme A to succinyl coenzyme A). A normal level excludes the possibility of B_{12} deficiency. Once B_{12} deficiency is confirmed, the next step is to determine the cause. In this regard, the initial test is to screen for the presence of intrinsic factor antibodies. If these antibodies are present, then a working diagnosis of pernicious anemia is made and additional testing may not be necessary. Otherwise, the Schilling test is performed. This particular test helps differentiate pernicious anemia from primary intestinal malabsorption disorders (tropical and celiac sprue, inflammatory bowel disease, amyloidosis, and intestinal lymphoma).

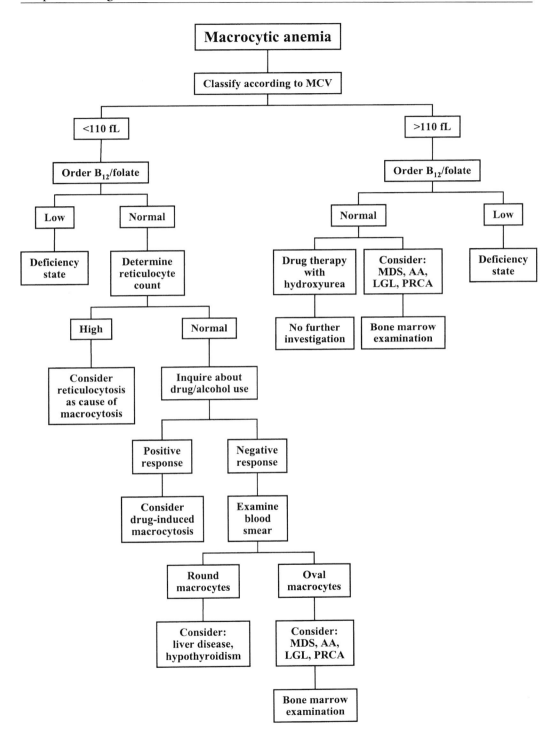

Fig. 5. A diagnostic approach to macrocytic anemia. AA, aplastic anemia; fL, femtoliters; LGL, large granular lymphocytic disorder; MCV, mean corpuscular volume; MDS, myelodysplastic syndrome; PRCA, pure red cell aplasia.

The Schilling Test

The Schilling test is performed in two stages. However, the second stage is performed only if the first stage is abnormal. In the first stage, the patient receives, simultaneously, 1 mg of unlabeled B_{12} (intramuscular injection) to saturate B_{12}-binding proteins and 1 μg of radiolabeled crystalline B_{12} (oral). A 24-hour urine collection follows immediately, and if detected radioactivity in the urine is more than 7% of the ingested load, the result is considered normal and the patient does not have problems absorbing crystalline B_{12}. Therefore, a normal stage 1 Schilling test rules out pernicious anemia but does not exclude the possibility of malabsorption from gastric atrophy (elderly patients may have difficulty absorbing food-bound B_{12}, which requires gastric acid and pepsin to release B_{12}). However, an abnormal stage 1 test suggests either pernicious anemia or a primary intestinal malabsorption disorder. Rare instances of intestinal bacterial overgrowth and pancreatic insufficiency also may cause abnormal stage 1 test results. Correction of an abnormal stage 1 result by the addition of intrinsic factor (60 mg) to the oral B_{12} dose (stage 2 Schilling test) establishes the diagnosis of pernicious anemia. However, an abnormal stage 2 test does not rule out the possibility of the anemia because the disease may secondarily affect the intestinal epithelium and mimic a primary malabsorption syndrome. Therefore, the best time to do the Schilling test is after 2 weeks of treatment with B_{12}, which allows healing of the absorptive surface.

Step 3: Nonnutritional Macrocytic Anemia That Is Not Drug-Induced

If neither vitamin deficiency nor drug (including ethyl alcohol) exposure can be implicated in a macrocytic process, it might be helpful to obtain detailed information from the peripheral blood smear before proceeding to additional diagnostic tests. Substantial polychromasia (indicative of reticulocytosis) suggests hemolysis as the cause of macrocytosis. Round morphology of the red cells, as opposed to oval macrocytosis, suggests liver disease (target cells are also evident) or hypothyroidism. In both reticulocytosis and round macrocytosis, the mean corpuscular volume is often less than 110 fL. However, it may exceed 110 fL in oval macrocytosis that is characteristic of hydroxyurea therapy, myelodysplastic syndrome, aplastic anemia, large granular lymphocytic leukemia, or pure red cell aplasia. Diagnosis of these disorders requires bone marrow examination with cytogenetic studies.

SUGGESTED READING

Hillman RS, Ault KA, eds. *Hematology in Clinical Practice: A Guide to Diagnosis and Management*, 2nd ed. McGraw-Hill, New York, 1998.

Hoffman R, Benz EJ Jr, Shattil SJ, Furie B, Cohen HJ, Silberstein LE, McGlave P, eds. *Hematology: Basic Principles and Practice*, 3rd ed. Churchill Livingstone, New York, 2000.

Schiffman FJ, ed. *Hematologic Pathophysiology*. Lippincott-Raven, Philadelphia, 1998.

2

Specific Anemia Syndromes and Their Management

Ayalew Tefferi, MD

Contents

NUTRITIONAL ANEMIAS

Iron Deficiency Anemia

BASIC CONCEPTS

Iron deficiency is the most common cause of anemia in the world. Therefore, it is appropriate to be familiar with some basic concepts of iron metabolism. The normal total amount of body iron is approximately 3 g in a woman and 4 g in a man. Approximately 2.5 g of the iron is in the form of hemoglobin, and the rest is stored in the form of ferritin and hemosiderin. A small amount is found in myoglobin and tissue heme enzymes (peroxidase, catalase, cytochromes). The iron cycle refers to the exchange of iron between the red cells and the storage iron. Stored iron is mostly in the monocyte-macrophage system of the liver, spleen, and bone marrow. There, it combines with the iron storage protein apoferritin and forms ferritin. The ferritin molecule is well structured and soluble and thus can circulate in the peripheral blood in amounts proportional to tissue iron stores. Hemosiderin is an insoluble form of storage iron that is made up of breakdown products of ferritin. The iron in both ferritin and hemosiderin is available for use in time of need.

Iron is introduced into the body either through intestinal absorption or during blood transfusion, in which each unit of blood (approximately 350 mL with a hematocrit of about 55%) contains 175 mg of iron. Dietary iron is in the form of either heme or inorganic iron. Absorption occurs in the duodenum and upper jejunum. Heme is absorbed intact (25% absorption rate), whereas inorganic dietary iron is usually in the ferric state, which is poorly absorbed (5% absorption rate). Therefore, the ferric iron is usually reduced to the ferrous state or is chelated to make it more absorbable. The factors

From: *Primary Hematology*
Edited by: A. Tefferi © Mayo Foundation for Medical Education and Research, Rochester, MN

facilitating this conversion include hydrochloric acid and reducing and chelating agents such as ascorbic acid. However, phytates and phosphates in vegetables, and tannates in tea and wine, decrease iron absorption. The absorbed ferrous iron is released into the circulation, where it is oxidized and binds to the plasma iron transporter protein transferrin. The transferrin-iron complex binds to specific cell receptors on erythroid cells and is then internalized and is either used for hemoglobin synthesis or stored as ferritin.

The iron requirement for heme production is almost completely met by iron reutilization (the iron cycle). This involves the mobilization of iron from ferritin, and to a lesser extent hemosiderin, in order to be used for hemoglobin synthesis and the redistribution of hemoglobin iron back to the storage forms during red cell attrition. However, the cycle is not completely closed, and approximately 1 mg of iron is lost per day in the form of, mostly, occult gastrointestinal blood loss. In addition, menstruating women lose about 30 mg each month, and pregnancy costs approximately 1 g of iron (iron transferred to the placenta and the fetus, and iron lost during bleeding at delivery). Growth spurts in children and adolescents also are associated with increased dietary iron requirements. When all these factors are considered, the average daily iron requirements become 1 mg/day for a man, 1.5 mg/day for a menstruating woman, and 2.5 mg/day during pregnancy.

In health, the amount of iron absorbed is equal to the amount lost over time. The normal American diet contains much more iron (10-20 mg per day) than is required for replenishing the iron deficit (i.e., 1 mg per day). As such, only a fraction (about 10%) of ingested iron is absorbed. Liver and meat products are rich sources of dietary iron, and vegetables and fruits are poor sources. In general, milk is a poor source of iron, although breast milk contains more iron than whole milk.

CLINICAL PRESENTATION

The generic symptoms and signs of anemia are also present in iron deficiency anemia and include fatigue, weakness, palpitations, light-headedness, somnolence, headache, tinnitus, angina in patients with coronary artery disease, shortness of breath, exercise intolerance, lack of ambition, decreased libido, pallor, tachycardia, and orthostatic hypotension. In addition, relatively specific clinical manifestations include pica (such as an unusual craving for ice [pagophagia], starch [amylophagia], clay [geophagia], or other items), glossitis (smooth and painful tongue from papillary atrophy), cheilitis (also known as angular stomatitis), Kelly-Paterson syndrome (the association of hypochromic anemia with cheilitis, glossitis, and solid food dysphagia from an upper esophageal mucosal web), and koilonychia (thinning, flattening, and spooning of the nails).

DIAGNOSIS

As detailed in Chapter 1, iron deficiency anemia usually presents as microcytic anemia with increased red cell distribution width (a measure of anisocytosis). However, these findings are neither sensitive nor specific to iron deficiency anemia. A few patients with iron deficiency anemia may present with normocytic anemia or normal red cell distribution width. Similarly, other causes of microcytic anemia, including thalassemia and sideroblastic anemia, may be accompanied by increased red cell distribution width. Therefore, although the red blood cell indices and the peripheral blood smear (elliptocytes and cigar-shaped red cells may be seen in iron deficiency anemia) may strongly suggest iron deficiency anemia, the diagnosis must be confirmed by demonstration of a low serum ferritin concentration. If it is low (< 10-20 µg/dL), then the diagnosis is confirmed and no additional tests are required. If the value is more than 60 µg/dL, then iron deficiency anemia is unlikely.

Table 1
Causes of Iron Deficiency

Gastrointestinal bleeding	Genitourinary bleeding	Other causes
Recurrent epistaxis	Menstrual bleeding	Inadequate nutrition
Esophageal varices	Uterine fibroids	Growth spurts, infancy
Hiatal hernia	Uterine neoplasia	Pregnancy, lactation
Use of aspirin and other	Cervical neoplasia	Blood donation
NSAIDs	Vaginal pathology	Recurrent hemoptysis
Gastric neoplasia	Urinary tract pathology	Pulmonary hemosiderosis
Gastritis or peptic ulcer	Urolithiasis	Intestinal malabsorption
disease	Renal cancer	Celiac disease
Hereditary hemorrhagic	Renal cyst	Inflammatory bowel
telangiectasia	Prostate pathology	disease
Angiodysplasia	Hemoglobinuria	Intestinal surgery
Hemobilia	Childbirth	Gastric surgery
Meckel's diverticulum	Schistosomiasis	Achlorhydria
Aortoenteric fistula		Self-induced (factitious)
Hookworm infection		
Inflammatory bowel disease		
Colon pathology		
Hemorrhoids		

Abbreviation: NSAID, nonsteroidal anti-inflammatory drug.

Because ferritin is an acute-phase reactant, serum ferritin levels between 20 and 60 µg/dL may not rule out the possibility of iron deficiency anemia in patients with inflammatory disorders. Also, a bone marrow examination, with a stain for iron particles, may provide a better estimate of body iron stores. However, these impressions are not based on convincing evidence, and this author questions the validity of considering bone marrow iron examination as the standard for evaluating iron deficiency anemia. In equivocal cases, a 2-month trial of iron supplementation may provide the necessary information and is preferred over bone marrow examination. Other serum iron measurements, including serum iron and iron-binding capacity, are usually not helpful for distinguishing iron deficiency anemia from anemia of chronic disease and are not recommended for evaluation of iron deficiency anemia.

CAUSES OF IRON DEFICIENCY

Iron deficiency is the most common form of anemia in the world. In developing countries, the major causes include inadequate nutrition and intestinal parasitosis (hookworm infestation). In the more developed countries, the most common causes include gastrointestinal and menstrual blood loss. Other causes of iron deficiency are listed in Table 1.

DETERMINING THE CAUSE OF IRON DEFICIENCY

In the presence of a confirmed iron-depleted state, the patient either is not obtaining adequate iron through intestinal absorption or is losing blood excessively. Inadequate dietary intake is easily determined from the history. The possibility of malabsorption is considered in the presence of previous gastrointestinal surgery, inflammatory bowel disease, or steatorrhea and weight loss. The clinical history also may identify the presence of nasal or oral bleeding, hematochezia, melena, excessive menstrual or nonmenstrual bleeding, hematuria, and blood donation.

In the absence of these clues, it is reasonable to start with the quantification of stool blood (HemoQuant) and urinalysis. Hematuria may be evaluated with excretory urography and cystoscopy. In the absence of hematuria, the gastrointestinal system is systematically examined to identify a possible source of bleeding. However, a bleeding site may not be detected in up to a third of patients undergoing an extensive gastrointestinal workup. The gastrointestinal investigation starts with colonoscopy in most patients. A negative result is usually followed by upper endoscopy (esophagogastroduodenoscopy). If both are negative, then a small intestinal barium study (small bowel follow-through) is performed to look for tumors or intestinal wall abnormalities. Enteroclysis (a contrast barium study of the small intestine by direct introduction via peroral intubation of the jejunum) may be more sensitive than "small bowel follow-through," but the yield remains very low.

A small number of patients may have no historical clue for celiac disease and may have negative results of upper and lower endoscopy and small intestinal barium study. In this situation, it should be remembered that the clinical presentation of sprue may be subtle and the measurement of serum carotene, stool fat, and serum antigliadin and antiendomysial antibodies is a reasonable next step. A positive antibody test is highly suggestive of sprue. A negative test, however, does not completely rule out the possibility of sprue, and a small bowel biopsy may still be necessary.

Additional evaluation techniques for a bleeding source include extended upper endoscopy (also known as push enteroscopy), endoscopic retrograde cholangiopancreatography (to look for a biliary source of bleeding), a technetium-labeled Meckel scan (to look for Meckel's diverticulum), a bleeding scan (technetium-tagged autologous red cells), angiography, and perioperative enteroscopy. In patients with active bleed, both the bleeding scan and angiography may be helpful. For those with intermittent bleeding, push (includes visualization of distal duodenum and proximal jejunum) or sonde (includes visualization of the entire small bowel) enteroscopy is preferred. If all these diagnostic tests are unrevealing, intraoperative enteroscopy may be considered. The indication for these additional tests depends on the clinical relevance of identifying the bleeding lesion.

MANAGEMENT

The treatment of the anemia itself, in iron deficiency anemia, is administration of oral iron supplements (Table 2). The three iron salts (sulfate, fumarate, gluconate) are roughly equivalent in both efficacy and side effects. In the available iron preparations, the amount of ascorbic acid that is combined with the vitamin may not be large enough to substantially increase absorption. Iron supplements are preferably taken before meals, two to four times a day. Side effects include gastrointestinal intolerance including nausea, abdominal cramps, constipation, and diarrhea. The gastric symptoms may be helped by taking the medication with meals, at the expense of markedly reduced absorption. Enteric-coated or sustained-release preparations are more expensive, and their possible benefit in reducing side effects is countered by reduced absorption due to retarded dissolution. The value of newer iron preparations, including polysaccharide-iron complexes, remains to be determined.

In patients with rapid intestinal transit, as a result of gastric resection or a Billroth II procedure (gastroenterostomy with duodenal bypass), and in those with achlorhydria, the

Table 2
Oral Iron Supplements

Preparation	Strength	Elemental iron	Ascorbic acid
Ferrous sulfate tablet	324 mg	65 mg	0
Ferrous sulfate elixir (Feosol)	220 mg/5 mL	44 mg/5 mL	0
Ferrous sulfate solution (Fer-In-Sol)	125 mg/mL	25 mg/mL	0
Ferrous fumarate tablet (Vitron-C)	200 mg	66 mg	125 mg
Ferrous gluconate tablet	300 mg	35 mg	0
Ferrous gluconate elixir (Fergon)	300 mg/5 mL	35 mg/5 mL	0
Polysaccharide-iron (Niferex)	150 mg	150 mg	0

use of an elixir preparation may be more effective (hydrochloric acid is needed to dissolve the tablet coat). For patients who cannot tolerate oral iron or for those who have intestinal malabsorption, a parenteral iron dextran preparation is available (InFed) and may be administered carefully. Treatment should continue until the serum ferritin level returns to normal.

Parenteral Iron Therapy

An iron dextran preparation (InFed) is available for both intramuscular and intravenous injection. Immediate anaphylactic (in up to 1% of patients) or delayed serum sickness reactions may occur with both methods of administration. Therefore, an intravenous test dose (0.5 mL) is initially infused over 5 to 10 minutes under supervision (epinephrine should be available on-site). If tolerated, 2.0 mL (100 mg) is infused intravenously over 5 minutes on a daily basis for a total of 1 to 2 g. Because of significant skin staining and development of sterile abscesses, intramuscular injections are not popular.

Vitamin B_{12} or Folate Deficiency

Leafy vegetables are rich in folate, whereas animal products are the only sources of dietary B_{12} (cyanocobalamin). The daily dietary requirement of folate necessary to replenish daily obligatory loss is 50 to 100 µg, and that of vitamin B_{12} is only 0.5 to 1 µg. The average daily Western diet contains approximately 5 to 10 times these amounts. The total body folate store is 5,000 to 10,000 µg, and that of vitamin B_{12} is 2,000 to 5,000 µg (the principal storage site for both vitamins is the liver). One can thus appreciate that it takes only 1 to 3 months to deplete the folate store, whereas it may take several years to deplete the vitamin B_{12} store. In general, diet is important in folate deficiency, whereas intestinal malabsorption is the usual cause of vitamin B_{12} deficiency (Table 3). Excessive cooking reduces available folate in the diet.

Dietary folic acid is in the polyglutamate form, which is deconjugated to the monoglutamate form during absorption. In the mucosa, folic acid undergoes complete reduction by dihydrofolate reductase into tetrahydrofolate. It is then methylated and released into the blood and transported (no specific carrier protein) into the target cells, where it transfers its methyl group to homocysteine to form methionine and tetrahydrofolate. This reaction is made possible by the enzyme methionine synthetase, which requires vitamin B_{12} as a cofactor. Tetrahydrofolate is used in the transfer of one-carbon fragments from donors such as serine to DNA bases (Fig. 1).

Table 3
Causes of Folate and B_{12} Deficiency

Causes of folate deficiency	Causes of B_{12} deficiency
Inadequate diet	Inadequate diet, only in strict vegetarians
Alcoholics and drug addicts	Malabsorption due to IF deficiency or
Malnourished elderly	achlorhydria
Parenteral nutrition	Pernicious anemia
Increased requirement	Gastric surgery
Hemolytic anemia	Proton pump inhibitor therapy
Exfoliative dermatitis	Food-bound B_{12} deficiency
Pregnancy	Malabsorption due to competing
Hemodialysis	intestinal flora
Malabsorption due to intestinal disease	*Diphyllobothrium latum* (fish
Sprue	tapeworm)
Inflammatory bowel disease	Bacterial overgrowth (blind loop
Small bowel resection (short bowel syndrome)	syndrome)
Drug-induced low serum folate levels	Malabsorption due to intestinal disease
Intracellular unavailability	Celiac sprue
Phenytoin (mechanism unknown)	Inflammatory bowel disease
Sulfasalazine (impairs intestinal deconjugation)	Small bowel resection
Oral contraceptives	Transcobalamin II deficiency
Alcohol (inhibits folate release from liver to bile)	Nitrous oxide (oxidizes B_{12})
Folate antagonists	Imerslund-Gräsbeck syndrome
Methotrexate (dihydrofolate reductase inhibitor)	(i.e., absence of B_{12} binders)
Pentamidine	
Trimethoprim	
Pyrimethamine	

Abbreviation: IF, intrinsic factor.

Vitamin B_{12} in food is bound to protein and must undergo peptic digestion in the acidic environment of the stomach to be released. In the stomach, the food-free form initially binds to salivary haptocorrin (a vitamin B_{12} binding protein formerly known as R-binder), only to be re-released in the duodenum after pancreatic enzymes degrade the haptocorrin. In the duodenum, the free vitamin B_{12} combines with another B_{12}-binder (intrinsic factor) secreted by the parietal cells of the stomach. Vitamin B_{12} is absorbed at the terminal ileum, and then only when it is bound to intrinsic factor. Idiopathic deficiency of intrinsic factor is called pernicious anemia. Once absorbed, vitamin B_{12} is freed from the B_{12}-intrinsic factor complex and released into the blood, where it is transported by a specific carrier protein, transcobalamin II. However, 80% of plasma vitamin B_{12} is bound to other serum haptocorrins (transcobalamin III and I). The transcobalamin II-B_{12} complex is carried to cells and is pinocytosed via transcobalamin II receptors. Intracellularly, vitamin B_{12} joins forces with folate and assists in DNA synthesis (Fig. 1).

CLINICAL MANIFESTATIONS

A deficiency in either folate or vitamin B_{12} results in impaired DNA synthesis, affecting all actively replicating cells. This is usually manifested clinically as megaloblastic

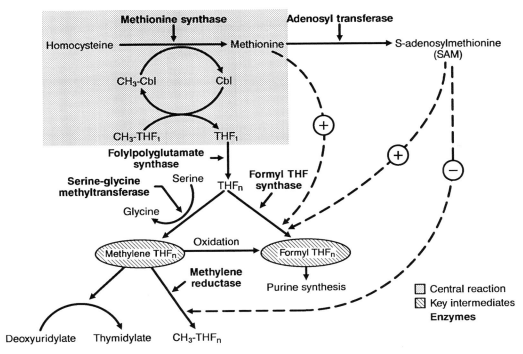

Fig. 1. Intracellular interdependent cofactor activity of cobalamin (*Cbl*) and folate. *CH3*, methyl group; *THF₁* and *THFₙ*, monoglutamated and polyglutamated forms of tetrahydrofolate. (From Tefferi A, Pruthi RK. The biochemical basis of cobalamin deficiency. *Mayo Clin Proc* 1994; 69: 181-186. By permission of Mayo Foundation for Medical Education and Research.)

anemia. In addition, the gastrointestinal system is often involved, and the pathologic lesions include atrophic tongue, glossitis, cheilosis, and secondary intestinal malabsorption (because of impaired replication of mucosal lining cells). The nervous system may be affected with vitamin B_{12} but not folate deficiency. The pathogenesis of B_{12} neuropathy is not known. Clinically, the process may affect the peripheral nerves (symmetrical mixed motor and sensory neuropathy), the spinal cord with demyelination of the posterior and lateral columns (subacute combined system disease), and the brain. The corresponding symptoms and signs include spastic paraparesis, gait apraxia, decreased proprioception (positive Romberg test) and vibration sense, dementia, personality changes, memory loss, and psychosis. The neuropathy may occur in the absence of anemia or macrocytosis.

Pernicious anemia is the most frequent cause of vitamin B_{12} deficiency. It is caused by idiopathic intrinsic factor deficiency. A possible autoimmune origin is suggested by the presence, in most but not all cases, of serum antibodies against both the parietal cells and intrinsic factor and the increased incidence of other autoimmune diseases (Hashimoto's thyroiditis, vitiligo). The disease is associated with gastric mucosal atrophy and achlorhydria (since the parietal cells also produce gastric acid). The disease has a typical onset after age 40 and affects all races.

DIAGNOSIS

The determination of serum folate and B_{12} levels is the initial step in the investigation of either megaloblastic anemia or a neurologic syndrome that is suggestive of vitamin B_{12}

deficiency. Serum folate assays may not always be accurate in assessing body folate status. Both false-positive and false-negative results may be due to recent dietary changes, alcohol intake (spuriously low levels), or concurrent hemolysis (spuriously high levels). Similarly, the sensitivity and specificity of red blood cell folate measurement are suboptimal despite the fact that they are less influenced by recent dietary changes. Spuriously low red blood cell folate values occur in vitamin B_{12} deficiency, pregnancy, and alcoholics.

Low serum B_{12} levels are not always indicative of B_{12} deficiency. Spuriously low values also may occur during pregnancy, with the use of oral contraceptives, and in leukopenia, plasma cell proliferative disease, folate deficiency, and advanced age. Conversely, vitamin B_{12}-deficient patients with spuriously normal levels have been reported and include patients with myeloproliferative diseases, liver disease, and congenital transcobalamin II deficiency. Patients with myeloproliferative diseases, such as polycythemia vera, may have increased levels of B_{12} because of increased production of serum haptocorrins (transcobalamin III and I) by the expanded granulocyte mass.

Thus, it is evident that serum levels of both folate and B_{12} may not reflect accurate tissue levels of the corresponding vitamins. Because of the co-participatory role of these vitamins in the formation of methionine from homocysteine, an increased plasma homocysteine level accompanies both folate and B_{12} deficiency (Fig. 2). Similarly, because vitamin B_{12}, and not folate, is required for the conversion of methylmalonyl-coenzyme A to succinyl-coenzyme A, serum methylmalonic acid is increased in B_{12} deficiency. Therefore, measurement of serum methylmalonic acid and plasma homocysteine is recommended in equivocal cases of B_{12} and folate deficiency, respectively. Normal values exclude true deficiency states. However, increased levels of both methylmalonic acid and homocysteine also may occur in renal insufficiency, hypo–volemia, and rare congenital disorders.

The detection of serum anti-intrinsic factor antibodies is diagnostic for pernicious anemia, and additional testing is not necessary. However, only 60% of affected patients are expected to be positive for anti-intrinsic factor antibody, and the Schilling test (described in Chapter 1) is recommended for the remaining patients to distinguish pernicious anemia from primary intestinal disease. Although sensitive (90% sensitivity), the detection of anti-parietal antibody or increased serum gastrin is not specific enough to be diagnostically useful.

The characteristic peripheral blood findings of megaloblastic anemia include oval macrocytosis and neutrophilic hypersegmentation (six-lobed or five-lobed nucleus in > 1% and 5% of the neutrophils, respectively). The typical bone marrow features include giant granulocyte precursors and erythroid nuclear immaturity (nuclear-cytoplasmic asynchrony). The erythroid nuclear immaturity results in ineffective erythropoiesis that is responsible for the increased lactate dehydrogenase in most patients and the indirect hyperbilirubinemia in some patients.

TREATMENT

It is critical that an accurate diagnosis be made before therapy is started because folate supplementation may mask underlying B_{12} deficiency by improving the anemia, but not the neurologic disease, associated with vitamin B_{12} deficiency and thus allowing the neuropathy to progress. Folate deficiency is usually treated with oral daily replacement (1 mg/day). B_{12} deficiency associated with pernicious anemia requires lifelong treatment. All patients should be started with intramuscular injection therapy at 100 to 1,000 µg/day,

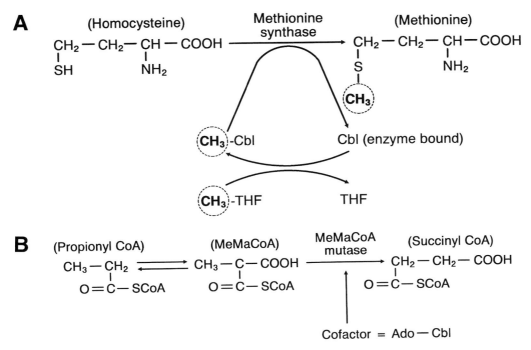

Fig. 2. *A,* Cofactor activity of methylcobalamin (*CH₃-Cbl*) in methionine synthesis. *THF,* tetrahydrofolate. *B,* Cofactor activity of adenosylcobalamin (*Ado-Cbl*) in succinyl-coenzyme A (*CoA*) synthesis. *MeMaCoA,* methylmalonyl-coenzyme A. (From Tefferi A, Pruthi RK. The biochemical basis of cobalamin deficiency. *Mayo Clin Proc* 1994; 69: 181-186. By permission of Mayo Foundation for Medical Education and Research.)

to be given every week for 1 month. Maintenance treatment may be administered intramuscularly, subcutaneously, orally, or intranasally (Table 4). In general, there is a dramatic improvement in well-being within a day of therapy with parenteral B$_{12}$. Reticulocytosis becomes apparent in 1 week, whereas anemia resolves in 2 months. Neurologic symptoms take longer to improve (6-12 months). Unfortunately, in up to 10% of patients with neurologic complications, and depending on the severity and duration of disease, the damage may be irreversible.

HEMOLYTIC ANEMIAS

Hereditary Spherocytosis

Hereditary spherocytosis is the most common inherited hemolytic anemia in the Western Hemisphere (a prevalence of 1 in 5,000). Inheritance is usually autosomal dominant, but both recessive inheritance and sporadic cases (20%) occur. Hereditary spherocytosis is characterized by chronic extravascular hemolytic anemia. The cause of hemolysis is a defect in the skeletal proteins (spectrin, ankyrin, band 3 protein, protein 4.2) of the red cell membrane which results in a spherocytic shape. These spherocytes are rigid and less deformable than the normal red cell, which has a biconcave shape. As a result, they are trapped in the microcirculation of the spleen and are destroyed by the macrophages of the spleen. This process leads to functional splenomegaly in most patients. Similarly, the chronically increased production of bilirubin results in clinical jaundice and pigmented gallstone formation. Additional clinical features include periods of severe hypoproliferative anemia from either folate deficiency (megaloblastic crisis) or parvovirus B19 infection (aplastic crisis). Rare complications have included secondary hemochromatosis and the development of extramedullary hematopoiesis.

DIAGNOSIS

The disease is suspected when laboratory features of extravascular hemolysis (increased reticulocyte count, indirect bilirubin, and lactate dehydrogenase and decreased haptoglobin) are accompanied by spherocytes in the peripheral blood. The differential diagnosis of peripheral blood spherocytosis includes hereditary spherocytosis and autoimmune hemolytic anemia (AIHA). Spherocytosis in AIHA results from the "erythroclasis" or "pitting" function of the spleen toward the antibody antigen-membrane complex on the red cell. Therefore, splenectomy corrects the spherocytosis in AIHA but not hereditary spherocytosis. Spherocytes have increased osmotic fragility (because of decreased distensibility associated with reduced surface membrane) in hypotonic saline, and this test (the osmotic fragility test) is positive in both hereditary spherocytosis and AIHA. The two are distinguished by the Coombs test, which is positive in AIHA and negative in hereditary spherocytosis. Once the diagnosis of hereditary spherocytosis is confirmed, ultrasonography of the abdomen is recommended to evaluate for the presence of biliary pigment stones.

TREATMENT

Because hemolysis in hereditary spherocytosis occurs primarily in the spleen, removal of the spleen often results in marked reduction of hemolysis. The question is whether everyone with hereditary spherocytosis requires splenectomy. The procedure is not without risk, and splenectomized patients have a small but real risk of overwhelming sepsis from encapsulated organisms. Therefore, the decision to remove the spleen should be individualized to each clinical situation.

Asymptomatic patients with well-compensated mild hemolytic anemia may be managed with oral folate therapy (1 mg/day) only. A more severe disease that results in substantial anemia or recurrent aplastic crisis should be managed with splenectomy. If splenectomy is indicated, it should be deferred until the patient reaches the age of 5 years. In addition, before splenectomy, all patients should receive vaccination against infection with *Pneumococcus*, *Meningococcus*, and *Haemophilus influenzae*. Furthermore, we usually treat all splenectomized patients with continuous daily oral penicillin (500 mg).

Glucose-6-Phosphate Dehydrogenase (G6PD) Deficiency

Red cell enzyme defects (enzymopathies) usually cause hemolysis either spontaneously or under red cell oxidant stress. Among the red cell enzymopathies, the most common is G6PD deficiency. G6PD deficiency is inherited as an X-linked recessive trait, but the less common enzymopathies (such as pyruvate kinase) are inherited as autosomal recessive traits. The deficiency in these enzymes results in ineffective neutralization of intracellular oxidants that oxidize sulfhydryl groups on hemoglobin and the cell membrane, resulting in both extravascular and intravascular hemolysis, respectively. The latter include superoxide (O_2^-) and hydrogen peroxide (H_2O_2). O_2^- is formed when oxyhe-

Table 4
Commercially Available Vitamin B_{12} Preparations

Vitamin B_{12} preparation	Dosage	Cost
Parenteral, given either intramuscularly or subcutaneously	1,000 µg/month	~$10.00 for 10 vials (each vial is 1 mL containing 1,000 µg)
Oral vitamin B_{12} tablets	500-1,000 µg/day	~$5.00 for 100 tablets of 500-µg dose
Nasal B_{12} (Nascobal)	500 µg/week	~$67.00 for 8 doses

moglobin is converted to methemoglobin. H_2O_2 is produced from intracellular oxidation reactions. Both processes are facilitated by certain drugs. The red cell uses O_2^- dismutase to convert O_2^- to H_2O_2, which is then eliminated by catalase.

Another mechanism of H_2O_2 elimination is the glutathione (GSH) antioxidant system. GSH peroxidase converts H_2O_2 to oxidized GSH (GSSG) and water. GSSG is then converted back to GSH by GSH reductase in the presence of nicotinamide adenine dinucleotide phosphate (NADPH). In the red cell, the only source of NADPH is the hexose monophosphate shunt that partly relies on G6PD for the formation of NADPH. Therefore, G6PD deficiency (which refers to the presence of a structural variant of the "normal" enzyme with low enzyme activity) results in increased susceptibility of a red cell to oxidant injury.

CLINICAL ASPECTS

G6PD synthesis is under an X-chromosome gene control and is therefore an X-linked trait affecting primarily males. Because of multiple mutations, there are more than 200 structural variants, some of which may not be associated with hemolysis. The normal G6PD in Caucasians is denoted as G6PD B+ (the wild type) and is found in 70% of African-American males. Fifteen percent of the latter have the variant G6PD A+. Both of these variants are functionally normal variants.

Twenty percent of African-American females carry a structural variant called G6PD A-. These women are rarely affected by the disease. However, 10% of African-American males carry the defective allele and experience intermittent episodes of hemolysis. The G6PD variant in people of Mediterranean origin is G6PD B-, which has even lower enzyme activity and causes more severe and sometimes chronic hemolysis. In the latter group, the ingestion of uncooked fava beans (broad beans) may cause acute hemolysis (favism).

G6PD deficiency is characterized by acute hemolysis, usually induced by drugs (sulfonamides, antimalarials, procainamide, high-dose aspirin, vitamin C, probenecid) or other oxidant stresses (such as infections and diabetic acidosis). In the African-American variant (the mild type), the hemolysis is self-limited because young red cells have higher enzyme activity (i.e., the sensitive old red cells are destroyed and the young resistant ones are left). Therefore, screening for enzyme activity during the hemolytic period may give spuriously normal values.

DIAGNOSIS

Both intravascular and extravascular hemolysis occur in G6PD deficiency. Intravascular hemolysis occurs as a result of oxidant injury to the red cell membrane. Extravascular hemolysis occurs because of oxidant injury to hemoglobin that is converted to methemoglobin and leads to hemoglobin denaturation. The precipitation of the denatured product on the red cell membrane (Heinz body inclusions) is sometimes noted on the peripheral smear under special basic stain. Furthermore, the presence of these inclusions causes "erythroclasis" and "pitting" by the spleen and results in spherocytosis.

Between episodes, hematologic findings including the peripheral blood are normal. During hemolysis, the laboratory features of intravascular hemolysis are observed, and red cell morphology may include spherocytosis and Heinz body formation. Laboratory detection is based on screening tests dependent on the ability of the red cells to generate NADPH from NADP. Enzyme assays also are available.

TREATMENT

Obviously, avoiding deleterious drugs and the ingestion of fava beans is critical. Daily intake of oral folic acid (1 mg) is advised for all patients. Splenectomy may be considered in patients with frequent hemolytic episodes and in those with symptomatic chronic disease. If splenectomy is indicated, the preoperative and postoperative measures that are outlined for patients with hereditary spherocytosis are to be taken.

Immune Hemolytic Anemia

Immune hemolytic anemia (IHA) results from the red cell binding of specific antibodies, complement, or immune complexes which results in either intravascular or extravascular hemolysis. Antibodies are always involved but may disconnect from the red cell membrane, leaving complement behind. Antibodies involved with IHA may be reactive to either non-self red cells (alloimmune) or self red cells (autoimmune).

ALLOIMMUNE IMMUNE HEMOLYTIC ANEMIA

Three clinical conditions illustrate alloimmune IHA (allo-IHA): hemolytic disease of the newborn (HDN), immediate hemolytic transfusion reaction (IHTR), and delayed HTR (DHTR). HDN results from extravascular hemolysis in neonates or fetuses which is mediated by IgG antibodies from the mother which cross the placenta. This occurs because the mother has been previously sensitized to the red cell antigen of the fetus, which is absent in the mother's red cells. The best known scenario is a Rhesus (Rh)-negative mother giving birth to an Rh-positive child. The best treatment is the prevention of allosensitization of the mother by the use of high-titered RhIg (300 µg within 72 hours of delivery).

IHTR occurs when patients are mistakenly (most frequently from clerical error) transfused with red cell antigen (ABO, Kell, Jk^a, Fy^a) mismatched blood. The recipient's preexisting, usually IgM, antibodies bind to the donor's red cells and cause a complement-mediated intravascular hemolysis. When IHTR is suspected (fever, chest or back pain during transfusion, shock, "hematuria"), transfusion should be stopped immediately and the blood bank and clinical service notified. In the meantime, the patient should be vigorously hydrated with intravenous fluids.

DHTR is characterized by the onset of anemia 5 to 10 days after red cell transfusion. DHTR is an extravascular hemolysis that results from an anamnestic response in a pre-sensitized patient in whom pretransfusion antibody testing missed identification because of low antibody titers.

AUTOIMMUNE HEMOLYTIC ANEMIA

Autoimmune hemolytic anemia (AIHA) results from the production of antibodies reacting against the patient's own red cell surface antigens. These antibodies may react best at body temperature (warm AIHA) or at temperatures between 4° and 30°C (cold AIHA). The antibody in warm AIHA is usually IgG and does not bind complement. As such, red cell destruction in warm AIHA is primarily extravascular and involves antibody-mediated phagocytosis by the reticuloendothelial system. Cold AIHA, in contrast, is usually IgM-mediated and involves complement fixation and complement-mediated intravascular red cell lysis. An important laboratory feature of AIHA is a positive direct antiglobulin test (direct Coombs test). The purpose of this test is to detect antibodies (IgG) or complement components (C3) on the red cell membrane.

WARM AUTOIMMUNE HEMOLYTIC ANEMIA

Warm AIHA may be idiopathic, drug-related, or associated with another underlying disease (connective tissue disease, chronic lymphocytic leukemia, lymphoma). As such, the drug history and physical examination are crucial in the initial assessment of warm AIHA. The diagnosis is considered when general indicators of hemolysis (increased lactate dehydrogenase, high reticulocyte count, low haptoglobin, indirect hyperbilirubinemia) are associated with peripheral blood spherocytosis and a positive Coombs test. Splenomegaly and jaundice may or may not be present. In the absence of a positive drug history, it is not unreasonable to perform computed tomography of the chest and abdomen, peripheral blood lymphocyte immunophenotyping by flow cytometry, serum protein electrophoresis, and serum antinuclear antibody test.

In drug-related warm AIHA, treatment is limited to discontinuation of the offending agent. In general, initial treatment of disease-associated AIHA is similar to that of idiopathic AIHA. Obviously, concomitant treatment of the underlying disorder is essential. Corticosteroids (prednisone, 1 mg/kg per day) are the usual agents of first-line therapy. Treatment is continued for 2 to 4 weeks, followed by a gradual taper in the following 2 to 4 weeks. If unmaintained remissions are not achieved in 2 months, splenectomy is considered (patients should be vaccinated against *Pneumococcus*, *Meningococcus*, and *H. influenzae* before splenectomy). Both corticosteroids and splenectomy have limited efficacy in IgM-mediated warm AIHA.

Warm AIHA that does not respond to splenectomy is difficult to treat. Various treatments have been used in this situation, including danazol (400-800 mg/day in two divided doses), oral (100 mg/day) or intravenous pulse therapy (1 g/m^2 every 3-4 weeks) with cyclophosphamide, high-dose intravenous gamma globulin (1 g/kg per day for 2-5 days), oral cyclosporine (starting dose 300 mg twice a day and blood drug levels kept between 100-300), oral azathioprine (150 mg/day), and anti-B-cell monoclonal antibody (rituxan 375 mg/m^2 intravenously weekly for 4-8 weeks). Regardless of the specific treatment used, all patients with AIHA should have supplementation with oral folate (1 mg/day).

MECHANISMS OF DRUG-RELATED AUTOIMMUNE HEMOLYTIC ANEMIA

If the mechanism is *drug adsorption (penicillin, cephalosporin)*, the drug in large doses binds firmly to the red cell membrane and antibody forms against the drug-membrane antigen complex. In *immune complex formation (quinidine, rifampin, para-aminosalicylic acid)*, the drug (behaving as a hapten) binds to a serum protein, and antibodies are formed directly against the drug. The antibody-drug immune complex attaches to the red cell membrane (which is the innocent bystander) and complement is fixed. In *drug-induced AIHA (methyldopa, L-dopa, procainamide)*, the hematologic and serologic findings are identical to those of idiopathic AIHA.

COLD AUTOIMMUNE HEMOLYTIC ANEMIA

Proteins that demonstrate in vitro reaction (precipitation, red cell agglutination) in cold (4°C) but lose their in vitro activity when warmed are called cryoproteins. Cryoproteins can be either immunoglobulins (cryoglobulins, cold agglutinins) or fibrinogen (cryofibrinogen). Cryofibrinogenemia is extremely rare and may be either idiopathic or associated with infectious or malignant disorders. Cryoglobulins are cold-precipitable and may occur without an identifiable cause (essential cryoglobulinemia) or in association with other diseases.

Cryoglobulins are classified as type I (monoclonal, associated with plasma cell proliferative disorders), type II (mixed monoclonal IgM and polyclonal IgG, associated with hepatitis C infection, lymphoma), and type III (no monoclonal component, associated with chronic infectious or inflammatory disorders). Clinical manifestations (such as vasculitis, acrocyanosis, digital ischemia) depend more on the thermal amplitude (the highest temperature at which red cell agglutination is observed) than on the concentration of cryoglobulins.

Cold agglutinins are antibodies that cause in vitro red cell agglutination at 4°C. Their concentration is measured by serially diluting the patient's serum and determining the lowest titration that maintains activity. If antibody specificity is sought, the patient's serum may be incubated with heterologous red cells of known antigenic profile. Most cold agglutinins have anti-I specificity (idiopathic cold agglutinin disease, *Mycoplasma pneumoniae*-associated cold AIHA), whereas some may have anti-i (infectious mononucleosis-associated cold AIHA) or anti-P (paroxysmal cold hemoglobinuria) specificity. In vitro, some cold agglutinins demonstrate potent hemolytic activity (paroxysmal cold hemoglobinuria), whereas others cause intense red cell agglutination (idiopathic cold agglutinin disease).

Cold AIHA may be either IgM-mediated or IgG-mediated. IgM-mediated cold AIHA may be idiopathic (idiopathic cold agglutinin disease) or be associated with infections (Epstein-Barr virus, *Mycoplasma*), lymphoma, or autoimmune diseases. In idiopathic cold agglutinin disease, the autoantibody is monoclonal, the degree of hemolysis is often mild, and the patients are more bothered by cold-induced acral cyanosis and dysesthesia. The Coombs test is positive (anti-complement only), and the blood smear may show red cell agglutination. The cold agglutinin titer is often more than 1:1,000. Idiopathic cold agglutinin disease may run a chronic course, but infection-associated AIHA is often self-limited.

IgG-mediated cold AIHA is represented by paroxysmal cold hemoglobinuria. The disease may be either idiopathic or associated with viral infections or syphilis. Clinical manifestations include cold-induced attacks of intravascular hemolysis that are associated with fever and back pain. The autoantibody and complement bind to the red cells in the cold (4°C) and cause hemolysis only when the complement is activated at 37°C. The direct Coombs test is positive (due to the presence of complement only) during or after an acute hemolytic episode. However, the test can be negative during remission. The cold agglutinin titer is usually low (< 1:64). The diagnosis of paroxysmal cold hemoglobinuria is confirmed by the Donath-Landsteiner test.

Treatment of Cold Autoimmune Hemolytic Anemia

Avoidance of cold exposure is central to the treatment of cold autoimmune hemolytic anemia (AIHA). Obviously, treatment of the underlying disorder, if present, is advised. Often, the degree of hemolysis in cold AIHA is mild enough not to warrant specific therapy. In general, treatment with corticosteroids or splenectomy is ineffective. However, occasional responses have been reported. On the basis of limited reports of success and anecdotal experiences, we use either oral danazol (200 mg twice a day) or subcutaneous interferon-α (5 million units three times a week) as initial therapy. Nonresponding patients may receive therapeutic trials with oral cyclophosphamide (100 mg/day) or chlorambucil (4 mg/day). In refractory cases, consideration may be given to treatment with vincristine, cyclosporine, antithymocyte immunoglobulin, or anti-B cell monoclonal antibody.

Microangiopathic Hemolytic Anemia

Microangiopathic hemolytic anemia (MAHA) is an intravascular hemolytic process that is a result of red cell injury by an abnormal endothelial surface. The abnormal endothelial surface may be a result of the introduction of a foreign substance (valvular prosthesis), endothelial injury (vasculitis, connective tissue disease, preeclampsia, malignancy, chemotherapy, organ transplantation, malignant hypertension), or an abnormal platelet-endothelial interaction (thrombotic thrombocytopenic purpura, hemolytic uremic syndrome, disseminated intravascular coagulation). Figure 3 outlines the causes of MAHA.

All patients with MAHA have evidence of red cell destruction (increased lactate dehydrogenase), intravascular hemolysis (decreased haptoglobin, hemosiderinuria), and schistocytes on a blood smear. In addition, patients with thrombotic thrombocytopenic purpura or hemolytic uremic syndrome often have accompanying thrombocytopenia.

INITIAL EVALUATION AND GENERAL MANAGEMENT

The first step in evaluating MAHA is to rule out the possibility of disseminated intravascular coagulation (DIC). This requires assessment of the clinical scenario and a DIC screen (prothrombin time, partial thromboplastin time, fibrinogen, D-dimer, fibrin monomer). A thorough history should reveal the presence of a prosthetic heart valve, infection, connective tissue disease, pregnancy, organ transplantation, or an offending drug. In the absence of DIC and a prosthetic heart valve, the diagnosis of thrombotic thrombocytopenic purpura/hemolytic uremic syndrome (TTP/HUS) is entertained (increased lactate dehydrogenase, decreased haptoglobin, schistocytosis, hemosiderinuria, thrombocytopenia, and a negative DIC screen). The management of DIC is discussed in Chapters 7 and 22. Valvular hemolysis may require surgical intervention to repair a malfunctioning valve. The management of TTP/HUS and TTP-like syndromes is discussed below. In general, patients with chronic or intermittent MAHA should receive daily oral folic acid (1 mg/day).

TTP/HUS

The pathologic hallmark of TTP/HUS is the occurrence of fibrin-coated platelet clumping (hyaline thrombi) in the microvasculature with endothelial proliferation and injury. In TTP, the pathogenesis has been linked to severe deficiency of the enzyme (protease) that cleaves the von Willebrand factor. The protease deficiency is due to a genetic muta-

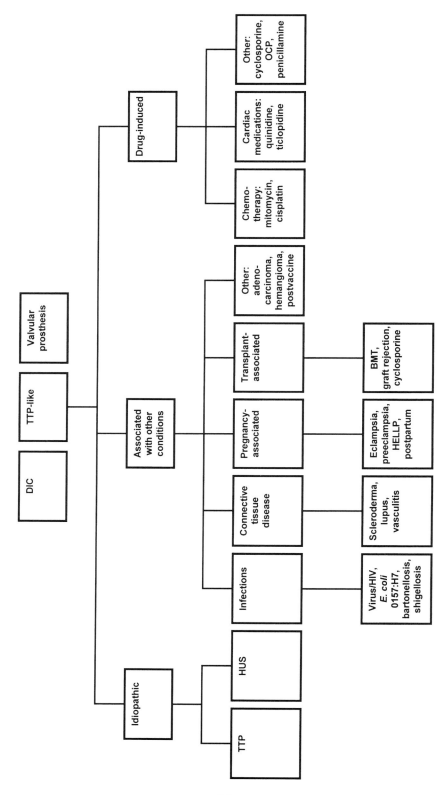

tion in familial TTP and an antibody-mediated inhibition of the enzyme in the sporadic form. A similar defect has not been found in patients with HUS. Similarly, protease activity may be normal in patients with TTP during remission. Others have shown increased endothelial apoptosis (programmed cell death) in both TTP and HUS, and plasma obtained from patients with TTP/HUS has been shown to induce apoptosis in cultured endothelial cells. These observations taken together suggest that uncleaved large von Willebrand protein in TTP and an unknown toxin in HUS may mediate the endothelial injury that triggers the disease process in affected patients.

All patients with TTP and HUS have schistocytosis, intravascular hemolysis (high lactate dehydrogenase, low haptoglobin), and thrombocytopenia. The degree of thrombocytopenia and schistocytosis may be less in HUS. In addition, approximately 70% of patients with TTP may have fluctuating neurologic changes (seizures, stroke, aphasia, altered mental status, stupor, coma), renal insufficiency, or fever. Patients with HUS have renal insufficiency without neurologic disease. HUS is more prevalent in children and has a close association with verotoxin-producing bacterial diarrhea, usually associated with consumption of poorly cooked contaminated meat (*Escherichia coli* 0157:H7, *Shigella dysenteriae*).

MANAGEMENT IN TTP/HUS

Plasma exchange (the combination of plasmapheresis and normal fresh frozen plasma infusion) is the cornerstone of therapy for both TTP and HUS. In the beginning, this should be done daily (2 plasma volumes; i.e., 3-4 liters in adults) until clinical manifestations have resolved and the thrombocytopenia and the increased lactate dehydrogenase are corrected. The interval between treatments can then be gradually increased (every 2 days for 1 week, then twice a week for 2 weeks, then weekly for 1 month). We usually use concurrent corticosteroid therapy (prednisone 2 mg/kg per day). The prednisone dosage is tapered gradually after remission is achieved. The additional value of platelet anti-aggregate therapy is not known. Platelet transfusion is best avoided unless the patient is bleeding. In general, plasma exchange works best for TTP, whereas corticosteroid therapy is essential in HUS.

Response to treatment is monitored by daily assessment of the hemoglobin level, platelet count, and serum creatinine and lactate dehydrogenase values. If adequate response to these initial measures is not achieved in 2 to 3 weeks, then additional therapy may be necessary. The options include the use of cryo-poor fresh frozen plasma (cryosupernatant) or intravenous vincristine (1-2 mg intravenously weekly). In vincristine-refractory cases, and in those with frequent disease relapse, splenectomy may be of benefit. Anecdotal reports of successful therapy in refractory cases have included the use of doxycycline (based on the assumption of occult bacterial infection in some patients), cyclosporine, intravenous high-dose gamma globulin, and cyclophosphamide. In TTP associated with chemotherapy, plasmapheresis with a staphylococcal protein A immunoperfusion column may work better. In TTP associated with pregnancy, optimal

---

Fig. 3. *(opposite page)* Causes of microangiopathic hemolytic anemia. BMT, bone marrow transplantation; DIC, disseminated intravascular coagulation; HELLP, *h*emolytic anemia, *e*levated *l*iver tests, *l*ow *p*latelets syndrome; HIV, human immunodeficiency virus; HUS, hemolytic uremic syndrome; OCP, oral contraceptive pills; TTP, thrombotic thrombocytopenic purpura.

management includes control of hypertension and prompt induction of delivery during the last trimester. During early pregnancy, standard TTP therapy may be tried.

ANEMIA OF CHRONIC DISEASE

Anemia of chronic disease (ACD) is usually normocytic but can be microcytic when it is associated with Hodgkin's disease, temporal arteritis, rheumatoid arthritis, Castleman's disease, and myelofibrosis with myeloid metaplasia. The pathogenesis is poorly understood. Current understanding suggests a cytokine-mediated process that inhibits red cell production or interferes with erythropoietin production or function. ACD is frequently associated with diabetes mellitus, connective tissue disease, chronic infections, and malignancy. However, any infectious or inflammatory process is capable of inducing ACD.

Diagnosis

The diagnosis of ACD is one of exclusion, and all other possibilities should be evaluated and excluded. The initial laboratory evaluation should include determination of serum ferritin, B_{12}, and folate levels (to exclude nutritional anemia), reticulocyte count, haptoglobin level, peripheral smear (to exclude hemolytic anemia), and serum creatinine level (to exclude anemia of renal insufficiency). The peripheral smear examination is also helpful for excluding a myelodysplastic syndrome (dimorphic red cells, dysgran–ulopoiesis, other cytopenias, monocytosis) or a marrow-infiltrating process (tear-drop-shaped and nucleated red cells, immature granulocytes).

It is reasonable to consider ACD when the peripheral smear is unremarkable, the serum creatinine level is normal, and the possibility of nutritional or hemolytic anemia is unlikely. ACD may be mistaken for iron deficiency anemia because low serum iron and decreased transferrin saturation occur in both conditions. Similarly, serum iron binding capacity may be low or normal in both conditions despite the fact that it is expected to be high in uncomplicated iron deficiency anemia. Therefore, serum ferritin determination is the single best noninvasive test to differentiate iron deficiency anemia from ACD. A low serum ferritin value is diagnostic of iron deficiency anemia, and it is unlikely in the presence of a serum ferritin value that is more than 60 μg/L. When the serum ferritin value is between 20 and 60 μg/L, the possibility of an acute-phase reaction is entertained. However, we do not recommend a bone marrow biopsy to resolve the issue. Instead, the patient may be empirically treated with iron therapy for 3 months and be reevaluated.

Another concern during the evaluation of ACD is the possible presence of a primary bone marrow disease. In this regard, the decision to do a bone marrow biopsy should consider the likelihood of discovering a primary bone marrow disease and the therapeutic and prognostic value of the information from the procedure. For example, it is not necessary to do a bone marrow biopsy in an elderly patient with mild anemia even if the peripheral smear suggests a primary hematologic disease because the result may not affect overall management decisions. However, a younger patient with a previous history of chemotherapy or a suggestive peripheral smear should have a bone marrow biopsy before a diagnosis of ACD is established.

Treatment

Obviously, optimal treatment of the underlying disease is crucial. In the absence of symptoms and if the hemoglobin value is more than 10 g/dL, specific treatment may not be necessary. Otherwise, a therapeutic trial with recombinant human erythropoietin (rhEPO) is reasonable. Currently, rhEPO treatment is approved for anemia associated with renal disease, prematurity, zidovudine therapy in patients with human immunodeficiency virus infection, cisplatin therapy, and certain groups with cancer. A wide range of dosages of rhEPO have been used in different settings. One can start with 10,000 units subcutaneously three times a week. Depending on the response, the dosage can then be either titrated down to 4,000 units subcutaneously once a week or increased to 20,000 units subcutaneously three times a week. If no response occurs in 6 to 8 weeks, continued treatment is not advised. Similarly, dosages more than 20,000 units three times a week may not be cost-effective. Baseline endogenous EPO levels more than 200 mU/mL suggest a low likelihood of response. Side effects are generally not observed in patients with ACD. Rare instances of influenza-like syndrome have been reported.

ANEMIA OF RENAL INSUFFICIENCY

Erythropoietin (EPO) is essential for the proliferation, differentiation, and survival of erythroid precursors and effective production of mature red cells. EPO acts at the level of late-stage burst-forming unit–erythroid and colony-forming unit–erythroid, and the density of EPO receptors diminishes with red cell maturation down to undetectable levels in reticulocytes. In humans, 90% of the hormone is produced by the kidneys (peritubular interstitial cells) and the rest by the liver. Therefore, EPO production is compromised in the presence of kidney disease. Although baseline production may not be substantially affected, the physiologically appropriate anemia-induced increase in EPO production is suboptimal and results in relative hypoerythropoietinemia.

Anemia of renal insufficiency is normocytic, and the peripheral blood smear picture is unremarkable. Although anemia is severe and symptomatic only with advanced kidney disease (serum creatinine, > 3 mg/dL), mild to moderate anemia may occur in moderate renal insufficiency (serum creatinine, 1.5-3 mg/dL), especially in diabetic patients with nephrotic syndrome. Therefore, a therapeutic trial with rhEPO (4,000 or 10,000 units subcutaneously once a week) is indicated in an otherwise unexplained anemia that is associated with any degree of renal insufficiency. The degree of increase in hemoglobin should not exceed 2 g/dL per month, and the target hemoglobin level in end-stage renal disease should be between 10 and 12 g/dL. These recommendations are meant to avoid the development of uncontrolled hypertension and seizures. Finally, the serum ferritin levels should be closely monitored in patients being treated with rhEPO to avoid treatment failure due to concomitant iron deficiency.

SIDEROBLASTIC ANEMIA

Sideroblastic anemia is characterized by the presence of ringed sideroblasts in bone marrow aspirate. Ringed sideroblasts are erythroid precursors whose mitochondria, which are located around the nucleus, are loaded with non-heme iron. Ringed sideroblastosis is due to defective iron utilization that results from a hereditary impairment of heme synthesis (aminolevulinic acid synthase deficiency in hereditary sideroblastic anemia) or an acquired abnormality that results from either chemical toxicity (lead, isoniazid, alcohol) or a clonal stem cell disease (refractory anemia with ringed sideroblasts). The hereditary variant is rare and inheritance is usually X-linked recessive. Patients with hereditary sideroblastic anemia present early in childhood with severe microcytic anemia and over many years develop hemochromatosis. Fifty percent of cases may respond to high doses of oral pyridoxine (200 mg/day). Microcytic anemia with red cell dimorphism also occurs in sideroblastic anemia associated with lead toxicity, isoniazid therapy, copper deficiency, and zinc overload. In contrast, refractory anemia with ringed sideroblasts is often macrocytic or normocytic and occurs late in life. There is no effective therapy for it.

SUGGESTED READING

Beutler E, Lichtman MA, Coller BS, Kipps TJ (editors). *Williams Hematology*, 5th ed. McGraw-Hill, New York, 1995.
Hoffman R, Benz EJ Jr, Shattil SJ, Furie B, Cohen HJ, Silberstein LE, McGlave P (editors). *Hematology: Basic Principles and Practice*, 3rd ed. Churchill Livingstone, New York, 2000.
Lee GR, Paraskevas F, Foerster J, Greer JP, Lukens J, Rodgers GM (editors). *Wintrobe's Clinical Hematology*, 10th ed, vol 1 and 2. Williams & Wilkins, Baltimore, 1999.

3

The Thalassemia Syndromes and the Hemoglobinopathies

Angela Dispenzieri, MD

Contents

INTRODUCTION

Advancements in the understanding of the hemoglobin molecule and its variants have been a driving force for medical and molecular genetics, making hemoglobin one of the best-characterized human proteins. These achievements in discovery and comprehension are indebted to the interplay between clinical and laboratory observations, to the abundance of nonlethal hemoglobin variants, and to the relative ease of obtaining large amounts of protein by simple venipuncture. As always, the productive application of science lags behind the discovery itself; hemoglobinopathies and thalassemia syndromes are no exception. However, each passing decade has held developments that have changed the natural history of these disorders.

This chapter addresses the clinical, laboratory, and management issues related to the thalassemia syndromes and several of the more common structural hemoglobinopathies. The rare structural variants causing unstable hemoglobin and altered oxygen affinity are covered briefly. Sickle cell disorders are discussed in Chapter 4.

HEMOGLOBIN NOMENCLATURE AND STRUCTURE

Hemoglobinopathies include the thalassemia syndromes and the inherited structural hemoglobin variants. "Thalassemia" refers to a genetic disorder in which there is inadequate synthesis of globin chain subunits of the hemoglobin tetramer; in α- and β-thalassemias, the globin chains produced—if any—are generally normal in structure.

From: *Primary Hematology*
Edited by: A. Tefferi © Mayo Foundation for Medical Education and Research, Rochester, MN

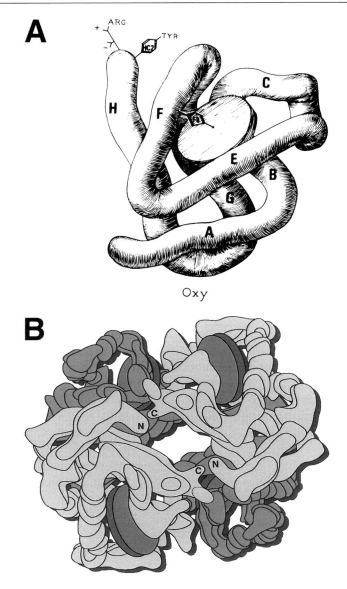

Oxy

In contrast, the structural variants, such as hemoglobins (Hb) S and C, are produced in normal quantities but have altered peptide sequence and function. Finally, variants such as Hb E and Lepore are both quantitatively and qualitatively abnormal. The hemoglobinopathies are most easily understood on the basis of an elementary understanding of hemoglobin structure.

Human hemoglobins are tetrameric molecules containing two pairs of globin chains, each of which is associated with an iron-containing heme group. The heme groups allow the hemoglobin molecules to perform their primary function, that is, the transport of oxygen to the tissues of the body. The normal adult hemoglobin tetramer (Hb A) is comprised of two pairs of $\alpha\beta$ heterodimers (Fig. 1 *A* and Fig. 1 *B*, Plate 1). The α and β chains are normally produced in nearly equal quantities and acquire heme groups rapidly. Each globin subunit forms a heterodimer with an unlike partner, such as $\alpha\beta^A$, $\alpha\beta^S$, $\alpha\gamma$,

C

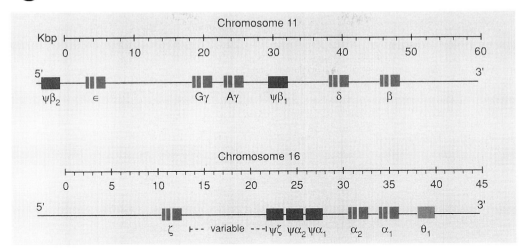

D

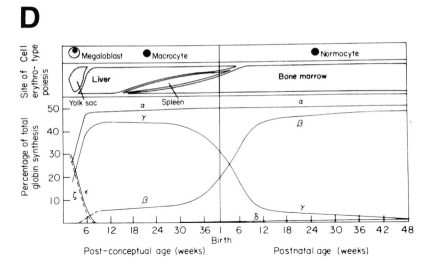

Fig. 1. *A (opposite page),* Globin molecule. The α-chain of hemoglobin. The iron of heme is attached to histidine F8. *B,* Plate 1 *(opposite page),* Hemoglobin molecule. The molecule is built from four subunits: two identical α chains (yellow) and two identical β chains (blue). "N" identifies the amino ends and "C" identifies the carboxyl ends of the two α chains. Each chain enfolds a heme group (red disk). *C,* Plate 2, Globin genes. *D,* Ontology of hemoglobin. (*A,* From Charache S. Haemoglobins with altered oxygen affinity. *Clin Haematol* 1974 June; 3: 357-381. By permission of WB Saunders Company. *B,* From Perutz MF. The hemoglobin molecule. *Sci Am* 1964, 211 no. 5: 64-76. *C,* From Steinberg MH, Benz EJ Jr. Hemoglobin synthesis, structure, and function, in *Hematology: Basic Principles and Practice* [Hoffman R, Benz EJ Jr, Shattil SJ, Furie B, Cohen HJ, Silberstein LE, eds], 2nd ed. Churchill Livingstone, New York, 1995, pp. 458-468. By permission of the publisher. *D,* From Weatherall DJ, Clegg JB. *The Thalassaemia Syndromes,* 3rd ed. Blackwell Scientific Publications, Oxford, 1981, p. 64. By permission of the publisher.)

or αδ. Like dimers finally associate into a tetramer, which is the finished hemoglobin product, that is, Hb A ($\alpha_2\beta_2^A$), Hb S ($\alpha_2\beta_2^S$), Hb F ($\alpha_2\gamma_2$), or Hb A_2 ($\alpha_2\delta_2$) (Table 1).

Table 1
Hemoglobin Nomenclature

	Hemoglobin	Genotype
Normal adult	A	$\alpha_2^A\beta_2^A$
	A_2	$\alpha_2^A\delta_2$
Fetal	F	$\alpha_2^A\gamma_2$
Embryonic	Portland	$\zeta_2\gamma_2$
	Gower I	$\zeta_2\varepsilon_2$
	Gower II	$\alpha_2\varepsilon_2$
Variants	S	$\alpha_2^A\beta_2^S$
	C	$\alpha_2^A\beta_2^C$
Thalassemias	See Tables 2 and 3	

The seven genes and pseudogenes of the α-chain family are located on chromosome 16, and the six of the β-chain cluster, on chromosome 11 (Fig. 1C, Plate 2). The globin genes and pseudogenes are believed to be products of ancient duplications and divergent mutations because they all are comprised of three similar exons and two intervening sequences. Per haplotype, there are two functioning α-globin gene copies, a single functioning β-globin gene, and two γ-globin genes. Mutations causing partially reduced globin product and total abrogation of globin product on a chromosome are referred to as α^+ (β^+) and α^0 (β^0), respectively.

The composition of hemoglobin changes through embryonic development and achieves constancy only after the first year of birth. During the first 8 weeks after conception, Hb Gower 1 ($\zeta_2\varepsilon_2$), Gower 2 ($\zeta_2\gamma_2$), and Portland ($\alpha_2\varepsilon_2$) are produced (Fig. 1 D). Fetal hemoglobin (Hb F, $\alpha_2\gamma_2$) predominates through the remainder of gestation, gradually replaced by adult hemoglobins, Hb A and Hb A_2, around the time of birth. Hemoglobin F production is incompletely extinguished in the adult, and a small proportion of red cells, called F cells, coexpress both fetal and adult globins. The nature of hemoglobin γ-gene regulation is not fully understood. Before the second year after birth, the normal adult complement of hemoglobins is present: 96% Hb A; 2% to 3% Hb A_2; and less than 1% Hb F.

GENETIC MECHANISMS OF ABNORMAL GLOBIN CHAIN SYNTHESIS

The general principles of the mechanism of mutation apply to the hemoglobinopathies. Deletion, substitution, or addition of nucleotide base(s) in DNA exons or surrounding sequences causes structural or regulatory abnormalities. The α-thalassemia mutations are most often large deletions of one or both α-globin genes on a given chromosome— the α^+ (or α-thalassemia-2) and α^0 (or α-thalassemia-1) determinants, respectively. In contrast to the α-thalassemia mutations, β-thalassemia mutations tend to involve one or a few bases. More than 125 mutations responsible for the β-thalassemia syndromes have been described, although only approximately 15 of them affect the majority of patients. Mutations disrupting every step in the β-globin synthesis pathway, including transcription, processing and cytoplasmic transport of RNA, and posttranslational integrity of the β-globin chain, have been reported. The mutations causing structural hemoglobinopathies are generally point mutations. Two of the more common of these variants are Hb

S and Hb C, which are the result of substitutions of the glutamic acid at position 6 by valine and lysine, respectively.

CLINICAL SYNDROMES

Hundreds of thalassemia mutations and hemoglobin variants exist, but only a minority occur with any regular frequency. The geographic distribution of most of the more common hemoglobinopathies—α- and β-thalassemia, Hb S, Hb E, and Hb C—coincides with that of endemic *Plasmodium falciparum*. The common hemoglobinopathies have been selected for and preserved over time in the Mediterranean basin and equatorial and near-equatorial regions of Asia and Africa because their simple heterozygous inheritance provides a selective advantage against dying of malaria. This section provides a framework in which these disorders and a few of the less common ones can be understood (Table 4), and the emphasis is on the conditions that are most frequent. Chapter 4 discusses Hb S and sickle cell disease.

Thalassemia Syndromes

Thalassemia is most common along the shores of the Mediterranean and in the Arabian peninsula, Turkey, Iran, India, Thailand, Cambodia, and southern China. The gene frequencies in these populations are 2.5% to 15%. The two most common thalassemia syndromes, α- and β-thalassemia, are due to decreased α- and β-globin chain production, respectively. Other mutations affecting *both* the structure and the quantity of either the α- or the β-globin products are assigned distinct names and cause particular syndromes. Two such variants are Hb Constant Spring—an α-globin variant—and Hb E—a β-globin variant (see page 55).

Although a multitude of potentially baffling labels (Tables 2 and 3) are used within the cadre of α- and β-thalassemia, the principles are straightforward:

1. Excluding double or compound heterozygosity, there is only one clinical disease of β-thalassemia, although the spectrum of severity has been arbitrarily divided into two clinical conditions—thalassemia intermedia and thalassemia major. Genotypic overlap between thalassemia intermedia and thalassemia major exists because of the phenotypic variability of β+-genotype and other coinherited determinants.
2. For α-thalassemia, also excluding compound heterozygosity, there is only one disease state compatible with life ex utero—Hb H disease.
3. The simple heterozygous states of α- or β-thalassemia are referred to as "trait" or "minor" and, with the exception of the potential for mild laboratory abnormalities, are clinically silent.

β-THALASSEMIA

Thalassemia Minor (Thalassemia Trait)

Thalassemia minor is a clinically silent condition (Table 3). Risks associated with this genotype are the potential for siring an offspring with thalassemia major or a compound heterozygous hemoglobinopathy and iatrogenic iron overload in the case of misdiagnosis of iron deficiency anemia. Patients with β-thalassemia minor have an increased erythrocyte count, hypochromia, and microcytosis (mean corpuscular volume, < 75 fL). There may be a mild anemia (hematocrit about 30% or more). The peripheral smear may reveal poikilocytosis, ovalocytes, and basophilic stippling (Fig. 2 *A*, Plate 3). Osmotic fragility is decreased. Features commonly distinguishing β-thalassemia minor from iron deficiency anemia include an increased erythrocyte count, a normal red cell distribution with

Table 2
Corresponding Phenotype, Genotype, Representation of Gene Map, and Abbreviation for Selected α-Thalassemia Syndromes

Phenotype	Genotype	α-Gene map[a]	Abbreviation
Normal	Normal	—■—■— / —■—■—	$\alpha\,\alpha$
Silent carrier of α-thalassemia	Heterozygous α^+	—■—■— / —■—	$\alpha\,\alpha^+$
α-Thalassemia trait	Heterozygous α^0	—■—■— / ———	$\alpha\,\alpha^0$
α-Thalassemia trait	Homozygous α^+	—■——— / —■———	$\alpha^+\alpha^+$
Hemoglobin H disease	Compound heterozygous $\alpha^+\alpha^0$	—■——— / ———	$\alpha^+\alpha^0$
Hemoglobin Bart's hydrops fetalis	Homozygous $\alpha^0\alpha^0$	——— / ———	$\alpha^0\alpha^0$

[a] ■, normal α-globin gene; —, deletion of gene.

Table 3
Corresponding Phenotype, Genotype, Representation of Gene Map, and Abbreviation for Selected β-Thalassemia Syndromes

Phenotype	Genotype	β-Gene map[a]	Abbreviation
Normal	Homozygous Hb A	——□—— / ——□——	$\beta^A\beta^A$
Thalassemia minor (thalassemia trait)	Heterozygous β^0 thalassemia	——□—— / ——⊡——	$\beta^A\beta^0$
	Heterozygous β^+ thalassemia	——□—— / ——⊞——	$\beta^A\beta^+$
Thalassemia intermedia[b]	Double heterozygous β-thalassemia	——⊞—— / ——⊡——	$\beta^+\beta^0$
	Homozygous β^+ thalassemia	——⊞—— / ——⊞——	$\beta^+\beta^+$
Thalassemia major ("Cooley's anemia")[b]	Homozygous β^0 thalassemia	——⊡—— / ——⊡——	$\beta^0\beta^0$

[a] —, deletion of gene; □, normal β-globin gene; ⊞ β^+-globin mutation; ⊡ β^0-globin mutation.
[b] Only a few of the genotypes for thalassemia major and thalassemia intermedia are represented (see text).

an increased Hb A_2 (in the absence of concurrent iron deficiency), and normal free erythrocyte porphyrins.

Thalassemia Intermedia

Thalassemia intermedia is the clinical appellation for patients with two β-thalassemia genes but whose phenotype is less severe than thalassemia major (Table 3). The most commonly associated genotypes are β^+/β^+ or β^+/β^0, with a relatively high β-globin producing β^+ mutation. The disease is extremely heterogeneous at the genotypic level. Coinheritance of α-thalassemia or hereditary persistence of fetal hemoglobin reduces disease severity and may transform what would have been a thalassemia major phenotype into thalassemia intermedia. Affected persons are typically asymptomatic, but the spectrum of disability is broad. The most frequent complications are hypersplenism, gallstones, and ankle ulcers. By definition, they are not transfusion-dependent, but they are still at risk for iron overload with its accompanying complications. Patients with thalassemia intermedia should be given folate supplementation and periodic red blood cell transfusions and be monitored for iron overload. Chelation therapy should be given as described on page 49.

Thalassemia Major

Thalassemia major is a severe clinical condition requiring chronic hypertransfusion therapy. The genotypes yielding this phenotype include β^0/β^0, β^+/β^0, and β^+/β^+ (Table 3). Much of the pathology in thalassemia is due to α- and β-globin chain imbalance (Fig. 3). The relative surplus of α-globin chains results in formation of insoluble α_4 tetramers, which poison proerythroblasts and erythrocytes, causing ineffective erythropoiesis and hemolysis, respectively. The attenuated syndrome observed with coinherited α-thalassemia is illustrative of this concept.

From ineffective erythropoiesis and chronic hemolysis stems reduced oxygen-carrying ability, futile increase in iron absorption, and red marrow expansion. The kidneys detect decreased oxygen-carrying capacity and produce increased erythropoietin, which causes massive bone marrow expansion, bony deformities, fractures, and extramedullary hematopoiesis. The spleen and liver are major sites of extramedullary hematopoiesis, and enlargement is common. Bone changes resulting from inadequate transfusion therapy include frontal bossing, flattening of the nose, prominent molar eminences, cortical thinning of the long bones (Fig. 4 A), premature closing of the epiphyses of the humerus and femur, and the classic "hair-on-end" appearance of skull radiographs. The increased gastrointestinal iron absorption triggered by chronic anemia and the defective iron utilization due to ineffective hematopoiesis result in hemosiderosis. Cirrhosis, cardiomyopathy (Fig. 4 B), and endocrine insufficiency are primarily due to iron deposition. Chronic hemolysis contributes to pigment gallstones, jaundice, leg ulcers, and splenomegaly—and sometimes hypersplenism.

Because of the normal production of Hb F in infants, thalassemia major is asymptomatic until approximately 6 months after birth. Without intervention, median survival is less than 4 years, and 80% of affected children die by the age of 5 years. Fortunately, with current management strategies, the natural history has been changed. Inherent disease modifiers include the specific β-globin mutation itself and coinheritance of α-thalassemia or hereditary persistence of fetal hemoglobin.

A myriad of laboratory abnormalities exist. There is marked anemia with a hemoglobin value in the range of 2.0 to 6.5 g/dL. The mean corpuscular volume, mean corpuscular hemoglobin, and mean corpuscular hemoglobin concentration are low. The peripheral blood smear reveals hypochromia, polychromasia, microcytosis, anisocytosis, poikilocytosis, target cells, basophilic stippling, and nucleated red blood cells (Fig. 2 B, Plate 4). The α_4 inclusions can be detected by special staining with methyl violet. Increases in transaminases represent both hemolysis and liver dysfunction. Increased bilirubin and lactate dehydrogenase and decreased haptoglobin are consistent with chronic hemolysis. Saturated iron-binding capacity is a function of ongoing iron overload, as is increased serum ferritin, which may in part be due to liver dysfunction. Hyposthenuria and proteinuria may be found. The diagnosis is made with hemoglobin electrophoresis (see page 60).

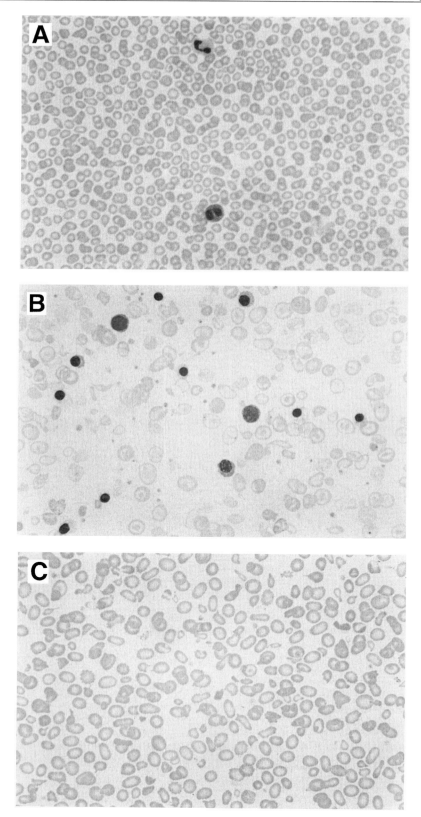

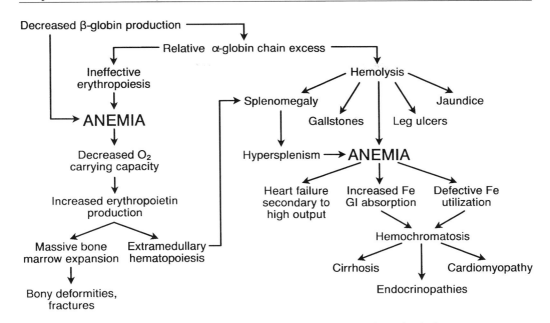

Fig. 3. Pathogenesis of β-thalassemia. Fe, iron; GI, gastrointestinal; O_2, oxygen.

The mainstays of treatment for thalassemia major are transfusion therapy plus chelation therapy and hematopoietic stem cell transplantation. Because these maneuvers are inconvenient and expensive, several preventive strategies exist. In high-risk populations, preventive programs based on mass education, heterozygote detection, nondirective counseling, fetal diagnosis, and elective termination of pregnancies have been effective for reducing the birth rate of infants with β-thalassemia major. For example, in Sardinia, the number of live infants born with β-thalassemia major has been reduced from 1 in 250 to 1 in 1,250 per year. Prenatal diagnosis can be made safely during the first 9 or 10 weeks of gestation through chorionic villus sampling and fetal DNA analysis by dot blot analysis or primer-specific amplification.

For persons born with thalassemia major, good—though physically, emotionally, and financially costly—therapeutic options exist. Hypertransfusion to a hemoglobin value of 9 to 10.5 g/dL not only improves symptomatic anemia, quality of life, and longevity but also prevents the red marrow expansion and resultant skeletal deformity, the high-output cardiomyopathy, and the growth retardation caused by severe chronic anemia. Adopted in the 1960s and 1970s, hypertransfusion with approximately 10 mL/kg every 2 to 3 weeks results in normal development until age 10, at which time stigmata of iron overload begin to become apparent. Without adequate chelation therapy, by the age of 20 the manifestations of secondary hemochromatosis are readily found: diabetes mellitus in 43%, hypothyroidism in 28%, liver disease in 26%, hypoparathyroidism in 22%, and cardiac disease in 20%. Once more than one of these complications manifest, the median survival is 10 years.

Fig. 2. *(opposite page)* Peripheral smears. *A*, Plate 3, β-Thalassemia minor: hypochromia, microcytosis, poikilocytosis, and ovalocytes. *B*, Plate 4, β-Thalassemia major: hypochromia, polychromasia, microcytosis, anisocytosis, poikilocytosis, target cells, basophilic stippling, and nucleated red blood cells. *C*, Plate 5, Hemoglobin H disease: marked hypochromia along with anisocytosis, poikilocytosis, basophilic stippling, polychromasia, and microcytosis.

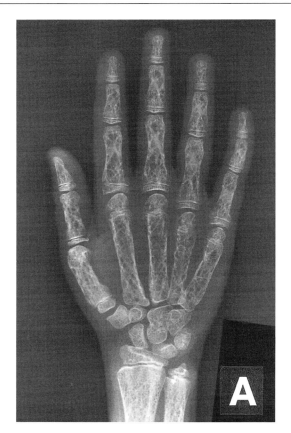

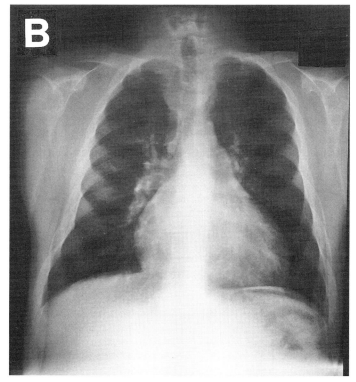

By the late 1970s, adequate chelation therapy with the drug deferoxamine had become routine. Deferoxamine, a parenteral chelator with a short half-life, is administered subcutaneously at a dose of approximately 40 mg/kg per day (upper limit of 2 g/day) over 10 to 12 hours 5 to 7 days per week. Treatment is commenced before the age of 5 or when the serum ferritin level is 1,000 to 1,500 ng/mL and the total iron-binding capacity saturation is more than 50%. For patients who have severe iron overload, large doses of continuous intravenous deferoxamine can reduce iron stores within 1 to 2 years. Care is taken not to use chelation when the iron burden is still low because there is a much higher risk of toxicity, including ophthalmic and ototoxicity complications. Yearly hearing and ophthalmologic testing are indicated. Infection with *Yersinia* spp. is not uncommon in deferoxamine-treated patients. It should be suspected in a patient who presents with abdominal complaints, fever, and sore throat while undergoing chelation therapy. L1 (1,2-dimethyl-hydroxypyrid-4-one) is an oral iron chelator that has not yet proved to be safe or effective.

Optimal chelation is possible when ascorbate levels are adequate, and supplementation with 60 to 100 mg per day is routine. Quantitating total body iron stores noninvasively is a challenge. Measurements of urinary or stool iron secretion, serum ferritin levels, and iron deposition in the liver by computed tomography or magnetic resonance imaging are used, but they correlate suboptimally with total body iron. Liver biopsy is considered the standard for quantitating total body iron stores.

Multiple strategies are implemented to increase the safety and effectiveness of erythrocyte transfusions. All patients should be immunized against hepatitis B. Because allosensitization of clinically important blood group antigens occurs in up to 25% of multiply transfused patients with thalassemia, their blood should always be matched with donor blood in ABO, Rhesus, and Kell systems. Leukocyte-reduced red cell products are administered to reduce HLA sensitization and urticarial and febrile transfusion reactions. Hypersplenism is a consequence of regular transfusion therapy, and splenectomy is generally recommended once transfusion requirements exceed 200 to 250 mL/kg of body weight per year. More than 3 to 4 weeks before elective splenectomy, patients should be immunized against *Streptococcus pneumoniae*, *Haemophilus influenzae*, and *Meningococcus*. After splenectomy, penicillin prophylaxis should be administered at least until the age of 5 to protect against overwhelming encapsulated organism sepsis.

Positive antibodies to hepatitis C virus are as high as 60%. Patients should be screened for the virus; if the results are positive, treatment with interferon-α should be considered. Predictors of response have included the degree of liver siderosis, hepatitis C virus serotype, and presence of cirrhosis. Response rates range from 30% to 41%.

The 1980s introduced allogeneic stem cell transplantation as a tool in the therapeutic armamentarium against homozygous β-thalassemia. Approximately 40% of patients with β-thalassemia major have an HLA-identical-matched relative who may serve as a donor. Certainly, transplantation is not without risk or expense. The intent, however, is cure. Morbidity and mortality due to acute and chronic graft-versus-host disease, graft failure, infection, multiorgan failure, and hemorrhage are possible. The largest experience with

Fig. 4. *(opposite page)* Radiographic changes due to β-thalassemia. *A*, Hand of 14-year-old boy with β-thalassemia. Note thinned cortex, thickened trabeculae, and widened marrow spaces. *B*, Chest of 21-year-old man with a history of β-thalassemia. Note increased bone width, coarse trabecular pattern, and cardiac enlargement due to high output failure.

allogeneic transplant for thalassemia has been in Pesaro, Italy. On the basis of this experience, patients are stratified into three classes of risk based on chelation therapy history, presence of hepatomegaly, and presence of portal fibrosis. Children with all favorable characteristics have close to a 100% survival rate, whereas those with one or two unfavorable characteristics have 87% and 54% survival rates, respectively. Patients older than 16 years have event-free survival rates of approximately 65%.

α-THALASSEMIA

Many of the principles of β-thalassemia apply to α-thalassemia, although three intrinsic characteristics set them apart: 1) the number of gene loci per haplotype, 2) the timing of globin gene switching during ontogeny, and 3) the solubility characteristics of the tetramers formed from the excess globin chains.

First, the number of gene loci per haplotype affects inheritance patterns and clinical severity. All normal individuals have two α-chain loci—but only one β-chain locus—per haploid genome. On any given chromosome, a mutation may occur that deletes either one or both α-globin genes, resulting in the α^+-thalassemia (-α/; α-thalassemia-2) and α^0-thalassemia (--/; α-thalassemia-1) haplotypes, respectively (Table 2). This has important clinical implications. Whereas loss of expression of two β-globin genes results in thalassemia major, the absence of one or two of four α-globin genes causes no *symptomatic* abnormality. Respectively, these two conditions are known as α-thalassemia silent carrier and α-thalassemia minor (trait).

Second, the timing of globin gene switching during development determines the timing of disease presentation. Recall that gene switching to the adult globin genes occurs at approximately 6 weeks and 6 months for the α-chains and β-chains, respectively (Fig. 1 D). Hence, persons homozygous for a β^0-thalassemia mutation do not manifest symptoms until approximately 6 months after birth; persons devoid of all four α-globin genes are affected by 6 weeks after conception.

Third, the solubility characteristics of the tetramers formed from excess globin chains determine the clinical spectrum of disease. Because the β_4 tetramers formed in the α-thalassemias are more soluble than the α_4 tetramers formed in β-thalassemia, they precipitate less readily. Fewer inclusions form in proerythroblasts, resulting in less ineffective hematopoiesis. The β_4 tetramers (Hb H) do, however, accumulate in erythrocytes and cause hemolysis.

α-Thalassemia Carrier States

The α^+-thalassemia carrier state may well be the single most common gene disorder in the world. The carrier states for α^+- and α^0-thalassemia do not produce symptoms. The α^+- and α^0-thalassemia deletions occur in both Asian and Mediterranean populations, although only the α^+-thalassemia deletions are common among Africans. The clinical implication is that the (--/-α) and (--/--) genotypes—hemoglobin H disease and hemoglobin Bart's hydrops fetalis, respectively—are possible among Asians but extremely rare among Africans, who in the homozygous state are (-α/-α).

From a routine laboratory perspective, an α^+-heterozygote—an α-thalassemia silent carrier—is usually undetectable. Affected persons have no anemia; only occasionally do they have minor erythrocyte changes such as microcytosis. Both the α^0-thalassemia heterozygote (αα/--) and the α^+-thalassemia homozygote (α-/α-) qualify as α-thalassemia trait. In these persons, the hemoglobin is normal to slightly decreased and the mean corpuscular volume is commonly decreased in the range of 60 to 75 fL. The red cell count may be increased. No easily identifiable abnormalities are present on electrophoresis for the α-thalassemia carrier states. Unlike the carrier state of β-thalassemia, the Hb A_2 is normal. The diagnosis of α-thalassemia carrier state is most easily made if microcytosis is present and there is a family history of Hb H disease. Globin-chain synthesis studies and DNA analysis can be used to obtain a definitive diagnosis, but they are rarely indicated. The differential diagnosis includes iron deficiency anemia, β-thalassemia trait, and sideroblastic anemia.

Hemoglobin Bart's Hydrops Fetalis Syndrome

The hemoglobin Bart's hydrops fetalis syndrome is due to homozygosity of the α^0-thalassemia haplotype (--/--). In utero, γ-globin tetramers form—Hb Bart's—because of the absence of α-globin. Affected infants have no Hb A and tiny amounts of Hb Portland and Hb H, and they die in utero or within hours after birth.

Hemoglobin H Disease

Hemoglobin H disease (--/-α) was the first recognized form of α-thalassemia. It occurs primarily in Southeast Asians and also, but to a far lesser degree, in persons from the Mediterranean basin and the Middle East. It is distinctly uncommon in people of African descent. The clinical phenotype is similar to that of thalassemia intermedia, although this is very variable.

The primary complications of this disorder are the anemia, skeletal changes due to marrow expansion, increased risk for infection, hepatomegaly, and splenomegaly with resultant hypersplenism. There is much less ineffective hematopoiesis in α-thalassemia than in β-thalassemia because of the different solubility characteristics of β_4 and α_4 tetramers, although there is still a moderate hemolytic anemia. Iron overload is less a problem in Hb H disease than in other forms of thalassemia. The chronic hemolytic anemia is sometimes exacerbated by oxidant drugs. Early development is normal, and longevity is not clearly compromised. Pregnancy frequently worsens the anemia, and hemoglobin concentrations may decrease to 4 to 5 g/dL.

The hematologic findings include an average hemoglobin value of 7.4 to 7.8 g/dL (range, 2.6 to 12.4 g/dL). The red cell count is relatively high, and the mean corpuscular hemoglobin and mean corpuscular volume are low. Marked hypochromia along with anisocytosis, poikilocytosis, basophilic stippling, polychromasia, and microcytosis are seen on the peripheral smear (Fig. 2 *C*, Plate 5). Most notable in Hb H disease, however, are the artifactual ragged red cell inclusions (precipitated Hb H) that can be seen after incubation with brilliant cresyl blue. After splenectomy, Heinz bodies are seen on supravital stain. The total amount of Hb H in the erythrocytes of patients with Hb H disease varies from 2% to 40% (mean, 8% to 9%); Hb Bart's is also present in small quantities, and Hb A_2 is always diminished.

Therapy is supportive and as needed. Transfusions are rarely required. Occasionally, splenectomy is useful if there is significant hypersplenism. Oxidant drugs should be avoided.

HPFH and $\delta\beta$-Thalassemia

Hereditary persistence of fetal hemoglobin (HPFH) and $\delta\beta$-thalassemia are the primary inherited conditions leading to persistently increased Hb F in adulthood. These conditions are heterogeneous, and the distinction between them is not always clear-cut, especially in deletional HPFH. Some of the more common genotypes leading to HPFH and $\delta\beta$-thalassemia are shown in Figure 5. Deletional HPFH is usually allelic with the

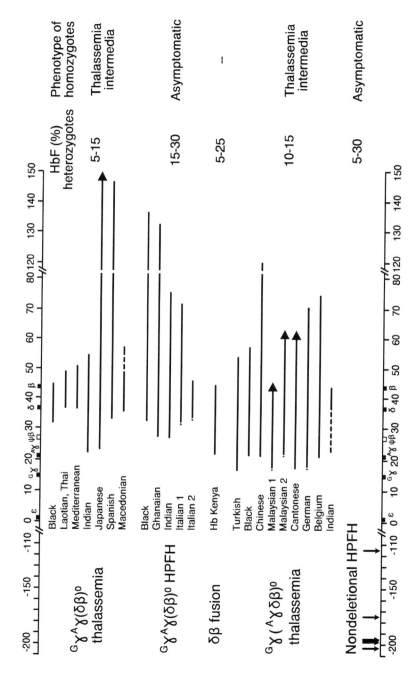

Fig. 5. Selected deletions and base substitutions resulting in δβ-thalassemia and hereditary persistence of fetal hemoglobin (HPFH) phenotypes. The extent of the deletion is shown by the solid line. Arrows indicate that the deletions continue for an unknown distance. Small regions of uncertainty at the ends of deletions are indicated by a dot. The dotted lines show the inverted region in the two inversion-deletion mutants. The scale is in kilobases measured from the 5' end of the ε-gene. Substitutions causing nondeletional HPFH conditions are marked by arrows. (Modified from Wood WG. Increased HbF in adult life. *Baillieres Clin Haematol* 1993; 6 no. 1: 177–213. By permission of WB Saunders Company.)

54

β-globin gene. In contrast, in nondeletional HPFH, the γ-globin and β-globin genes situated next to each other (cis-configuration) are usually produced in inverse proportions. In the classic form of HPFH, heterozygosity is characterized by an absence of microcytosis and levels of Hb F of 15% to 25%. Homozygous inheritance is clinically asymptomatic, although the red cells are microcytic and hypochromic. In contrast, δβ-thalassemia heterozygotes usually have levels of Hb F of 5% to 15% and microcytosis, and homozygotes have a phenotype similar to that of thalassemia intermedia or major. Compound heterozygosity of β-thalassemia with HPFH produces mild disease, whereas with δβ-thalassemia, there is clinically moderate to severe disease. The number and nature of all the genetic factors both within and outside the β-globin gene cluster are yet to be determined.

Thalassemia Variants

The most common thalassemic structural variants include Hb E, Hb Constant Spring, and Hb Lepore. These variants share the characteristics of decreased globin production, but they differ from simple α- and β-thalassemia in that the globin product is abnormal.

HEMOGLOBIN E

Found almost exclusively in peoples of Southeast Asian and Indian subcontinent ancestry, hemoglobin E is the second most common abnormal hemoglobin in the world. It results from a mutation at codon 26 of the β-globin gene. The mutant DNA sequence is transcribed into an mRNA that can either be translated into a β-globin chain with a glutamic acid to lysine substitution at position 26—Hb E—or be alternatively spliced into a structurally abnormal, untranslatable mRNA. The alternative splicing region is a function of the Hb E DNA mutation doubling as a new cryptic RNA splice region. This alternative splicing occurs 40% to 50% of the time. Fifteen to 30% of the Cambodian, Thai, Chinese, and Vietnamese populations carry the Hb E mutation. Clinically, both heterozygotes and homozygotes are asymptomatic, although their erythrocytes are microcytic. In homozygous Hb E "disease," there is only minimal anemia. The peripheral smear is notable for the absence of polychromasia and reticulocytosis and for the presence of microcytosis, hypochromia, and target cells. In dramatic contrast, compound heterozygotes for Hb E and β-thalassemia have a clinical syndrome akin to β-thalassemia intermedia or major.

HEMOGLOBIN CONSTANT SPRING

Hemoglobin Constant Spring is an α-chain variant. The mutation occurs at the 3'-terminus of the α-globin gene and results in alteration of the normal translation termination codon. The α-globin output of this gene is only about 1% of normal, and its α-globin product is 31 amino acids longer than normal. The phenotype is similar to that of α+-thalassemia.

HEMOGLOBIN LEPORE

Hemoglobin Lepore (Hb Lepore) results from fusion of the 5' portion of the δ-gene and the 3' portion of the β-gene. Because production of this globin chain is controlled by the δ-gene promoter, only small amounts are transcribed—hence, the thalassemia classification. This hemoglobin migrates in the Hb S position. Hemoglobin Lepore contributes to 5% to 10% of the clinical cases of β-thalassemia in Greeks and Italians.

Structural Hemoglobinopathies

The structural hemoglobinopathies are categorized separately in Table 4, but there is considerable overlap. More than 1,000 structural variants have been described. Table 4

Table 4
Classification of Qualitative and Quantitative
Hemoglobin Variants, With a Few Representative Examples

Thalassemia syndromes
  α-Thalassemia
  β-Thalassemia
Hereditary persistence of fetal hemoglobin and δβ-thalassemia
Thalassemic structural variants
  Hemoglobin E ($\beta^{26Glu \to Lys}$)
  Hemoglobin Lepore (δ–β fusion)
  Hemoglobin Constant Spring (α variant)
Structural hemoglobinopathies
  Hemoglobins with altered solubility characteristics
    Hemoglobin S ($\beta^{6Glu \to Val}$)
    Hemoglobin C ($\beta^{6Glu \to Lys}$)
  Unstable hemoglobins
    Hemoglobin Köln ($\beta^{98Val \to Met}$)
    Hemoglobin Olmsted ($\beta^{141Leu \to Arg}$)
    Hemoglobin H (β_4 in individuals with α-thalassemia)
  Hemoglobins associated with altered oxygen affinity
    Increased affinity: associated with erythrocytosis
      Hemoglobin Malmö ($\beta^{97His \to Gln}$)
      Hemoglobin Chesapeake ($\alpha^{92Arg \to Leu}$)
      Methemoglobin (see below)
    Reduced affinity: associated with cyanosis
      Hemoglobin Kansas ($\beta^{102Asp \to Thr}$)
  Methemoglobin
    Hemoglobin M-Boston ($\alpha^{58His \to Tyr}$)
    Hemoglobin Saskatoon ($\beta63^{His \to Tyr}$)

is not intended to be comprehensive; rather, it is meant to facilitate an understanding of the hemoglobinopathies and thalassemias. Among the structural variants, hemoglobins S, E, and C are the three most common. Hemoglobin E was discussed under "Thalassemia Variants" (page 55).

HEMOGLOBINS WITH ALTERED SOLUBILITY CHARACTERISTICS

Both Hb S and Hb C demonstrate altered solubility characteristics, and they occur in persons of African heritage. For more about Hb S, see Chapter 4.

Hemoglobin C

Hemoglobin C was the second variant hemoglobin to be recognized. It results from substitution of a glutamic acid by a lysine at position 6 of the β-globin peptide. Hemoglobin C trait occurs in about 3% of African-Americans and is a harmless condition characterized by the presence of increased target cells. There are no symptoms and no anemia. Homozygous hemoglobin C disease is also relatively benign. Affected persons are generally asymptomatic, although they usually have splenomegaly. Once at a critical concentration, Hb C forms crystals, making red cells rigid, resulting in a mild hemolytic anemia with reticulocytosis and striking target cell formation. The compound heterozygous state for Hb C and Hb S is more common than homozygous CC disease, and it is associated with serious clinical disease. This disease occurs in approximately 1 of every 1,000 births among African-Americans, a prevalence nearly half that of homozygous hemoglobin S disease. See Chapter 4 for more information. In contrast, persons who are compound heterozygotes for β^0-thalassemia and Hb C are phenotypically similar to Hb C homozygotes.

Rare Functional Variants

Although the functional variants discussed in this section—the unstable hemoglobins, the altered oxygen-affinity hemoglobins, and the methemoglobins—are rare, multiple clinical scenarios exist in which they should be considered. Most of these variants produce in vitro phenomena, providing insight into the physical properties of the hemoglobin molecule, without producing any significant clinical manifestions. These hemoglobinopathies are expressed in an autosomal dominant fashion.

Two points worthy of emphasis regarding these variants are 1) hemoglobin electrophoresis should *not* be the initial laboratory test when one of these conditions is suspected, because many of these abnormalities are electrophoretically silent, and 2) lack of a family history does not exclude any of these diagnoses, given their relative rarity and the potential for spontaneous mutation.

UNSTABLE HEMOGLOBINS

More than 100 unstable hemoglobin variants have been described. The vast majority are without clinical significance; those that cause congenital hemolytic anemia are usually well compensated, although exacerbations may occur with the stress of infection or oxidant drugs. Hemoglobin Köln is the most common of these variants and is among the most common hemoglobinopathies for persons of French and German ancestry.

Mutations causing unstable hemoglobin cause weakening of the molecular interactions between the globin and heme molecules. Denatured fragments of globin subunits and heme precipitate, forming Heinz bodies, which can be seen on supravital stain with new methylene blue or brilliant cresyl blue. The Heinz bodies interact with the erythrocyte membrane, thereby impairing red cell deformability. Splenic trapping by reticuloendothelial cells results in "bite cells," extravascular hemolysis, and frequently complete removal of circulating Heinz bodies. The two most useful diagnostic tests are the heat instability and the isopropanol instability tests, either of which will cause denaturation of an unstable hemoglobin. Hemoglobin electrophoresis is optional because many mutations are electrophoretically neutral. Supportive transfusional therapy during times of stress may be indicated. If the chronic hemolysis is severe, splenectomy may be considered as a therapeutic strategy.

HEMOGLOBINS ASSOCIATED WITH ALTERED OXYGEN AFFINITY

Although altered oxygen-affinity variants are also rare, they should be considered in the setting of rubor and erythrocytosis or cyanosis. As shown in Figure 6, the test of choice is measurement of the P_{50}, the partial pressure of oxygen at which hemoglobin is 50% saturated with oxygen.

Increased-Affinity Hemoglobins

A history of lifelong erythrocytosis should trigger suspicion of an increased-affinity hemoglobin (Fig. 6). See Chapter 8 for the differential diagnosis of erythrocytosis. Hemoglobin Malmö is one such variant. Increased oxygen-affinity hemoglobins bind

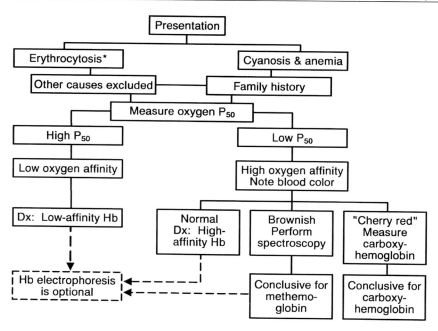

Fig. 6. Algorithm for abnormal oxygen-affinity hemoglobins. *Note that the absence of a family history does not exclude the diagnosis because the rate of spontaneous mutation is fairly high. *See Chapter 8 for erythrocytosis and text of this chapter for differential diagnosis of cyanosis. Dx, diagnosis; Hb, hemoglobin; P_{50}, partial pressure of oxygen at which hemoglobin is 50% saturated with oxygen.

oxygen more tightly than normal hemoglobin, and the oxygen dissociation curve is shifted to the left, resulting in a low P_{50} (Fig. 7). Note, however, that the most common cause of a low P_{50} is carboxyhemoglobin as a result of carbon monoxide exposure. Under normal atmospheric oxygen conditions, no more oxygen than normal is extracted from the lungs. At the peripheral capillary beds, where Po_2 is about 40 mm Hg, normal hemoglobin (P_{50}, 27 mm Hg) readily releases oxygen, whereas a high-affinity hemoglobin does not.

Despite an increased hematocrit value, patients are effectively "anemic" in that half of their hemoglobin—all of their increased-affinity hemoglobin—does not release oxygen. Most are asymptomatic, although some may experience mild fatigability. Usually the erythrocytosis is mild, and no intervention is required. When hematocrit values exceed 55% to 60%, phlebotomy may be considered. Smoking must be emphatically discouraged because carboxyhemoglobin compounds the erythrocytosis and reduces the "effective hematocrit."

Reduced-Affinity Hemoglobins

The hallmarks of reduced oxygen-affinity hemoglobins are asymptomatic, lifelong anemia and cyanosis. These hemoglobins bind oxygen less tightly than normal hemoglobin, and the oxygen dissociation curve is shifted to the right. The P_{50} is high (Fig. 6 and 7). The capacity to extract oxygen from the lungs is reduced, but under normal atmospheric oxygen conditions most of the hemoglobin molecules become fully saturated. At the peripheral capillary beds, the low oxygen-affinity hemoglobins efficiently release oxygen and become more desaturated than normal hemoglobin. When the concentration

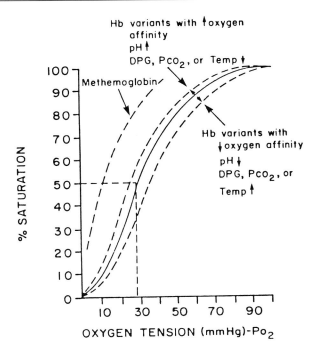

Fig. 7. Oxygen dissociation curve of hemoglobin. The normal curve is depicted by the solid sigmoidal curve. The P_{50} is represented by the dotted lines and is defined as the oxygen tension at which the hemoglobin molecule is 50% saturated with oxygen. 2,3-DPG, diphosphoglycerate; Hb, hemoglobin; P_{CO_2}, partial pressure of carbon dioxide; Temp, temperature. (From Benz EJ Jr. Synthesis, structure, and function of hemoglobin, in *Textbook of Internal Medicine* [Kelly WN, DeVita VT Jr, DuPont HL, Harris ED Jr, Hazzard WR, Holmes EW, Hudson LD, Humes HD, Paty DW, Watanabe AM, Yamada T, eds]. JB Lippincott Company, Philadelphia, 1989, pp. 1373-1379. By permission of the publisher.)

of deoxyhemoglobin exceeds 5 g/dL, patients appear cyanotic. Because of the efficiency with which these hemoglobins release oxygen, adequate tissue oxygenation is achieved at lower than normal hematocrit values. No treatment is indicated.

METHEMOGLOBIN

Methemoglobin is a hemoglobin whose heme molecules have been oxidized from the ferrous (Fe^{2+}) to the ferric (Fe^{3+}) state and therefore cannot carry oxygen. Despite normal Pa_{O_2} levels, values more than 1.5 g/dL result in cyanosis and a brownish tinge to venous blood. Small amounts of methemoglobin are normally formed in all persons because of the interaction of hemoglobin with superoxide ion. Levels are maintained at less than 1% by several mechanisms, one of which includes the reduced nicotinamide adenine dinucleotide (NADH) dehydrogenase (or the cytochrome b_5 reductase) system. In general, aside from cyanosis, methemoglobinemia is asymptomatic until levels exceed 30% to 50%. This condition may be inherited or acquired.

The M hemoglobins result from an amino acid substitution in either the α- or the β-globin gene in the region of the heme pocket that allows for formation of a stable methemoglobin. Hemoglobins M-Boston and M-Saskatoon are examples. The homozygous state is incompatible with life. Heterozygotes have about 20% to 30% methemoglobin. Another congenital form of methemoglobinemia is not due to a mutation of the globin genes but to a mutation in the gene for NADH dehydrogenase. In the homozygous state, most persons have methemoglobin levels of approximately 20% to 45%. Persons with congenital methemoglobinemia require no treatment. For the purpose of cosmesis, oral methylene blue and ascorbic acid can abrogate the cyanosis in NADH dehydrogenase deficiency.

Acquired methemoglobinemia is due to drugs or toxins. Infants, whose erythrocyte methemoglobin-reducing capacity is normally not fully developed, are at greatest risk. Large doses of oxidant drugs such as nitrites, sulfonamides, local anesthetics such as benzocaine and lidocaine, phenacetin, antimalarials, hydrogen peroxide, pyridium, and dapsone can all cause lethal methemoglobinemia. Nitrates, like those found in some well water, are converted to nitrites in the gut and can lead to methemoglobinemia. Sufficient exposure can be life-threatening. Symptoms of oxygen deprivation such as malaise and mental status changes occur as levels exceed 30%; loss of consciousness, coma, and death may occur as levels exceed 50%. Emergency treatment is intravenous methylene blue.

SPECIALIZED TESTING

The tools most frequently used clinically to identify hemoglobinopathies include cellulose acetate gel and citrate agarose gel electrophoresis, high-pressure liquid chromatography, and the sickle solubility test. For patients presenting with cyanosis or erythrocytosis, Po_2 and P_{50} measurements are the more appropriate first steps. In particular instances, isoelectric focusing, hemoglobin functional studies, and DNA testing also may be required. Reverse oligonucleotide hybridization, primer-specific amplification, single-strand conformation polymorphism analysis, and direct sequencing are among the techniques used in research laboratories rather than for routine clinical use.

Before specialized testing is used, several questions should be addressed. 1. What is the indication for testing? Clinical symptoms, family history, complete blood cell count, and peripheral blood smear abnormalities all contribute to the selection and sequence of laboratory investigations. 2. What is the patient's age? Hematocrit, erythrocyte indices, and Hb F levels are all age-dependent. 3. What is the individual's ethnic heritage? The prevalence of variants differs in different ethnic groups. 4. Have any transfusions been administered recently, or is iron deficiency present? Either will likely confound the results. Once a case is placed in the proper clinical context and other causes of anemia have been excluded, general algorithms may be followed, as outlined in Figures 6, 8, and 9 and Fig. 3 in Chapter 4. The importance of excluding iron deficiency before proceeding with hemoglobin electrophoresis cannot be overemphasized. Levels of Hb A_2, E, and H are reduced in the presence of iron deficiency; until replacement has occurred, diagnoses—most commonly, carrier states—may be missed.

Hemoglobin Electrophoresis

Hemoglobin electrophoresis separates molecules on the basis of their charge at a given pH. Cellulose acetate electrophoresis is performed at a pH of 8.6, whereas acid citrate agar electrophoresis is performed at a pH of 6.2. Because some hemoglobin variants have charge differentials as a result of their amino acid substitutions, they migrate at different rates under these particular conditions (Fig. 10).

Figure 8 outlines the approach for evaluating a person suspected of having either thalassemia or a structural variant other than an unstable or altered oxygen-affinity

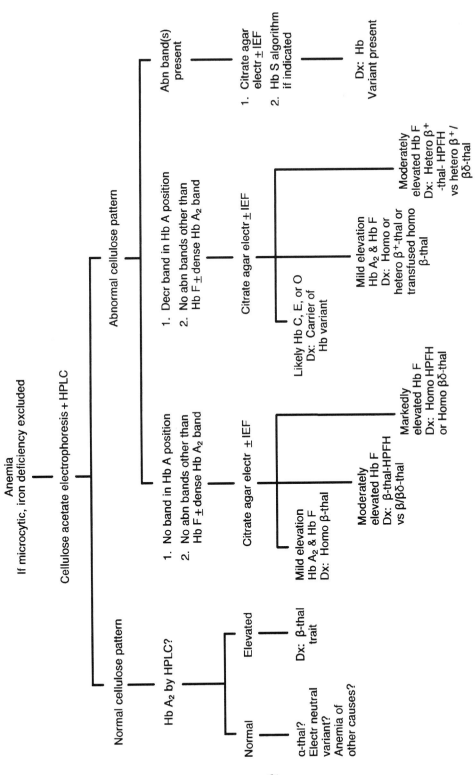

Fig. 8. Algorithm for detecting thalassemia or hemoglobin variant. Abn, abnormal; Decr, decreased; Dx, diagnosis; Electr, electrophoresis; Hb, hemoglobin; hetero, heterozygous; homo, homozygous; HPFH, hereditary persistence of fetal hemoglobin; HPLC, high-pressure liquid chromatography; IEF, isoelectric focusing; thal, thalassemia.

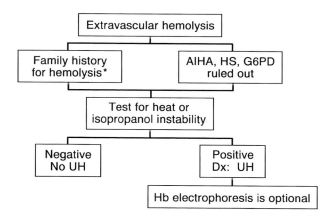

Fig. 9. Algorithm for unstable hemoglobin. AIHA, autoimmune hemolytic anemia; Dx, diagnosis; G6PD, glucose-6-phosphate dehydrogenase deficiency; Hb, hemoglobin; HS, hereditary sphero-cytosis; UH, unstable hemoglobin. *Absence of family history does not exclude diagnosis because the rate of spontaneous mutation is fairly high. For details on the extravascular hemolysis workup, see Chapters 1 and 2.

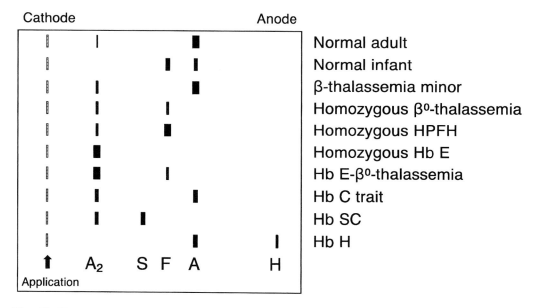

Fig. 10. Hemoglobin electrophoresis on cellulose acetate for selected hemoglobinopathies. Hb, hemoglobin; HPFH, hereditary persistence of fetal hemoglobin.

hemoglobin. It begins with cellulose acetate electrophoresis. If the pattern appears normal or if there is a slight increase in the band in the Hb A_2 region, Hb A_2 quantification by high-pressure liquid chromatography should be done. Hemoglobin A_2 of more than 3% to 6% in the presence of a mild microcytic anemia is consistent with β-thalassemia trait. A grossly normal cellulose acetate electrophoresis and a normal Hb A_2 in the absence of other causes for mild microcytic anemia, including iron deficiency, may represent α-thalassemia trait. There is usually no need to pursue globin chain synthesis studies or DNA testing to verify the α-thalassemia trait diagnosis.

Complete absence of the Hb A band implies homozygous β^0-thalassemia or homozygosity of a variant hemoglobin. Absence of additional bands with the exception of mild increases of Hb F and A_2 implies homozygous β^0-thalassemia. A moderate increase of Hb F suggests heterozygosity for HPFH or $\delta\beta$-thalassemia, whereas markedly increased levels of Hb F are consistent with homozygous HPFH or $\delta\beta$-thalassemia. A markedly reduced concentration in the Hb A position in the absence of abnormal bands, except for mild increases in the Hb F and A_2 positions, suggests homozygous β^0-thalassemia with a recent transfusion or a form of β^+-thalassemia. Additional bands in other positions require further evaluation with citrate agar electrophoresis and possibly isoelectric focusing. The presence of the fast-running Hb H (β_4) band along with a microcytic anemia establishes the diagnosis of Hb H disease—α-thalassemia. A band detected in the Hb S position is usually Hb S, but not always. Hemoglobins D-Punjab, G-Philadelphia, and Lepore migrate in this position, and a positive sickle solubility test easily excludes these three diagnoses. (See Chapter 4 for more on Hb S.) Trace amounts of Hb A with mild increases of Hb F and A_2 suggest a form of β^+-thalassemia. A moderate increase in density at the Hb A_2 position on cellulose acetate implies the presence of a variant hemoglobin migrating at this position, most commonly Hb C, Hb E, and Hb O-Arab. Erythrocyte indices, acid citrate agar electrophoresis, and sometimes isoelectric focusing are useful in this circumstance.

Evaluation of Hemoglobin F

The quantification of Hb F is important in the diagnosis and management of the various forms of β-thalassemia and sickle cell disease. The most useful methods of quantitating Hb F include high-pressure liquid chromatography and the Kleihauer-Betke test. The former gives the percentage of Hb F present in the hemolysate. The latter allows for microscopic evaluation of the relative Hb F content of individual erythrocytes. Defining the distribution of Hb F in the red cells distinguishes among the various forms of $\delta\beta$-thalassemia and HPFH.

Evaluation of Unstable Hemoglobins and the Altered Oxygen-Affinity Hemoglobins

Algorithms for evaluation of the altered oxygen-affinity hemoglobins and the unstable hemoglobins are in Figures 6 and 9, respectively. Hemoglobin electrophoresis should *not* be the initial laboratory test when one of these conditions is suspected, because many of them are electrophoretically silent. For the unstable hemoglobins, the two most useful diagnostic tests are the heat instability and the isopropanol instability tests. With either of these tests, an unstable hemoglobin will denature, yielding the diagnosis.

Measurement of the P_{50}, the partial pressure of oxygen at which hemoglobin is 50% saturated with oxygen, determines whether an abnormal oxygen-affinity hemoglobin, including a methemoglobin, is present (Fig. 7). Methemoglobinemia—either congenital or acquired—can be detected with spectrophotometry. Hemoglobin M, an inherited form of methemoglobinemia, often can be appreciated with altered electrophoretic mobility, especially after exposure to ferricyanide in vitro.

FUTURE DIRECTIONS

Much progress has been made in understanding the molecular mechanisms of the hemoglobin gene clusters and the pathogenesis of the hemoglobinopathies and thalassemia syndromes. Better implementation of screening and prevention strategies is yet to come. As the fund of knowledge and technologic abilities continue to grow, more options will be available to patients with symptomatic disease. Although pharmacokinetic modulation of Hb F expression has not yet met with success for patients with β-thalassemia, other strategies appear promising. Efforts to produce a more convenient iron chelator continue. Advances in hematopoietic stem cell transplant technology, including cord blood, HLA mismatched, and unrelated donor transplantation, will make transplantation safer and more available for affected patients without HLA-identical related donors. Slow but consistent progress is being made in the realm of gene therapy, and with time perhaps it will be the intervention of choice.

SUGGESTED READING

Bollekens JA, Forget BG. δβ Thalassemia and hereditary persistence of fetal hemoglobin. *Hematol Oncol Clin North Am* 1991; 5 no. 3: 399-422.

Bunn HF, Forget BG. *Hemoglobin: Molecular, Genetic and Clinical Aspects.* WB Saunders, Philadelphia, 1986.

Fairbanks VF, ed. *Hemoglobinopathies and Thalassemias: Laboratory Methods and Case Studies.* Brian C. Decker, New York, 1980.

Higgs DR. α-Thalassemia. *Baillieres Clin Haematol* 1993; 6 no. 1: 117-150.

Higgs DR, Weatherall DJ, eds. The haemoglobinopathies. *Baillieres Clin Haematol* 1993; 6 no. 1.

Kazazian HH Jr, Boehm CD. Molecular basis and prenatal diagnosis of β-thalassemia. *Blood* 1988; 72: 1107-1116.

Lucarelli G, ed. *Bone Marrow Transplant* 1997; 19 Suppl 2.

Nagel RL, ed. *Hematol Oncol Clin North Am* 1991; 5 no. 3.

Weatherall DJ, Clegg JB. *The Thalassaemia Syndromes*, 3rd ed. Blackwell Scientific Publications, Oxford, 1981.

4 Sickle Cell Disorders

Angela Dispenzieri, MD

Contents

INTRODUCTION

The evolution of the understanding of sickle cell anemia has paralleled and driven that of medical and molecular genetics. The eventual discovery that a single amino acid substitution was responsible for the inheritable condition known as sickle cell anemia provided the first direct evidence that genes are expressed as polypeptides of specific sequence and that gene mutations can produce altered polypeptide products.

The term "sickle cell disease" refers to the collection of multisystem conditions defined by inheritance of at least one sickle hemoglobin gene. Hemolytic anemia, clinically painful crises, and multisystem complications characterize these disorders. Inheritance of the sickle cell gene in homozygosity results in **sickle cell anemia**; in simple heterozygosity, **sickle cell trait**, a clinically silent condition; and in compound heterozygosity with other mutant β-globin genes, **other forms of sickle cell disease**, including hemoglobin SC disease and sickle cell-thalassemia (Table 1). The clinical heterogeneity of these conditions is due to both genetic modulation and environmental factors.

The prevalence of the sickle cell gene is highest in equatorial Africa, Arabia, India, Israel, Turkey, Greece, and Italy. Endemic *Plasmodium falciparum* appears to be the force in preserving and selecting for the sickle cell trait in that carriers of sickle cell trait have innate partial resistance to dying of *P. falciparum* malaria. In African-American newborns the prevalence of sickle cell trait is 8% to 10%; sickle cell anemia, 0.17% to 0.25%; and sickle cell disease, 0.2% to 0.5%. Taken as a group, compound heterozygotes of β^S along with other β-globin mutations are almost as common as sickle cell anemia.

From: *Primary Hematology*
Edited by: A. Tefferi © Mayo Foundation for Medical Education and Research, Rochester, MN

Table 1
Laboratory Values

Diagnosis	Hemoglobin (Hb) pattern, %$^\alpha$			Hemoglobin, g/dL	Mean corpuscular volume, fL	Sickle cell crises
	Hb S	Hb A	Other			
Sickle cell trait	40	60		Normal	Normal	None
Sickle cell anemia	100	0		6-9	Normal to ↑	4+
Compound heterozygote Hb S-Hb C or sickle cell disease	57	0	Hb C 42	10-12	Normal to ↓	2+ to 3+
Sickle with HPFH	73-78	0	Hb F 20-25	Normal to ↓	Normal	1+ to 2+
Sickle-α-thalassemia	100	0	Hb A$_2$ 1-3	8-10	↓↓	3+
Sickle-β^0-thalassemia	100	0	Hb A$_2$ 4-6	7-10	↓↓	3+ to 4+
Sickle-β$^+$-thalassemia	70-94	3-25	Hb A$_2$ 3-6	9-11	↓	2+ to 3+

$^\alpha$Percentages are approximate.
Abbreviation: HPFH, hereditary persistence of fetal hemoglobin.

The goal of this chapter is to review the pathophysiology, diagnosis, clinical features, and management of the sickle cell syndromes. The primary emphasis is on sickle cell anemia, that is, the homozygous inheritance of hemoglobin (Hb) S. When distinctions between sickle cell anemia and the other forms of sickle cell disease need to be made, they are emphasized.

PATHOPHYSIOLOGY

An understanding of sickle cell disease requires a basic understanding of hemoglobin structure (see Chapter 3). Recall that hemoglobin is a tetrameric molecule and that the normal adult hemoglobin tetramer (Hb A) is comprised of two pairs of αβ heterodimers. The sickle cell mutation, a GAG → GTG transversion at codon 6 of the β-globin gene, results in the replacement of a glutamic acid by a valine at position 6 in the β-globin protein (Fig. 1). Hemoglobin S has distinctive chemical properties that alter the rheologic properties and the membrane function of the sickle erythrocyte. The continuous cycling of sickle hemoglobin between the oxy- and deoxy-conformations contributes to the damage done to the red cell membrane and to the vaso-occlusion that occurs in the capillaries.

Unlike deoxygenated Hb A, totally or partially deoxygenated Hb S is capable of aggregating into rigid polymers. These polymers form highly ordered fiber aggregates that essentially fill the cell, distorting it into the classic sickle shape or other elongated forms. The exquisite dependence of polymer formation on Hb S concentration accounts for the usual lack of polymerization, and therefore symptoms, in carriers (heterozygotes, Hb AS), newborn SS homozygotes (presence of significant amounts of Hb F for first 6 months after birth), and other persons with persistent Hb F expression. Other factors that play a role in solubility characteristics of Hb S are pH and temperature.

Although sickle cell anemia is not a "red cell membrane disorder," the red cell membranes are damaged by mechanical and oxidative injury imposed on them by the Hb S polymers and Hb S breakdown products. There is chronic hemolysis, and the injured

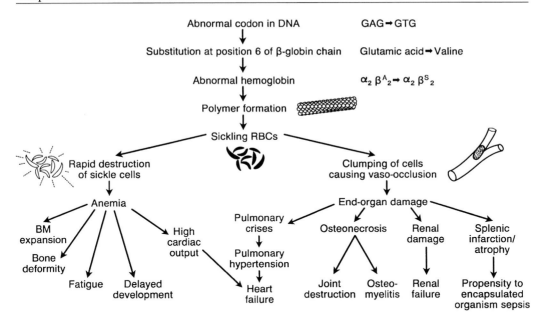

Fig. 1. Pathogenesis of sickle cell anemia. BM, bone marrow; RBCs, red blood cells.

membrane less effectively controls intracellular concentration and presents an abnormal surface to other cells and proteins in the plasma and along the vascular endothelium.

Vaso-occlusion is a function of decreased erythrocyte deformability, increased whole blood viscosity, and increased erythrocyte adherence to endothelium. Acute events of vaso-occlusion occur sporadically, erratically, and at various levels of clinical severity. Subacute and chronic subclinical events also contribute to end-organ damage. Sickling of red cells is sufficient to precipitate vaso-occlusion in certain situations; however, vaso-occlusion may also be due to other antecedent events, such as hemostatic activation, endothelial adhesivity, and increased vascular tone, with sickling then occurring as a secondary event.

A red cell containing a normal complement of Hb A undergoes passive deformation during passage through the microvasculature. The combination of decreased deformability of Hb S-containing erythrocytes and of low oxygen tension in the capillaries can cause a reduced rate of erythrocyte entry into, a reduction in flow rates through, and a mechanical trapping of these erythrocytes in these capillaries. Further conversion of oxy-Hb S to deoxy-Hb S may occur under these conditions, fueling a cyclic process of slowed transit time, deoxygenation, and progressive occlusion. Tissue hypoxia and damage result.

Blood viscosity is a function of four separate components: plasma viscosity, hematocrit, red cell aggregation, and red cell deformability. Decreased sickle erythrocyte deformability and increased plasma viscosity—which facilitate red cell aggregation—contribute to increased blood viscosity, whereas a low hematocrit decreases blood viscosity.

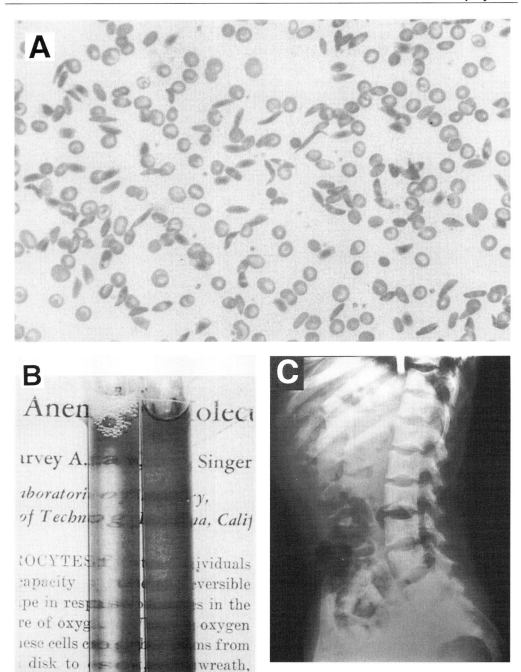

DIAGNOSTIC TESTS

The multisystem nature of sickle cell disease guarantees that a myriad of laboratory abnormalities will exist. The degree of abnormality depends on features of the individual, including genotype, age, and coexisting environmental factors.

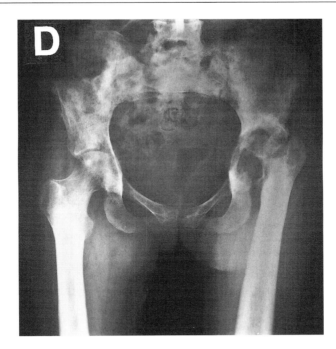

Fig. 2. *(opposite page and above)* Sickle cell composite findings. *A*, Plate 6, Sickle cell disease (peripheral smear): irreversibly sickled red cell forms, other elongated forms, nucleated red blood cells (not shown), Howell-Jolly bodies, polychromasia, target cells, mild leukocytosis (not shown), and thrombocytosis. *B*, Sickle solubility test. *C*, Sickle cell disease of spine. Note increased density of bones and the "fish-mouth" appearance of the vertebrae. *D*, Sickle cell disease of hips. Note marked deformity and resorption of left femoral head and neck and deformity of left acetabulum due to aseptic necrosis of femoral head. (*B*, From Fairbanks, VF. Hemoglobin, hemoglobin derivatves, and myoglobin, in *Fundamentals of Clinical Chemistry* [Tietz NW, ed] 2nd ed. W.B. Saunders Company, Philadelphia, 1976, pp. 401-454. By permission of the publisher.)

Routine Laboratory Tests

Persons with sickle cell trait do not have sickle cell disease, and their complete blood cell counts, peripheral smears, and serum chemistry values are normal. Under conditions of low oxygen pressure, sickling can be induced in vitro.

In contrast, patients with isolated homozygous sickle cell anemia have characteristic laboratory abnormalities. Their hemoglobin levels range from 6 to 9 g/dL (Table 1). In the absence of coexistent iron deficiency or thalassemia, the mean corpuscular volume is normal to high as a result of constitutive hemolysis and reticulocytosis. Reticulocytosis (reticulocyte value of 3% to 15%) is common. Irreversibly sickled red cell forms, other elongated forms, nucleated red blood cells, polychromasia, mild leukocytosis, and thrombocytosis also occur. Howell-Jolly bodies, Pappenheimer bodies, and Heinz bodies also may be found and are due to functional asplenia (Fig. 2 *A*, Plate 6). Unconjugated hyperbilirubinemia and increased lactate dehydrogenase and low haptoglobin levels are all a function of chronic hemolysis. In all genotypes, aspartate aminotransferase, alanine aminotransferase, and alkaline phosphatase levels are often increased; creatinine levels increase with age, presumably from declining renal function.

The presence of microcytosis with sickle forms suggests a compound heterozygous form of sickle cell disease. Such conditions include associated thalassemia or Hb C or Hb

E trait. The peripheral smear in these disorders is similar to that of sickle cell anemia, with the exception of the absence of leukocytosis and thrombocytosis. Persons with Hb SC disease have a mild anemia and microcytosis and sometimes thrombocytopenia secondary to hypersplenism. Because many of these patients are not asplenic, Howell-Jolly bodies, Pappenheimer bodies, and Heinz bodies may not be present. The serum bilirubin value is lower in Hb SC disease and sickle cell-β+-thalassemia than in sickle cell anemia as a result of a lower hemolytic rate. In all of these conditions, the lactate dehydrogenase value is increased and the haptoglobin value is low as a function of chronic hemolysis.

Methods of Hemoglobin Identification

The basic methods of identifying hemoglobinopathies include cellulose acetate gel and citrate agarose gel electrophoresis, high-pressure liquid chromatography, and the sickle solubility test (Fig. 3). Because the Hb S tetramer contains two more positive charges than does Hb A, its migration is slower on agarose gel electrophoresis (Fig. 4). For patients older than 1 to 2 years, cellulose acetate is adequate to exclude the presence of Hb S. In newborns, however, about 80% of the hemoglobin is Hb F. Because Hb F migrates between Hb A and Hb S on cellulose acetate, distinguishing Hb F from Hb A and Hb S in this age group may be difficult. Citrate agar gel electrophoresis is used in this circumstance because it clearly separates these three forms of hemoglobin. High-performance liquid chromatography is another method that can be used to separate hemoglobins.

The sickle solubility test (Fig. 2 B) is a very useful adjunct to cellulose acetate electrophoresis, because it can distinguish the presence of Hb S from other nonsickling hemoglobins that migrate in the Hb S position, such as Hb D-Punjab, G-Philadelphia, and Lepore. Hemoglobin S is insoluble and precipitates in high-molarity phosphate buffer solution when reduced with sodium hydrosulfite. Alone, the sickle solubility test cannot distinguish sickle cell trait from sickle cell anemia or sickle β-thalassemia. The test is also negative in newborns, given their high protective concentrations of Hb F.

Prenatal and Newborn Hemoglobin Testing

Safe prenatal testing and screening procedures are in routine use at many centers. The scientific, ethical, and legal discussions are beyond the scope of this chapter. The purpose of newborn hemoglobin testing is to identify affected individuals and begin early intervention programs. Newborn hemoglobin testing for hemoglobinopathies has been incorporated into newborn screening programs for metabolic disorders and is currently done in most states in the United States.

CLINICAL MANIFESTATIONS

Natural History

The natural history of the disease is variable and modulated by fixed factors (including coinheritance of other traits, among which are other hemoglobinopathies) and by environmental stressors. Chronic anemia, clinically painful crises, and multisystem complications characterize sickle cell anemia (Fig. 1 and 5). From 1973 to 1994, the mean duration of survival for patients with sickle cell disease increased from 14.3 years to 42 years for men and to 48 years for women with sickle cell anemia. This improvement is the result of improved general medical care.

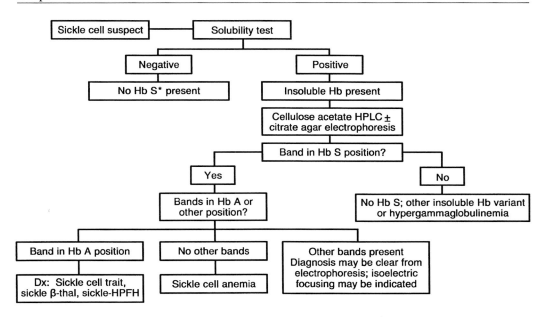

Fig. 3. Algorithm for diagnosing the presence of sickle hemoglobin. *Persons with a high level of Hb F will have a negative result of sickle solubility test despite the presence of Hb S. (See text for exceptions and explanation.) HPFH, hereditary persistence of fetal hemoglobin; HPLC, high-pressure liquid chromatography.

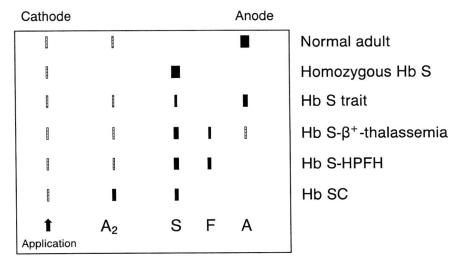

Fig. 4. Representation of hemoglobin electrophoresis on cellulose acetate. HPFH, hereditary persistence of fetal hemoglobin.

The importance of early identification and specialized routine health maintenance and education cannot be overemphasized. Immunizations, penicillin prophylaxis, education of parents and patients about maintaining hydration in heat and in illness, prompt attention to febrile illnesses, care for perimaleolar injuries, and follow-up in sickle cell centers have reduced early mortality rates and improved quality of life for many patients. Edu-

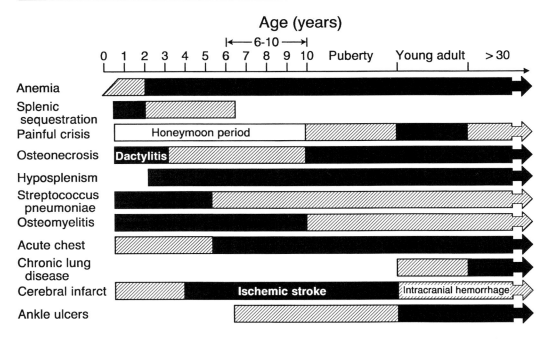

Fig. 5. Manifestations of sickle cell anemia. Clear area, rare; hatched, more common; black, most common.

cation of physicians about adequate pain management and specialized psychosocial support are also imperative.

Hematologic Complications

Anemia, the result of chronic hemolysis, is a typical feature of homozygous sickle cell anemia and of the compound heterozygous sickle syndromes other than sickle cell trait; in sickle cell trait, there is no anemia or hemolysis. The degree of hemolysis correlates with the number of irreversibly sickled cells, which is a function of the intracellular concentration of Hb S and the heterogeneous distribution of fetal hemoglobin. The anemia is detectable 2 to 3 months after birth, and in any given patient the hemoglobin concentration, reticulocyte count, and magnitude of hemolysis are relatively constant. Exacerbations may be due to aplastic crises, splenic sequestration crises, hepatic sequestration crises, folic acid deficiency, iron deficiency, chronic renal disease, or bone marrow necrosis.

Aplasia due to infection with B19 parvovirus, the most common cause of transient aplasia in children with sickle cell anemia, is less common in adults. The diagnosis is made by detection of B19 parvovirus particles or of IgM anti-B19 antibodies. Salmonella, *Streptococcus pneumoniae*, and Epstein-Barr virus infections have all been implicated in transient aplastic crises. Although the duration of aplasia is short, usually lasting only a few days, the severity may be extreme given the continued chronic hemolysis in the absence of compensatory erythropoiesis. The decision to transfuse should be based on the degree of anemia and cardiopulmonary distress because spontaneous reticulocytosis occurs within a few days of presentation.

Acute splenic sequestration crises are due to the acute intrasplenic trapping of blood, which leads to severe anemia, hypovolemia, and splenomegaly. The generally accepted criteria for this diagnosis are a decrease in the steady-state hemoglobin concentration of more than 2 g/dL, evidence of a compensatory marrow response, and an acutely enlarging spleen. Attacks may be mild (resolving spontaneously) or severe (causing shock and death). The inciting event for sequestration is unknown. The vast majority of cases occur before 2 years of age and almost all before 6 years. Splenic sequestration is less common in Hb SC disease, although it may occur beyond childhood in this population. Red cell transfusions and correction of hypovolemia are the mainstays of treatment. Recurrent splenic sequestration occurs in about 50% of children who survive the first episode. Strategies to prevent recurrence include a chronic transfusion program or splenectomy. Hepatic sequestration also has been described, but it is much less common. Management is akin to that of splenic sequestration.

Exacerbations due to folate and iron deficiency are uncommon in the United States. Normal erythropoiesis is dependent on an adequate folic acid store, and most patients with sickle cell anemia are folate-deficient, although deficiency has not been shown to correlate with hematologic changes or clinical course. Regardless, a prophylactic prescription of 1 mg/day of folic acid is common. Because sickle cell anemia is generally associated with an increase in total body iron stores as a result of enhanced gastrointestinal absorption of iron and red blood cell transfusion, iron deficiency is rare. Individuals with poor socioeconomic status, however, may become iron-deficient. They should be screened and treated appropriately.

Other causes for worsening anemia include drug or toxin exposure and erythropoietin deficiency arising from renal insufficiency.

Painful Crises

Second only to anemia, vaso-occlusive pain is the most common problem in patients with sickle cell disease. Painful crisis is typically defined as pain in the extremities, back, abdomen, chest, or head for which there is no other explanation. Only about 5% of patients with sickle cell disease have frequent (> 3 per year) pain episodes; approximately 80% have an average of 1 or fewer painful episodes per year. Pain syndromes and rates are also a function of age. Dactylitis occurs in patients younger than 2 to 3 years. From birth to the age of 10, there is a "honeymoon period" during which painful crises are less common. Pain rates are highest between 19 and 39 years. The frequency of painful crisis varies directly with the hemoglobin level and inversely with the percentage of Hb F. Cold, dehydration, infection, stress, or menses may precipitate a painful crisis, but the vast majority of episodes have no identifiable stimulus. Pain may be localized, multifocal, generalized, or migratory and lasts an average of 10 days (range, hours to weeks).

Few reliable objective signs of painful crisis exist. Clinical objective signs, which are present in about half of presenting patients, include fever, tenderness and swelling of an involved area, hypertension, tachypnea, tachycardia, nausea, and vomiting. Mild episodes can be managed at home. Episodes prompting medical attention, however, demand a thorough history and physical examination, a complete blood cell count, reticulocyte count, and measurement of lactate dehydrogenase for comparison with baseline values. Relative to the steady state, there is an increase in dense cells, a decrease in erythrocyte deformability, increased leukocytosis, and an increase in the red cell distribution width. Plasma viscosity, levels of serum lactate dehydrogenase, C-reactive protein, and fibrinogen, and fibrin D-dimer fragments are often increased over baseline. If the pain is not typical of a patient's usual crisis, an aggressive search for other causes such as infection, cholelithiasis, osteonecrosis, delayed transfusion reaction, and abdominal emergencies should be pursued as indicated.

Painful episodes of mild severity can be treated at home with bed rest, hydration, massage, relaxation, heating pads, and tub baths. Nonnarcotic analgesics, such as nonsteroidal anti-inflammatory drugs, or weak or strong narcotics are used as needed. For more severe episodes, a workup should proceed as outlined above. Oral or intravenous hydration, a heating pad, laxatives, muscle relaxants, and antiemetics may all provide benefit. Unless there are pulmonary problems, oxygen inhalation has not been shown to improve the course of the crisis.

The pain itself should be characterized for optimal management; fear of addiction should not interfere with prescribing narcotics. Most patients do not become addicted; reported rates of addiction range from 0% to 11%. Narcotics should be given on a scheduled basis with liberal rescue doses. Antihistamines such as hydroxyzine and diphenhydramine provide adjuvant analgesia. Tissue damage that accompanies the painful crisis results in histamine release, and antihistamines antagonize histamine effects at H_1 receptors. Nonpharmacologic methods to treat pain, such as cognitive-behavioral techniques, physiotherapy, and acupuncture, may be useful adjuncts.

Infectious Complications

Patients with sickle cell disease are at increased risk for bacterial infection because of their functional hyposplenism and their tendency for frequent tissue ischemia and infarct. Bacterial sepsis due to encapsulated organisms is the most common cause of death in infants and children with sickle cell disease. Infants and young children are subject to both an impaired reticuloendothelial system because of their sickle cell anemia and the normal age-dependent deficiency of immunoglobulins observed in this age group. Because the splenic red pulp environment is conducive to sickling—sluggish blood flow, increased viscosity, and a hypoxic, acidic milieu—local vaso-occlusion is common in sickle cell anemia. Resultant loss of reticuloendothelial function and intrasplenic shunting cause functional hyposplenism and a marked impairment in the ability to control infections caused by encapsulated microorganisms.

The use of prophylactic antibiotic therapy has been among the greatest advancements in managing sickle cell anemia. Childhood morbidity and mortality have been significantly reduced with oral penicillin therapy, beginning no later than 4 months of age to at least 3 years. *Haemophilus influenzae,* type b, conjugated vaccine and polyvalent pneumococcal vaccine should be given at 2 months and at 24 months of age, respectively. The pneumococcal vaccine may be repeated every 3 to 5 years. If there is any indication of chronic lung problems, the influenza vaccine should be administered yearly.

Any illness in a 6-month-old to 3-year-old associated with a temperature of more than 38.5°C should be treated as a medical emergency. After a thorough physical examination, blood, cerebrospinal fluid, and urine cultures and a chest roentgenogram should be obtained and empiric intravenous antibiotic therapy begun. Pneumococcal sepsis can present with nonspecific upper respiratory symptoms or diarrhea and a low-grade fever and deteriorate into high fever, rigors, shock, disseminated intravascular coagulation, and death within hours. If symptoms of an upper respiratory infection or pulmonary infiltrates are present, antibiotic coverage for *Mycoplasma pneumoniae* should be included. *M. pneumoniae* has been implicated as a possible precipitant of acute chest syndrome. *Chlamydia pneumoniae* and viral infections also may play a role in the acute chest syndrome (see Pulmonary Complications, see below).

The milieu provided by the relatively frequent bony tissue ischemia and infarct serves as a fertile environment for acute and chronic infection (see Bones and Joints, page 76). The most common pathogen is *Salmonella* spp., followed by *Staphylococcus aureus* as a distant second. Osteomyelitis more commonly occurs in children 10 years or younger. Presentation may be acute or insidious. It may be multifocal and even mimic acute dactylitis in infants and young children. The differential diagnosis is bone infarction, which is at least 50 times more common. Osteomyelitis is associated with high fever, chills, an increased erythrocyte sedimentation rate, a left shift in the leukocyte count, and positive blood culture; in contrast, osteonecrosis is associated with low-grade fever, a less increased erythrocyte sedimentation rate, negative cultures, and no left shift. When osteomyelitis is suspected, the bone should be aspirated for culture before instituting antibiotic therapy.

The risk for viral infection is no greater in patients with sickle cell disease than in individuals without a hemoglobinopathy. They do, however, have greater exposure to transfusion-transmitted viruses. Patients with sickle cell disease should, therefore, be vaccinated against hepatitis B. Sequelae of viral infection also may differ in patients with sickle cell disease, such as parvovirus-related aplastic crisis and the marked hyperbilirubinemia associated with viral hepatitis.

Pulmonary Complications

ACUTE CHEST SYNDROME

Beyond the age of 5, the major causes of mortality and morbidity are pulmonary. The acute chest syndrome occurs in 15% to 43% of patients with sickle cell disease and is responsible for up to 25% of deaths. Event death rates of 1.1% for children and 4.3% for adults have been described. Infectious agents (including viruses, typical and atypical bacteria), thromboembolism, and bone marrow and fat embolism have all been implicated as potential precipitants, but the cause of acute chest syndrome remains unclear and is likely multifactorial. Fever, chest pain, cough, hypoxemia, leukocytosis, and new pulmonary infiltrate(s)—most commonly in the lower lobes—characterize the syndrome. The course may progress to acute respiratory failure with an acute respiratory distress syndrome-like picture.

Treatment of acute chest syndrome includes 1) maintenance of normal arterial oxygen tension; 2) empiric antibiotic therapy, including coverage for community-acquired and atypical pneumonia; 3) cautious hydration with hypotonic saline to maintain euvolemia; 4) adequate analgesia; 5) simple transfusion for progressive anemia or hypoxemia; and 6) exchange transfusion for acute respiratory failure, the goal being reduction of the Hb S concentration to 20% to 30% while not exceeding a hematocrit value of 30%.

CHRONIC LUNG DISEASE

Chronic lung disease develops in some older children and adults after years of recurrent, often asymptomatic, vaso-occlusive events. It is characterized by progressive disabling dyspnea, exercise limitation, hypoxemia, chest pain, increased interstitial markings, a restrictive pattern on pulmonary function tests, pulmonary hypertension, and cor pulmonale. Interval chest roentgenography, ventilation-perfusion scanning, and blood gas and pulmonary function tests can identify early stages of sickle cell chronic lung disease. Because no randomized trials have examined the management of sickle cell chronic lung disease, interventions are empiric. Options include transfusion therapy or hydroxyurea (see pages 80 and 81).

Bones and Joints

Bone complications include osteonecrosis, osteomyelitis, joint damage, and disruption of normal bone architecture as a result of erythroid hyperplasia.

OSTEONECROSIS OF BONE

Infarcts occur in the red marrow of long bones, ribs, sternum, vertebrae, pelvic bones, and occasionally in the skull and facial bones (Fig. 2 *C* and *D*). Dactylitis, which occurs in early childhood, is caused by infarction in the small long bones of the hands or feet; it rarely occurs after the age of 2 years. Localized infarcts may produce swelling, excruciating tenderness, and rubor, making the clinical distinction from osteomyelitis difficult. Acute onset suggests infarction, whereas marked fever favors osteomyelitis. Compensated disseminated intravascular coagulation and fat emboli may occur. Long bone infarcts are rare in patients with Hb SC or Hb S-β^+ thalassemia.

Radiologic tools that may clarify the diagnosis include magnetic resonance imaging and bone, gallium, and bone marrow scanning. On magnetic resonance imaging, infarcted areas are best seen on intermediate and T2-weighted images, where they produce an increased signal. Congruent areas of increased uptake on both technetium Tc 99m-diphosphonate bone scan and gallium scan are consistent with osteomyelitis. A bone marrow scan may be helpful if the bone scan is not informative. In this clinical scenario, a defect in the marrow scan is highly specific for necrosis; a normal bone marrow scan strongly suggests osteomyelitis. Blood culture and bone culture should support this diagnosis.

Therapy is supportive for osteonecrosis, whereas osteomyelitis requires antibiotics with or without debridement (see page 75).

JOINT COMPLICATIONS

The incidence of osteonecrosis of the femoral and humeral heads tends to increase with advancing age and usually leads to progressive joint damage and destruction. Moderately high levels of Hb F or the presence of concomitant α-thalassemia does not protect patients from this complication. Total hip replacement may be considered for pain control or to regain function as the process advances over time. The prognosis for hip replacement has not been good; the rate of hip revision within 4 to 5 years is 30%. Core decompression of the adult femoral head may be a useful treatment option for patients with painful early-stage osteonecrosis. Osteonecrosis of the humeral head is less of a problem. Conservative strategies should be tried first, with joint replacement as a last resort.

Neurologic Complications

Cerebral vascular thrombosis is possibly the most catastrophic complication. Subtle neurologic damage is seen in many patients with sickle cell anemia, likely due to chronic insult to the cerebral microvasculature. Intracranial hemorrhage also may occur as a complication of cerebral infarction, as a result of a ruptured aneurysm, or in the setting of occlusive vasculopathy. The incidence of stroke per year during the first 2 decades of life is approximately 0.7%, and 79% to 80% of these strokes are cerebral infarctions. Abnormal results of transcranial Doppler study are predictive of a higher risk for stroke. The probability of remaining stroke-free at 40 months in the presence of an abnormal transcranial Doppler study is only 60%. Prophylactic transfusion to maintain Hb S below

30% reduced the incidence of stroke in high-risk children from 11/67 to 1/63 at a median follow-up of 21 months. Whether the cost and complications of prophylactic transfusion warrant the widespread application of this strategy is yet to be determined.

Acute treatment of a proved or suspected cerebral infarction consists of immediate partial or complete exchange transfusion and intravenous hydration with isotonic fluids. There are no randomized data to support this practice, but it is standard. Exchange is instituted as quickly as possible, the goal being to decrease the Hb S level to less than 30% without increasing the hematocrit to more than 33% to 35%. Care is taken to avoid hemodynamic instability. Typically, patients make good recovery from motor deficits. Cognitive deficits, however, are demonstrable on neuropsychological testing, especially if multiple infarcts have occurred.

The rate of recurrent stroke without chronic transfusion therapy is 46% to 90%. With chronic transfusion, maintaining Hb S at less than 30%, the risk of recurrent stroke is less than 10%. There are data to suggest that maintaining the Hb S at 50% is likely equally effective. Controversy exists about the timing of safe discontinuation of chronic transfusion.

Hepatobiliary and Gastrointestinal Complications

Hepatobiliary and gastrointestinal complications occur in sickle cell disease. Although biliary conditions are more common, intestinal and liver abnormalities also may exist. For example, bowel involvement is manifested by the paralytic ileus seen during some painful crises. Furthermore, hepatomegaly is present in 40% to 80% of patients in clinical series and in 80% to 100% in autopsy series. In addition, chronically transfused patients are at risk for infectious hepatitis and hemochromatosis.

There are multiple presentations of cholestasis. For example, mild cholestasis is common during acute painful syndromes. More significant biliary abnormality, however, may relate to the pigmented gallstones present in 30% to 70% of patients with sickle cell anemia. Right upper quadrant pain may represent acute cholecystitis, although the constellation of right upper quadrant pain, fever, leukocytosis, and mild increase in the transaminase level alternatively may be due to hepatic crisis. Hepatic crisis usually resolves in 1 to 3 weeks with supportive and transfusion therapy, but occasionally it may progress. Increases in total serum bilirubin and alkaline phosphatase values may reach 100 to 150 times the upper limits of normal; renal failure, coagulopathy, and death may follow. Fever, leukocytosis, and hyperbilirubinemia are not helpful for distinguishing acute cholecystitis from painful crisis. For this reason, the general recommendation for patients who have symptomatic cholelithiasis is to have elective laparoscopic cholecystectomy (see "Surgery," page 80).

Leg Ulcers

Leg ulcers are a very common cause of morbidity in patients with sickle cell anemia; the vast majority occur at the malleoli. Rates range from 25% to 75%. Characteristically, they are painful, slow to heal, and prone to recur. They may arise after trauma or spontaneously. Involvement of the subcutaneous tissues is not uncommon. Infection may contribute to enlargement and maintenance of these ulcers; *Staphylococcus aureus,* *Pseudomonas*, and *Streptococcus* are the organisms recovered most commonly. Subcutaneous fibrosis, joint deformity, chronic periostitis, and chronic osteomyelitis may develop. Management of chronic ulcers is similar to that of any chronic ulcer and includes gentle debridement and control of edema and infection.

Genitourinary Complications

RENAL

The entire nephron is affected by sickle cell disease. The environment of the normal renal medulla is one of hypertonicity, relative hypoxemia, and local acidemia—an environment that readily fosters sickling. Even persons with sickle cell trait, who are otherwise normal, have evidence of medullary damage. Patients are incapable of concentrating urine adequately. With advanced disease, tubular atrophy and focal infarction occur. An incomplete form of distal renal tubular acidosis with impaired potassium metabolism may develop. Papillary necrosis may develop and manifest as hematuria. In these extreme cases, the best therapy appears to be conservative, including bed rest, maintenance of a high urinary flow to prevent clots, alkalinization of the urine, and blood transfusion if anemia becomes severe. Glomerulosclerosis with resultant nephrotic syndrome is not uncommon. Renal insufficiency has been reported to occur in 4% to 18% of patients with sickle cell disease. Once renal failure occurs, patients generally do poorly. Dialysis with erythropoietin support is probably preferable to renal transplantation, even though 2-year survival after instituting dialysis is only about 60%.

PRIAPISM

The erection of priapism is that of persistent, usually painful, engorgement of the penis. Most episodes are self-limited and last less than 3 hours. If tumescence persists, partial exchange transfusion therapy can be tried. Injection of α-adrenergic agents, including phenylephrine and epinephrine, has met with variable success. Surgical intervention may be considered if there is no detumescence after 12 to 24 hours. The most frequent complications include persistence and recurrence. Some degree of impotence is common after a major episode of priapism.

Ophthalmic Complications

Retinopathy with neovascular malformations, vitreous hemorrhage, retinal tear, and retinal detachment are all potential complications of sickle cell disease. Hyphema, which often spontaneously resolves in patients without sickle cell disease, can lead to decreased vascular perfusion of the entire eye and irreversible blindness. Vitreous hemorrhage and retinitis proliferans are more common in Hb SC disease.

Growth and Development and Psychosocial Issues

Delays in somatic growth and sexual maturation occur and are related to the severity of the hemolytic anemia. Most patients are within 2 standard deviations of the mean; those below that range should have a more thorough endocrine and nutritional evaluation. The psychosocial stress of small stature and delayed sexual development can contribute further to the psychological hardship experienced by some affected children and young adults.

COMPOUND HETEROZYGOTES

Sickle Cell Trait

Sickle cell trait is benign clinically. The erythrocytes polymerize only when both dehydration and severe deoxygenation occur. There is a slightly increased risk for the following: hyposthenuria, hematuria, pulmonary embolism, splenic infarction at high altitudes, glaucoma due to hyphema, and pyelonephritis during pregnancy.

Hemoglobin SC Disease

In African-Americans, the prevalence of the double heterozygous state of Hb S and Hb C (Hb SC disease) is nearly half that of homozygous hemoglobin S disease. Almost all of the clinical manifestations of sickle cell anemia also occur in Hb SC disease, although usually in a milder form. Autosplenectomy occurs at an older age than in sickle cell anemia, and ophthalmic complications are more common.

Concurrent Thalassemia

About 15% of African-Americans have an α^+ deletion. Because a reduction of intracellular hemoglobin concentration decreases Hb S polymer formation, affected patients have slightly milder disease and potentially greater longevity.

Compound heterozygous sickle cell-β^0-thalassemia occurs infrequently. In contrast, sickle cell-β^+-thalassemia (Hb S-β^+-thalassemia) is more common and is subclassified according to the percentage of Hb A present: type I has 3% to 5%, type II has 8% to 14%, and type III has 18% to 25%. Eighty percent of African-American β^+-thalassemia mutations are due to the promoter region mutations that result in a type III phenotype. Clinically, Hb S-β^+-thalassemia tends to be less severe than sickle cell anemia. Splenomegaly may be present.

Sickle Cell Anemia With Hereditary Persistence of Fetal Hemoglobin

Sickle cell anemia with hereditary persistence of fetal hemoglobin (Hb S-HPFH) is a condition in which one β-globin gene is affected with the sickle mutation and the other with the HPFH mutation. No Hb A is produced. The most classic form of HPFH results from one of several large deletions of the δ- and β-globin genes that retard the switch from the production of Hb F to Hb A or from one of many point mutations that up-regulate the expression of the γ-globin gene. Because the Hb F tetramer and the $(\alpha\beta^S)(\alpha\gamma)$ mixed tetramer are virtually never incorporated into the Hb S polymer, the presence of Hb F very effectively decreases Hb S polymerization. Patients with Hb S-HPFH are usually asymptomatic; some may have aseptic necrosis of bone or minor joint or abdominal pains. They are rarely anemic.

SPECIAL MANAGEMENT ISSUES
Pregnancy

Pregnancy in women with sickle cell anemia is potentially fraught with complications, including urinary tract infection, pneumonia, painful crises, progressive anemia, spontaneous abortion, eclampsia, premature delivery, intrauterine growth retardation, and perinatal mortality for mother or child. Perinatal mortality was as high as 25% to 50% in prior decades, but improvements in prenatal care have reduced maternal perinatal mortality to 5% to 8%.

Pregnancies are high-risk, and patients should be monitored for preeclampsia and indications of preterm labor. Asymptomatic bacteriuria is common and should be treated. At the time of labor and delivery, oxygen and fluid replacement should be administered. Fetal monitoring should be continuous. Although prophylactic exchange transfusions were used previously, several randomized prospective studies have shown that they have no role. Transfusions are typically given, however, for toxemia, twin pregnancy, previous infant perinatal mortality, septicemia, acute renal failure, severe anemia, acute chest syndrome, hypoxemia, anticipated surgery, and angiography.

Surgery

Patients with sickle cell anemia require special perioperative care. Management with scrupulous attention to adequate hydration, oxygenation, pulmonary toilet, and analgesia before, during, and after operation is essential.

For many years, the standard preparation was simple transfusion or exchange transfusion 1 to 2 weeks preoperatively to a hemoglobin level of more than 8 to 10 g/dL and less than 50% Hb S. Data now support conservative preoperative simple transfusion to a hemoglobin concentration of 10 g/dL irrespective of the Hb S concentration. Hydration is begun at least 12 hours preoperatively.

Intraoperatively, excellent general anesthesia standards should be adhered to, that is, maintenance of a normal pH, oxygenation, and body temperature and avoidance of circulatory stasis. Hemoglobin levels are maintained at around 10 g/dL. Cardiopulmonary bypass requires special consideration. As temperature decreases, the rate of intracellular Hb S polymerization decreases in vitro. Intraoperative hypothermia can be well tolerated as long as regional vasoconstriction is prevented with vasodilators.

In general, for elective surgery using conservative transfusion strategy, a mortality rate of less than 1% and a total serious complication rate of 30% to 39% can be expected. Complications may include acute chest syndrome in about 10%, transfusion-related problems in about 10%, fever or infection in about 7%, painful crisis in about 7%, and neurologic and renal complications in less than 1% of patients each.

MANAGEMENT STRATEGIES

Specific therapeutic strategies for particular clinical scenarios were discussed previously. This section reviews strategies that potentially alter the overall disease process.

Transfusion Therapy

In patients with sickle cell anemia, the benefits of increased oxygen-carrying capacity provided by simple transfusion can be offset by the adverse effect of increased viscosity, which thwarts oxygen delivery and promotes vascular occlusion. Blood flow is jeopardized at hematocrit levels more than 35%. Hemoglobin S fractions of less than 30% have been recommended for life-threatening complications, but it is not known whether this approach is superior to levels of less than 50%. The level of anemia that patients tolerate is impressive. If the patient is asymptomatic, a hemoglobin level of 5 g/dL can be tolerated.

Methods of transfusion include simple transfusion, partial exchange transfusion, and exchange transfusion. Simple transfusion is a regular packed red blood cell transfusion. Partial exchange transfusion is manual phlebotomy, followed by normal saline replacement, followed by phlebotomy, followed by simple transfusion. Exchange transfusion is automated extracorporeal exchange.

Simple transfusion is usually adequate as long as posttransfusion increases of hemoglobin to more than 10 g/dL can be avoided. Potential indications for simple transfusion include symptomatic anemia, sequestration crisis, aplastic crisis, accelerated hemolysis, blood loss, and preoperative preparation. Emergencies such as cerebrovascular disease, arterial hypoxemia syndrome, acute chest syndrome, priapism, retinal arterial vasoocclusion, hepatic failure, septic shock, metabolic acidosis, and cerebral angiography are indications for exchange transfusions.

Blood transfusion has risk and should not be taken lightly. Risks include transfusion reaction, infectious complications, alloimmunization, and iron overload. Iron overload is a real and potentially life-threatening problem in patients undergoing chronic transfusion therapy, although it appears to be less of a problem in sickle cell disease than in thalassemia. Each unit of transfused red cells adds 200 to 250 mg of iron to the recipient's iron stores. Chronic transfusion therapy by erythrocytopheresis reduces the extent of iron overload that one would have with simple transfusion therapy.

Reducing Crises With Hydroxyurea

As in patients with Hb S-HPFH, higher levels of Hb F inhibit Hb S polymerization and result in a more benign course. Randomized placebo-controlled trials have demonstrated that the drug hydroxyurea (HU) augments production of Hb F and reduces the crisis rate by almost half in patients with very symptomatic sickle cell disease. Increases of Hb F levels may be only one of the mechanisms by which HU causes clinical benefit. Patients with the highest baseline neutrophil and reticulocyte counts seem to have the best responses to HU. Fifty percent of HU-assigned patients have long-term increments in Hb F.

HU is recommended only for patients with severe morbidity due to sickle cell anemia, given its potential leukemogenic risk. Therapy is usually begun at a dosage of 10 to 15 mg/kg a day as a single oral dose. Weekly blood cell counts, including a reticulocyte count and Hb F determination, are obtained for the first 2 weeks or after any dose adjustment and then monthly. Hepatic and renal function are monitored periodically. The dose may be increased by 5 mg/kg every 8 weeks as long as no significant myelosuppression develops.

Allogeneic Hematopoietic Stem Cell Transplantation

As a treatment for sickle cell anemia, allogeneic hematopoietic stem cell transplantation is controversial. Although it is a potentially curative procedure in patients with sickle cell anemia, the possibility of procedure-related morbidity and mortality fuels the controversy. Selecting patients for transplantation is difficult, given the unpredictable course of the disease and the lack of valuable prognostic markers. With appropriate medical attention, many patients with sickle cell anemia can have normal lives with limited morbidity and potentially near-normal life spans. Patient selection, donor availability, and cost are also issues. For a group of 100 patients undergoing transplantation in Europe, the current Kaplan-Meier estimates of overall survival, event-free survival, and disease-free survival rates are 90%, 79%, and 81%, respectively.

Future Strategies

Many other therapies designed to interrupt the pathophysiologic changes in sickle cell anemia are being explored. They include gene therapy, hemoglobin ligands, and membrane-active drugs.

SUGGESTED READING

Adams DM, Schultz WH, Ware RE, Kinney TR. Erythrocytapheresis can reduce iron overload and prevent the need for chelation therapy in chronically transfused pediatric patients. *J Pediatr Hematol Oncol* 1996; 18: 46-50.

Adams RJ, McKie VC, Hsu L, Files B, Vichinsky E, Pegelow C, Abboud M, Gallagher D, Kutlar A, Nichols FT, Bonds DR, Brambilla D. Prevention of a first stroke by transfusions in children with sickle cell anemia and abnormal results on transcranial Doppler ultrasonography. *N Engl J Med* 1998; 339: 5-11.

Charache S. Mechanism of action of hydroxyurea in the management of sickle cell anemia in adults. *Semin Hematol* 1997; 34 Suppl 3: 15-21.

Embury S, Hebbel RP, Mohandas N, Steinberg MH, eds. *Sickle Cell Disease: Basic Principles and Clinical Practice*. Raven Press, New York, 1994.

Haberkern CM, Neumayr LD, Orringer EP, Earles AN, Robertson SM, Black D, Abboud MR, Koshy M, Idowu O, Vichinsky EP. Preoperative Transfusion in Sickle Cell Disease Study Group. Cholecystectomy in sickle cell anemia patients: perioperative outcome of 364 cases from the National Preoperative Transfusion Study. *Blood* 1997; 89: 1533-1542.

Powars D, Weidman JA, Odom-Maryon T, Niland JC, Johnson C. Sickle cell chronic lung disease: prior morbidity and the risk of pulmonary failure. *Medicine (Baltimore)* 1988; 67: 66-76.

Steinberg MH, Lu ZH, Barton FB, Terrin ML, Charache S, Dover GJ. Multicenter Study of Hydroxyurea. Fetal hemoglobin in sickle cell anemia: determinants of response to hydroxyurea. *Blood* 1997; 89: 1078-1088.

Steinberg MH. Sickle cell disease: present and future treatment. *Am J Med Sci* 1996; 312: 166-174.

Vermylen C, Cornu G. Hematopoietic stem cell transplantation for sickle cell anemia. *Curr Opin Hematol* 1997; 4: 377-380.

Vichinsky EP, Styles LA, Colangelo LH, Wright EC, Castro O, Nickerson B. Cooperative Study of Sickle Cell Disease. Acute chest syndrome in sickle cell disease: clinical presentation and course. *Blood* 1997; 89: 1787-1792.

Wayne AS, Kevy SV, Nathan DG. Transfusion management of sickle cell disease. *Blood* 1993; 81: 1109-1123.

Weil JV, Castro O, Malik AB, Rodgers G, Bonds DR, Jacobs TP. NHLBI Workshop Summary. Pathogenesis of lung disease in sickle hemoglobinopathies. *Am Rev Respir Dis* 1993; 148: 249-256.

5

Practical Aspects in the Diagnosis and Management of Aplastic Anemia

Rafael Fonseca, MD

Contents

INTRODUCTION

Aplastic anemia (AA) is a rare bone marrow failure state (2–6 cases/million persons per year). Pancytopenia and severe marrow hypoplasia characterize the disease. The disease has wide geographic distribution, with a reported high incidence in Latin America and Southeast Asia. The increased rate of the disease in people of low socioeconomic status likely represents a surrogate marker of exposure to causative environmental or toxic factors.

The pathogenetic mechanisms are heterogeneous and mostly undefined. Because of successful reconstitution of hematopoiesis after allogeneic or syngeneic bone marrow transplantation (BMT) and the failure of hematopoietic progenitor cells of patients with AA to thrive in an allogeneic stromal environment, defects in the stem cell are thought to be of primordial importance. The reason for this failure is usually not evident, but occasionally causative agents can be identified. The late development of related stem cell disorders such as paroxysmal nocturnal hemoglobinuria, myelodysplastic syndrome, and acute myeloid leukemia suggests that in some cases AA may be a disorder of clonal hematopoiesis. In other cases, autoimmunity appears to lead to AA, as initially described after a treatment response to antilymphocyte globulin and other immunosuppressive agents. The pathogenetic role of lymphocytes in AA is further supported by the clinical observation that T-cell and natural killer cell disorders are sometimes associated with severe pancytopenia and marrow hypoplasia.

AA may result from several other pathogenetic mechanisms, including chemotherapy and radiation injury. However, only a small number of patients have a history of drug or chemical exposure. Many anecdotal case reports of agents thought to be associated with AA exist in the literature; however, a true causative relationship has been proved for only a few. Viral causes have been implicated in a subset of patients with AA, and although several agents are suspected of being capable of producing aplasia, none do so in a

From: *Primary Hematology*
Edited by: A. Tefferi © Mayo Foundation for Medical Education and Research, Rochester, MN

reproducible manner. The incidence of AA after hepatitis is low (< 1%), although a higher incidence has been noted after liver transplantation (Table 1).

DIAGNOSIS

The results of peripheral blood examination usually are nonspecific, with variable degrees of hypoproliferative pancytopenia. Patients are usually anemic, but most clinical manifestations are derived from either the thrombocytopenia or the leukopenia. Examination of a bone marrow biopsy specimen and aspirate is the most important laboratory study in the diagnosis of AA. It usually reveals hypoplasia (< 25% cellularity), with the rest of the marrow filled with fat spaces. In some instances, elements of dyserythropoiesis, relative lymphocytosis, and occasional islands of normal or increased cellularity may be noted. Severe dysplastic changes should alert the clinician because the hypocellular variant of myelodysplastic syndrome can be clinically indistinguishable from AA. Before AA is diagnosed, other hematologic disorders should be considered and excluded (Table 2).

> Consultation with an expert hematopathologist is mandatory in cases of suspected AA. The findings of myelodysplasia may be subtle and apparent only to the trained eye. Similarly, procurement of cytogenetic studies in patients with pancytopenia is highly recommended to avoid the need for obtaining additional samples.

Paroxysmal nocturnal hemoglobinuria can present with pancytopenia and a hypocellular marrow. The use of flow cytometry analysis for the presence of the cell surface markers CD59 and CD58 will result in a sensitive and objective evaluation to exclude paroxysmal nocturnal hemoglobinuria in patients with AA. If this test is unavailable, the sucrose lysis test and the acidified serum lysis test (Ham's test) can help exclude the possibility of paroxysmal nocturnal hemoglobinuria. Almost half of patients can have varying degrees of deficiency of cell surface markers CD58 and CD59 in bone marrow reticulocytes. Regardless, the treatment of paroxysmal nocturnal hemoglobinuria with bone marrow failure is generally similar to that of AA.

As mentioned, myelodysplastic syndrome may present as a hypocellular variant, with bone marrow cellularity less than 20% in up to 10% of patients. The differential diagnosis may be difficult because of the presence of some degree of dyserythropoiesis in AA. However, dysplastic cellularity is usually limited to the erythroid lineage in AA, and the presence of clonal cytogenetic abnormalities favors the diagnosis of myelodysplastic syndrome rather than AA. The differentiation between myelodysplastic syndrome and AA is critical for treatment, because consideration of BMT in myelodysplastic syndrome requires conditioning regimens used for acute leukemia instead of those used in AA.

Fanconi's anemia is an inherited disease associated with AA and congenital musculoskeletal and cutaneous abnormalities. AA may not develop until later in life, and up to a third of patients with Fanconi's anemia may not have any detectable physical stigmata. The consequences of misdiagnosing Fanconi's anemia as AA are dire. Because the treatment of choice for both disorders is BMT, donor cytogenetic analysis is mandatory in Fanconi's anemia to exclude the presence of the congenital defect in the sibling donor. Furthermore, post-BMT complications in patients with Fanconi's anemia include increased susceptibility to cyclophosphamide toxicity, which requires avoidance or dose modifications of this drug in the conditioning regimens for BMT. Therefore, in all patients with AA, the possibility of Fanconi's anemia should be addressed by testing peripheral

Table 1
Causes of Aplastic Anemia

Acquired aplastic anemia
   Primary
      Idiopathic
   Secondary
      Physical and chemical agents
         Regularly produce disease at sufficient dose:
            Radiation
            Chemotherapeutic agents
            Benzene
         Idiosyncratic
            Chloramphenicol
            Quinacrine
            Anticonvulsants
            Phenylbutazone
            Gold
            D-Penicillamine
            Insecticides
            Estrogens in high doses
   Other causes
      Idiopathic, including autoimmune
      Viral
         Non-A, non-B hepatitis
         Human immunodeficiency virus
         Epstein-Barr virus
      Miscellaneous (including severe pancytopenias)
         Other autoimmune disorders
            Eosinophilic fasciitis
            Graft-versus-host disease
            Large granular lymphocytes
            Thymoma and thymic carcinoma
         Pregnancy
         Preceding acute lymphoblastic leukemia
         Organochlorines and organophosphates
Constitutional aplastic anemia
   Fanconi's anemia
Other
   Paroxysmal nocturnal hemoglobinuria

blood lymphocytes for increased chromosome fragility induced by DNA cross-linking agents.

Other lymphoproliferative disorders, including clonal proliferations of large granular lymphocytes, can be associated with bone marrow hypoplasia and thus need to be excluded by flow cytometry analysis of peripheral blood lymphocytes. Suspected cases should be pursued further with T-cell receptor gene rearrangement studies, also of the peripheral blood.

Because of the aforementioned diagnostic possibilities, initial laboratory testing in all patients with AA should include evaluation of the bone marrow and peripheral blood

Table 2
Differential Diagnosis for Patients With
Pancytopenia and Hypocellular Bone Marrow

Aplastic anemia
Myelodysplastic syndrome
T-cell clonal disorders
Paroxysmal nocturnal hemoglobinuria
Fanconi's anemia

smear, cytogenetic studies including fragility testing, flow cytometry of peripheral lymphocytes including testing specific for paroxysmal nocturnal hemoglobinuria, B_{12} and folate levels, and viral serologic testing, including tests for hepatitis, human immunodeficiency virus, and the Epstein-Barr virus.

MANAGEMENT

Initial Measures

The degree of cytopenia and its consequences dictate current management guidelines (Table 3). Patients with AA should undergo immediate HLA typing while they still have an adequate number of circulating lymphocytes. In suitable candidates, work-up for possible BMT should be started, and platelet products need to be used judiciously to prevent alloimmunization. A search for unrelated HLA-matched donors can be considered in patients younger than 30 years without an HLA-matched sibling, because unrelated BMT is a reasonable consideration for such young patients if immunosuppressive therapy fails (see below and page 87).

Use of blood products should be minimized to prevent alloimmunization and to reduce the risk of graft failure after BMT. However, for the patient in need of blood components, they will have minimal impact on the probability of engraftment; the use of 40 or fewer transfusion units has had minimal impact on the rates of graft rejection. In addition, the impact of previous transfusions when higher intensity immunosuppressive agents are used for conditioning is not well defined. Blood products from family members should not be used so as to avoid sensitization to minor histocompatibility antigens, and the prophylactic transfusion of packed red blood cells and platelets should be restricted for hemoglobin levels less than 7 g/dL and platelet levels less than 10×10^9/L, respectively. The use of leukocyte-depleted and single-donor products is recommended. Blood products that are cytomegalovirus (CMV)-negative should be used in candidates for BMT until the CMV status of the patient and donor is determined. If the patient is CMV-negative, CMV-negative blood products should continue to be used until the CMV status of the marrow donor is determined.

Infections need aggressive and appropriate treatment. If the response to antibiotics is not optimal, myeloid growth factors may be used. It cannot be overemphasized that the use of growth factors is for the transient corrrection of cytopenias but is not a definitive treatment option. As in any other neutropenic patient, the use of empiric antifungal treatment is indicated when fever persists after 48 hours. The benefit of prophylactic treatment with antibiotics or growth factors is not well substantiated. Such treatment may be more appropriate for patients with recurrent and frequent infections. There is no proven benefit for strict isolation techniques or for the sterilization of food.

Table 3
Aplastic Anemia Prognostic Groups$^{\alpha}$

Severe aplastic anemia	
Blood	
Neutrophils	$< 0.5 \times 10^9/L$
Platelets	$< 20 \times 10^9/L$
Reticulocytes	$< 1\%$ (corrected)
Marrow	
Severe hypocellularity, $< 25\%$ cellularity	
Moderate hypocellularity, with $< 30\%$ of cells being hematopoietic	
Very severe aplastic anemia	
As above, plus granulocytes $< 0.2 \times 10^9/L$	

$^{\alpha}$Two of the peripheral blood criteria plus one of the bone marrow criteria are required for diagnosis.

Definitive Therapy

Definitive treatment options for AA are either BMT or immunosuppression. Long-term survival rates range from 40% in older series to up to 90% in the most recent figures. Certain subsets of patients derive superior benefits from one or the other treatment. For initial treatment, several factors should be considered, including age, availability of HLA-matched sibling donors, and severity of the disease (Table 3). Patients should be well informed of the procedure-related risks, including graft-versus-host disease and secondary solid tumors in BMT and the development of clonal myeloid disorders in long-term survivors of immunosuppressive therapy (Table 4).

In the absence of HLA-matched sibling donors, immunosuppressive therapy is the obvious initial treatment of choice, even in very young patients. Reported survival rates are superior to those with unrelated BMT. For patients older than 40, immunosuppression is the treatment of choice. The controversy is in regard to middle-aged patients (between ages 20 and 40) with matched sibling donors. Several retrospective studies have compared the two treatments, and the results suggest that BMT is superior in patients younger than 20 years but that in older patients the overall outcome is comparable for the two treatments. In patients older than 40 years, toxicity is such that most physicians recommend immunosuppression.

The use of more immunosuppressive conditioning regimens and cyclosporin A-based prophylaxis for graft-versus-host disease has considerably decreased the risk of graft rejection and graft-versus-host disease associated with BMT. Recently reported survival rates for patients up to age 40 years with severe AA exceed 70% and are thought to be superior to those reported for immunosuppressive therapy. With the exception of children younger than 20 years, there is no conclusive evidence that BMT is superior to immunosuppression. Because the long-term survival curves do not reflect the benefit of the better prophylaxis for graft-versus-host disease and conditioning regimens used recently, a survival advantage for patients between 20 and 40 years may exist.

Although not appreciated with short-term follow-up, the long-term complications of immunosuppressive therapy, including recurrence rates of up to 35% and development of clonal myeloid disorders in up to 40% of patients, may further diminish the long-term survival. Furthermore, early mortality rates of patients with severe AA or very severe AA treated with immunosuppression are significantly increased.

In view of the preceding discussion, we recommend BMT from related donors as the initial treatment of choice for patients younger than 20 years. This treatment is also

Table 4
Incidence of Clonal Hematologic Disorders in Long-Term Survivors
After Immunosuppressive Therapy for Aplastic Anemia

	No. of patients	MDS/AML		PNH	
		No.	%	No.	%
Manchester Royal Infirmary	37	13	35	4	11
Fred Hutchinson Cancer Research Center	30	6	20	3	10
Kantonsspital, Basel, Switzerland	75[a]	8	11	13[b]	17
European BMT-SAA Working Party	860	MDS 52 AML 47	12	NA	NA

[a]Risk of developing a hematologic complication was 57% at 8 years.
[b]Nine of the 13 patients with PNH had clinical signs of hemolysis; 4 had only positive laboratory test results. One patient had PNH and acute leukemia.
Abbreviations: AML, acute myeloid leukemia; MDS, myelodysplastic syndrome; PNH, paroxysmal nocturnal hemoglobinuria.

preferred for patients 20 to 40 years old with severe and very severe AA. In young patients with AA that is not severe and in all patients older than 40 years, a strategy of initially using immunosuppressive therapy, followed by BMT in patients without a response, is reasonable, with documented benefits. In addition, management preferences should consider the individual risk profiles associated with the potential development of both acute and chronic graft-versus-host disease.

IMMUNOSUPPRESSIVE TREATMENT

Effective immunosuppressive regimens can improve hematopoiesis in some patients. It is now common practice to initiate immunosuppressive therapy with a combination of cyclosporin A, methylprednisolone, and antithymocyte globulin, which has resulted in better response and survival rates than the use of single agents. In a randomized study, the combination of these three agents was superior to the combination of antithymocyte globulin and methylprednisolone (70% vs. 46% remission rates at 6 months), and the survival rate of patients with severe AA was improved. The National Institutes of Health has achieved response rates of up to 78% in patients with severe AA treated with combination antithymocyte globulin and cyclosporin A. The series of 51 patients had a median age of 28 years and median follow-up time of 912 days. They had a survival rate of 72% at 2 years and a probability of relapse of 36%.

A pilot study from the European Bone Marrow Transplant Severe Aplastic Anemia Working Party evaluated the addition of growth factors to the immunosuppressive regimen. Patients treated with the combination of antithymocyte globulin, cyclosporin A, and granulocyte colony-stimulating factor had an 82% response rate at 1 year and a 92% survival at 34 months. These patients had a median neutrophil count of 0.185×10^9/L (range, $0.03–0.5 \times 10^9$/L) at diagnosis. Although the data are confounded by the fact that 20 patients were re-treated with antithymocyte globulin, there is no reason to believe that repeated courses of this agent are beneficial.

Transient short-term side effects of antithymocyte globulin therapy include anaphylaxis, urticaria, fever, chills, thrombocytopenia, and serum sickness (rash, arthralgias, and fever). Although an epicutaneous test dose of 50 mg/mL has been advocated to identify patients who are sensitive to the medication, some patients will have a severe reaction to this small amount of the medication, and there is no accepted way of assessing for severe subsequent response to the treatment. The progressive desensitization of patients to antithymocyte globulin has been achieved with increasing doses and concentrations of the medication. Similarly, although used routinely, the concomitant use of corticosteroids has not been studied enough to be able to conclude that the risk of serum sickness is reduced, a disease that in itself is self-limited. Chronic use of cyclosporin A may result in the development of high blood pressure, seizures, hypomagnesemia, and renal insufficiency. Thus, periodic monitoring of serum levels of cyclosporin A, magnesium, creatinine, and blood pressure is advised.

Currently, the immunosuppressive therapy we prefer is the combination of antithymocyte globulin (40 mg/kg for 4 days), cyclosporin A (10–12 mg/kg daily for 6 months and taper afterward), and methylprednisolone (2 mg/kg daily for 5 days and taper afterward). Because patients undergoing intensive immunosuppression are at significant risk of opportunistic infections similar to what develops in CD4 deficiency states, the use of a nonmyelosuppressive *Pneumocystis carinii* prophylaxis regimen such as pentamidine can be considered.

Used separately, antithymocyte globulin and cyclosporin A have a comparable response rate (50%), which is superior to that of androgen therapy. Prolonged duration of antithymocyte globulin therapy or repeated courses have not resulted in improved responses. Because antithymocyte globulin may not be readily available in all parts of the world, the combination of cyclosporin A with prednisone has been tried; some results have been promising (survival of 68% at 3 years). The use of cyclosporin A alone is a reasonable and convenient therapeutic option for a select group of patients with nonsevere AA in an outpatient setting. Significant responses have been observed, even in patients who are otherwise refractory to antithymocyte globulin (up to 50% response rate). Although high doses of methylprednisolone alone (1 g/day for 10 days) may be used as an alternative immunosuppressive method, this regimen has inferior response rates and is associated with more severe side effects.

BONE MARROW TRANSPLANT

Allogeneic BMT from related donors is an effective treatment of AA. Early series of transplants had substantial rates of graft rejection and graft-versus-host disease. As discussed, the careful use of blood component transfusions before transplantation, the appropriate selection of patients, the application of stronger immunosuppressive conditioning regimens, and the use of cyclosporin A-based prophylaxis for graft-versus-host disease have decreased transplant-related mortality. Patients undergoing allogeneic BMT in Seattle between 1988 and 1993, conditioned with cyclophosphamide and antithymocyte globulin and receiving methotrexate and cyclosporin A for graft-versus-host prophylaxis, had a graft failure rate of 5%, acute graft-versus-host disease rate of 15%, and chronic rate of 34%. In patients reported to the International Bone Marrow Transplant Registry between 1980 and 1987, the rate of graft failure was 10% and the rates of acute and chronic graft-versus-host disease were 40% and 45%, respectively. This series, however, lacks the homogeneity of induction regimens and graft-versus-host prophylaxis of the Seattle series. Both acute and chronic graft-versus-host disease have an important effect on survival after BMT in patients with AA. Acute graft-versus-host disease is a very sensitive indicator of the subsequent development of chronic disease.

> The only hematologic condition in which BMT is considered an urgent procedure is AA. The process of screening for possible BMT should be expedited to minimize blood product use and prevent the development of infections. Both could jeopardize a subsequent successful transplantation. For that reason, a patient with possible AA should be referred to specialized medical centers.

Cyclophosphamide alone or in combination with radiation or antithymocyte globulin has been used in most preparative regimens; graft rejection rates have been significantly decreased and survival improved (survival rates of 60%–70%). The use of radiation has been associated with an increased risk of interstitial pneumonia, growth impairment, and development of secondary solid tumors (22% vs. 3.8% for immunosuppressive therapy at 15 years) and is now not included in most preparative regimens. Graft rejection is a dreaded complication because only 30% of patients who receive a second transplant achieve engraftment, and most of them have poor reconstitution of hematopoiesis.

The combined use of cyclophosphamide and antithymocyte globulin has resulted in excellent short-term survival rates of up to 90%, with a significant decrease in both graft rejection and chronic graft-versus-host disease. The encouraging results obtained with use of this combination also have been observed in patients who previously had transfusion. Therefore, our current preparative regimen of choice is cyclophosphamide (50 mg/kg daily for 4 days, on days 5, 4, 3, and 2) in combination with antithymocyte globulin (30 mg/kg daily for 3 days, on days 5, 4, and 3, given 12 hours after the infusion of cyclophosphamide).

Age is a major determining factor in the rate of success of BMT. The results of the International Bone Marrow Transplant Registry show that at 5 years the overall survival is 68% in patients who had transplantation before age 30 and 43% in those 30 to 50 years. The Seattle study reported a 3-year actuarial survival rate of 92% for 39 patients with a median age of 24.5 years who had transplantation between 1988 and 1993. However, with improving experience in large transplant series, it is possible that older patients will be further considered for transplantation. Clearly, when possible, BMT should be performed in children and adults up to the age of 40 years, with the understanding that patients between the ages of 20 and 40 years will be at higher risk from transplant-related complications. Available information suggests that transplantation in older patients will be more successful as better prophylaxis and treatment of graft-versus-host disease are established.

Patients treated for severe AA and undergoing BMT have a high risk of development of a secondary malignancy (14%) at 20 years. In multivariable analysis, the use of azathioprine therapy and the diagnosis of Fanconi's anemia were significant for the development of a secondary malignancy. For patients not affected by Fanconi's anemia, age and irradiation were significant factors.

ALTERNATIVE MANAGEMENT OPTIONS

Androgens have been shown to be of inferior value in comparison with BMT or immunosuppression in the treatment of AA. Hematopoietic growth factors, including granulocyte-macrophage colony-stimulating factor, granulocyte colony-stimulating factor, interleukin-3, and the combination of granulocyte colony-stimulating factor and erythropoietin, have not shown durable trilineage improvement in AA and are not recommended. The responses are transient and dependent on continuous use of the growth factor. There is no evidence that they correct the underlying defect in AA. Their use should be thought of as supportive only. The role of BMT from matched unrelated donors is being investigated. Current results of unrelated BMT show that one-third of the patients can survive with or without residual disease. Immunosuppression is still thought to be a better initial definitive treatment alternative for the patient without a matched donor.

SUGGESTED READING

Bacigalupo A, Broccia G, Corda G, Arcese W, Carotenuto M, Gallamini A, Locatelli F, Mori PG, Saracco P, Todeschini G, Coser P, Iacopino P, van Lint MT, Gluckman E, for the European Group for Blood and Marrow Transplantation (EBMT) Working Party on SAA. Antilymphocyte globulin, cyclosporin, and granulocyte colony-stimulating factor in patients with acquired severe aplastic anemia (SAA): a pilot study of the EBMT SAA Working Party. Blood 1995; 85: 1348-1353.

Frickhofen N, Kaltwasser JP, Schrezenmeier H, Raghavachar A, Vogt HG, Herrmann F, Freund M, Meusers P, Salama A, Heimpel H, for the German Aplastic Anemia Study Group. Treatment of aplastic anemia with antilymphocyte globulin and methylprednisolone with or without cyclosporine. N Engl J Med 1991; 324: 1297-1304.

Gluckman E, Devergie A, Poros A, Degoulet P. Results of immunosuppression in 170 cases of severe aplastic anaemia. Report of the European Group of Bone Marrow Transplant (EGBMT). Br J Haematol 1982; 51: 541-550.

Gluckman E, Socie G, Devergie A, Bourdeau-Esperou H, Traineau R, Cosset JM. Bone marrow transplantation in 107 patients with severe aplastic anemia using cyclophosphamide and thoraco-abdominal irradiation for conditioning: long-term follow-up. Blood 1991; 78: 2451-2455.

Marsh JC, Socie G, Schrezenmeier H, Tichelli A, Gluckman E, Ljungman P, McCann SR, Raghavachar A, Marin P, Hows JM, Bacigalupo, for the European Bone Marrow Transplant Working Party for Severe Aplastic Anaemia. Haemopoietic growth factors in aplastic anaemia: a cautionary note. Lancet 1994; 344: 172-173.

Young NS, Alter BP. Aplastic Anemia: Acquired and Inherited. W. B. Saunders Company, Philadelphia, 1994.

Young NS, Barrett AJ. The treatment of severe acquired aplastic anemia. Blood 1995; 85: 3367-3377.

6

Differential Diagnosis of Neutropenia

Costas L. Constantinou, MD

Contents

DEFINITION

Neutropenia (or granulocytopenia) is a depression of the absolute neutrophil count to less than 1,500/mm^3. Leukopenia is a related term, denoting the depression of the total leukocyte count. Although neutropenia is the most frequent cause of leukopenia, a marked lymphocytopenia can depress the total leukocyte count in the "penic" range with a normal neutrophil count. However, a severe leukopenia always implies neutropenia. The absolute neutrophil count (ANC) is derived by multiplying the total leukocyte count by the percentage of band neutrophils and segmented neutrophils:

$$ANC = \text{leukocyte count} \times (\% \text{ bands} + \% \text{ segmented neutrophils}) \times 0.01$$

Cells less mature than bands are not included in the calculation because they are rare in the circulation, and even when present they do not display the biologic function of neutrophils. There is some epidemiologic variability of the normal range for the leukocyte count. Although neutrophil counts of less than 2,000/mm^3 are uncommon in the general white U.S. population, some individuals of African or Yemenite Jewish descent may have counts as low as 1,000/mm^3 without an apparent cause. Neutropenia can be subclassified as mild, moderate, or severe based on the absolute neutrophil count: mild, 1,000 to 1,500/mm^3; moderate, 500 to 1,000/mm^3; severe, less than 500/mm^3. Agranulocytosis is a term that refers to severe neutropenia, usually implying a hypoplastic marrow. Physicians of different specialties tend to have varying working definitions of neutropenia. Although a count less than 1,500/mm^3 technically constitutes neutropenia, oncologists almost always use this term to refer to counts less than 500/mm^3.

From: *Primary Hematology*
Edited by: A. Tefferi © Mayo Foundation for Medical Education and Research, Rochester, MN

NEUTROPHIL PRODUCTION, STORAGE, AND KINETICS

An understanding of neutrophil kinetics is important for clarifying the pathophysiology of the different causes of neutropenia. For the purpose of simplification, neutrophils and their precursors in bone marrow can be divided into two types: mitotic and postmitotic. The earliest recognizable neutrophil precursor is the myeloblast that together with the promyelocyte and the myelocyte forms the mitotic, or production, pool. The postmitotic pool consists of metamyelocytes, bands, and segmented neutrophils. Within the postmitotic pool, there is no division but a continuous maturation process. The average cell spends 10 to 14 days in the maturation and storage pool before it is released into the circulation. Under normal conditions, the storage pool contains 10 to 20 times as many segmented neutrophils and bands as are present in the periphery. This dynamic equilibrium can be influenced by several physiologic or pathologic processes. Although neutropenia can be associated with many kinetic changes, it is most often due to decreased production. Several homeostatic mechanisms exist in an effort to maintain a normal peripheral neutrophil level. The mechanism that is most useful, in a diagnostic sense, is that the peripheral destruction of neutrophils leads to an increased production, which can be found on bone marrow examination.

CLASSIFICATION OF NEUTROPENIA

Neutropenia can be due to reduced production, peripheral destruction, shift of neutrophils from the circulating pool to the storage or marginated pool (maldistribution), or a combination of these causes. It is perhaps useful to draw some analogies among the causal mechanisms of anemia, thrombocytopenia, and neutropenia because pathophysiologically they are similar. When neutropenia coexists with anemia or thrombocytopenia or both, the term "pancytopenia" is used. In pancytopenia, a common pathogenetic mechanism is usually responsible for all abnormalities. This mechanism is usually a production defect, even though other causes are possible.

Neutropenia also can be classified into genetic and acquired syndromes. Several genetic intrinsic defects, which can be associated with neutropenia, are listed in Table 1. For the practicing internist, most causes of genetically determined neutropenia should be of academic interest only because adults presenting with neutropenia of new onset almost always have an acquired defect. It is thus more useful to develop a pathophysiologic approach to the diagnosis, workup, and management of neutropenia (Table 2).

Reduced Production

DRUG-INDUCED NEUTROPENIA

This is by far the most common cause of neutropenia. The two major causes of isolated neutropenia are iatrogenic. The use of cytotoxic chemotherapy produces a predictable neutropenia, whereas several other drugs may give rise to idiosyncratic neutropenia related to reduced production or peripheral destruction or both. Although some agents are more common offenders than others (Table 3), it is important to realize that any drug can be associated with this effect and no list can be complete. Drug-induced neutropenia usually manifests a few weeks after initial exposure, or sooner after a repeat exposure. However, neutropenia may develop even after chronic administration, and thus the time since exposure should not serve as a diagnostic criterion in determining the cause of

Table 1
Congenital Defects Associated
With Neutropenia

Reticular dysgenesis
Kostmann's syndrome
Shwachman-Diamond syndrome
Dyskeratosis congenita
Cartilage-hair hypoplasia
Lazy leukocyte syndrome
Chédiak-Higashi syndrome

Table 2
Causes of Neutropenia

Reduced production
    Congenital defects
    Drug-induced
        Antineoplastic agents
        Other drugs
    Postinfectious
    Ineffective granulocytopoiesis
        B_{12} deficiency
        Folate deficiency
        Drugs[a]
    Bone marrow replacement-myelophthisis
    Acquired precursor damage
        Leukemias
        Myelodysplastic syndromes
        Aplastic anemia
    Suppressor T-cell-induced (Tγ lymphocytosis)
    Associated with collagen vascular diseases[a]
    Cyclic neutropenia
    Benign familial neutropenia (normal variant)[a]
Increased destruction
    Autoimmune neutropenia
    Isoimmune neutropenia
    Drugs[a]
    Systemic lupus erythematosus and other collagen
        vascular diseases[a]
    Hypersplenism[a]
Abnormal distribution
    Hypersplenism[a]
    Pseudoneutropenia
    Benign familial neutropenia[a]

[a]These may cause neutropenia on the basis of one or
more pathophysiologic mechanisms.

neutropenia. Neutropenia that is due to cytotoxic chemotherapy is predictable and associated with other cytopenias.

Table 3
Drugs That Can Cause Neutropenia

Cytotoxic agents of several classes
Antibiotics (penicillins, cephalosporins, sulfonamides, chloramphenicol)
Nonsteroidal anti-inflammatory agents (phenylbutazone)
Antithyroid agents (propylthiouracil, methimazole)
Anticonvulsants
Phenothiazines
α-Methyldopa
Diuretics (spironolactone, chlorothiazide, ethacrynic acid)
Clozapine
Cimetidine
Allopurinol
Penicillamine
Many other drugs

Note: Many drugs can cause neutropenia either by bone marrow suppression or by peripheral destruction. Because no list is complete, physicians are encouraged to consult the *Physicians' Desk Reference* and package inserts. Even if no information regarding neutropenia is found, a drug could still be considered potentially responsible and its use discontinued if it is not essential.

A more challenging diagnostic situation faced by the general internist is the unpredictable neutropenia caused by several nonchemotherapeutic drugs. Drug-induced neutropenia is more common in women and older persons. Patients who have had hypersensitivity reactions are more likely to develop drug-induced neutropenia. Even though antibiotics such as the penicillins, cephalosporins, and sulfonamides are relatively common offenders, the neutropenia is often clinically silent because of the short duration of therapy with these agents. Clinically more significant is the neutropenia associated with medications that are used for chronic conditions, such as antithyroid agents, certain cardiac antiarrhythmic drugs, anticonvulsants, and nonsteroidal anti-inflammatory agents. As a general principle, when faced with a list of medications, a drug that has recently been added is more likely to be the offender, especially if it is associated with a considerable risk for neutropenia. However, neutropenia can be caused by almost any drug at any interval, and this principle should sometimes guide management decisions.

POSTINFECTIOUS

A neutropenia can develop after viral infections. It is more common in children and young adults because of the increased incidence of the implicated viral infections in this population. These infections include infectious mononucleosis, cytomegalovirus, hepatitis A and B, varicella, measles, rubella, and parvovirus. In addition, human immunodeficiency virus (HIV) infection can cause a neutropenia immediately after infection as a result of production suppression. The neutropenia that is common in the more advanced stages of acquired immunodeficiency syndrome (AIDS) is multifactorial, and all mechanisms of neutropenia are implicated.

A wide range of infectious pathogens can produce neutropenia during the acute phase of the illness as a result of production suppression and peripheral destruction and redistribution. These include infections with rickettsia (especially *Rickettsia rickettsii*, the cause of Rocky Mountain spotted fever), tularemia, *Salmonella typhi*, ehrlichiosis, and

Staphylococcus aureus. Several other bacterial, mycobacterial, and viral agents can rarely induce neutropenia in the acute infectious setting. Usually neutropenia is a consequence of the underlying infection and does not predispose to more serious complications, except in the setting of sepsis.

Nutritional Deficiencies

Vitamin B_{12} and folate deficiency can cause mild to moderate neutropenia (absolute neutrophil count, > 1,000/mm³) because of granulocytopoiesis. Anemia is almost always present. Megaloblastosis (macrocytosis), although diagnostically useful, is not always present because it can be masked by iron deficiency. Trace element deficiency, such as copper, also can cause a mild neutropenia.

Marrow Replacement by Neoplasms or Other Space-Occupying Lesions

Many solid and hematologic malignancies and, less commonly, nonmalignant diseases can infiltrate and replace the marrow. This process is sometimes called myelophthisis. Neutropenia as a result of myelophthisis occurs in advanced disease processes and does not usually present a diagnostic challenge. A peripheral smear showing leukoerythroblastic features is characteristic of this condition. Thrombocytopenia and anemia of varying degree are usually present.

Hematologic Diseases Directly Affecting Neutrophil Precursors

Several hematologic neoplasms directly involve the hematopoietic precursor cells. Such diseases are the myelodysplastic syndromes (preleukemias), the various leukemias, and aplastic anemia. The neutropenia can be severe and is almost always associated with anemia and thrombocytopenia. Pancytopenia, except in a few specific circumstances, is an indication for a bone marrow examination. A rarer syndrome is pure white cell aplasia, which is associated with thymoma in most cases. Like its counterpart, pure red cell aplasia, the diagnosis of thymoma can predate, coincide with, or antedate the diagnosis of pure white cell aplasia. A marrow examination shows complete absence of early myeloid precursors, as opposed to Kostmann's syndrome, in which the defect occurs after the early myeloid stage.

Suppressor T-Cell-Induced Neutropenia

This is a clinical syndrome of neutropenia, usually mild to moderate, associated with T-cell lymphocytosis. This disease, also known as large granular lymphocytic disorder (leukemia), consists of proliferation of large lymphocytes with cytoplasmic granules. These cells are phenotypically of either the cytotoxic/suppressor type (T8) or natural killer cell type (NK). This disorder sometimes occurs in association with rheumatoid arthritis and Felty's syndrome. Although affected patients may have recurrent infections, the disease usually runs an indolent course.

Cyclic Neutropenia

This disorder, although genetically determined and usually presenting in childhood, may not be diagnosed until early or sometimes late adulthood. Affected patients have symptoms such as fatigue, mouth sores, cervical adenopathy, and, less commonly, fever every 3 to 4 weeks lasting for 3 to 4 days. Between the episodes, the patients are generally well. Such a recurrent pattern should lead to a determination of the leukocyte count twice a week for 7 to 8 weeks in an effort to establish the periodicity and identify the nadir neutrophil count. This entity is thought to result from a regulatory defect of the stem cell.

Benign Familial Neutropenia or Leukopenia

This condition is not a disorder but rather a genetically determined variation in the control of proliferation and distribution of neutrophils. The bone marrow has normal cellularity. A lower than normal leukocyte count has been found in several ethnic groups, such as African and American blacks, West Indians, and Yemenite Jews. There is no predisposition to infection. The finding is usually incidental. If isolated mild to moderate neutropenia is found in the appropriate setting and population, no further diagnostic workup is indicated other than an examination of the peripheral smear and a repeat complete blood cell count in 4 to 8 weeks to establish the stability of this condition.

Increased Peripheral Destruction

Drugs

Many drugs (Table 3) can cause neutropenia by decreasing neutrophil survival in the periphery. The operating mechanism is the production of antineutrophilic antibodies. These antibodies are produced when a complex between the drug (hapten) and a leukocyte surface protein becomes antigenic. Other pathways leading to antibody production are less common. The coating of the neutrophil surface with antineutrophilic antibodies may cause complement activation and subsequent intravascular destruction or removal by the reticuloendothelial system. Although the mechanisms involved are very similar to the ones responsible for most immune hemolytic anemias, procedures for the detection of leukocyte antibodies are not as reliable and widely available as the Coombs test. In addition, there is lack of a practical leukokinetic parameter, as compared with the reticulocyte count, as a measurement of erythrokinetic activity. For these reasons, it is more difficult to elucidate the specific mechanism of neutropenia related to a drug (decreased production vs. increased destruction). However, the differentiation is not clinically important, because the required action, independent of the mechanism, is to discontinue use of the offending drug.

Collagen Vascular Disease

Antineutrophilic antibodies can be detected in autoimmune diseases such as systemic lupus erythematosus, rheumatoid arthritis, and its variant, Felty's syndrome. When neutropenia is found in a patient with a collagen vascular disease, it is usually mild to moderate in severity and is associated with anemia or thrombocytopenia. In these diseases, the cause of neutropenia can be multifactorial and frequently correlates with the activity of the underlying disease. Treatment is generally directed toward the disease.

Hypersplenism

Neutropenia of usually mild to moderate severity can occur in hypersplenism, in association with variable anemia and thrombocytopenia. Hypersplenism is almost never the cause of isolated neutropenia in the absence of other contributing factors. Reduced neutrophil survival does not correlate well with the spleen size, and it can occur with a nonpalpable spleen. There are different causes of hypersplenism, of which the most common is congestive splenomegaly in liver disease.

Sepsis

Overwhelming sepsis can accentuate peripheral utilization and destruction of neutrophils, with resultant neutropenia. This effect is more pronounced in patients with reduced bone marrow reserves such as the very old and the nutritionally deprived.

ISOIMMUNE NEUTROPENIA

This condition is of only academic interest to internists because it affects neonates. The pathogenesis of this disease is similar to Rh hemolytic disorder. Prenatal sensitization to neutrophil antigens results in production of IgG antibodies, which then cross the placenta and coat the neonate's neutrophils. When a newborn presents with neutropenic sepsis, it is difficult to distinguish between cause and effect because overwhelming sepsis not uncommonly results in neutropenia in neonates.

Abnormal Distribution

HYPERSPLENISM

Sequestration in a large spleen can cause neutropenia even without accentuated destruction in the splenic sinusoids. Without a significant functional component (destruction), hypersplenism usually causes only a mild neutropenia because of the compensatory acceleration of neutrophil production by the bone marrow.

PSEUDONEUTROPENIA

In this condition a portion of the circulating neutrophils transfers to the marginated pool. This phenomenon is the opposite of epinephrine-induced demargination. The shifts between the two pools are temporary and usually caused by hypersensitivity reactions or hemodynamic changes.

BENIGN CHRONIC NEUTROPENIA

Permanent increased margination is probably responsible for some of the familial forms of benign chronic neutropenia that occur in certain ethnic populations. Stimulation with epinephrine in affected patients produces a prompt increase in the neutrophil count. On the contrary, the variant caused by a dysregulation at the precursor level will not respond to an epinephrine injection. This test is seldom used in the routine evaluation of patients with neutropenia.

PRACTICAL APPROACH TO THE PATIENT WITH NEUTROPENIA

The most common cause of predictable neutropenia is the use of cytotoxic agents; the degree of severity depends on the agents used, the intensity of treatment, and the nature of the underlying disease. For patients presenting with unexpected neutropenia, the clinical history and examination and examination of the peripheral smear are the most important parts of the diagnostic evaluation. Examination of the oral cavity, perianal region, and skin is necessary to assess the clinical impact of chronic neutropenia. The presence of gingivitis, ulcers, and abscesses implies clinically significant neutropenia. New-onset neutropenia in children and young adults is usually of benign cause, most likely postinfectious.

If a mild to moderate neutropenia occurs in the otherwise well adult not taking any medications and whose peripheral smear does not show other abnormalities, a period of observation is suggested. A repeat complete blood cell count in about a month is useful to document improvement. If a medication known to be associated with neutropenia has recently been prescribed, its use should be discontinued. For the patient with long-term use of several medications, none of which stands out as a common offender, all essential medications should be substituted and use of nonessential medications should be discontinued. Drugs can depress the absolute neutrophil count by reduced production and peripheral destruction. When the mechanism is peripheral destruction, recovery of the absolute neutrophil count is usually prompt (within a few days), whereas in the case of marrow suppression, the count may be slower to recover (usually weeks). Although serum can be tested for antineutrophilic antibodies, the results of this test should not affect the clinical decision in most cases, and therefore it mainly remains of academic interest.

When the history suggests a collagen vascular disorder, an immunologic evaluation can be done. However, in the absence of relevant signs and symptoms, an undirected search will likely lead to incidental and confounding findings, especially with the considerable prevalence of nonspecific immunologic markers in the general population.

In an otherwise unexplained isolated neutropenia, peripheral blood immunophenotyping of lymphocytes is recommended to entertain the possibility of a large granular lymphocyte disorder. It is also recommended that a T-cell receptor gene rearrangement study be performed to evaluate for the occult presence of a T-cell clonal disorder. When neutropenia is associated with peripheral stool smear abnormalities (circulating blasts, Pelger-Huët anomaly, red cell dimorphism, oral macrocytosis), a bone marrow examination is recommended to evaluate for the possible presence of a myelodysplastic syndrome or other clonal hematologic disorder.

TREATMENT OF NEUTROPENIA

Even though an absolute neutrophil count of less than 1,500/mm^3 is defined as neutropenia, it does not usually become clinically significant until the count is less than 500/mm^3 (Table 4). In most cases, isolated neutropenia does not require any specific therapy other than maintenance of low threshold for intervention if fever or other symptoms develop. The previously widespread practice of strict isolation of the patient with neutropenia is no longer considered necessary or advisable. In fact, most infections in patients with neutropenia are of endogenous origin. Commonsense avoidance of persons with obvious viral or bacterial infections should apply. Masks should be worn in enclosed, crowded places but are not necessary in the home environment. Thorough hand washing should be practiced by the patient, visitors, and care providers.

Attention to dental care should include careful, nonvigorous brushing with a soft toothbrush. Elective invasive procedures should be postponed. The diet should be high in fiber, and a stool softener should be prescribed to avoid disruption of the rectal mucosa as much as possible. Fresh fruits and vegetables should be avoided. Particular attention should be paid to the care of venous access devices, for which meticulous aseptic technique is warranted. For hospitalization, a private room is recommended. Selective decontamination of the skin and bowel flora is no longer advisable.

The prophylactic use of antibiotics is a controversial issue. In general, most hematologists prescribe an oral antibiotic for expected protracted and severe neutropenia resulting from the effect of chemotherapy. The antibiotic chosen is primarily directed against gram-negative organisms, which have been the most frequent bacteremic isolates. Commonly prescribed antibiotics are the quinolones. Although this practice has resulted in a decrease in the incidence of gram-negative bacterial infections and, to a lesser extent, some decrease in morbidity, a resultant decrease in mortality has not occurred. An adverse effect of this practice has been the emergence of quinolone resistance among some gram-negative isolates such as *Escherichia coli*. In addition, the incidence of gram-positive infections has increased because of preferential selection.

Table 4
Clinical Significance of Neutrophil Counts

Count, mm^3	Clinical significance
> 1,500	Normal
1,000-1,500	No significant tendency for infection. Outpatient management of fever
500-1,000	Moderate increase in risk for infection. The count alone should not determine decision for hospitalization of the febrile patient
< 500	Marked increase in risk for fever and serious infection. The count alone may serve as a strong determining factor in deciding the need for hospitalization. Clinical signs and symptoms may be deceiving

In terms of prophylactic antifungal therapy, data support the role of fluconazole in reducing the incidence of *Candida* infections in patients undergoing allogeneic bone marrow transplantation. However, the role of antifungal therapy is less clearly established in other settings.

Patients with anticipated short-lived neutropenia (a few days) should probably not be given prophylactic antibiotics. Such patients are those receiving moderate-intensity chemotherapy and patients with neutropenia caused by a medication after discontinuing use of the offending agent. Patients with postinfectious and infectious neutropenia and patients with chronic idiopathic neutropenia also belong in the same category.

FEBRILE NEUTROPENIA

"Febrile neutropenia" and "neutropenic fever" are terms that are used interchangeably. By far, the condition is most common in the context of therapy of malignant disease with cytotoxic agents. The incidence of neutropenic fever has increased in recent years because of the intensification of chemotherapeutic regimens, which in turn has been partially allowed by improvement in supportive measures.

The morbidity associated with neutropenia is a function of its severity and duration and the nature of the underlying disease. In general, a protracted severe neutropenia (weeks) is more likely to be associated with a life-threatening infection than a short period of neutropenia (days) with a similar or even lower nadir neutrophil count. Among patients with an equal absolute neutrophil count, those with a low marrow reserve (production defect) because of either chemotherapy or a hematologic disease are more likely to have a serious infection than patients with neutropenia due to peripheral destruction or a distribution problem. A useful analogy is that among thrombocytopenias of equal severity, the one caused by a defective marrow is more likely to be associated with bleeding than the one caused by peripheral destruction (immune thrombocytopenic purpura) or sequestration. The physiologic explanation for this phenomenon is that in the case of defective marrow, the absence of neutrophils is rather static. In the case of peripheral destruction or margination, the neutrophils are more functional and more available in a dynamic sense than their mere number implies.

The patient with neutropenia who presents with a single episode of fever (> 38.5°C) requires immediate intervention and institution of broad-spectrum empiric antibiotic therapy. Patients with repeated low-grade fever also should be evaluated and treated. Prompt evaluation is needed for the patient with neutropenia who does not have fever but does have symptoms compatible with infection. Although it is appropriate to delay therapy in the nonneutropenic patient until the source of infection is identified, such a delay in the severely neutropenic patient may be associated with deleterious effects. Infections in patients with severe neutropenia are often characterized by lack of significant symptoms and clinical findings, probably due to the absence of an adequate inflammatory response. As a result, the severity of the infection can sometimes be underestimated.

In most cases, hospitalization is indicated for the febrile patient with neutropenia. However, in the past few years, there has been some tendency toward outpatient management for patients thought to be at low risk. One of the criteria used for risk stratification is the duration of neutropenia. Although a few antibiotic choices are acceptable, a third-generation cephalosporin with antipseudomonal coverage (ceftazidime) has been confirmed in randomized clinical trials to be effective empiric monotherapy for the patient without an identifiable source. Double-antibiotic therapy has been shown in some studies to result in faster resolution of fever; however, it has not produced better eventual outcomes. Including vancomycin in the primary empiric treatment, which previously has been common practice, is currently discouraged because of emerging resistance patterns. The addition of vancomycin or an antistaphylococcal semisynthetic penicillin to the existing coverage is still the most frequent modification for the patient with persistent fever. The identification of a particular source of infection should guide the choice of antibiotic therapy. Some general guidelines regarding the workup of the febrile patient with neutropenia are shown in Table 5.

The source of fever is definable in the minority of cases, and cultures are positive in 20% to 30% of cases even when repeated several times. The responsible organisms usually are derived from endogenous flora (gastrointestinal tract and skin). If fever and neutropenia persist for more than a few days with use of broad-spectrum antibiotics, consideration should be given to the addition of antifungal therapy. The most important risk factor for the development of invasive fungal infection is protracted severe neutropenia. Such infections are rare when the neutropenia lasts for less than a week. Most commonly, protracted neutropenia is the result of serious hematologic malignancies or intensified cytotoxic therapy for these diseases.

USE OF HEMATOPOIETIC GROWTH FACTORS

Growth factors such as granulocyte colony-stimulating factor (G-CSF) and granulocyte-monocyte colony-stimulating factor (GM-CSF) have been available for the past few years. Several studies have shown their efficacy in terms of decreasing the duration of neutropenia and, to a lesser extent, the incidence of febrile neutropenia and duration of hospitalization when used as prophylaxis, immediately after the administration of chemotherapy. Only a few studies have shown a limited benefit in specific subsets of patients in terms of a decrease in serious morbidity and mortality. No study has shown benefit in terms of mortality for patients given growth factors after they present with neutropenic fever. Also, no benefit in terms of mortality has been shown for the afebrile patient with neutropenia who receives hematopoietic growth factor at the onset of neutropenia. Outside the context of chemotherapy-induced neutropenia, administration of growth factors has been shown to benefit patients with cyclic neutropenia and some other forms of severe chronic neutropenia only in cases of previously established recurrent pyogenic infections.

Table 5
Diagnostic and Therapeutic Workup for Febrile Neutropenia

Blood cultures from two peripheral sites
Blood cultures from any intravenous catheters (all lumens)
Urinalysis and culture
Chest radiograph
Site-specific diagnostic approach directed by signs and symptoms (i.e.,
  sinus films)
Institution of broad-spectrum intravenous antibiotics (i.e., ceftazidime)
Restrict use of vancomycin to documented methicillin-resistant
  Staphylococcus aureus infections, gram-positive infections before
  identification of the organism, when suspicion is high, and in neutropenic
  septic shock
Add antifungal therapy for refractory fever after 2 to 4 days of broad-
  spectrum antibiotics
Discontinue use of antibiotics when both neutropenia and fever resolve, if
  the source of fever remains unknown
Continue use of antibiotics for the appropriate interval for documented
  infections

This chapter is not intended to provide a comprehensive discussion of the indications for use of growth factors. As an example, the 1996 American Society of Clinical Oncology guidelines regarding growth factors in patients receiving chemotherapy recommend primary prophylaxis when the expected incidence of febrile neutropenia is higher than 40%. In several special circumstances, patients may benefit from the administration of these agents. However, it is important to realize that the increase in neutrophil count does not always translate into clinical benefit. Therefore, alterations of absolute neutrophil counts and duration of neutropenia as surrogate markers should not be used by clinicians in making decisions about the use of these agents. Rather, physicians should base their decisions on results of randomized clinical trials that are designed to examine important clinical end points such as morbidity and mortality. Pharmacoeconomic advantage is also an acceptable force in driving decisions if the other, more important clinical end points are similar in outcome.

SUGGESTED READING

Bodey GP. The treatment of febrile neutropenia: from the Dark Ages to the present. *Support Care Cancer* 1997; 5: 351-357.

Chanock SJ, Pizzo PA. Fever in the neutropenic host. *Infect Dis Clin North Am* 1996; 10: 777-796.

De Pauw BE, Raemaekers JMM, Schattenberg T, Donnelly JP. Empirical and subsequent use of antibacterial agents in the febrile neutropenic patient. *J Intern Med* 1997; 242 Suppl 740: 69-77.

Elting LS, Rubenstein EB, Rolston KV, Bodey GP. Outcomes of bacteremia in patients with cancer and neutropenia: observations from two decades of epidemiological and clinical trials. *Clin Infect Dis* 1997; 25: 247-259.

Engels EA, Lau J, Barza M. Efficacy of quinolone prophylaxis in neutropenic cancer patients: a meta-analysis. *J Clin Oncol* 1998; 16: 1179-1187.

Escalante CP, Rubenstein EB, Rolston KV. Outpatient antibiotic therapy for febrile episodes in low-risk neutropenic patients with cancer. *Cancer Invest* 1997; 15: 237-242.

Gotzsche PC, Johansen HK. Meta-analysis of prophylactic or empirical antifungal treatment versus placebo or no treatment in patients with cancer complicated by neutropenia. *BMJ* 1997; 314: 1238-1244.

Hartmann LC, Tschetter LK, Habermann TM, Ebbert LP, Johnson PS, Mailliard JA, Levitt R, Suman VJ, Witzig TE, Wieand HS, Miller LL, Moertel CG. Granulocyte colony-stimulating factor in severe chemotherapy-induced afebrile neutropenia. *N Engl J Med* 1997; 336: 1776-1780.

Hathorn JW, Lyke K. Empirical treatment of febrile neutropenia: evolution of current therapeutic approaches. *Clin Infect Dis* 1997; 24 Suppl 2: S256-S265.

Kyle RA. Natural history of chronic idiopathic neutropenia. *N Engl J Med* 1980; 302: 908-909.

Ozer H. American Society of Clinical Oncology guidelines for the use of hematopoietic colony-stimulating factors. *Curr Opin Hematol* 1996; 3: 3-10.

Pizzo PA. Management of fever in patients with cancer and treatment-induced neutropenia. *N Engl J Med* 1993; 328: 1323-1332.

Rubenstein EB, Rolston K, Benjamin RS, Loewy J, Escalante C, Manzullo E, Hughes P, Moreland B, Fender A, Kennedy K, Holmes F, Elting L, Bodey GP. Outpatient treatment of febrile episodes in low-risk neutropenic patients with cancer. *Cancer* 1993; 71: 3640-3646.

7

Causes and Management of Isolated Thrombocytopenia

Gerardo Colon-Otero, MD

Contents

INTRODUCTION

The inclusion of platelet count determination as part of a routinely ordered automated blood cell count has led to the frequent recognition of asymptomatic thrombocytopenia in adult patients. Physical signs of thrombocytopenia are limited to easy bruising as long as the platelet count remains more than 20,000/µL. Patients with platelet counts less than 10,000/µL frequently present with mucosal bleeding (gum bleeding, nosebleeds, heavy menses), petechiae, and ecchymoses (Fig. 1, Plate 7). Less frequently, life-threatening gastrointestinal bleeding and central nervous system hemorrhage may be associated with severe thrombocytopenia. Bleeding diathesis in thrombocytopenia is significantly increased in the presence of an underlying structural lesion (gastric ulcer), uremia, and treatment with anticoagulants (heparin, warfarin) or nonsteroidal anti-inflammatory drugs.

CAUSES OF ISOLATED THROMBOCYTOPENIA

For practical purposes, the causes of isolated thrombocytopenia can be broadly classified into six categories: spurious, immune-mediated, intravascular consumption, splenic sequestration (hypersplenism), hereditary, and ineffective bone marrow production (Table 1).

Spurious Thrombocytopenia

The first step in the evaluation of isolated thrombocytopenia is to confirm that the thrombocytopenia is real and not a laboratory artifact due to EDTA-induced platelet clumping. EDTA is an anticoagulant added to the purple-top vacuum tubes used for the

From: *Primary Hematology*
Edited by: A. Tefferi © Mayo Foundation for Medical Education and Research, Rochester, MN

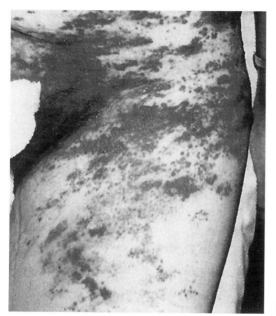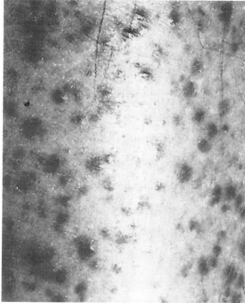

Fig. 1, Plate 7. Ecchymoses (*Left*) and petechiae (*Right*) from severe thrombocytopenia. (From Hoffbrand AV, Pettit JE. *Color Atlas of Clinical Hematology*, 2nd ed. Mosby-Wolfe, London, 1994. By permission of the publisher.)

collection of blood for cell counting. Some platelets either clump or adhere to neutrophils in the test tube in the presence of EDTA, leading to falsely low automated platelet counts. The presence of EDTA-induced platelet clumping can be appreciated by examining the peripheral smear (Fig. 2, Plate 8). If the phenomenon of EDTA-induced platelet clumping is suspected, a true platelet count may be obtained by redrawing the blood and using an alternative anticoagulant (sodium citrate, blue-top tube).

Immune-Mediated Thrombocytopenia

Most cases of thrombocytopenia are due to increased platelet destruction, most commonly from immune-mediated mechanisms. In most of these cases, the cause is unknown, and the process is referred to as idiopathic immune thrombocytopenic purpura (ITP). The remaining cases may be related to drugs such as heparin (heparin-induced thrombocytopenia, HIT), autoimmune disorders (systemic lupus erythematosus), hematologic malignancies (lymphoproliferative disorders), infections (human immunodeficiency virus infection, sepsis), and alloimmune mechanisms (posttransfusion purpura, neonatal purpura). ITP is operationally classified as acute or chronic; the acute form predominates in children, whereas the chronic form usually occurs in adults. In HIT, the antigen inducing the production of antibody is a multimolecular complex between heparin and platelet factor 4 (PF4).

Intravascular Consumption of Platelets

Intravascular consumption is the main mechanism in the thrombocytopenia of thrombotic thrombocytopenic purpura/hemolytic-uremic syndrome (TTP/HUS), valvular heart

Table 1
Causes of Isolated Thrombocytopenia

Spurious thrombocytopenia
Immune-mediated
    Drug-related (heparin, antibiotics, quinine, valproic acid, sulfa drugs)
    Autoimmune (systemic lupus erythematosus, rheumatoid arthritis)
    Hematologic malignancies (chronic lymphocytic leukemia, lymphoma)
    Infections (human immunodeficiency virus, cytomegalovirus, sepsis, malaria)
    Alloimmune (posttransfusion purpura, neonatal purpura)
    Idiopathic thrombocytopenic purpura
Intravascular consumption
    Thrombotic thrombocytopenic purpura/hemolytic-uremic syndrome
    Valvular heart disease
    Disseminated intravascular coagulation
    Systemic inflammatory response syndromes
    Hemangioma-thrombocytopenia (Kasabach-Merritt) syndrome
Hypersplenism
    Chronic liver disease
    Lymphomas, hairy cell leukemia, amyloidosis
Hereditary
    May-Hegglin anomaly
    Thrombocytopenia with absent radius
    Gray platelet syndrome
    Bernard-Soulier syndrome
    Alport's syndrome
    Wiskott-Aldrich syndrome
Bone marrow production problems
    Drugs
    Myelodysplastic syndrome
    Vitamin B_{12} or folate deficiencies
    Acute alcohol intoxication
    Amegakaryocytic thrombocytopenia

disease, disseminated intravascular coagulation (DIC), systemic inflammatory response syndromes (bacterial sepsis, acute pancreatitis, acute rickettsial or viral infections), and the hemangioma-thrombocytopenia (Kasabach-Merritt) syndrome. Microangiopathic hemolysis is usually present in these cases (schistocytes in the peripheral blood, reticulocytosis, decreased plasma haptoglobin levels, hemosiderinuria, and increased lactate dehydrogenase enzyme levels).

Hypersplenism

Hypersplenism is most commonly due to chronic liver disease. The possibility of cryptogenic cirrhosis and associated hypersplenism should be entertained in all patients with thrombocytopenia. Liver function tests, physical stigmata of liver disease, and historical data should be examined carefully, and imaging studies (ultrasonography or plain radiography of the abdomen) may sometimes be necessary to assess spleen size and the liver parenchyma. Other causes of splenomegaly, including lymphoma, amyloidosis, and hairy cell leukemia, also should be considered.

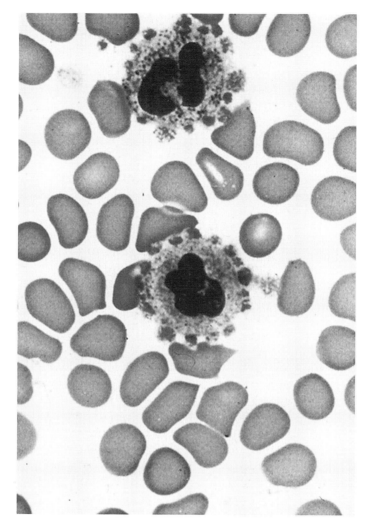

Fig. 2, Plate 8. Platelet rosetting in the presence of EDTA. (From Hoffbrand AV, Pettit JE. *Color Atlas of Clinical Hematology*, 2nd ed. Mosby-Wolfe, London, 1994. By permission of the publisher.)

Hereditary Causes of Thrombocytopenia

Hereditary thrombocytopenias are rare disorders that may escape diagnosis until the patient reaches adulthood. One of these conditions diagnosed in adulthood is the May-Hegglin anomaly, in which patients have moderately severe thrombocytopenia, giant platelets, and neutrophilic cytoplasmic inclusions (Döhle bodies). Other inherited thrombocytopenia syndromes include thrombocytopenia with absent radius, gray platelet syndrome (alpha granule deficiency), Bernard-Soulier syndrome, Alport's syndrome (nerve deafness, nephritis, thrombocytopenia), and the X-linked Wiskott-Aldrich syndrome (eczema, immune deficiency, and thrombocytopenia).

Ineffective Bone Marrow Production of Platelets

Most patients with bone marrow production problems have pancytopenia rather than isolated thrombocytopenia. This is especially true for bone marrow infiltrative processes such as metastatic cancer, myelofibrosis, and lymphoma. Isolated thrombocytopenia is rarely the presenting manifestation of a myelodysplastic syndrome. Toxic chemical exposure usually affects all cell lines. However, drugs such as alcohol, thiazide diuretics, and antibiotics can cause isolated thrombocytopenia by inhibiting platelet production. A rare condition, amegakaryocytic thrombocytopenia, is caused by immunologically mediated inhibition of megakaryocyte and platelet production.

EVALUATION OF THROMBOCYTOPENIA AND DIFFERENTIAL DIAGNOSIS

A stepwise diagnostic process during the evaluation of thrombocytopenia is outlined in Table 2. The most important steps, and the ones that should always be done, are listed below.

Evaluation of Thrombocytopenia

- Screen for any drug therapy that might be causally related.

- Exclude the possibility of TTP/HUS and DIC.

- Entertain the possibility of hypersplenism.

The medication history is critical. Drug-related immune thrombocytopenia has been described with many of the currently available agents. The most common culprits are antibiotics (penicillin and its analogs, cephalosporins, sulfa derivatives), cardiac medications (quinidine, procainamide), diuretics (thiazide derivatives), quinine, and heparin. Heparin-induced thrombocytopenia (HIT, also known as heparin-associated thrombocytopenia) may be associated with acute arterial thrombotic events and requires immediate discontinuation of the use of heparin, including heparin flushes. The date of onset of thrombocytopenia can be elicited by reviewing previous platelet counts, and their relationship with initiation of the use of new medications could establish the possibility of a drug-related phenomenon. It is always reasonable to consider discontinuing use of any medication that is temporally related to onset of the thrombocytopenia. If the observed thrombocytopenia could be related to medications, then no further investigation is warranted unless the thrombocytopenia persists despite discontinuation of the "offending" drug.

Thrombotic thrombocytopenic purpura (TTP) is a potentially fatal disorder. Therefore, it is very important to recognize and treat this condition early. Traditionally, five cardinal manifestations are attributed to TTP: fever, altered mental status, microangiopathic hemolytic anemia (presence of fragmented red cells with associated hemolysis), thrombocytopenia, and renal insufficiency. However, the presence of all five features is not required to make the diagnosis. Table 3 outlines clinical conditions that might be associated with TTP. The demonstration of microangiopathic hemolysis and thrombocytopenia in the absence of DIC is adequate to make a working diagnosis of TTP. In the presence of significant renal involvement and absence of central nervous system involvement, the process is referred to as hemolytic-uremic syndrome (HUS). HUS is more prevalent in children. TTP/HUS is potentially treatable with total plasma exchange, which should be started immediately.

Although the cause of TTP/HUS is often unknown, several conditions have been associated with the syndrome (Table 3). A bone marrow biopsy is not necessary in the evaluation of TTP. Instead, initial evaluation and follow-up tests include peripheral

Table 2
Initial Evaluation of Isolated Thrombocytopenia

First step:	Rule out EDTA-induced platelet clumping
	Tests: Citrated platelet count
	Peripheral blood smear
Second step:	Screen for medications and alcohol use
Third step:	Entertain the possibility of liver disease and hypersplenism
	Tests: Liver function tests
	Plain abdominal radiography, ultrasonography of the spleen
Fourth step:	Exclude the possibility of TTP/HUS and DIC[a]
	Tests: Peripheral blood smear
	PT, PTT, d-dimer, fibrinogen, LDH, serum creatinine[b]
Fifth step:	Proceed with additional tests to establish correct diagnosis
	Tests:

- Asymptomatic: human immunodeficiency virus serology, antinuclear antibody, serum vitamin B_{12} and folate levels, platelet antibody testing
- Acutely ill patient with fevers: fibrinogen, FSP, PT, APTT, chest radiography, blood and urine cultures[c]
- Patient with polyarthritis or serositis: anti-native DNA, rheumatoid factor, complement levels
- Patient with adenopathy: computed tomography of the body
- Patient with abnormal liver function studies, chronic liver stigmata, or history of hepatitis or blood transfusions: hepatitis serologic tests, serum iron studies, ceruloplasmin, α_1-antitrypsin, computed tomography of abdomen

[a]DIC, disseminated intravascular coagulation; TTP/HUS, thrombotic thrombocytopenic purpura/hemolytic-uremic syndrome.
[b]LDH, lactate dehydrogenase; PT, prothrombin time; PTT, partial thromboplastin time.
[c]APTT, activated partial thromboplastin time; FSP, fibrin split products.

Table 3
Associated Conditions in Thrombotic
Thrombocytopenic Purpura

Toxigenic *Escherichia coli* (O157:H7)-associated diarrhea
Human immunodeficiency virus infection
Drugs (ticlopidine, quinine, mitomycin C, cisplatin, cyclosporin A)
Pregnancy
Bone marrow transplant
Metastatic carcinomas

smear, determination of lactate dehydrogenase and serum creatinine levels, and complete blood cell count. Schistocytes are appreciated in the peripheral blood smear, and the lactate dehydrogenase level is often increased. Alternatively, prothrombin time, partial thromboplastin time, d-dimer, and blood fibrinogen levels are usually normal; these values help discriminate the process from DIC.

We emphasize the need to entertain occult liver disease and hypersplenism as a cause of thrombocytopenia. Usually, hypersplenic thrombocytopenia is moderate (platelet count, 50,000-100,000/µL) and not progressive. Patients should be investigated for alcohol consumption, history of hepatitis or other liver disease, the use of hepatotoxic drugs, and the presence of right heart failure or large vessel thrombosis. Physical stigmata of liver disease, including palpable splenomegaly, should be sought. At times, ultrasound assessment of spleen size and endoscopic evaluation for the detection of esophageal varices may be indicated.

Once drug-induced thrombocytopenia, microangiopathic hemolytic anemia, and hypersplenism are ruled out, an immune-mediated process becomes the major contender in the differential diagnosis. An immune-mediated thrombocytopenia may be either idiopathic (ITP) or associated with other conditions (Table 1). A history of polyarthritis, serositis, and malar skin eruption should raise the suspicion of a connective tissue disorder. Serologic testing for human immunodeficiency virus infection is highly recommended for most patients. The presence of constitutional symptoms, splenomegaly, and lymphadenopathy suggests lymphoma or chronic lymphocytic leukemia. It should be noted that splenomegaly is unusual in uncomplicated ITP.

The specific evaluation of ITP requires a careful evaluation of the peripheral smear to exclude the possibility of spurious thrombocytopenia, TTP/HUS, DIC, and hereditary thrombocytopenia. Although "large" platelets are mentioned in conjunction with ITP, they also are found in other platelet-destructive processes and lack specificity. Determination of platelet antigen-specific or platelet-associated antibodies, although not inappropriate, is not recommended because the tests lack both sensitivity and specificity. Bone marrow biopsy is not indicated in the workup of most patients with ITP. When a bone marrow examination is indicated, it can be performed safely even with very low platelet counts (< 10,000/µL). The bone marrow examination may reveal the presence of lymphoma or other marrow infiltrating process, a myelodysplastic process, or "adequate" or "increased" megakaryocyte number that would be consistent with a diagnosis of ITP.

Bleeding Time and Platelets

- In the presence of fully functional platelets, the bleeding time is usually normal when the platelet count is more than 75,000/µL.

- Avoid ordering a bleeding time test when the platelet count is less than 50,000/µL. The bleeding time, in this case, will be prolonged because of the low platelet count and not necessarily from platelet dysfunction.

- Bleeding time is not helpful and should not be ordered during treatment with nonsteroidal anti-inflammatory drugs.

- A prolonged bleeding time with a normal platelet count suggests either the intake of nonsteroidal anti-inflammatory drugs or a functional platelet or von Willebrand factor abnormality.

MANAGEMENT OF THROMBOCYTOPENIA

Obviously, treatment depends on the cause of the problem. In general, there is no urgency in treating the asymptomatic patient with a platelet count of 10,000/µL or more. Spontaneous bleeding complications are rare when the platelet count is more than 10,000/µL. Therefore, initial diagnostic evaluation, including laboratory tests, should be completed before treatment is planned for the asymptomatic patient with a platelet count of more than 10,000/µL. However, platelet transfusions may be needed if the platelet count is less than 50,000/µL in bleeding patients. The need for platelet transfusion in the asymptomatic patient with a platelet count less than 10,000/µL depends on several factors. If the problem is chronic and is anticipated to continue (such as a patient with chronic ITP or myelodysplastic syndrome), then platelet transfusion should be reserved for bleeding episodes only. If the problem is newly recognized, then prophylactic platelet transfusion is reasonable while diagnostic evaluation is being performed.

Treatment of TTP/HUS

Definitive therapy in TTP is daily plasma exchange (plasmapheresis combined with infusion of fresh frozen plasma or cryosupernatant) until the platelet count and lactate dehydrogenase level are significantly improved. Initially, most patients require 5 to 10 daily plasma exchanges. A program of tapering can then be instituted with an every-other-day schedule for 1 to 2 weeks followed by weekly exchange for 1 to 2 months. No additional therapy is indicated for patients showing response in the first few days. If response is not adequate after the first 3 days of therapy, oral corticosteroids (prednisone, 1 mg/kg per day) and low-dose aspirin (81 mg/day) may be added. Platelet transfusions are not recommended. In treatment-refractory patients, vincristine (1 to 2 mg/day intravenously weekly) may be used before considering splenectomy. In patients with chronic TTP, intermittent plasma exchange, chronic corticosteroid therapy, and splenectomy have all been reported to be useful.

Treatment of DIC

In the nonbleeding patient with DIC, platelet transfusions are not necessary unless the platelet count is less than 10,000/µL or there is an associated comorbid condition, such as uremia, that predisposes the patient to bleeding. In general, the patient should be supported with infusion of cryoprecipitate (if the fibrinogen level is < 100 mg/dL), fresh frozen plasma if the prothrombin time is significantly increased (> twofold), and platelet transfusion (if the platelet count is < 10,000/µL). The bleeding patient should receive platelet transfusions for a platelet count less than 50,000/µL and infusion of fresh frozen plasma for any degree of prolongation in the prothrombin time. Heparin may be indicated in the presence of clinically evident arterial or venous thrombosis.

Treatment of Drug- or Heparin-Induced Thrombocytopenia (HIT)

Patients with drug-induced thrombocytopenia or HIT require immediate discontinuation of use of the offending drug(s). Management in most cases is otherwise supportive. The most common cause of drug-induced thrombocytopenia is heparin. HIT occurs in approximately 1% of patients receiving heparin therapy, and the incidence is less with the use of porcine (instead of bovine) products and low-molecular-weight heparin. Associated thrombosis occurs in approximately 10% of patients with HIT. In previously unexposed patients, thrombocytopenia develops in 3 to 5 days of heparin therapy.

Prevention of HIT is much more successful than treatment of HIT. The use of low-molecular-weight heparin is associated with a significantly lower incidence of HIT. It is good practice to obtain daily platelet counts in patients starting on heparin therapy. Use of all heparin products, including heparin flushes, should be discontinued as soon as the diagnosis is suspected. Because discontinuation of heparin may place the patient at risk of thrombosis, it is recommended that warfarin therapy be initiated early to allow adequate coagulation with warfarin at the time of discontinuation.

The diagnosis of HIT may be confirmed by in vitro testing to detect heparin-dependent platelet antibodies. One functional assay involves serotonin release of normal donor platelets incubated with heparin and patient plasma (serotonin-release assay). A positive test is fairly specific and is attained in more than 90% of clinically diagnosed cases. Other functional assays include platelet aggregation studies and flow cytometry for detecting platelet-derived microparticles. An antigen assay (enzyme-linked immunosorbent assay) that detects antibodies against heparin/PF4 complex is currently the most frequently used diagnostic method. In patients with HIT who require continued anticoagulation, either a heparinoid (danaparoid sodium, Orgaran, 750 anti-Xa units subcutaneously twice a day) or a thrombin inhibitor (lepirudin, Refludan) may be used. Anti-factor Xa levels may be used for monitoring anticoagulant activity of danaparoid, and activated partial thromboplastin time is used to monitor lepirudin therapy.

Treatment of Posttransfusion Purpura

Posttransfusion purpura is a rare complication of blood transfusion. A history of blood component transfusion a few days (7-14 days) before the onset of thrombocytopenia should suggest the diagnosis. Posttransfusion purpura is due to an anamnestic production of platelet alloantibodies (anti-PL^{A1}), and it usually occurs in multiparous women. Platelet transfusions are usually discouraged unless the patient is bleeding. The process is self-limited, and treatment with intravenous immunoglobulin (IgG) or corticosteroids is needed occasionally.

Treatment of Immune Thrombocytopenic Purpura (ITP)

Management of ITP in adults depends on the severity of the thrombocytopenia. Specific therapy may not be needed if the platelet count remains more than 30,000/μL. Instead, patients are advised to avoid the use of nonsteroidal anti-inflammatory drugs or excess alcohol. If the platelet count is less than 30,000/μL, then an initial treatment trial with oral corticosteroids (prednisone, 1 mg/kg per day) is reasonable. The usual corticosteroid side effects should be emphasized. An adequate (platelet count, > 50,000/μL) and durable response may be achieved in up to 50% of patients. However, long-term and unmaintained remissions are infrequent (< 10%). If the severe thrombocytopenia does not respond, or responds minimally (platelet count, < 50,000/μL), to a 4-week trial of corticosteroids or recurs during steroid taper (which should be commenced after 4-6 weeks of therapy), then splenectomy is recommended. In patients who are not eligible for splenectomy, intravenous or oral cyclophosphamide is an option. We usually give pneumococcal, meningococcal, and *Haemophilus influenzae* vaccinations well before the time of splenectomy and penicillin prophylaxis (Pen VK 250 mg twice a day or erythromycin 250 mg twice a day) indefinitely after splenectomy.

Splenectomy results in durable and adequate remissions in approximately two-thirds of patients. If ITP recurs after splenectomy, the first step is to rule out residual accessory spleen. Evaluation for accessory spleen should include both peripheral smear examination (to look for Howell-Jolly bodies, the presence of which suggests a hyposplenic state) and computed tomography of the abdomen. The presence of Howell-Jolly bodies does not rule out the existence of an accessory spleen. Accessory spleen should be surgically removed. In the absence of accessory spleen, we use danazol (400 mg twice a day) as second-line drug therapy. Before treatment with danazol is instituted, men should be screened for prostate cancer and women have to be briefed about the virilizing side

Table 4
Salvage Therapy for Refractory
Idiopathic Thrombocytopenic Purpura

Treatment	Dosage
Colchicine	0.6 mg orally three times a day
Dapsone	100 mg orally daily
Vincristine	1-2 mg intravenously weekly
Vinblastine	5-10 mg intravenously every 2-4 weeks
High-dose dexamethasone	40 mg/day orally for 4 days; repeat cycle monthly for 6 months
Azathioprine	150 mg/day orally
Intravenous cyclophosphamide	1 g intravenously every 2 weeks
Oral cyclophosphamide	100-200 mg/day
Cyclosporine	300 mg orally twice a day; starting dose to be adjusted according to drug level and toxicity
Interferon-α	3 million units subcutaneously three times a week

effects. In addition, patients receiving danazol therapy should have liver function tests periodically.

Treatment of the patient with ITP in whom both splenectomy and drug therapy (with either corticosteroids or danazol) fail is difficult and often unsuccessful. In general, the use of intravenous IgG (1.0 g/kg a day for 2 days) or Rh immune globulin (250 IU/kg intravenously for Rh-positive individuals) does not provide durable remission. Treatment with intravenous IgG is expensive and may be associated with severe headaches. However, these agents can increase the platelet count promptly and may be useful in urgent situations. Drugs that have been reported to be of use to some patients with refractory thrombocytopenia are outlined in Table 4. The reader is encouraged to examine the original reports before instituting salvage therapy to patients. Plasmapheresis with staphylococcal protein A column may benefit some patients with drug-refractory disease. When nothing works, significant mucocutaneous bleeding may be alleviated by the careful use of antifibrinolytic agents (aminocaproic or tranexamic acid).

Management of Thrombocytopenia During Pregnancy

Approximately 7% of healthy women experience mild to moderate thrombocytopenia (platelet count, 75,000-150,000/µL) during pregnancy (incidental thrombocytopenia of pregnancy). In general, a diagnostic workup and treatment are not indicated for incidental thrombocytopenia of pregnancy. A similar degree of thrombocytopenia may occur in association with preeclampsia and is treated as such. The management of ITP in the pregnant patient should be as conservative as possible. In general, a maternal platelet count of more than 30,000/µL is considered safe for both mother and child and does not require specific therapy. In the presence of a lower platelet count or at the time of delivery, either prednisone (1 mg/kg a day) or intravenous IgG (1 g/kg a day for 2 days) may be used. Cesarean section is not routinely recommended.

SUGGESTED READING

Bell WR, Braine HG, Ness PM, Kickler TS. Improved survival in thrombotic thrombocytopenic purpura-hemolytic uremic syndrome. Clinical experience in 108 patients. *N Engl J Med* 1991; 325: 398-403.

Berchtold P, McMillan R. Therapy of chronic idiopathic thrombocytopenic purpura in adults. *Blood* 1989; 74: 2309-2317.

George JN, Woolf SH, Raskob GE, Wasser JS, Aledort LM, Ballem PJ, Blanchette VS, Bussel JB, Cines DB, Kelton JG, Lichtin AE, McMillan R, Okerbloom JA, Regan DH, Warrier I. Idiopathic thrombocytopenic purpura: a practice guideline developed by explicit methods for the American Society of Hematology. *Blood* 1996; 88: 3-40.

Menke DM, Colon-Otero G, Cockerill KJ, Jenkins RB, Noel P, Pierre RV. Refractory thrombocytopenia. A myelodysplastic syndrome that may mimic immune thrombocytopenic purpura. *Am J Clin Pathol* 1992; 98: 502-510.

II PRIMARY AND SECONDARY MYELOPROLIFERATIVE DISORDERS

8

An Approach to the Patient With Erythrocytosis

Ayalew Tefferi, MD

Contents

INTRODUCTION

The main objective during the evaluation of an increased hematocrit or hemoglobin value is to ascertain the presence or absence of polycythemia vera (PV). However, PV is not the only cause of an increased red cell mass (RCM), and a seemingly increased hematocrit value does not always indicate a true increase in RCM. "Relative polycythemia" refers to a state of reduced plasma volume which secondarily increases the hematocrit level without an associated increase in RCM (Fig. 1). True erythrocytosis is due to either an autonomous (growth factor-independent) proliferation of erythroid cells (as in PV) or an erythropoietin (EPO)-driven secondary process, as in secondary erythrocytosis. EPO production in secondary erythrocytosis may be oxygen-sensitive (as in hypoxic conditions) or oxygen-insensitive (as in EPO-producing tumors). Oxygen-sensitive EPO production may be physiologically appropriate, as in patients with chronic lung disease, or inappropriate, as in patients with renal artery stenosis. Finally, the hematocrit level in PV may remain in the normal range because of an associated increase in plasma volume (inapparent polycythemia) (Fig. 1).

From: *Primary Hematology*
Edited by: A. Tefferi © Mayo Foundation for Medical Education and Research, Rochester, MN

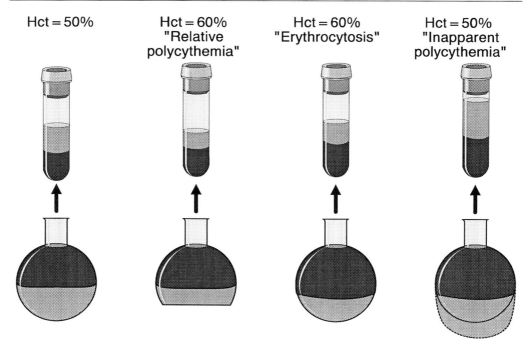

Fig. 1. Correlations of hematocrit (Hct, dark shading), red cell mass, and plasma volume (lighter shading).

RELATIVE POLYCYTHEMIA

It is important to differentiate absolute erythrocytosis from relative polycythemia because the latter condition may not require further evaluation or treatment. True erythrocytosis, however, may signify a serious blood disorder (PV) or may be a marker of an underlying disease process that secondarily increases RCM through an EPO-mediated mechanism (secondary erythrocytosis). Conventionally, the distinction between erythrocytosis and relative polycythemia has involved the laboratory measurement of RCM and plasma volume (Fig. 2). These measurements also have been incorporated in the diagnostic criteria for PV published by the Polycythemia Vera Study Group more than 23 years ago (Table 1).

Although relative polycythemia can be appreciated during acute intravascular fluid depletion, there is controversy regarding the existence of chronic states of contracted plasma volume in association with either hypertension (Gaisböck's syndrome) or anxiety (stress polycythemia). The original studies regarding relative polycythemia included patients with normal hemoglobin values, and the observations were based on estimates of plasma volume indirectly derived from measurements of RCM and did not correct for lean body mass or for the difference between venous and whole body hematocrit values. The latter point refers to the systematic underestimation of RCM because of the higher concentration of red cells in venous blood than in arterial blood. In a recent study of 109 consecutive measurements of RCM and plasma volume at the Mayo Clinic, not a single case of relative polycythemia was found. Similarly, other studies have suggested that abnormally low body:venous hematocrit ratios, and not reduced plasma volume, accounted for the relative polycythemia observed in patients with hypertension (so-called Gaisböck's syndrome).

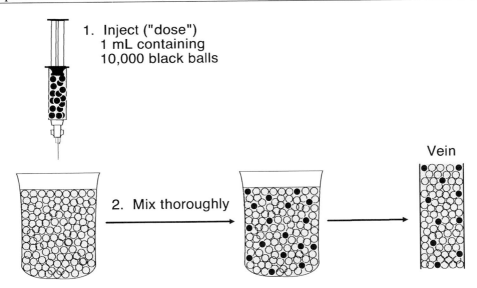

Fig. 2. The principle behind the measurement of blood volumes. The black balls represent radio-actively tagged red cells. The total blood volume is estimated by dividing the concentration of the black balls in the injected solution by that in the vein. The red cell mass is then calculated by multiplying the total estimated blood volume by the hematocrit value.

In general, measurements of RCM and plasma volume are costly, time-consuming, and not readily available to the general practitioner. They also are subject to methodologic inaccuracies, and meaningful data require that the measurements be done under controlled and standard conditions. Also, RCM correlates well with the hemoglobin (or hematocrit) level, and the additional information obtained from measurement of RCM may not always be necessary. For example, in patients with a hemoglobin value of 18.5 g/dL or more (16.5 g/dL in women), measurement of RCM may be redundant because this degree of increase in hemoglobin, in the absence of a clinically obvious dehydrated state, is almost always associated with absolute erythrocytosis.

INAPPARENT POLYCYTHEMIA

As mentioned earlier, the term "inapparent polycythemia" is used to describe the situation in which both the RCM and the plasma volume are increased to an equal degree, thus resulting in a "normal" hematocrit value (Fig. 1). However, the situation is not different from that of patients with true PV who have "normal" RCM because of associated bleeding, iron deficiency, or latent disease. Furthermore, an isolated RCM value that is within the normal reference interval does not take into account the possibility of a lower baseline value in a particular patient. Therefore, the presence of a PV-related feature (Fig. 3) dictates the subsequent measurement of more specific biologic parameters regardless of the calculated RCM. Alternatively, overreliance on RCM measurement may result in overdiagnosis for part of the normal population because of the statistically narrow limits of the reference interval.

PHYSIOLOGY OF ERYTHROPOIESIS

Similar to all other blood cells, red blood cells are derived from the pluripotent hematopoietic stem cell after a hierarchical process of lineage commitment and differentiation.

Table 1
The Polycythemia Vera Study Group
Diagnostic Criteria for Polycythemia Vera[a]

Major criteria	Minor criteria

1. Increased red cell mass
    Males: $\geq$ 36 mL/kg
    Females: $\geq$ 32 mL/kg
2. Normal arterial oxygen
    saturation, $\geq$ 92%
3. Splenomegaly
	1. Platelets > 400,000/mL
	2. Leukocytes >12,000/mL
	3. Leukocyte alkaline phosphatase > 100
	    or vitamin B_{12} > 900 pg/mL
	    or unbound B_{12} binding capacity > 2,200 pg/mL

[a]Diagnosis of polycythemia vera requires the presence of all three major criteria or the presence of the first two major criteria and any two minor criteria.

From Tefferi A, Silverstein MN. Myeloproliferative disease, in Cecil Textbook of Medicine (Goldman L, Bennett JC, eds), 21st ed. WB Saunders Company, Philadelphia, 2000, pp. 935-941. By permission of the publisher.

Under normal conditions, the earliest erythroid-committed progenitor cells depend on EPO to differentiate further and effectively produce red blood cells. In humans, 90% of the circulating EPO is synthesized by the kidneys in response to a hypoxic signal. The hypoxic signal to the EPO-producing renal cells may be a result of decreased red blood cell concentration (anemia), decreased oxygen saturation (hypoxemia), decreased oxygen release (high-oxygen–affinity hemoglobinopathies), or decreased blood flow (renal stenosis). A negative feedback inhibition mechanism exists which down-regulates EPO production with erythrocytosis. Accordingly, an EPO-independent erythrocytosis suppresses production of EPO and usually results in low serum EPO levels. However, an EPO-driven erythrocytosis characterizes secondary erythrocytosis and is associated with high or normal serum EPO levels.

DIAGNOSIS OF POLYCYTHEMIA
VERA: PAST AND PRESENT

It is imperative to apply the sex- and race-adjusted normal reference intervals before considering erythrocytosis on the basis of hemoglobin concentration (Fig. 4). It is also important to recognize that the stated normal range usually refers to the lower and upper limits observed in 95% of the normal population and does not necessarily imply that outlying values are always abnormal (Fig. 4). Therefore, initial evaluation should start with review of previous laboratory records (to document interim change) and determination of the presence or absence of any PV-related feature (Fig. 3). In the absence of a PV-related feature, there should be no further investigation of a hemoglobin level within the appropriate normal range unless a persistent change from a previous baseline value is documented.

The Polycythemia Vera Study Group diagnostic criteria for PV are outlined in Table 1. According to these criteria, the measurement of RCM is an absolute requirement. However, RCM measurement is associated with a few shortcomings (described in previous sections). An alternative approach to the diagnosis of PV is possible because the disease differs from all other causes of erythrocytosis in its pathogenesis and therefore influences, in a unique fashion, the production of EPO. Similarly, because of the clonal, EPO-independent nature of the disease, endogenous (without the addition of EPO) eryth-

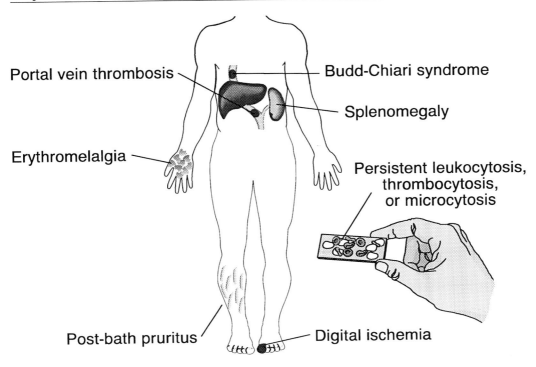

Fig. 3. Polycythemia vera-related clinical and laboratory features.

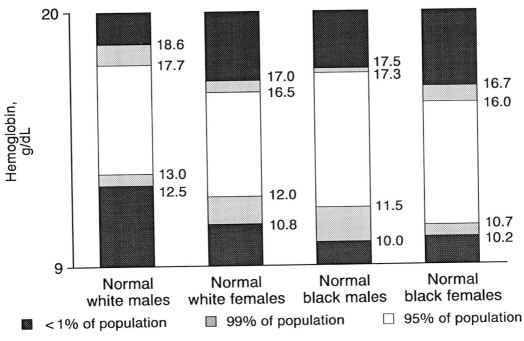

Fig. 4. Dependence of normal hemoglobin values on sex and race (adult values).

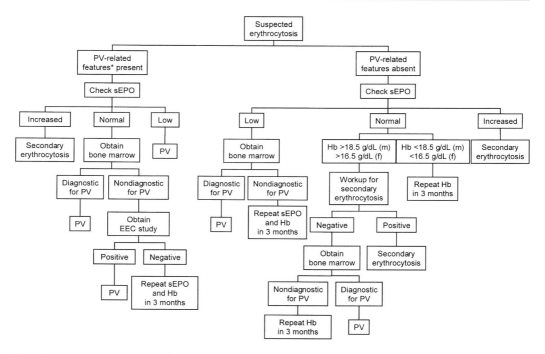

Fig. 5. A diagnostic approach to suspected erythrocytosis. EEC, endogenous erythroid colony; f, female; Hb, hemoglobin; m, male; PV, polycythemia vera; sEPO, serum erythropoietin level.*See Figure 3 for PV-related features.

roid colony growth is a relatively specific manifestation associated with PV. Therefore, the measurement of these biologic parameters may allow an alternative approach to the evaluation of erythrocytosis.

DIAGNOSTIC UTILITY OF SERUM ERYTHROPOIETIN LEVEL IN ERYTHROCYTOSIS

It is reasonable to start the investigation of erythrocytosis by determining the serum EPO level (Fig. 5); low levels are relatively specific to PV and levels above normal are unusual in PV. Therefore, PV is a diagnostic possibility only when the serum EPO level is low or normal.

Low Serum Erythropoietin Level

A low serum EPO level, in the appropriate clinical context, is highly suggestive of PV and should prompt a bone marrow examination with cytogenetic studies. The diagnosis is confirmed if the bone marrow reveals consistent morphologic or cytogenetic abnormalities. In the absence of a PV-related feature (Fig. 3), a confirmatory re-determination of the serum EPO level is advised before proceeding with a bone marrow biopsy. If the bone marrow is nondiagnostic in an asymptomatic patient, one can either proceed with an endogenous erythroid colony assay or repeat measurement of the hemoglobin and serum EPO levels in 3 months (Fig. 5). Rarely, an EPO-receptor mutant may result in congenital pure erythrocytosis with a low serum EPO level. The family history, the age at disease onset, and the associated clinical findings should provide adequate information to distinguish this familial disorder from PV.

Normal Serum Erythropoietin Level

Investigative decisions regarding suspected erythrocytosis with a normal serum EPO level depend primarily on the presence or absence of a PV-related feature (Fig. 3). In the presence of any such feature, it is reasonable to proceed with a bone marrow examination with cytogenetic studies. If the results are not consistent with PV, either an endogenous erythroid colony study (if available) is obtained or the patient may be observed and repeat determinations of the hemoglobin and serum EPO levels are done in 3 months. Multiple determinations of serum EPO have increased the diagnostic sensitivity for PV. If available, an endogenous erythroid colony study may provide further insight.

In the absence of any PV-related feature, a normal serum EPO level associated with a hemoglobin level of less than 18.5 g/dL (16.5 g/dL in women) may represent either a physiologic outlier value or relative polycythemia. Accordingly, repeat determinations of these values in 3 months may be a reasonable initial approach to such cases. However, if the hemoglobin level is 18.5 g/dL or more (16.5 g/dL in women), the possibility of either PV or a feedback-sensitive secondary erythrocytosis is higher. In this instance, an initial workup for secondary erythrocytosis (see below) is recommended, and a negative evaluation may be followed by a bone marrow examination, especially if the hemoglobin increase is recently recognized (Fig. 5).

ENDOGENOUS ERYTHROID COLONY ASSAY IN ERYTHROCYTOSIS

Occasionally, the results obtained from both measurement of the serum EPO level and examination of the bone marrow are nondiagnostic. In this event, depending on the presence or absence of a PV-related feature (Fig. 3), one may proceed with obtaining an endogenous erythroid colony assay. Many investigators have repeatedly demonstrated the specificity of endogenous erythroid colony growth to clonal myeloid disorders, especially to PV. Therefore, in the context of erythrocytosis, in vitro endogenous erythroid colony growth strongly suggests PV. However, endogenous erythroid colony assays are not available in many hematology laboratories, and the alternative is to determine the hemoglobin and serum EPO levels periodically. Furthermore, endogenous erythroid colony growth rarely has been observed in EPO-dependent congenital erythrocytosis because of a physiologic upward adjustment of the threshold for EPO production. However, it is more usual for these rare forms of congenital erythrocytosis to demonstrate in vitro EPO hypersensitivity (rather than EPO independence) because of mutations of the EPO receptor.

EVALUATION OF SECONDARY ERYTHROCYTOSIS

Erythrocytosis associated with an increased serum EPO level is very unlikely to represent PV and, instead, a working diagnosis of secondary erythrocytosis is made. Secondary erythrocytosis could be either congenital (Table 2) or acquired (Table 3). In both situations, the increase in the EPO level may be an appropriate response to generalized hypoxia. Examples include erythrocytosis in a patient with chronic obstructive lung disease (acquired) or high-oxygen–affinity hemoglobinopathy (congenital). Serum EPO

Table 2
Causes of Congenital Erythrocytosis

Low P_{50}[a]
    High-oxygen–affinity hemoglobins
    2,3-Diphosphoglycerate deficiency
Normal P_{50}[a]
    Autosomal dominant (benign) familial erythrocytosis
    Autosomal recessive familial erythrocytosis

[a]P_{50}, oxygen pressure at 50% hemoglobin saturation.
From Tefferi A, Silverstein MN. Myeloproliferative disease, in Cecil Textbook of Medicine (Goldman L, Bennett JC, eds), 21st ed. WB Saunders Company, Philadelphia, 2000, pp. 935-941. By permission of the publisher.

Table 3
Causes of Acquired Secondary Erythrocytosis

Oxygen-sensitive erythropoietin response to tissue hypoxia
    Appropriate response to generalized hypoxia
        Chronic lung disease or pickwickian syndrome
        Arteriovenous or intracardiac shunts
        High-altitude habitat
        Chronic carbon monoxide exposure (smoking)
    Inappropriate response to localized tissue anoxia
        Renal vascular disease
Pathologic unregulated erythropoietin production
        Tumors (hepatoma, hypernephroma, cerebellar
            hemangioblastoma, endocrine tumors)
        Renal cysts and hydronephrosis
        Uterine fibroids
        Post-renal transplant
Drugs
        Androgen preparations
        Exogenous erythropoietin administration

levels may be normal in this instance because the appropriate EPO response is negative feedback-sensitive to the subsequent increase in hemoglobin. However, erythrocytosis associated with tumors usually is associated with persistently increased serum EPO levels (inappropriate EPO production by tumor cells).

Congenital Erythrocytosis

Congenital erythrocytosis is suspected in the presence of disease onset at an early age or a family history of erythrocytosis. Laboratory investigation begins with determination of the oxygen pressure at 50% hemoglobin saturation (P_{50}) (Table 2). A low P_{50} suggests either a high-oxygen–affinity hemoglobinopathy (autosomal dominant) or familial 2,3-diphosphoglycerate deficiency (autosomal recessive). In both of these disorders, serum EPO levels may be normal because of the negative feedback inhibition of EPO production by the resultant erythrocytosis.

A normal P_{50} in congenital erythrocytosis is consistent with either autosomal dominant (benign) familial erythrocytosis or autosomal recessive familial erythrocytosis. Benign familial erythrocytosis is associated with a low or normal serum EPO level and erythroid progenitor EPO hypersensitivity. EPO-receptor mutations have been recognized in some patients with benign familial erythrocytosis. Recessive familial erythrocytosis is the most frequent form of familial erythrocytosis and is prevalent in Russia. EPO levels in recessive familial erythrocytosis are usually increased.

Acquired Secondary Erythrocytosis

Acquired secondary erythrocytosis is an EPO-driven process initiated by either an oxygen-sensitive EPO response to hypoxia or an unregulated pathologic production of EPO by tumors (Table 3). Oxygen-sensitive EPO response is further classified as being appropriate or inappropriate depending on the hypoxic stimulus being generalized or regional, respectively (Table 3). The degree of increase of the serum EPO level may differ among the various conditions associated with secondary erythrocytosis. In general, serum EPO levels are highest in patients with congenital heart disease or after renal transplantation.

The initial workup of patients suspected of having secondary erythrocytosis should include measurement of the arterial oxygen tension, hemoglobin saturation, and carboxyhemoglobin level. If these values are normal, then further investigation depends on assessment of the particular clinical situation and the degree of increase in the serum EPO. Obviously, in the presence of particular symptoms and signs, the appropriate clinical studies are pursued. Otherwise, a significant increase despite high hemoglobin values suggests unregulated EPO production and may require abdominal ultrasonography and a renal vascular study.

SUMMARY

To utilize the serum EPO level for both the evaluation of erythrocytosis and the diagnosis of PV, an accurate assay for the measurement of serum EPO should be available to the physician. Often, additional supporting clinical characteristics are present to help in the diagnostic process. In certain instances, the physician may feel obligated to obtain RCM and plasma volume studies, and I do not consider the practice inappropriate. Furthermore, I advise against overreliance on the serum EPO level and underscore the primary importance of the clinical circumstances, including family history, age at disease onset, clinical presentation, presence or absence of other hematologic abnormalities, splenomegaly, thrombohemorrhagic manifestations, vasomotor symptoms (including erythromelalgia), or post-bath pruritus. However, strict adherence to the original criteria of the Polycythemia Vera Study Group should no longer be considered a prerequisite to the diagnosis of PV.

Not infrequently, spurious polycythemia reflects clinicians' misperceptions as to what are normal values for hemoglobin and hematocrit. Normal ranges for these red cell parameters have been carefully defined in extensive studies. Yet, for various reasons, lower normal ranges have been adopted in some medical centers and have led to unnecessary investigations in otherwise hematologically normal patients with high-normal hemoglobin or hematocrit values. Similarly, associated conditions, including high-altitude habitat, chronic diuretic therapy, and dehydration from the fasting required before having blood tests, occasionally may influence these values. The use of realistic normal ranges adjusted for altitude and awareness of the potential causes for mild dehydration may avoid unnecessary and costly diagnostic procedures.

SUGGESTED READING

Birgegard G, Wide L. Serum erythropoietin in the diagnosis of polycythaemia and after phlebotomy treatment. *Br J Haematol* 1992; 81: 603-606.

Cotes PM, Dore CJ, Yin JA, Lewis SM, Messinezy M, Pearson TC, Reid C. Determination of serum immunoreactive erythropoietin in the investigation of erythrocytosis. *N Engl J Med* 1986; 315: 283-287.

Fairbanks VF, Klee GG, Wiseman GA, Hoyer JD, Tefferi A, Petitt RM, Silverstein MN. Measurement of blood volume and red cell mass: re-examination of ^{51}Cr and ^{125}I methods. *Blood Cells Mol Dis* 1996; 22: 169-186.

Fessel WJ. Odd men out: individuals with extreme values. *Arch Intern Med* 1965; 115: 736-737.

Messinezy M, Westwood NB, Woodcock SP, Strong RM, Pearson TC. Low serum erythropoietin—a strong diagnostic criterion of primary polycythaemia even at normal haemoglobin levels. *Clin Lab Haematol* 1995; 17: 217-220.

Najean Y, Schlageter MH, Toubert ME, Podgorniak MP. Radioimmunoassay of immunoreactive erythropoietin as a clinical tool for the classification of polycythaemias. *Nouv Rev Fr Hematol* 1990; 32: 237-240.

Prchal JT, Sokol L. "Benign erythrocytosis" and other familial and congenital polycythemias. *Eur J Haematol* 1996; 57: 263-268.

Remacha AF, Montserrat I, Santamaria A, Oliver A, Barcelo MJ, Parellada M. Serum erythropoietin in the diagnosis of polycythemia vera. A follow-up study. *Haematologica* 1997; 82: 406-410.

Weinreb NJ. *Relative polycythemia, in Polycythemia Vera and the Myeloproliferative Disorders* (Wasserman LR, Berk PD, Berlin NI, eds). WB Saunders Company, Philadelphia, 1995, pp. 226-258.

Westwood NB, Pearson TC. Diagnostic applications of haemopoietic progenitor culture techniques in polycythaemias and thrombocythaemias. *Leuk Lymphoma* 1996; 22 Suppl 1: 95-103.

9

Differential Diagnosis and Management of Thrombocytosis

Lawrence A. Solberg, Jr., MD, PHD

Contents

THE INITIAL APPROACH TO THROMBOCYTOSIS

The clinician should attempt to understand any platelet count increased above the normal range of values and confirmed on two blood tests. One pitfall in leaving chronic thrombocytosis unexplained is the later development of a thrombotic complication and an oversight in the diagnosis of an underlying myeloproliferative disorder.

One way to approach thrombocytosis is for the clinician to work toward answering two questions with simple information from the history, a complete blood cell count, and a peripheral smear. First, is this thrombocytosis reactive and thus not needing significant evaluation or treatment? Second, what is the immediate risk to the patient from the thrombocytosis?

After answering these two questions, the clinician should make one of three decisions: 1) monitor the increased platelet count while treating any underlying medical condition, 2) have the patient seen by a hematologist in routine consultation for help in diagnosing or managing a possible myeloproliferative disorder, or 3) obtain emergency consultation for evaluation and treatment of thrombocythemia.

From: *Primary Hematology*
Edited by: A. Tefferi © Mayo Foundation for Medical Education and Research, Rochester, MN

Table 1
Causes of Reactive Thrombocytosis

Acute conditions
    The immediate postsurgical period
    Acute bleeding
    Acute hemolysis
    Infections
    Tissue damage (acute pancreatitis, myocardial infarction, trauma, burns)
    Coronary artery bypass grafting
    Rebound effect from chemotherapy or immune thrombocytopenia
Chronic conditions
    Iron deficiency anemia
    Surgical or functional asplenia
    Metastatic cancer, lymphoma
    Inflammations (rheumatoid arthritis, vasculitis, allergies)
    Renal failure, nephrotic syndrome

From Tefferi A, Silverstein MN. Myeloproliferative disease, in *Cecil Textbook of Medicine* (Goldman L, Bennett JC, eds), 21st ed. WB Saunders Company, Philadelphia, 2000, pp. 935-941. By permission of the publisher.

CLINICAL FINDINGS SUGGESTING
THE THROMBOCYTOSIS IS REACTIVE

Three findings favor reactive thrombocytosis (Table 1).

First, a recent normal platelet count before a current illness known to be associated with a reactive thrombocytosis makes an underlying myeloproliferative disorder very unlikely. The clinician can treat the basic medical condition, follow the thrombocytosis without further investigation, and document its reversal to baseline value.

Second, the patient has an identified clinical condition commonly causing reactive thrombocytosis (Table 1). Examples of such conditions include patients in intensive care units with trauma, sepsis, or postsurgical complications and patients with chronic inflammation such as inflammatory bowel disease or rheumatoid arthritis. Patients may have had splenectomy or have acquired functional hyposplenism due to sprue. They may have a clinical picture suggesting an underlying occult malignancy. Many such clinical situations suggest reactive thrombocytosis.

Third, the patient with reactive thrombocytosis typically does not have clinical features suggesting a myeloproliferative disorder. Table 2 summarizes these features.

CLINICAL FEATURES SUGGESTING THE
THROMBOCYTOSIS IS FROM A PRIMARY MARROW DISORDER

Patients with thrombocytosis due to primary marrow disorders typically have not recently had normal blood cell counts, do not have a clearly identifiable cause of reactive thrombocytosis, and usually have one or more clinical features suggesting a myeloproliferative disorder (Table 2). Primary marrow disorders that commonly cause thrombocytosis include essential thrombocythemia, polycythemia vera, chronic myelocytic leukemia, and agnogenic myeloid metaplasia. Patients with acute leukemia or myelodysplasia also may present with thrombocytosis.

Table 2
Clinical Features Suggesting Thrombocytosis
Is From a Primary Bone Marrow Disorder

Feature	Significance
Symptoms	Post-bathing pruritus suggests polycythemia vera; erythromelalgia (painful, red, ischemic digits) can be seen with polycythemia vera and essential thrombocythemia
Physical examination	Splenomegaly always suggests a myeloproliferative disorder; plethora can be striking in untreated polycythemia vera. Unusual thrombotic complications such as Budd-Chiari syndrome and portal vein thrombosis
Peripheral blood cell counts and smear	Antecedent sustained thrombocytosis or leukocytosis with immature white cells (e.g., metamyelocytes or myelocytes). A high percentage of myelocytes suggests chronic myelocytic leukemia. A leukoerythroblastic blood smear (this is required to diagnose AMM[a] but can occur with any myeloproliferative disorder; it can also occur with stroke, trauma, sepsis, etc., so is not entirely specific for a myeloproliferative disorder). A high erythrocyte count, particularly if associated with microcytosis, suggests polycythemia vera; oval macrocytes can be associated with various clonal stem cell disorders. Pancytopenia or blasts in the peripheral blood count raise the possibility of underlying myelodysplasia or leukemia

[a]AMM, agnogenic myeloid metaplasia.

ASSESSING THE RISK OF ADVERSE
EVENTS FROM THROMBOCYTOSIS

As already implied, there is no significant risk attributed to reactive thrombocytosis except in rare case reports, for example, the healing of skin flaps. The underlying clinical condition should be treated.

If the patient has clinical features suggesting a myeloproliferative disorder, the clinician should assess the risk of the thrombocytosis. One way of doing this is to evaluate four clinical factors that are often analyzed for their potential contribution to the risk of thrombosis: age, a history of antecedent thrombosis or the presence of active ischemic disease, the presence or absence of cardiovascular risk factors, and the platelet count. These are discussed in Table 3.

PLANNING FURTHER EVALUATION
AND INITIAL TREATMENT

After evaluating the likelihood of primary or secondary thrombocytosis and the risk to the patient of the thrombocytosis, the clinician should be able to undertake one of three approaches.

Table 3
Risk Factor Assessment in Essential Thrombocythemia

Factor	Significance
Age	Typical series reports increased risk of strokes beginning at 60 to 65 years
Thrombosis history	A history of deep venous thrombosis increases risk. Active or unstable angina, recent or current transient ischemic attacks, gastrointestinal hemorrhage not responding well to therapy, evolving stroke, and priapism are all major risk factors that favor immediate intervention
Cardiovascular risk factors	The contribution of hypertension, smoking, diabetes, and hyperlipidemia to the thrombotic risk associated with clonal thrombocytosis is controversial
Platelet count	There is not a good correlation between thrombohemorrhagic complications of thrombocythemia and the absolute platelet count. Life-threatening complications such as Budd-Chiari syndrome have occurred in patients with essential thrombocythemia who have platelet counts in the normal range or only slightly increased. Platelet counts in excess of 1 million/μL in symptomatic patients can reasonably be thought of as emergencies, but symptomatic patients with platelet counts between 600,000 and 1 million/μL may need urgent attention if they are symptomatic and if there is strong supporting evidence that their thrombocytosis is due to a myeloproliferative disorder

Thrombocytosis With Clinical Features Suggesting Reactive Thrombocytosis and No Features Suggesting a Myeloproliferative Disorder

In this case, patients typically have evidence of recent normal blood cell counts and are being treated for readily identifiable other intercurrent medical conditions such as trauma, sepsis, or diseases with inflammation. The underlying condition can be treated and a follow-up platelet count obtained 1 month after the primary condition has resolved or stabilized.

Thrombocytosis With Clinical Features Suggesting Primary Marrow Disorder But Low Risk of Adverse Events

Patients have one or more of the features listed in Table 2, raising the possibility of an underlying marrow disorder. They do not have active ischemic symptoms or a history of recent thrombosis, nor do they have underlying medical conditions that might be associated with increased risk. They may be young, that is, less than 60 years. Platelet counts may be as high as 1.5 million/μL. It is reasonable to obtain routine hematology consultation for these patients within 2 to 4 weeks.

Thrombocytosis With Clinical Features Suggesting an Underlying Primary Marrow Disorder and Significant Risk of Adverse Events

Patients have angina, recent or ongoing transient ischemic attacks or subacute evolving stroke, uncontrolled gastrointestinal bleeding, deep venous thrombosis or pulmonary embolism, arterial occlusion, or priapism. They may have very high platelet counts (> 1 million/µL) and may have one or more factors suggesting that platelet count increases may be due to an underlying myeloproliferative disorder rather than a secondary cause. These patients should have emergency hematology consultation, and platelet apheresis to lower the platelet count should be considered.

LABORATORY EVALUATION OF THROMBOCYTOSIS

For the initial classification of the patient, the physician primarily needs the history, physical examination, recent laboratory records, a complete blood cell count, a peripheral smear, and the serum ferritin value.

A normal serum ferritin value excludes the possibility of iron deficiency being the cause of thrombocytosis. Similarly, the absence of Howell-Jolly bodies in the peripheral smear excludes hyposplenism as a cause of thrombocytosis. We have found a low C-reactive protein value to be more consistent with clonal thrombocytosis, and most causes of reactive thrombocytosis are associated with increased levels of C-reactive protein.

If a myeloproliferative disorder is suspected, a bone marrow examination with an aspirate, biopsy, and cytogenetics studies should be obtained. It is important to obtain a cytogenetic study of the bone marrow aspirate to exclude chronic myelocytic leukemia. One should realize, however, that some presentations of chronic myelocytic leukemia require DNA-based testing with probes for the *bcr-abl* gene rearrangement. Some reference laboratories will be able to automatically proceed to appropriate DNA-based testing if this arrangement is made in advance.

If erythrocytosis is present, a low serum erythropoietin level can provide evidence for polycythemia vera.

Many of the primary marrow conditions causing thrombocytosis are readily diagnosed after a bone marrow examination. If a diagnosis remains uncertain, hematology consultation should be obtained.

LONG-TERM MANAGEMENT OF ESSENTIAL THROMBOCYTHEMIA

In general, patients with essential thrombocythemia have a near-normal life expectancy and the disease transformation rate to acute leukemia or myelofibrosis is less than 5%. Therefore, the primary purpose of specific therapy is to prevent thrombosis and hemorrhage.

Thrombotic events are unusual in patients younger than 60 years and in patients without a history of thrombosis (Table 3). As such, these patients can be followed without specific therapy. In particular, we discourage the use of drugs in pregnant women and in women who are of childbearing age.

Young women with essential thrombocythemia experience an increased risk of recurrent miscarriages. Specific therapy, including the use of acetylsalicylic acid, does not seem to influence this complication.

Older patients and those with a previous history of thrombosis derive benefit from a specific platelet-lowering agent. Hydroxyurea is the current treatment of choice for these patients. It is started at a dosage of 500 mg orally twice a day, and a platelet count less than 400,000/µL is desired. One must follow the leukocyte count and make sure that it does not decrease to less than 2,000/µL. The side effects of hydroxyurea are outlined in Table 4.

Although not proved, a concern exists regarding a possible leukemogenic potential with hydroxyurea in patients with essential thrombocythemia. As such, some investigators use alternative platelet-lowering agents, including anagrelide and interferon-α.

Table 4
Side Effects of Hydroxyurea

Neutropenia
Anemia
Gastrointestinal (nausea, cramps)
Oral ulcers
Skin pigmentary changes
Leg ulcers

Table 5
Side Effects of Anagrelide

Headaches
Palpitations and forceful heartbeats
Gastrointestinal (nausea, diarrhea)
Fluid retention
Congestive heart failure

Anagrelide is a new agent that has a specific platelet-lowering ability. It is a costly drug and has several side effects (Table 5). Anagrelide is started at a dosage of 0.5 mg orally four times daily. It is currently the alternative drug used in patients who cannot tolerate hydroxyurea. It is also a reasonable alternative drug when there is a major concern about the long-term use of hydroxyurea (i.e., very young patients).

Both hydroxyurea and anagrelide should be avoided in pregnant women. Interferon-α has been used in pregnant women without complications.

Finally, some patients may have functional symptoms, including headaches, dizziness, visual symptoms, or erythromelalgia (Table 2). Low-dose acetylsalicylic acid (81 mg) is often successful in treating these conditions.

SUMMARY

The clinician should attempt to determine whether newly encountered thrombocytosis is reactive or possibly due to an underlying primary marrow disorder. If clearly reactive, thrombocytosis need not be addressed but should be followed to be sure it resolves. If a myeloproliferative disorder is suspected, the clinician should evaluate the risk that the thrombocytosis poses to the patient. This is done by considering age, prior history of thrombosis, active symptoms of ischemia, and the degree of increase of the platelet count. After this process, the clinician should be able to classify patients into those who can receive routine consultation or evaluation for their possible myeloproliferative disorders and those for whom emergency consultation or urgent therapy with platelet apheresis might be needed.

SUGGESTED READING

Buss DH, O'Connor ML, Woodruff RD, Richards F II, Brockschmidt JK. Bone marrow and peripheral blood findings in patients with extreme thrombocytosis. A report of 63 cases. *Arch Pathol Lab Med* 1991; 115: 475-480.
Cortelazzo S, Finazzi G, Ruggeri M, Vestri O, Galli M, Rodeghiero F, Barbui T. Hydroxyurea for patients with essential thrombocythemia and a high risk of thrombosis. *N Engl J Med* 1995; 332: 1132-1136.

Kessler CM, Klein HG, Havlik RJ. Uncontrolled thrombocytosis in chronic myeloproliferative disorders. *Br J Haematol* 1982; 50: 157-167.

Messinezy M, Pearson TC. ABC of clinical haematology. Polycythaemia, primary (essential) thrombocythaemia and myelofibrosis. *BMJ* 1997; 314: 587-590.

Michiels JJ, van Genderen PJ, Lindemans J, van Vliet HH. Erythromelalgic, thrombotic and hemorrhagic manifestations in 50 cases of thrombocythemia. *Leuk Lymphoma* 1996; 22 Suppl 1: 47-56.

Murphy S, Peterson P, Iland H, Laszlo J. Experience of the Polycythemia Vera Study Group with essential thrombocythemia: a final report on diagnostic criteria, survival, and leukemic transition by treatment. *Semin Hematol* 1997; 34: 29-39.

Ravandi-Kashani F, Schafer AI. Microvascular disturbances, thrombosis, and bleeding in thrombocythemia: current concepts and perspectives. *Semin Thromb Hemost* 1997; 23: 479-488.

Tefferi A, Silverstein MN, Hoagland HC. Primary thrombocythemia. *Semin Oncol* 1995; 22: 334-340.

10 Chronic Myeloproliferative Diseases: Polycythemia Vera and Agnogenic Myeloid Metaplasia

Ayalew Tefferi, MD

Contents

INTRODUCTION

Hematopoiesis

Blood cells can be operationally classified as being lymphocyte-derived (lymphoid precursors, B lymphocytes, T lymphocytes, natural killer cells, plasma cells) or myeloid-derived (red cells, platelets, neutrophils, eosinophils, basophils, monocytes, and the precursors of these cells). All blood cells are derived from a common ancestor in the bone marrow: the hematopoietic stem cell. Because the stem cell is capable of differentiating into various cell types, it is referred to as being pluripotent. The hematopoietic pluripotent stem cell is capable of both self-renewal and a stepwise differentiation into either the lymphoid or the myeloid lineage. Accordingly, during normal hematopoiesis, there exists a cellular hierarchy headed by a stable population of pluripotent stem cells that generate lineage-specific progenitors differentiating into the various types of mature blood cells. Effective hematopoiesis is facilitated by the interactive functions of hematopoietic growth factors, various sets of receptors, and the bone marrow microenvironment.

Hematologic Malignancies

Parallel to the above-mentioned classification of blood cells, hematologic malignancies are organized into lymphoid or myeloid processes (Fig. 1). Each of these are in turn classified as being acute or chronic depending on the proportion of morphologically and immunophenotypically immature precursors (blasts) in the bone marrow. Accordingly, the myeloid hematologic malignancies are divided into acute myeloid leukemia (bone marrow blasts more than 30%) and the chronic myeloid disorders (bone marrow blasts less than 30%). The lymphoid malignancies are similarly divided into acute lymphocytic leukemia and chronic lymphoproliferative disorders. The latter include chronic lymphoid leukemia, lymphoma, and plasma cell proliferative disorders.

From: *Primary Hematology*
Edited by: A. Tefferi © Mayo Foundation for Medical Education and Research, Rochester, MN

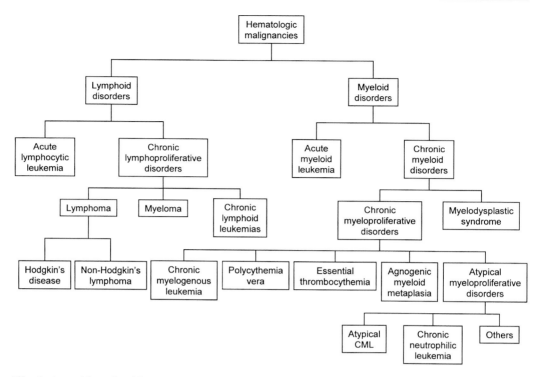

Fig. 1. A working classification of hematologic malignancies. CML, chronic myelogenous leukemia.

The chronic myeloid disorders encompass several clinicopathologic entities. Conceptually, they can be organized into those that demonstrate morphologic dysplasia (the myelodysplastic syndromes) or those that do not (chronic myeloproliferative disorders, CMPDs). The myelodysplastic syndromes are characterized by dysplastic bone marrow hyperplasia associated with variable degrees of peripheral blood pancytopenia with or without monocytosis. Unlike the myelodysplastic syndromes, the CMPDs usually exhibit leukocytosis, thrombocytosis, or erythrocytosis in the peripheral blood.

Chronic Myeloproliferative Disorders

The CMPDs are classified into several subgroups, among which four are well characterized. These include chronic myelogenous leukemia (CML), polycythemia vera (PV), agnogenic myeloid metaplasia (AMM), and essential thrombocythemia (ET). Among these, only CML is genetically characterized by the reciprocal chromosome translocation between chromosomes 9 and 22, t(9;22) (the Philadelphia chromosome). Specific genetic lesions have not been recognized for the other CMPDs. The distinction among these is based on the presence or absence of particular clinical and laboratory features. As such, an increased red cell mass defines PV, whereas the presence of substantial bone marrow fibrosis is characteristic of AMM. ET is a diagnosis of exclusion, representing clonal thrombocytosis not classifiable as PV, AMM, CML, or myelodysplastic syndromes. Although most of the chronic myeloid disorders are classifiable as myelodysplastic syndromes, CML, PV, ET, or AMM, some are difficult to categorize and may be referred to as atypical CMPDs. Included in this latter group are atypical CML, chronic neutrophilic leukemia, mast cell disease, and chronic eosinophilic leukemia.

Table 1
Polycythemia Vera-Related Clinical
and Laboratory Features

Persistent leukocytosis
Persistent thrombocytosis
Microcytosis due to iron deficiency
Splenomegaly
Generalized pruritus (post-bath)
Unusual thrombosis
Erythromelalgia (acral dysesthesia and erythema)

As a group, the CMPDs are all preleukemic and are predisposed to indigenous disease transformation. The propensity to acute leukemic transformation differs among the subgroups and is highest for CML (more than 90%) and least for ET (less than 5%). Similarly, patients with PV have a 10% to 25% chance of having transformation into a myelofibrotic stage at 10 to 25 years of follow-up. Another biologic complication shared among the CMPDs is the significant risk of thrombohemorrhagic complications, which is pronounced in patients with PV and ET. Because of the variable risks to blastic transformation and thrombosis-associated deaths, overall survival in the CMPDs ranges from a "near-normal" life expectancy in patients with ET to a median of less than 5 years in patients with AMM. In this chapter, PV and AMM are discussed. ET and CML are discussed in other chapters.

POLYCYTHEMIA VERA

Epidemiology

PV occurs in approximately 2.3/100,000 persons per year. As is true for most hematologic malignancies, the incidence rates are significantly higher in the older age groups. However, as many as 7% of patients are younger than 40 years, and the disease occasionally occurs in children. There is a slight male preponderance, and the median age at diagnosis is approximately 60 years. In general, the connection between disease incidence and exposure to environmental factors has not been strong.

Pathogenesis

Studies based on analyses of glucose-6-phosphate dehydrogenase isoenzyme patterns and X-linked DNA analyses have supported the stem cell origin of the clonal process in PV. As such, the disease represents a growth factor-independent proliferation of not only red cell precursors but also other myeloid precursors. So far, genetic lesions involving the erythropoietin (EPO) gene or the gene for the EPO receptor have not been recognized. The usually low serum EPO level in patients with PV supports the autonomic nature of the erythrocyte proliferation. Similarly, erythroid precursors (BFU-E and CFU-E) can grow in tissue culture without the exogenous addition of EPO. A detailed discussion on the physiology of erythropoiesis and the relationship of serum EPO levels to the different causes of erythrocytosis is outlined in Chapter 8.

Clinical Features and Prognosis

At presentation, patients may have symptoms and signs related to hyperviscosity and splenomegaly. Characteristic PV-related symptoms and signs are illustrated in Table 1.

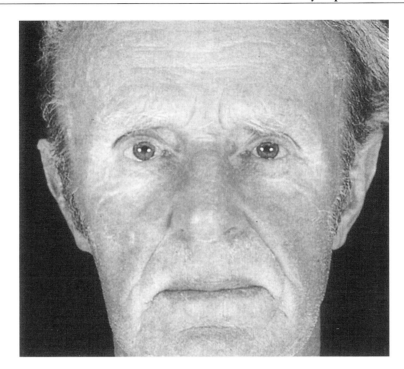

Fig. 2, Plate 9. Facial plethora in a patient with polycythemia vera. Notice the ruddy skin appearance. (From Hoffbrand AV, Pettit JE. *Color Atlas of Clinical Hematology*, 2nd ed. Mosby-Wolfe, London, 1994. By permission of the publisher.)

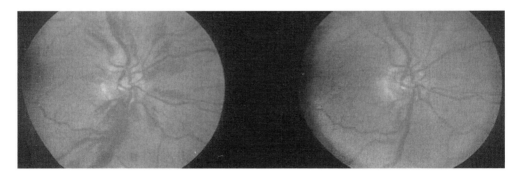

Fig. 3, Plate 10. Retinal vein distention in a patient with polycythemia vera, before and after phlebotomy. Notice the thickened "sausage-shaped" appearance of the retinal veins and fundal hemorrhage. (From Hoffbrand AV, Pettit JE. *Color Atlas of Clinical Hematology*, 2nd ed. Mosby-Wolfe, London, 1994. By permission of the publisher.)

The absolute increase in red cell mass increases whole blood viscosity, which impairs the delivery of oxygen to vital organs. Some of the symptoms of hyperviscosity include headaches, dizziness, visual symptoms, paresthesias, and fatigue. The symptoms of marked splenomegaly include abdominal discomfort, weight loss, and night sweats. Post-bath pruritus is a poorly understood, frequent complaint. Clinical examination may reveal plethora (facial fullness and erythema) (Fig. 2, Plate 9), retinal vein distention (Fig. 3, Plate 10), and palpable splenomegaly. More than half of patients have associated

Table 2
The Polycythemia Vera Study Group
Diagnostic Criteria for Polycythemia Vera[a]

Major criteria	Minor criteria

1. Increased red cell mass
    Males: ≥ 36 mL/kg
    Females: ≥ 32 mL/kg
2. Normal arterial oxygen
    saturation, $\geq 92\%$
3. Splenomegaly
	1. Platelets > 400,000/mL
	2. Leukocytes > 12,000/mL
	3. Leukocyte alkaline phosphatase > 100
	    or vitamin B_{12} > 900 pg/mL
	    or unbound B_{12} binding capacity > 2,200 pg/mL

[a]Diagnosis of polycythemia vera requires the presence of all three major criteria *or* the presence of the first two major criteria and any two minor criteria.

From Tefferi A, Silverstein MN. Myeloproliferative diseases, in *Cecil Textbook of Medicine* (Goldman L, Bennett JC, eds), 21st ed. WB Saunders Company, Philadelphia, 2000, pp. 935-941. By permission of the publisher.

leukocytosis or thrombocytosis. Microcytosis is frequent and indicates iron deficiency from phlebotomy or occult gastrointestinal blood loss. Nonspecific additional laboratory abnormalities include increases of leukocyte alkaline phosphatase score and serum vitamin B_{12} and uric acid levels.

Thrombotic events are frequent (20%) in PV and include cerebrovascular accident, transient ischemic attack, retinal vein thrombosis, central retinal artery occlusion, myocardial infarction, angina, pulmonary embolism, hepatic and portal vein thrombosis, deep vein thrombosis, and peripheral arterial occlusion. Thrombotic risk is correlated with advanced age and a history of thrombosis. In addition, the increased blood viscosity associated with the increased red cell mass contributes to thrombosis. Bleeding is less frequent and occurs in the gastrointestinal system. In addition, patients may experience vasomotor disturbances such as erythromelalgia (acral dysesthesia and erythema), headaches, and visual symptoms. In addition to the increased risk of thrombosis, patients with PV have an approximately 10% long-term risk of having transformation into acute leukemia. The risk of transformation into the fibrotic stage of the disease (post-polycythemic myeloid metaplasia) is even higher (approximately 20%).

Differential Diagnosis

Once PV is suspected, the initial step is to exclude the possibility of relative or secondary erythrocytosis (see the tables and figures in Chapter 8). In view of the current availability of accurate assays for measurement of serum EPO and culture methods to demonstrate endogenous erythroid colonies, we no longer require the absolute attainment of the criteria of the Polycythemia Vera Study Group to diagnose PV (Table 2). Unlike all other causes of erythrocytosis, the erythroid proliferation in PV is EPO-independent and down-regulates the production of EPO. As a result, serum EPO levels are usually low, occasionally normal, but never increased in PV. Similarly, endogenous erythroid colony growth is specific to PV. If the initial evaluation does not suggest relative or secondary erythrocytosis, then a bone marrow examination with cytogenetic studies and a reticulin stain is recommended. The bone marrow examination in PV may show overall hypercellularity, megakaryocyte clusters, or reticulin fibrosis. Cytogenetic abnormalities are detected in approximately 12% of chemotherapy-naïve patients with PV.

General Management

All patients should undergo phlebotomy with the goal of keeping the hematocrit value less than 45% in men and 42% in women. Approximately 500 mL of blood may be removed daily (in symptomatic patients) or weekly (in asymptomatic patients) until the target hematocrit level is reached. Thereafter, the frequency is adjusted to maintain the required hematocrit level at all times. No additional therapy may be required in patients who are at low risk for thrombosis (age less than 60 years, no history of thrombosis). In patients at high risk, the current preference is to use hydroxyurea (starting dosage 500 mg orally twice a day) as a supplement to phlebotomy.

For patients who do not tolerate hydroxyurea because of either side effects or neutropenia, interferon-α (3 million units subcutaneously 3 times a week) is a reasonable alternative. Interferon-α also may be considered as an alternative to hydroxyurea in women of childbearing age and in young patients (age less than 50 years), in whom years of therapy with hydroxyurea are anticipated. ^{32}P (2.3 mCi/m^2) may be considered if life expectancy in a particular patient is less than 10 years and when compliance to medication is an issue. Low-dose acetylsalicylic acid (81 mg a day) is effective for alleviating vasomotor symptoms and is to be used if there are other treatment indications.

Management of Thrombosis and Bleeding

THROMBOSIS

- Start intravenous heparin, 5,000 units loading dose followed by a continuous infusion of 1,000 units/h (partial thromboplastin time, 1.5 to 2.5 times normal).
- Start oral warfarin, 5 mg/day, as soon as partial thromboplastin time is in the therapeutic range.
- Start oral hydroxyurea 1 g 4 times a day for 3 days if platelet count is more than 1 million/μL, 1 g 2 times a day if the count is more than 600,000/μL, and 500 mg 2 times a day if the count is more than 400,000/μL.
- Blood bank should be contacted for immediate platelet apheresis if the platelet count is more than 800,000/μL.
- Phlebotomy should be performed daily until the hematocrit level is less than 45% in men and 42% in women.
- Start oral allopurinol, 300 mg/day (100 mg/day if creatinine value is more than 2 mg/dL), if leukocyte count is more than 30,000/μL.

Heparin therapy is discontinued after a 5-day overlap with warfarin. In general, thrombocytosis and erythrocytosis are considered reversible risk factors for thrombosis, and warfarin therapy is continued for 3 months (target international normalized ratio [INR], between 2.0 and 3.0) after the thrombotic event. After the first 3 days, the dose of hydroxyurea is adjusted to keep the platelet count less than 400,000/μL without reducing the leukocyte count to less than 3,000/μL.

BLEEDING

The first step in the management of bleeding complications is to discontinue the use of any platelet antiaggregating agent. If the platelet count is less than 100,000/μL, platelet transfusion is recommended. Initial laboratory evaluation should include a workup for disseminated intravascular coagulation and coagulation factor deficiency. Acquired factor V deficiency is treated with fresh frozen plasma infusion or platelet concentrates. Occasionally, extreme thrombocytosis is associated with an acquired type II von

Willebrand disease because of an abnormal platelet adsorption of circulating von Willebrand factor multimers. As such, platelet apheresis is recommended for bleeding associated with thrombocytosis. Concomitantly, therapy with a platelet-lowering agent should be started (see above guidelines for using hydroxyurea).

Summary Points in Polycythemia Vera

- Phlebotomy is the cornerstone of therapy, and the hematocrit level should be kept below 45% in men and 42% in women at all times.

- In patients older than 60 years and in those with a history of thrombosis, phlebotomy should be supplanted with chemotherapy (hydroxyurea, 500 mg orally 2 or 3 times a day).

- The dose of hydroxyurea is titrated to keep the platelet count less than 400,000/μL and the leukocyte count more than 3,000/μL.

- Avoid use of high doses of aspirin or nonsteroidal agents.

- Low-dose aspirin (81 mg/day) is safe and effective for treating vasomotor symptoms.

- Avoid smoking.

AGNOGENIC MYELOID METAPLASIA

Epidemiology and Nomenclature

The incidence of AMM approaches 1.3/100,000, as estimated from a predominantly white North American population. Similar to PV, the disease is slightly more prevalent in males, and the median age at diagnosis is approximately 60 years. AMM has been known by several names, including myelofibrosis, myeloid metaplasia with myelofibrosis, idiopathic myelofibrosis, primary myelofibrosis, and myeloid metaplasia. We prefer to use the term AMM and reserve use of the broader term of myeloid metaplasia with myelofibrosis to include AMM and the fibrotic stages of both PV (post-polycythemic myeloid metaplasia) and ET (post-thrombocythemic myelofibrosis).

Pathogenesis

Similar to PV, AMM is also a stem cell disease. In addition, the clonal megakaryocytes in myeloid metaplasia with myelofibrosis abnormally secrete growth factors, which stimulate the normal neighboring fibroblasts to both proliferate and overproduce collagen, resulting in substantial bone marrow fibrosis. The growth factor that is primarily implicated in the pathogenesis of bone marrow fibrosis is transforming growth factor-β.

Clinical Features and Prognosis

The median survival in AMM may be as long as 8 years or as short as 1 year, depending, respectively, on the absence or presence of anemia and leukocytosis. Causes of death include heart failure, infection, and leukemic transformation, which occur in approximately 10% of patients. Most patients experience massive hepatosplenomegaly and progressive anemia requiring frequent red blood cell transfusions (Fig. 4, Plates 11 and 12) associated with the hypercatabolic symptoms of profound fatigue, weight loss, night sweats, and low-grade fever. In addition, in some patients, extramedullary hematopoiesis may develop in the spinal cord, the pleural and peritoneal cavity, and other organs. At

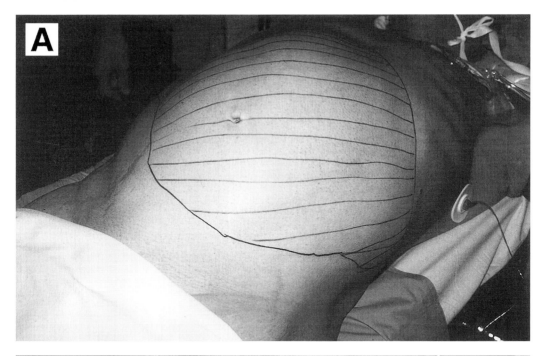

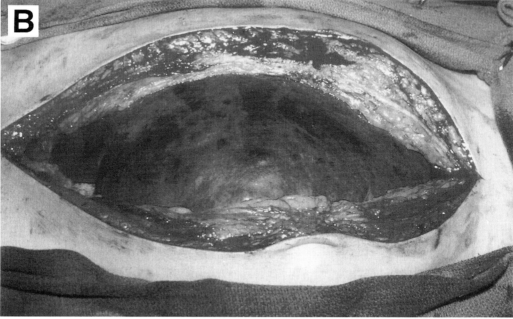

Fig. 4. *A* (Plate 11) and *B* (Plate 12), Massive splenomegaly in a patient with myelofibrosis. (*A* from Tefferi A, Silverstein MN. Myeloproliferative diseases, in *Cecil Textbook of Medicine* [Goldman L, Bennett JC, eds], 21st ed. WB Saunders Company, Philadelphia, 2000, pp. 935-941. By permission of the publisher.)

presentation, 45% of patients have a hemoglobin level of less than 10 g/dL, and 25% may have thrombocytopenia, thrombocytosis, or leukocytosis.

Table 3
Causes of Bone Marrow Fibrosis

Myeloid disorders
    Chronic myeloproliferative diseases
    Myelodysplastic syndrome
    Acute myelofibrosis
    Acute myeloid leukemia
    Mast cell disease
    Malignant histiocytosis
Lymphoid disorders
    Lymphomas
    Hairy cell leukemia
    Multiple myeloma
Nonhematologic disorders
    Metastatic cancer
    Connective tissue disease
    Infections
    Vitamin D-deficiency rickets
    Renal osteodystrophy
    Gray platelet syndrome

Modified from Tefferi A, Silverstein MN. Myeloproliferative diseases, in *Cecil Textbook of Medicine* (Goldman L, Bennett JC, eds), 21st ed. WB Saunders Company, Philadelphia, 2000, pp. 935-941. By permission of the publisher.

Differential Diagnosis

The presence of bone marrow fibrosis requires exclusion of other causes of the fibrosis before AMM is diagnosed (Table 3). Bone marrow fibrosis may accompany both non-malignant and malignant conditions. Within the context of a chronic myeloproliferative disease, the possibilities of both CML and PV should be excluded. The demonstration of the Philadelphia chromosome, t(9;22), is diagnostic of CML. The presence of t(9;22) is not always detected by karyotypic analysis. A peripheral blood fluorescence in situ hybridization study may identify cytogenetically occult cases of CML. Myelodysplastic syndrome is characterized by dyserythropoiesis. A particular subtype of myelodysplastic syndromes may present with significant bone marrow fibrosis. Because the prognosis and management of myelodysplastic syndrome are different from those of AMM, the distinction is clinically relevant.

General Management

In young patients, allogeneic bone marrow transplantation may provide durable remissions to some. Otherwise, most patients are treated palliatively. The combination of an androgen preparation (fluoxymesterone, Halotestin, 10 mg orally twice a day) and a corticosteroid (prednisone, 30 mg orally) improves anemia in a third of patients. After 1 month of therapy, the dosage of corticosteroid is tapered. All patients treated with androgens should have periodic liver function tests, and male patients should be screened for prostate cancer before initiating therapy. In addition, the virilizing side effects should be emphasized to female patients. However, in most patients, periodic red cell transfusion remains the major supportive therapy in AMM.

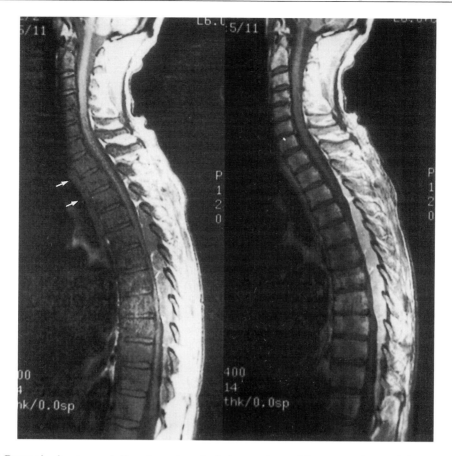

Fig. 5. Paraspinal extramedullary hematopoiesis in a patient with agnogenic myeloid metaplasia.

Splenectomy may provide benefit to approximately half of patients with symptomatic splenomegaly (mechanical discomfort, refractory thrombocytopenia, hypercatabolic symptoms, portal hypertension). At experienced centers, the mortality rate with the procedure should be less than 10%. Postsurgical complications include intra-abdominal bleeding, subphrenic abscess, sepsis, large vessel thrombosis, extreme thrombocytosis, and accelerated hepatomegaly. In poor surgical candidates, the alternative to splenectomy is splenic irradiation (200 to 300 cGy delivered in 10 to 15 daily fractions), which usually provides a transient (3 to 6 months) benefit.

Management of Extramedullary Hematopoiesis

Extramedullary hematopoiesis can occur at several locations, including the spleen, liver, lymph nodes, peritoneum (causing ascites), pleura (causing pleural effusions), lung, bladder, and paraspinal and epidural spaces (causing spinal cord and nerve root compression). New-onset back pain with or without associated tenderness on palpation or neurologic findings should be evaluated for possible spinal cord compression. Neurologic symptoms and signs of spinal cord compression include paresthesia, motor weakness, hyperreflexia, and bladder or bowel incontinence. We currently prefer spinal magnetic resonance imaging with gadolinium as the initial diagnostic test (Fig. 5). If the clinical data are highly suggestive of cord compression, the patient should receive 10 mg of oral dexamethasone even before the test is performed. If the test supports the diagnosis, then the use of dexamethasone should be continued at a dosage of 4 mg orally 4 times a day until definitive treatment with radiation is started. Extramedullary hematopoiesis is best treated with low-dose irradiation (1,000 cGy) in 5 to 10 fractions. Occasionally, a laminectomy may be required.

Summary Points in Agnogenic Myeloid Metaplasia

- Other causes of bone marrow fibrosis should be excluded.

- Major clinical problems are anemia, massive splenomegaly, and cachexia.

- Bone marrow transplantation may be considered for young patients.

- Anemia is initially treated with androgen preparations.

- Splenectomy is a reasonable option to palliate symptoms of significant abdominal discomfort, refractory cytopenia, and profound cachexia.

- Extramedullary hematopoiesis is best treated with low-dose irradiation.

SUGGESTED READING

Berk PD, Wasserman LR, Fruchtman SM, Goldberg JD. Treatment of polycythemia vera: a summary of clinical trials conducted by the Polycythemia Vera Study Group, in *Polycythemia Vera and the Myeloproliferative Disorders* (Wasserman LR, Berk PD, Berlin NI, eds). WB Saunders Company, Philadelphia, 1995, pp. 166-194.

Cortelazzo S, Finazzi G, Ruggeri M, Vestri O, Galli M, Rodeghiero F, Barbui T. Hydroxyurea for patients with essential thrombocythemia and a high risk of thrombosis. *N Engl J Med* 1995; 332: 1132-1136.

Dameshek W. Some speculations on the myeloproliferative syndromes (editorial). *Blood* 1951; 6: 372-375.

Rozman C, Giralt M, Feliu E, Rubio D, Cortes MT. Life expectancy of patients with chronic nonleukemic myeloproliferative disorders. *Cancer* 1991; 67: 2658-2663.

Schafer AI. Bleeding and thrombosis in the myeloproliferative disorders. *Blood* 1984; 64: 1-12.

Tefferi A, Elliott MA, Solberg LA Jr, Silverstein MN. New drugs in essential thrombocythemia and polycythemia vera. *Blood Rev* 1997; 11: 1-7.

Tefferi A, Silverstein MN, Hoagland HC. Primary thrombocythemia. *Semin Oncol* 1995; 22: 334-340.

Tefferi A, Silverstein MN, Noel P. Agnogenic myeloid metaplasia. *Semin Oncol* 1995; 22: 327-333.

11

An Approach to the Patient With Myelodysplasia

Pierre Noël, MD

Contents

INTRODUCTION

A myelodysplastic syndrome (MDS) is a clonal hemopathy characterized by ineffective hematopoiesis and cellular dysfunction. Most patients die of complications of marrow failure or acute leukemia.

Confirming a diagnosis of MDS can be challenging because several diseases are associated with marrow dysplasia. In the absence of karyotypic abnormalities, it is often difficult to be confident of a diagnosis of refractory anemia.

Bone marrow transplantation and high-dose chemotherapy are currently the only potential curative treatments.

CLINICAL FEATURES

The incidence of MDS has been estimated at 1 or 2 cases per 100,000. In a general hospital, 16% of patients undergoing a bone marrow evaluation for pancytopenia had MDS. The incidence of MDS is higher in men than in women, the median age of patients ranges from 65 to 75 years, and less than 15% of patients are younger than 45 years.

The course of MDS is complicated by hemorrhage in 20% of cases and infection in 40%. Lower respiratory tract bacterial infections and skin abscesses are the most com-

From: *Primary Hematology*
Edited by: A. Tefferi © Mayo Foundation for Medical Education and Research, Rochester, MN

Table 1
Classification of the Myelodysplastic Syndromes,
as Proposed by the French-American-British
Cooperative Group

Subtype	Monocytes, PB, μL	Ringed sideroblasts, marrow, %	Myeloblasts, %		Auer rods, PB/marrow
			PB	Marrow	
RA	< 1,000	< 15	< 1	< 5	–
RARS	< 1,000	> 15	< 1	< 5	–
RAEB	< 1,000	NA	< 5	5–20	–
RAEBIT	NA	NA	>, < 5	20–30	+/–
CMML	> 1,000	NA	< 5	< 20	–

Abbreviations: CMML, chronic myelomonocytic leukemia; NA, not applicable; PB, peripheral blood; RA, refractory anemia; RAEB, RA with excess blasts; RAEBIT, RA with excess blasts in transformation; RARS, RA with ringed sideroblasts.

mon infections. The risk of infection is directly related to the severity of the neutropenia. Splenomegaly occurs in 5% to 30% of patients and hepatomegaly in 10% to 40%.

Autoimmune disorders occur in association with MDS, most often in chronic myelomonocytic leukemia and refractory anemia with excess blasts. Cutaneous vasculitis, Sweet's syndrome, eosinophilic fasciitis, chronic nonsuppurative panniculitis, and relapsing polychondritis have been described in association with MDS.

CLASSIFICATION

MDSs have been classified by the French-American-British (FAB) Cooperative Group into five categories: refractory anemia (RA), refractory anemia with ringed sideroblasts (RARS), refractory anemia with excess blasts (RAEB), refractory anemia with excess blasts in transformation (RAEBIT), and chronic myelomonocytic leukemia (CMML). This classification applies to primary MDS and is based on the percentage of peripheral and bone marrow myeloblasts and on the presence or absence of ringed sideroblasts or Auer rods (Table 1).

Many patients with MDS do not have a marrow disorder that fits in the FAB classification scheme, including patients with MDS associated with myelofibrosis, isolated neutropenias and thrombocytopenias, and syndromes having features of MDS and myeloproliferative syndromes.

DIFFERENTIAL DIAGNOSIS

For the diagnosis of MDS, it is important to realize that several diseases can mimic it. Vitamin B_{12} or folic acid deficiency was the cause of pancytopenia in 7.5% of patients undergoing a bone marrow examination for evaluation of the pancytopenia. Cytopenias and trilineage dysplasia are common in patients with acquired immunodeficiency syndrome.

Bone marrow dysplasia occurs in paroxysmal nocturnal hemoglobinuria, and it is most often accompanied by the absence of stainable iron. In patients with MDS, iron stores are most often normal or increased.

In patients with pancytopenia and splenomegaly, hairy cell leukemia, agnogenic myeloid metaplasia, hypersplenism, and Felty's syndrome need to be considered. Large granular lymphocyte leukemias are associated with cytopenias and erythroid dysplasia. Alcohol toxicity, heavy metal poisoning, and drug-induced cytopenia, postviral cytopenia, and immunocytopenia also need to be considered before establishing a diagnosis of MDS.

Clues to the Diagnosis of Myelodysplastic Syndrome

- A history of chemotherapy or radiation therapy
- Unexplained macrocytosis with or without anemia
- Peripheral blood monocytosis
- Unexplained anemia or pancytopenia in an elderly person

LABORATORY FEATURES
Peripheral Blood

The hemoglobin value is less than 7 g/dL in 30% of patients, between 7 and 10 g/dL in 50%, and more than 10 g/dL in 20%. The neutrophil value is less than 500/µL in 10%, between 500 and 1,000/µL in 15%, and more than 1,000/µL in 75%. The platelet value is less than 25,000/µL in 15%, between 25,000 and 100,000/µL in 30%, and more than 100,000/µL in 55%.

The peripheral blood typically has a dimorphic erythroid population with an increased red cell distribution width on the automated cell counter. Oval macrocytes are common. Neutrophil granules are often deficient or abnormal, and pseudo–Pelger-Huët and ring-shaped nuclei are frequent. Platelets may be large and have abnormal granules. Thrombocytosis has been found in some patients with RARS.

Bone Marrow

The erythroid lineage on the bone marrow aspirate may show megaloblastoid maturation, multinuclearity, nuclear bridging, impaired hemoglobinization, and cytoplasmic vacuoles. Erythroid precursors are most often increased. Prussian blue staining may show the presence of pathologic ringed sideroblasts, which are defined as having in excess of five large iron-containing granules encircling one-third or more of the nucleus. These iron granules are localized in the mitochondria.

Granulocytic abnormalities on the bone marrow aspirate include left-shifted myeloid maturation with an increase in myeloblasts, pseudo–Pelger-Huët cells, ring-shaped nuclei, hypersegmentation, and abnormal or absent staining of the primary and secondary granules. Iron-laden macrophages are frequent and reflect ineffective erythropoiesis.

Dysmegakaryopoiesis is often observed in the aspirate; the most frequent findings are hypogranulation, large hypolobulated megakaryocytes, megakaryocytes with multiple separate nuclei, and micromegakaryocytes.

The bone marrow biopsy specimen is in general hypercellular; hypocellularity is found in 10% to 20% of patients. Islands of left-shifted erythroblasts and clusters of immature myeloid cells localized between bony trabeculae can be seen histologically. Myelofibrosis is occasionally found in the marrow biopsy specimens of patients with MDS (Fig. 1, Plate 13; Fig. 2, Plate 14; Fig. 3, Plate 15).

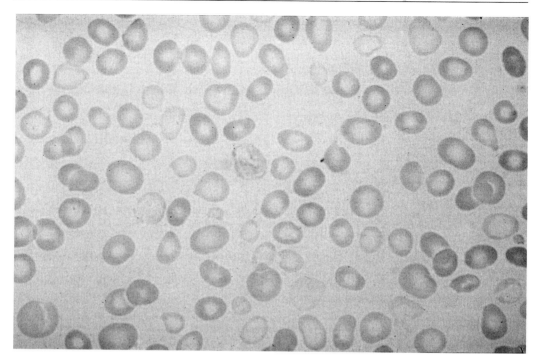

Fig. 1, Plate 13. Dimorphic red cells.

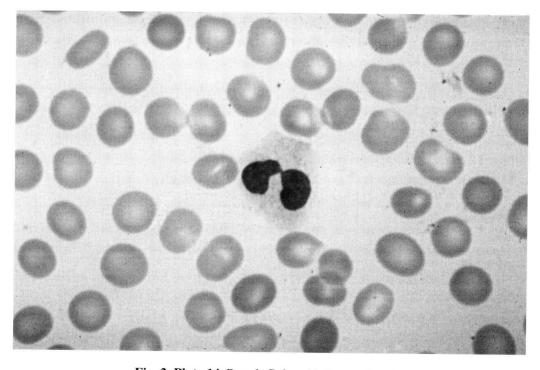

Fig. 2, Plate 14. Pseudo Pelger-Huët granulocyte.

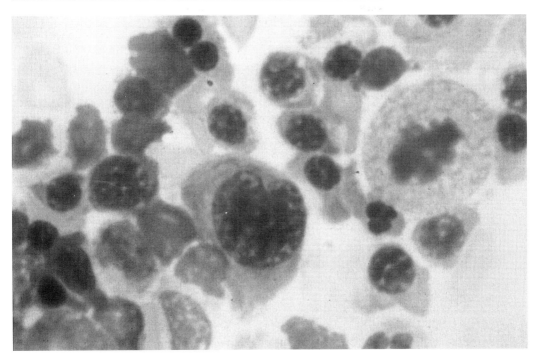

Fig. 3, Plate 15. Dyserythopoiesis seen in bone marrow aspirate.

Cellular Dysfunction

A sugar-water test or Ham-Crosby test is occasionally positive. Hemoglobin F is increased in approximately 8% of patients.

Abnormal granulocyte adhesion, chemotaxis, phagocytosis, and microbicidal activity are described. Granulocytes may show reduced myeloperoxidase activity and abnormal esterase cytochemistry. Leukocyte alkaline phosphatase levels are decreased in 20% of patients.

Bleeding time is frequently abnormal and is correlated with a dense-granule storage-pool defect. An acquired Bernard-Soulier platelet glycoprotein defect has been described. Collagen adhesion, adenosine diphosphate, and collagen aggregation are often abnormal.

Hypergammaglobulinemia is present in 32% of patients, monoclonal gammopathies in 12.5%, positive direct Coombs test in 8%, and autoantibodies in 22%.

Cytogenetics

The rate of chromosome abnormalities in MDS varies from 30% to 70%. Technical factors influence the rate of karyotypic abnormalities, which was reported to be 55% at the Sixth International Workshop on Chromosomes in Leukemia. The rate of karyotypic abnormalities in the different FAB subtypes was 31% in RA, 39% in RARS, 60% in RAEB, 40% in CMML, and 57% in RAEBIT. The most frequent karyotypic abnormalities in MDS include deletion of the long arm of chromosome 5, deletions of the long or short arm of chromosome 7, monosomy 7, trisomy 8, deletions or translocations involving the long arms of chromosome 11 and 12, and deletions of the long arm of chromosome 20.

The presence of trisomy 8, monosomy 7, or complex chromosome anomalies is associated with a poor prognosis.

A Practical Approach to Anemia in the Elderly Person

- Always rule out nutritional causes first; check serum ferritin, B_{12}, and folate levels.

- Always entertain the possibility of hemolysis; check reticulocyte count and indirect bilirubin, haptoglobin, and lactate dehydrogenase values.

- Always obtain a peripheral smear, which should help with both of the above considerations and, in MDS, may show oval macrocytes, dimorphic red cell popula tions, and pseudo Pelger-Huët cells.

- Do not forget to review the peripheral blood monocyte count; an increased level is strongly suggestive of MDS.

- Always check the erythrocyte sedimentation rate and serum creatinine value to entertain the possibility of anemia of chronic disease and renal insufficiency, respectively.

- A bone marrow biopsy is not always necessary in an elderly person because the information may not alter treatment decisions; if you do a bone marrow biopsy, do not forget to order cytogenetic studies and iron stain.

PROGNOSIS

The median duration of survival varies from 18 to 50 months in RA, 21 to 76 months in RARS, 9 to 18 months in RAEB, 9 to 60 months in CMML, and 5 to 7 months in RAEBIT.

A significant proportion of patients with MDS die of cytopenic complications and their disease does not transform to acute leukemia. The rate of leukemic transformation is approximately 10% in RA, 5% in RARS, 30% in RAEB, 60% in RAEBIT, and 15% in CMML.

THERAPY
Supportive Care

Patients with MDS usually do not benefit from vitamin supplementation unless they are vitamin-deficient. Rare patients with RARS respond to pyridoxine supplementation.

Patients with MDS are frequently red-cell-transfusion–dependent. The need for red cell transfusions should not be based only on the hemoglobin concentration but rather on the cardiopulmonary and functional status of the patient. Iron overload and secondary end-organ damage occur when the cumulative transfusion burden exceeds 50 to 75 units of red blood cells. Iron chelation therapy with desferoxamine may slow iron accumulation and delay end-organ damage. A daily dosage of 20 to 40 mg/kg should be administered over 8 to 12 hours with a small portable pump capable of providing continuous mini-infusion. Iron chelation is considered a difficult solution by many patients. Orally administered iron chelators are not yet approved for this indication.

Platelet transfusions should be given to patients with a bleeding problem. The use of prophylactic platelet transfusions is controversial.

The early and aggressive management of infections and the use of growth factors in patients unresponsive to appropriate antibiotics often prevent early mortality.

Glucocorticoids

A 9% response rate has been described with the use of glucocorticoids. The clinical response to glucocorticoids can be predicted by their in vitro effect on myeloid colony growth. Because of the side effects and further immunosuppression associated with glucocorticoids, their use is generally not recommended.

Androgens

Androgens increase the hemoglobin concentration in some patients with RA. In patients with RAEB, androgens do not prolong survival. In general, the use of androgens in MDS is not recommended.

Danazol

Danazol is a synthetic attenuated androgen. It is believed to decrease the monocyte Fc receptor number and improve thrombocytopenia in patients with positive cell-bound platelet antibodies. Very few patients have had clinically significant responses.

Retinoic Acid and Trans-Retinoic Acid

13-*cis*-Retinoic acid induces differentiation of leukemic cells in vitro. No significant difference is noted between patients receiving supportive care and those treated with 13-*cis*-retinoic acid.

The administration of *trans*-retinoic acid in MDS has failed to demonstrate any significant clinical activity. The combination of *trans*-retinoic acid and granulocyte colony-stimulating factor leads to an improvement in neutrophils in most patients and to an increase in platelets and hemoglobin in a minority of patients. The role of *trans*-retinoic acid in this combination remains unclear.

Trans-retinoic acid in combination with cytarabine cannot be recommended for the management of MDS.

Vitamin D

Human leukemic cell lines have been shown to differentiate terminally in the presence of 1,25-dihydroxyvitamin D_3. Clinical responses to 1,25-dihydroxyvitamin D_3 are rare, and treatment often is complicated by hypercalcemia.

New analogues of vitamin D with more hematopoietic differentiation ability and fewer effects on calcium metabolism are being evaluated in clinical trials.

Erythropoietin

A clinically significant stimulation of erythropoiesis occurs in 15% to 20% of patients with MDS. The improvement usually occurs in the first 8 weeks of treatment. Patients with RA and RAEB have a higher response rate than patients with RARS. Transfusion-dependent patients with RARS and an erythropoietin level in excess of 200 U/L are unlikely to respond to erythropoietin. The optimal dosage of erythropoietin has not been defined; a commonly used regimen is 50 U/kg per day 3 days a week.

Using granulocyte colony-stimulating factor or granulocyte-macrophage colony-stimulating factor in combination with erythropoietin increases clinically significant responses up to 30% to 40%. The cost of this treatment strategy may render it impractical.

Granulocyte Colony-Stimulating Factor (G-CSF)

G-CSF increases the absolute neutrophil count in more than 90% of patients with MDS. The hemoglobin value rarely increases, and the platelet count occasionally may increase or decrease. G-CSF is used in febrile neutropenic patients to promote rapid increase in neutrophils. G-CSF is not used prophylactically. Adverse effects include thrombocytopenia, bone pain, fluid overload, and Sweet's syndrome. The number of myeloblasts may increase, especially in patients with RAEB, RAEBIT, and CMML. The usual dosage is 5 µg/kg daily.

Granulocyte-Macrophage Colony-Stimulating Factor (GM-CSF)

GM-CSF increases the absolute neutrophil count in more than 80% of patients with MDS. There is no clinically significant stimulation of eythropoiesis, and the platelet value increases in 6% of patients and decreases in 6%. Lymphocyte, monocyte, and eosinophil values increase with GM-CSF treatment.

Adverse effects include fever, bone pain, erythema at the subcutaneous injection site, and phlebitis at the site of intravenous infusion. In patients receiving more than $250 \, \mu g/m^2$, pleuritis and thrombocytopenia have been described. Leukemic transformation has been described in patients treated with a percentage of bone marrow blasts in excess of 14%.

Interferons

The response rate to interferons in MDS has been very low. Myelosuppression is the dose-limiting factor with interferons. Weight loss is a frequent adverse effect in MDS.

Low-Dose Cytarabine

The rationale for the use of cytarabine in MDS is induction of terminal differentiation with minimal cytoreduction. In a trial conducted by the Eastern and Southwest Oncology Groups, patients were randomized to receive either cytarabine ($10 \, mg/m^2$ subcutaneously every 12 hours for 21 days) or supportive care. The complete response rate to a single cycle was 8%, and the partial response rate was 16%. The median survival was not different between the two groups—8.7 months in the cytarabine group and 6.9 months in the supportive-care group.

5-Azacytadine

5-Azacytidine causes DNA hypomethylation through inhibition of DNA methyl-transferase; this action correlates with differentiation of leukemic cells in vitro. At a dosage of $75 \, mg/m^2$ daily for 7 days every 28 days, the complete remission rate is approximately 10%. The role of 5-azacytidine in the management of MDS is currently being evaluated by cooperative groups.

Conventional Antileukemic Therapy

Antileukemic chemotherapy is used in patients with MDS who have severe cytopenias, progressive increases in bone marrow blasts, and transformation to acute leukemia. Patients treated during the preleukemic phase of the disease had a complete remission rate of 47% to 66%, a treatment-related mortality of 14% to 33%, and a median survival of 5 to 11 months.

Patients treated after leukemic transformation had a complete remission rate of 24% to 41%, a treatment-related mortality of 21% to 44%, and a median survival of less than 6 months.

P-glycoprotein expression is correlated with multidrug resistance. It is present in the bone marrow myeloblasts of 22% of patients with MDS and 57% of patients who have had transformation to acute leukemia.

New chemotherapy regimens, including drugs that are not affected by multidrug resistance, may improve these results. Clinical trials with topoisomerase I inhibitors such as topotecan show promising results.

Transplantation

Allogeneic sibling-donor marrow transplantation is currently done in patients with a poor prognosis. Candidates are usually younger than 60 years and have a neutrophil count of less than 1,000/μL and a platelet count of less than 50,000/μL. Patients who have a progressive increase in myeloblasts in the marrow and patients with secondary myelodysplasia are also candidates. The disease-free survival at 3 years varies from 30% to 45%, the transplant-related mortality from 25% to 45%, and the relapse rate from 10% to 35%.

Unrelated donor allogeneic transplantations are increasingly being performed in patients younger than 55 years. Transplant-related mortality is increased compared with the mortality in sibling allogeneic transplantation, but the relapse rates remain similar.

High-dose chemotherapy and autologous peripheral blood stem cell rescue are being evaluated in MDS. Stem cells are harvested during the first complete remission after antileukemic chemotherapy. Transplantation-related mortality is less than in allogeneic transplantation, but the relapse rate is higher. The role of autologous transplantation in MDS remains to be defined.

Experimental Approaches

Cyclosporine and antithymocyte globulin are being evaluated in the management of MDS, with promising preliminary results. It has been known since the early 1980s that subsets of T lymphocytes inhibit hematopoiesis in MDS.

Amifostine is a cytoprotective agent that decreases the toxicities of chemotherapy. In vitro, it promotes the formation and survival of primitive hematopoietic progenitors. Clinically significant responses have occurred in a significant proportion of patients. Amifostine is administered by intravenous infusion three times a week. Ongoing trials are evaluating different routes of administration and combinations with other growth factors and drugs.

General Management Recommendations in Myelodysplastic Syndrome

1. If the patient is younger than 50 years and has a histocompatible related donor, then consider allogeneic bone marrow transplantation.
2. Otherwise, the main purpose of treatment should be palliative unless there is an experimental treatment protocol for which the patient might be eligible.
3. If the patient is not on a protocol, one has to decide what needs palliation:
   a. If anemia is the problem, measure serum erythropoietin (EPO) level. If EPO level is less than 200 U/L, then try exogenous EPO administration at 10,000 units subcutaneously three times a week for 2 months. If there is a response, continue EPO. If there is no response, then discontinue EPO and proceed with red cell transfusions as necessary. If there is a partial response to EPO or failure from initial response, it is then reasonable to consider increasing the EPO dose or adding myeloid growth factor (granulocyte colony-stimulating factor, G-CSF) therapy at either 300 or 450 mg (depending on body weight) subcutaneously daily.
   b. If thrombocytopenia is the problem, then try oral danazol at 400 mg twice a day bleeding, the use of oral tranexamic acid at 1 to 2 g three times a day may alleviate

the symptoms and signs without increasing the platelet count. Similarly, a short course of corticosteroid therapy (prednisone, 1 mg/kg daily) may be tried for symptomatic severe thrombocytopenia. However, many precautions have to be taken.

    i. Digital rectal examination should be done and prostate-specific antigen levels should be checked before the patient is started on danazol therapy.

    ii. Liver function tests should be monitored periodically during danazol therapy.

    iii. The virilizing side effects of danazol must be emphasized to female patients.

    iv. Disseminated intravascular coagulation and urogenital bleeding must be excluded before considering treatment with tranexamic acid. Also, tranexamic acid should be given under the supervision of a hematologist, and dosing requires adjustment in renal insufficiency.

  c. If the problem is neutropenia that is not associated with infection, nothing needs to be done. If neutropenia is associated with infection, then G-CSF at either 300 or 450 mg subcutaneously daily is appropriate. Use of G-CSF should be stopped after the infection is controlled. If the patient has recurrent infections, continuous therapy with G-CSF may be considered. Current data do not support the notion that G-CSF promotes leukemic transformation.

  d. If RAEB or RAEBIT is accompanied by symptomatic refractory cytopenia(s) or severe constitutional symptoms, then one may consider chemotherapy, as is used for acute myeloid leukemia.

Therapy-Related Myelodysplasia (t-MDS)

t-MDS precedes 10% to 20% of all cases of acute myeloid leukemia (AML). A preleukemic phase precedes 70% of the cases of therapy-related AML (t-AML). The median duration of the preleukemic phase is 11 months in patients exposed to alkylators. Patients in whom t-AML develops after treatment with a DNA-topoisomerase II inhibitor (etoposide, tenoposide) do not, in general, have a preleukemic phase.

Cytogenetic abnormalities are thought to occur in 80% of patients with t-MDS and t-AML. The most common abnormality in patients who have received alkylators is loss of either all or part of chromosome 5 or 7. Other frequent chromosome changes involve loss or abnormalities of chromosomes 3, 17, and 18. Patients who have received epipodophyllotoxins often have balanced translocations involving either band 11q23 or band 21q22.

The median latent period to the development of t-MDS or t-AML is 4 to 5 years. The incidence is higher in patients who have received high doses of alkylators or epipodophyllotoxins. The risk may vary according to the schedule of drug administration.

The mainstay of treatment of t-MDS is supportive care. The treatments available to patients with t-MDS are identical to those available to patients with primary MDS. The overall treatment outcome in t-MDS and t-AML is worse than in primary MDS or AML. Allogeneic bone marrow transplantation is the only treatment option that can provide a chance for long-term survival. Transplant-related mortality is higher in t-MDS and t-AML than in primary MDS. The median disease-free survival for patients undergoing allogeneic transplantation for t-MDS or t-AML can be expected to be 25% to 30% at 2 years.

SUMMARY

Our understanding of the biology of myelodysplasia is incomplete. This lack of understanding of the disease affects our capacity to treat it with specificity and effectiveness. Supportive care remains the backbone of the medical management of this disorder.

Antileukemic chemotherapy and marrow transplantation prolong survival in young patients. The development of new differentiation agents and clinical trials with amifostine, cyclosporine, and antithymocyte globulin may broaden our therapeutic armamentarium.

SUGGESTED READING

De Witte T, Van Biezen A, Hermans J, Labopin M, Runde V, Or R, Meloni G, Mauri SB, Carella A, Apperley J, Gratwohl A, Laporte JP, for the Chronic and Acute Leukemia Working Parties of the European Group for Blood and Marrow Transplantation. Autologous bone marrow transplantation for patients with myelodysplastic syndrome (MDS) or acute myeloid leukemia following MDS. *Blood* 1997; 90: 3853-3857.

Ganser A, Hoelzer D. Clinical use of hematopoietic growth factors in the myelodysplastic syndromes. *Semin Hematol* 1996; 33: 186-195.

Gassmann W, Schmitz N, Loffler H, De Witte T. Intensive chemotherapy and bone marrow transplantation for myelodysplastic syndromes. *Semin Hematol* 1996; 33: 196-205.

Jonasova A, Neuwirtova R, Cermak J, Vozobulova V, Mockikova K, Siskova M, Hochova I. Cyclosporin A therapy in hypoplastic MDS patients and certain refractory anaemias without hypoplastic bone marrow. *Br J Haematol* 1998; 100: 304-309.

Karp JE. Molecular pathogenesis and targets for therapy in myelodysplastic syndrome (MDS) and MDS-related leukemias. *Curr Opin Oncol* 1998; 10: 3-9.

Karp JE, Smith MA. The molecular pathogenesis of treatment-induced (secondary) leukemias: foundations for treatment and prevention. *Semin Oncol* 1997; 24: 103-113.

List AF, Brasfield F, Heaton R, Glinsmann-Gibson B, Crook L, Taetle R, Capizzi R. Stimulation of hematopoiesis by amifostine in patients with myelodysplastic syndrome. *Blood* 1997; 90: 3364-3369.

Molldrem JJ, Caples M, Mavroudis D, Plante M, Young NS, Barrett AJ. Antithymocyte globulin for patients with myelodysplastic syndrome. *Br J Haematol* 1997; 99: 699-705.

Noël P, Solberg LA Jr. Myelodysplastic syndromes. Pathogenesis, diagnosis and treatment. *Crit Rev Oncol Hematol* 1992; 12: 193-215.

Park DJ, Koeffler HP. Therapy-related myelodysplastic syndromes. *Semin Hematol* 1996; 33: 256-273.

Parker JE, Mufti GJ. Ineffective haemopoiesis and apoptosis in myelodysplastic syndromes. *Br J Haematol* 1998; 101: 220-230.

12 The Eosinophil and Eosinophilia

Joseph H. Butterfield, MD

Contents

INTRODUCTION

Because of the eosinophil's association with unusual disorders, few discoveries on the peripheral blood smear elicit as much trepidation as that of an increased eosinophil count. Despite the ease of eosinophil quantitation afforded by automated leukocyte differential counts, it is important to remember that eosinophils reside mainly in the tissues. In humans, the ratio of bone marrow:blood eosinophils is 3.7-5.1 to 1. In the adult rat, the ratio of tissue:blood eosinophils is about 200-300 to 1. It is here, in the organs themselves, that this cell works both to protect and to damage the host. The eosinophil numbers in the peripheral blood represent an equilibrium among bone marrow production, trafficking in the circulation, and a final destination in tissue, where eosinophil function, apoptosis, and death transpire. The half-life of eosinophils in the circulation is approximately 18 hours, and their total life span is about 6 days.

NORMAL EOSINOPHIL NUMBERS

The eosinophil is a rare granulocyte. Therefore, even a small sampling error on a 100 leukocyte differential count can make a significant change in the total eosinophil number. The range for a normal morning eosinophil count is broadly defined as $40/mm^3$ to $500-600/mm^3$. The consistent finding of an eosinophil value higher than the upper end of this range constitutes a working definition of eosinophilia. Nonatopic subjects have a significantly lower mean total eosinophil count ($99.6/mm^3$; range, 34-257) than do patients with positive skin test reactivity ($201.6/mm^3$; range, 81-427).

The peripheral eosinophil count also fluctuates in a diurnal pattern. Numbers peak during the hours between midnight and 4 a.m. and decrease at least 20% between 6:30

From: *Primary Hematology*
Edited by: A. Tefferi © Mayo Foundation for Medical Education and Research, Rochester, MN

a.m. and 9:30 a.m. to reach a nadir during the morning hours. This pattern holds true for both normal volunteers and for patients with bronchial asthma not treated with glucocorticoids. Therefore, it is important to establish a consistent monitoring time when following a patient with eosinophilia.

EOSINOPHIL STAINING AND QUANTITATION

Wright-Giemsa stains of peripheral blood leukocytes serve to readily identify eosinophils by the presence of their brilliant orange or red-orange refractile granules. Eosinophil nuclear segmentation (80% bilobed, heavily condensed chromatin) is also a defining characteristic.

Several dyes have been utilized to stain eosinophils in the peripheral blood. A leukocyte-diluting solution of phloxine and methylene blue dissolved in a 50% aqueous solution of propylene glycol has allowed clear staining of eosinophils for quantitation in counting chambers. In recent years, however, automated leukocyte differential counts enumerate eosinophils and other cell types by a combination of direct measurements of aperture impedance, aperture conductance, and laser light scatter. This information is used to generate a three-dimensional scatterplot from which eosinophils (and other granulocyte types) are quantitated. Agreement with manual differential counts is generally excellent.

CAUSES OF EOSINOPHILIA

When faced with a new case of undiagnosed eosinophilia, it is helpful for the clinician to consider not only the potential causes of the eosinophilia but also the degree of the eosinophilia. Causes of prolonged, sustained, *hyper*eosinophilia are few. The patient's ethnicity, sex, and current country of residence may give clues for insightful questions to elicit the potential cause of eosinophilia. Considering the mobility of our society and the frequency of international travel, it is not inconceivable that a physician in the continental United States may have a patient from Southeast Asia who presents with eosinophilia.

The number of both common and uncommon disorders that have been associated with eosinophilia exceeds 60; however, ailments *commonly* accompanied by eosinophilia number about 30, and approximately 15 afflictions are associated with sustained *hyper*eosinophilia (>1,500/mm^3). Eosinophil-associated diseases can be grouped into seven or eight broad categories for ease of clinical differential diagnosis. A suggested workup for patients with eosinophilia is presented in Table 1. On a mechanistic level, eosinophilia can more simply be categorized as either 1) reactive, that is, due to (in)appropriate stimulation of eosinophil colony-forming cells by interleukin-5 (IL-5) and other eosinophil-active cytokines, or 2) clonal, in which eosinophils may be part of a malignant clonal population, such as in acute myeloid leukemia.

Parasites

Eosinophilia is common only in **helminthic** infestations (angiostrongyliasis, ascariasis, capillariasis, clonorchiasis, coenurosis, cysticercosis, dicroceliasis, dirofilariasis, dracunculiasis, echinococcosis, fascioliasis, fasciolopsiasis, filariasis, gnathostomiasis, hookworm infection, hymenolepiasis, metagonimiasis, opisthorchiasis, paragonimiasis, schistosomiasis, trichinosis, trichostrongyliasis, trichuriasis, visceral larval migrans), and it is not common in protozoan infestations, except for the intestinal coccidian parasite *Isospora belli*.

Table 1
Workup of Patients With Idiopathic Eosinophilia

Focused history and physical examination
Complete blood cell count and leukocyte differential count, erythrocyte sedimentation rate
Midstream urinalysis and Gram stain
13-Channel serum chemistry group
Vitamin B_{12} and folate determinations
Quantitative immunoglobulin levels, including IgE
Serum protein electrophoresis
Serum interleukin-5 determination
AM and PM cortisol levels
Skin tests for common inhalants, molds, and foods
Electrocardiography and echocardiography
Fresh stool examination for ova and parasites (×3)
Parasite serologic tests (*Strongyloides, Trichinosis, Toxocara* [*canis, cati*], *Echinococcus,*
    Entamoeba histolytica, and others as clinically warranted)
Computed tomography of the chest and abdomen
Bone marrow aspirate and biopsy with chromosome studies and stains for mast cells
Tissue biopsy (fascia, muscle, skin, lung, tumor) with staining for eosinophils and eosinophil
    proteins, when indicated
Molecular genetic studies for B- and T-cell gene rearrangements of peripheral blood
    lymphocytes
Clinical circumstances or laboratory availability may warrant or allow one or more of the
    following tests: urinary drug screen, rheumatoid factor, serum complement determinations,
    serum eosinophil protein levels, quantitation of urinary *N*-methylhistamine

The diagnosis of parasitic infection depends on careful questioning about current residence, travel to regions where parasites are endemic, and appropriate laboratory testing: tissue biopsy, fresh stool analysis, and in vitro assays, including serologic and polymerase chain reaction-based tests.

Eosinophilia is more common during early infection and during parasitic migration than during later stages of infestations. The migration of filariae through the pulmonary vascular bed with lodging of microfilariae in alveolar capillaries leads to **tropical pulmonary eosinophilia**. Patients may be asymptomatic or experience malaise, fever, and sporadic bronchial asthma. Complement fixation testing is positive for filaria. Response to diethylcarbamazine is rapid and favorable. Eosinophilia may be prolonged in many of the disorders, especially in schistosomiasis (which can establish a self-perpetuating autoinfection cycle). The eosinophil value associated with these infestations frequently exceeds 3,000/mm³, yet even more extreme levels occasionally have been reported. The eosinophilia of parasitic diseases is IL-5-driven. Serum levels of eosinophil cationic protein and eosinophil-derived neurotoxin are increased in patients with onchocerciasis, bancroftian filariasis, and intestinal schistosomiasis when compared with controls. Deposition of toxic eosinophil granule proteins onto microfilariae of *Onchocerca volvulus* and other parasites also has been demonstrated in vivo. Yet, the absolute necessity of eosinophils for resistance to parasites is not firmly established. For example, anti-IL-5 treatment of mice infected with *Schistosoma mansoni* or with *Trichinella spiralis* does not seem to decrease resistance to these parasites.

The importance of detecting parasitic disorders as the cause of eosinophilia is twofold: 1) curative treatment is now available for most parasitic infestations, and 2) administration of glucocorticoids to patients with undiagnosed parasitism in an effort to suppress eosinophilia may lead to a potentially serious (or fatal) superinfection.

Asthma and Other Atopic Disorders

ASTHMA

Several lines of evidence implicate the eosinophil as a central and highly significant cell in the inflammatory pathogenesis of asthma. Since the 1960s, the relationship between asthma in relapse and the total peripheral eosinophil count has been recognized. In the eosinophilia of uncomplicated bronchial asthma, the eosinophil count is generally less than 800/mm^3. A higher value in a patient with symptoms of bronchial asthma should raise the possibility of another eosinophilic disorder such as Churg-Strauss syndrome, allergic bronchopulmonary aspergillosis, chronic eosinophilic pneumonia, Löffler's syndrome, sarcoidosis, or tropical pulmonary eosinophilia.

Several authors have noted the utility of following the total eosinophil count as a measurement of the response to glucocorticoid treatment of asthma. Total eosinophil counts of more than 350/mm^3 in patients not receiving glucocorticoids and more than 85/mm^3 in those receiving glucocorticoids were associated with active intrinsic asthma.

Eosinophil adhesion to bronchial epithelium is regulated by cytokines and suppressed by dexamethasone. By their secretion of toxic granule proteins, eosinophils contribute to the pathophysiology of asthma. Eosinophil granule major basic protein has been examined thoroughly, and in several systems it has been shown to increase bronchial hyperreactivity. This effect results from the action of major basic protein on lung M_2 muscarinic receptors and from its toxic, desquamative effect on respiratory epithelium. In allergic asthma, serum levels of eosinophil cationic protein and eosinophil-derived neurotoxin increase during pollen season. Bronchial wash and serum levels of these proteins decrease in response to prednisone therapy.

OTHER ATOPIC DISORDERS

Other common atopic disorders that commonly have been associated with eosinophilia include **seasonal allergic rhinitis, urticaria,** and **atopic dermatitis**. Nonetheless, allergic rhinitis and chronic urticaria are important examples of **tissue** eosinophilia, which may or may not have an accompanying peripheral blood eosinophilia in the range of 4% to 12%. Studies of allergic rhinitis have utilized nasal biopsy, nasal scrapings, or nasal lavage to demonstrate increased nasal eosinophil counts during allergy season or after nasal antigen provocation. An increased percentage of hypodense eosinophils has been discovered in the **circulation** at the onset of allergic nasal symptoms. Nasal lavage fluid levels of eosinophil major basic protein and eosinophil cationic protein, as well as leukotriene C4, are increased after nasal allergen challenge. Immunotherapy with short ragweed causes a dose- and duration-dependent reduction of eosinophil infiltration into the nasal mucosa. In chronic urticaria, peripheral eosinophilia is not common. As detected by the presence of free eosinophil granules and extracellular major basic protein, eosinophil degranulation occurs in lesional skin, where eosinophils migrate under the influence of inflammatory cytokines.

Disease severity in atopic dermatitis correlates with the number of hypodense eosinophils in the circulation. Serum levels of toxic eosinophil granule proteins, such as major basic protein, eosinophil-derived neurotoxin, and eosinophil-cationic protein are all increased in atopic dermatitis, and there is a close correlation between the number of hypodense eosinophils and the serum level of eosinophil cationic protein. Furthermore, major basic protein deposition has been demonstrated in lesional (but not uninvolved) skin. The eosinophilia of atopic dermatitis results in part from a combination of increased sensitivity of eosinophils for eosinopoietic cytokines and a delay in programmed cell death mediated by autocrine production of growth factors by eosinophils.

Drug-Induced Eosinophilia

The thoughtful clinician is always alert to the possibility of drug-induced eosinophilia. It is prudent to question a patient with eosinophilia about not only changes in prescription medications but also any recent use of over-the-counter, nontraditional, holistic, or herbal preparations. Leading contenders for prescription drug-induced eosinophilia include penicillin, cephalosporins, nitrofurantoin, para-aminosalicylic acid, phenytoin, hydralazine, chlorpromazine, warfarin, and carbamazepine. "Cutting-edge" regimens such as interleukin-2/lymphocyte-activated killer cell therapy for cancer also may have unintended consequences, such as eosinophilia. Other therapy-associated causes of eosinophilia include infected ventriculoperitoneal shunts and, occasionally, radiation therapy. Often, drug-induced eosinophilia presents as drug-induced eosinophilic pneumonia with symptoms of dry cough, fever, chills, and dyspnea occurring 2 hours to 10 days after initiation of drug therapy. This type of reaction is typified by acute reactions to nitrofurantoin. Unfortunately, although the number of new drugs available to clinicians continually increases, penicillin G is the only medication for which a standardized skin test preparation is available. Discontinuing use of a suspected drug should result in resolution of eosinophilia if it is indeed the underlying cause.

Malignant Disorders

For more than 100 years, eosinophilia has been a well-described feature of both clonal and certain nonclonal neoplasms. In some cases of clonal eosinophilia, the eosinophils are part of the malignant clone itself, whereas in other cases cytokine production by leukemic cells may stimulate eosinophil production indirectly. Because eosinophils themselves can secrete many cytokines, including IL-1 and IL-5, persistence of eosinophilia via self-perpetuating autocrine loops then becomes possible. Clonal disorders with eosinophilia include acute and chronic eosinophilic leukemia, chronic granulocytic leukemia, polycythemia rubra vera, essential thrombocythemia, acute myeloid leukemia, myelodysplastic syndrome, systemic mastocytosis, T-lymphoblastic lymphoma, and acute lymphoblastic leukemia. Methods of establishing clonality have been reviewed recently.

Both local and peripheral blood eosinophilia have been reported with numerous nonhematologic neoplasms, including Hodgkin's disease, non-Hodgkin's lymphoma, angioimmunoblastic lymphadenopathy, lymphomatoid granulomatosis, Omenn's syndrome, vascular tumors, gastrointestinal tract neoplasms and lymphomas, breast cancer, renal tumors, female genital tract neoplasms, and lung cancer.

The significance of tissue eosinophilia associated with solid tumors and the role of eosinophils in the immune response to these neoplasms are often difficult to judge. In many instances, eosinophilia results from cytokine production by the tumor. Eosinophilia also may be present in various necrotic or metastatic malignancies, perhaps as an immune response to the tumor. For example, 88% of breast cancer cases in one series had eosinophil peroxidase deposits within or around the tumor. This finding may indicate participation in an anti-tumor response because of the ability of eosinophil peroxidase to induce production of large amounts of tissue necrosis factor and to enhance the release of phorbol 12-myristate 13-acetate-triggered hydrogen peroxide by human macrophages. The association of eosinophilia with metastatic disease has led some investigators to conclude that this is an unfavorable sign. A generalized conclusion may not be possible regarding the significance of tumor-associated eosinophilia, and the relevance may vary on a tumor-to-tumor basis.

Autoimmune Causes

Several rare autoimmune diseases may be associated with eosinophilia. Initially, it may be difficult to differentiate these disorders from early hypereosinophilic syndrome (see page 168). The more common autoimmune disorders to consider are eosinophilic fasciitis, the eosinophilia-myalgia syndrome, eosinophilic myositis, eosinophilic gastroenteritis, eosinophilic cystitis, Löffler's endocarditis, chronic hepatitis, and, less frequently, ulcerative colitis, regional enteritis, and rheumatoid arthritis.

Eosinophilic fasciitis may be difficult to distinguish from scleroderma. Symptoms include fatigue, myalgias, sclerodermatous skin changes, and swelling in the distal extremities and occasionally the abdomen and thorax. In contrast to scleroderma, however, eosinophilic fasciitis has an acute onset after periods of physical (over)exertion, spares the hands and feet, and does not have associated Raynaud's phenomenon, calcinosis, or visceral involvement. Eosinophilic fasciitis responds to treatment with corticosteroids, often in low doses, and cimetidine. Peripheral blood findings include increased erythrocyte sedimentation rate, hypergammaglobulinemia, increased levels of eosinophil chemotactic factor, and prominent eosinophilia. Staining of tissue for eosinophils gives variable results. A biopsy of deep fascia is helpful for diagnosis and shows inflammation of collagen bundles of deep fascia and perivascular infiltration with plasma cells, lymphocytes, and occasional eosinophils. In some cases of eosinophilic fasciitis, the organism *Borrelia burgdorferi* has been detected in involved tissue.

In 1989, the **eosinophilia-myalgia syndrome**, a complex of intense myalgias, weakness, fatigue, rash, fever, edema, alopecia, arthralgias, skin tightening, distal paresthesias, and eosinophilia associated with ingestion of L-tryptophan, was reported. This syndrome occurred as the result of specific tryptophan-manufacturing conditions at one bulk producer. Biopsy showed histopathologic changes of scleroderma in the dermis and subcutaneous tissue with inflamed and fibrotic fascia and perifascicular inflammation of adjacent muscle. Increases in serum and urine levels of major basic protein and eosinophil-derived neurotoxin and extracellular deposits of major basic protein in affected tissues were reported. Although the associated eosinophilia was responsive to prednisone, the long-term severity and duration of disease were not affected by steroid treatment, and a protracted phase of symptom resolution was common. In some series, patients developed eosinophilic fasciitis.

Eosinophil infiltration into muscle, **eosinophilic myositis**, is uncommon, but it may occur as a manifestation of the hypereosinophilic syndrome. Localized pseudotumorous swelling and tenderness of involved muscles may be confused with parasitic muscular invasion by trichinella or cysticercosis. Eosinophilic myositic involvement often has been reported as cyclic, relapsing eosinophilia. Increases in levels of eosinophilic cationic protein and IL-5 parallel disease activity.

Symptoms of **eosinophilic gastroenteritis** are cramping abdominal pain, vomiting, and diarrhea, which may be disabling. Histologically, an eosinophil infiltrate involves the mucosa or muscularis and rarely the serosal surface of the bowel. Thickening, induration, and necrosis have all been reported as pathologic findings. A useful classification of eosinophilic gastroenteritis based on the layer of bowel involvement has been suggested: 1) patients who have mucosal involvement, with attendant protein wasting, malabsorption, and gastrointestinal blood loss, often have atopy, increased IgE levels, and food allergy; 2) patients with primarily muscularis involvement lack specific food sensitivity and have normal IgE levels, and the diagnosis of muscularis disease depends on a full-thickness bowel biopsy; 3) serosal disease may occur as an isolated finding or as a component of transmural disease. Eosinophilic ascites has been associated with serosal disease. Eosinophilic gastroenteritis may occur as a predominant clinical component of Churg-Strauss syndrome, and, conversely, in isolated cases pathologic features of necrotizing granulomas identical to those of Churg-Strauss syndrome may be found. Glucocorticoids given in high-dose, short-term courses are effective therapy for all forms of eosinophilic gastroenteritis. In some cases, recurrent or prolonged treatment with prednisone is necessary. Food elimination diets generally have not been helpful.

Eosinophilic cystitis is a rare disease of unknown cause. Patients present with hematuria, frequency, dysuria, and suprapubic pain. In some patients, this disorder has been ascribed to a food allergic reaction. At the time of presentation, eosinophilic cystitis may mimic bladder cancer. Treatment has consisted of glucocorticoids, antihistamines, and nonsteroidal anti-inflammatory drugs.

Löffler's endocarditis is now thought to represent a cardiovascular manifestation of the idiopathic hypereosinophilic syndrome (see page 168).

Eosinophil-induced chronic active hepatitis most commonly has been associated with the hypereosinophilic syndrome, but it may occur as an isolated disorder. Liver involvement in this syndrome occurs in about 30% of cases; however, the clinical manifestations, consisting chiefly of hepatomegaly and mildly abnormal results of liver function studies, may not be clinically important. Patients present with cholestasis, malaise, fatigue, myalgias, and eosinophilia. Liver biopsy shows an eosinophilic infiltrate with biliary damage but no cirrhosis. Treatment with oral glucocorticoids leads to marked clinical improvement, and maintenance treatment with low-dose prednisone in combination with azathioprine can maintain stable remissions with no progression to the hypereosinophilic syndrome.

Dermatologic Disorders

Reference has already been made to atopic dermatitis and chronic urticaria. Other dermatologic disorders associated with eosinophilia are not numerous. 1. The syndrome of **episodic angioedema and eosinophilia** first described by Gleich et al. *(1)* consists of recurrent attacks of angioedema with associated weight gain, fever, urticaria, leukocytosis, and marked eosinophilia. This syndrome readily responds to glucocorticoid administration, which induces a rapid diuresis and resolution of eosinophilia. Low-dose interferon-α can be used to prevent recurrence. In contrast to the hypereosinophilic syndrome, cardiac sequelae are rare in the syndrome of episodic angioedema with eosinophilia. 2. In about 15% of cases, **bullous pemphigoid** may have an accompanying hypereosinophilia. The eosinophilia responds to treatment of the underlying skin ailment. 3. **Kimura's disease** has an accompanying hypereosinophilia in approximately 50% of cases. Kimura's disease should be suspected in young Chinese or Japanese males with angiolymphoid proliferation of the head and neck. Before treatment, semi-quantitative reverse transcription-polymerase chain reaction analysis has shown increased levels of IL-4, IL-5, and IL-13 mRNA but normal levels of interferon-γ mRNA in peripheral blood mononuclear cells. After therapy with operation and radiation, levels of IL-4, IL-5, and IL-13 mRNA, IgE, and eosinophil numbers all decrease. Cyclosporin A also causes a dose-dependent decrease in these parameters. 4. **Wells syndrome**, or eosinophilic cellulitis, is a rare dermatologic condition with marked eosinophilia in about 50% of cases. Wells syndrome is characterized by recurrent cutaneous swellings resembling bacterial cellulitis. Skin lesions have a dermal eosinophilic infiltrate, and the characteristic "flame figures" consist of collagen bundles onto which eosinophil major basic protein has been deposited. Various triggering factors such as myeloproliferative disorders, lymphoma, insect bites, and drugs have been described. Albendazole treatment of two patients with Wells syndrome, who had increased antibody titers to the excretory-secretory antigen of *Toxocara canis*, resulted in clearance of skin lesions.

Idiopathic Hypereosinophilic Syndrome

The hypereosinophilic syndrome is a continuum of disorders of unknown cause whose formal criteria were previously established: 1) sustained eosinophil count of more than 1,500/mm^3 for longer than 6 months (or death before 6 months with signs and symptoms of hypereosinophilic disease), 2) absence of other recognized causes of eosinophilia, and 3) signs and symptoms of organ system involvement (hepatosplenomegaly, anemia, pulmonary fibrosis, central nervous system abnormalities, fever, congestive heart failure) which are otherwise unexplained in the clinical setting.

Hypereosinophilic syndrome is generally a disorder of men between the ages of 20 and 50 years. The eosinophilia of the syndrome is comprised of cells having a prolonged blood half-life. Only rarely has an increase in the serum level of IL-5 been demonstrated, but T-cell clones producing eosinophil colony-stimulating factor have been established from the peripheral blood of some patients. Generally, no chromosome abnormalities are found on bone marrow examination. The differential diagnosis in patients with a sustained eosinophil count of more than 1,500/mm^3 includes 1) (untreated) bullous pemphigoid, 2) Churg-Strauss syndrome, 3) drug reactions, 4) eosinophilic leukemia, 5) eosinophilia-myalgia syndrome, 6) eosinophilic cellulitis (Wells syndrome), 7) eosinophilic fasciitis, 8) eosinophilic pneumonia, 9) eosinophilic gastroenteritis, 10) eosinophilic vasculitis, 11) episodic angioedema with eosinophilia syndrome, 12) infection with helminthic parasites, 13) Kimura's disease, 14) lymphoid or myeloid hematologic malignancies, 15) metastatic or necrotic tumors, and 16) tropical eosinophilia.

The prognosis in untreated hypereosinophilic syndrome is poor—the average survival is only 9 months. Control of organ damage caused by eosinophils is a primary goal of treatment. Generally, this can be achieved by lowering the total eosinophil count to less than 1,000/mm^3. Patients who often respond to prednisone alone have favorable prognostic findings, including an increased IgE level and the presence of urticaria or angioedema. First-line treatment of hypereosinophilic syndrome now includes interferon-α alone or in combination with prednisone or hydroxyurea. Recently, several reports of successful allogeneic bone marrow transplantation for resistant disease have been published.

Cardiovascular disease associated with the hypereosinophilic syndrome remains a cause of significant morbidity and mortality in untreated patients. The risk of cardiac damage does not correlate with the absolute number of peripheral blood eosinophils or with the duration of eosinophilia but rather with the presence of vacuolated or degranulated eosinophils. In addition to agents for lowering the total eosinophil count, patients with cardiovascular disease are commonly treated with warfarin and antiplatelet drugs to prevent thromboembolic complications; however, controlled studies to establish the benefit of anticoagulants are lacking. Patients with congestive heart failure have benefited from bed rest, diuretics, and digitalis. Patients with irreversible cardiac structural damage may benefit from valve replacement. Bioprosthetic valves seem to work well in these patients. Ventricular decortication also may be needed for patients with obliterative disease. It is of paramount importance in all cases of cardiovascular disease to continue measures to control eosinophilia in addition to treating the cardiac symptoms because failure to control eosinophilia will lead to inevitable deterioration and death.

Pulmonary Eosinophilic Disorders

In addition to asthma, tropical pulmonary eosinophilia from migrating parasites (filaria), drug-induced pulmonary eosinophilias, and several idiopathic eosinophilic pulmonary disorders warrant mention.

Churg-Strauss syndrome is characterized by tissue infiltration by eosinophils, necrotizing vasculitis, and extravascular granulomas; however, simultaneous occurrence of these three histologic changes is unusual. Asthma may occur simultaneously with or precede the clinical presentation of Churg-Strauss syndrome. The eosinophilia of Churg-Strauss syndrome (often > $1,500/mm^3$ and frequently > $5,000/mm^3$) greatly exceeds that of uncomplicated asthma. Bronchoalveolar lavage fluid eosinophilia in Churg-Strauss syndrome may exceed that of chronic eosinophilic pneumonia (33.6% ± 14.5% vs. 28.9% ± 27.4%). Additional clinical findings commonly include fever, weakness, weight loss, malaise, peripheral neuropathy, anemia, and increased sedimentation rate. The vasculitis of Churg-Strauss syndrome affects small arteries and veins, and typical fibrinoid necrosis of vessel walls occurs. The granulomas contain a central eosinophilic core with necrotic eosinophils (eosinophilic abscesses) and altered collagen fibers with fibrinoid swelling. Churg-Strauss syndrome generally responds well to glucocorticoids (prednisone, 40-60 mg/day); however, a subset of patients may additionally require adjunctive treatment with azathioprine or cyclophosphamide or both.

Allergic bronchopulmonary aspergillosis, a pulmonary hypersensitivity response to spores of the mold *Aspergillus fumigatus*, occurs in 1% to 2% of patients with asthma and 10% of patients with cystic fibrosis. T-cell activation, as demonstrated by increased levels of soluble IL-2 receptor in the peripheral blood, can be documented when the condition is flaring clinically. Mononuclear and T cells of affected patients produce heightened amounts of eosinophil colony-stimulating factor but not neutrophil colony-stimulating factor. This suggests one mechanism both for activation of the eosinophils and for the eosinophilia itself. Serotyping has shown a significant increase in the frequency of HLA-DR2 and HLA-DR5 antigens. Clinical features include peripheral blood and pulmonary eosinophilia, asthma, recurrent pulmonary infiltrates or mucoid impactions, and central, saccular bronchiectasis. A staging system for clinical disease has been proposed. Patients with allergic bronchopulmonary aspergillosis have precipitating antibodies and increased IgA serum levels to *Aspergillus fumigatus*. Patients show positive immediate and late skin test reactivity to *Aspergillus fumigatus*; however, a standardized skin test extract is needed because of variable skin test response to available reagents. These patients should not receive immunotherapy to *Aspergillus fumigatus*. Rather, treatment consists of prednisone to control flares of disease activity and to prevent development of bronchiectasis. The serum IgE levels are used as a guide to disease activity and prednisone dosage. Increasing IgE levels herald a flare of activity, whereas decreasing or stable IgE levels indicate disease remission. Recently, adjunctive use of the antifungal agent itraconazole has proved beneficial for treatment.

Löffler's syndrome is a self-limited condition, usually lasting weeks, characterized radiographically by migratory pulmonary infiltrates and moderate eosinophilia. Clinical symptoms are usually caused by pulmonary transit of larvae of the *Ascaris* species, although Löffler's syndrome may be drug-induced in some cases or idiopathic (30%). Symptoms include low-grade fever, blood-streaked sputum, cough, wheeze, substernal chest pain, and shortness of breath. The brief duration of symptoms and moderate degree of eosinophilia serve to distinguish this disorder from hypereosinophilic syndrome.

Chronic eosinophilic (Carrington's) pneumonia is a disorder of middle-aged women who present with high fever, night sweats, weight loss, and dyspnea. Interstitial and intra-alveolar eosinophilic infiltration, bronchiolitis, and eosinophilic abscesses on biopsy illustrate the intensity of the eosinophilic involvement in this disorder. Bronchiolar lavage fluid eosinophilia may exceed 40% and is comprised of hypodense, presumably activated eosinophils. Documentation of eosinophil degranulation has come from several lines of evidence. Patients have a uniformly excellent response to systemic glucocorticoids; however, relapse, necessitating re-treatment, occurs in up to a third of cases.

Bronchocentric granulomatosis may be a nonspecific hypersensitivity response to *Aspergillus* species or other intrabronchial antigens. The diagnosis is one of exclusion; about half of the cases have a history of asthma. Open lung biopsy shows massive infiltration of bronchi and bronchioles by eosinophils, lymphocytes, mononuclear cells, and multinucleated giant cells. Necrotic granulomas surrounded by epithelial cells involve the small bronchioles, but pulmonary vessels are usually spared. Extensive necrosis can lead to bronchostenosis and bronchiectasis. Clinical symptoms are similar to those of chronic eosinophilic pneumonia. Extrapulmonary involvement does not occur. Chest radiography may show atelectasis, segmental or lobar consolidation, large nodules, or mass lesions, but findings are variable. Oral glucocorticoid therapy is effective. Surgical resection of involved segments also has been used and has a high cure rate.

SUMMARY

Although, at first glance, workup of a patient with eosinophilia may seem daunting, keeping in mind a brief list of seven or eight major disease categories greatly simplifies matters. Insightful questioning about occupation, travel history, atopic disease, drug use, and major associated symptoms usually helps to narrow the list of differential possibilities. In addition, close monitoring of appropriate laboratory values and evolving clinical findings will generally focus the diagnosis. Correct diagnosis of eosinophilic disorders is important because effective treatment is available.

REFERENCE

1. Gleich GJ, Schroeter AL, Marcoux JP, Sachs MI, O'Connell EJ, Kohler PF. Episodic angioedema associated with eosinophilia. *N Engl J Med* 1984; 310: 1621-1626.

SUGGESTED READING

Brito-Babapulle F. Clonal eosinophilic disorders and the hypereosinophilic syndrome. *Blood Rev* 1997; 11: 129-145.

Butterfield JH. Hypereosinophilic syndromes. Established and new treatment options. *Biodrugs* 1997; 7: 341-355.

Butterfield JH, Leiferman KM, Gleich GJ. Eosinophil-associated diseases, in Samter's Immunologic Diseases (Frank MM, Austen KF, Claman HN, Unanue ER, eds.), 5th ed, vol 1. Little, Brown and Company, Boston, 1995, pp. 501-527.

Carrington CB, Addington WW, Goff AM, Madoff IM, Marks A, Schwaber JR, Gaensler EA. Chronic eosinophilic pneumonia. *N Engl J Med* 1969; 280: 787-798.

Denning DW, Van Wye JE, Lewiston NJ, Stevens DA. Adjunctive therapy of allergic bronchopulmonary aspergillosis with itraconazole. *Chest* 1991; 100: 813-819.

Frigas E, Loegering DA, Solley GO, Farrow GM, Gleich GJ. Elevated levels of the eosinophil granule major basic protein in the sputum of patients with bronchial asthma. *Mayo Clin Proc* 1981; 56: 345-353.

Imbeau SA, Nichols D, Flaherty D, Dickie H, Reed C. Relationships between prednisone therapy, disease activity, and the total serum IgE level in allergic bronchopulmonary aspergillosis. *J Allergy Clin Immunol* 1978; 62: 91-95.

Klein NC, Hargrove RL, Sleisenger MH, Jeffries GH. Eosinophilic gastroenteritis. *Medicine (Baltimore)* 1970; 49: 299-319.

Nicolas L, Scoles GA. Multiplex polymerase chain reaction for detection of *Dirofilaria immitis* (Filariidea: Onchocercidae) and *Wuchereria bancrofti* (Filarioidea: Dipetalonematidae) in their common vector *Aedes polynesiensis* (Diptera: Culicidae). *J Med Entomol* 1997; 34: 741-744.

Peters MS, Schroeter AL, Kephart GM, Gleich GJ. Localization of eosinophil granule major basic protein in chronic urticaria. *J Invest Dermatol* 1983; 81: 39-43.

Sen P, Gil C, Estrellas B, Middleton JR. Corticosteroid-induced asthma: a manifestation of limited hyperinfection syndrome due to *Strongyloides stercoralis*. *South Med J* 1995; 88: 923-927.

Silver RM, Heyes MP, Maize JC, Quearry B, Vionnet-Fuasset M, Sternberg EM. Scleroderma, fasciitis, and eosinophilia associated with the ingestion of tryptophan. *N Engl J Med* 1990; 322: 874-881.

Uhrbrand H. The number of circulating eosinophils: normal figures and spontaneous variations. *Acta Med Scand* 1992; 160: 99-104.

van Haelst Pisani C, Kovach JS, Kita H, Leiferman KM, Gleich GJ, Silver JE, Dennin R, Abrams JS. Administration of interleukin-2 (IL-2) results in increased plasma concentrations of IL-5 and eosinophilia in patients with cancer. *Blood* 1991; 78: 1538-1544.

Weller PF, Bubley GJ. The idiopathic hypereosinophilic syndrome. *Blood* 1994; 83: 2759-2779.

III LEUKEMIAS AND HEMATOPOIETIC STEM CELL TRANSPLANTATION

13 Leukocytosis and the Chronic Leukemias

Ayalew Tefferi, MD

Contents

INTRODUCTION

The peripheral blood contains three principal types of white blood cells (leukocytes): granulocytes, monocytes, and lymphocytes. The granules in the granulocytes may stain neutral (neutrophils), acidic (eosinophils), or basic (basophils) under special staining procedures. In addition, neutrophils in normal peripheral blood are usually terminally differentiated (polymorphonuclear neutrophils [PMNs]), and only few immediate precursors to the PMNs (band neutrophils) are appreciated. The total white blood cell count (WBC) is determined by an automated electronic counter and is reported as cells per microliter. The differential count, which determines the percentage of each white cell subtype, is estimated by either an automated counter or by a direct morphologic examination of a peripheral blood smear (Table 1).

LEUKOCYTOSIS

The first step in evaluating an increased WBC is to examine the white cell differential to determine which white cell type is in excess. The differential is usually reported along with the WBC at no extra charge. The next step is to obtain a peripheral blood smear study, which will help exclude the possibility of acute leukemia (leukemic blasts may be reported as lymphocytes or monocytes by the electronic counter or the inexperienced observer). The peripheral blood smear examination also will confirm the process as granulocytosis, lymphocytosis, or monocytosis and provide additional information on cell morphology and whether immature precursors are present or absent. The final step of the initial approach to leukocytosis is to determine whether the process represents a reactive state or a neoplastic (clonal) blood disorder.

From: *Primary Hematology*
Edited by: A. Tefferi © Mayo Foundation for Medical Education and Research, Rochester, MN

Table 1
Normal Peripheral White Blood Cell Count
(WBC) and Differential (Adult Values)

Total WBC	$3.5\text{-}10.5 \times 10^9/L$
Polymorphonuclear neutrophils, %	45-65
Band neutrophils, %	0-5
Eosinophils %	0-5
Basophils, %	0-3
Lymphocytes, %	15-40
Monocytes, %	2-8

Table 2
Conditions Causing Reactive Granulocytosis

Demargination	Release of marrow storage pool	Stimulation of granulocyte production
Exercise	Corticosteroid therapy	Acute infection
Stress	Sepsis	Myeloid growth factors
Psychiatric disorders	Heatstroke	Chronic inflammation
Epinephrine injection		Lithium
β-Agonists		Hemolytic anemia
Surgery		Immune thrombocytopenia
Myocardial infarction		Sickle cell anemia
Postictal state		Solid tumors
Acute illness		Lung cancer
Hyposplenism		Gastric cancer
		Breast cancer

Granulocytosis

There are several causes of reactive granulocytosis (neutrophilia) (Table 2). Half of the intravascular granulocytes circulate freely in the peripheral blood (the circulating pool), whereas the other half marginate along the endothelium of the blood vessels (the marginal pool). The WBC does not take the marginal pool into account and, as such, factors causing demargination may cause a modest increase in granulocytes (Table 2). Similarly, a mature granulocyte pool is also found in the bone marrow (the reserve pool), which is recruited to the peripheral blood during corticosteroid therapy or sepsis (endotoxin-mediated), causing granulocytosis. Also, several nonhematologic disease states can secondarily stimulate the bone marrow to produce excess granulocytes (cytokine-mediated) (Table 2).

Because the significant increase in neutrophils and their precursors associated with reactive granulocytosis resembles leukemia, the process has been called a leukemoid reaction. Alternatively, a neoplastic (clonal) proliferation of granulocytes or monocytes is responsible for a group of disorders that are collectively classified as chronic myeloid leukemias (Table 3).

Table 3
The Chronic Myeloid Leukemias and Their Peripheral Blood Features

Subtype	Ph^1	LAP score	Monocyte, %	Monocyte count (absolute)	Basophil count (absolute)	Myelocytes and metamyelocytes
CML	+	↓	N or ↓	N or ↑	↑ or N	Present
ACML	-	N or ↓	N or ↑	↑ or N	↓ or N	Present
CMML	-	N or ↓	↑	↑	↓ or N	Absent
CNL	-	↑	N or ↓	N or ↓	↓ or N	Absent
JMML	-	N or ↓	N or ↑	↑ or N	↓ or N	Present

Abbreviations: ACML, atypical CML; CML, chronic myelocytic leukemia; CMML, chronic myelo-monocytic leukemia; CNL, chronic neutrophilic leukemia; JMML, juvenile myelomonocytic leukemia; LAP, leukocyte alkaline phosphatase; N, normal; Ph^1, Philadelphia chromosome; ↑, increased; ↓, decreased; +, positive; -, negative.

Differentiating a Leukemoid Reaction From Chronic Leukemia

A leukemoid reaction must be differentiated from the chronic myeloid leukemias (Table 3). The degree of granulocytosis and left shift (the presence of immature granulocyte precursors such as band neutrophils and myelocytes) is more pronounced in the latter but is not definitive for distinguishing the two. Similarly, the leukocyte alkaline phosphatase (LAP) score is not definitive for differentiating a leukemoid reaction from a clonal process. It is true that the LAP score is usually low in chronic myelocytic leukemia (CML) and high in a leukemoid reaction. However, chronic myeloid leukemias other than CML also may display an increased LAP score (Table 3). Therefore, although it is still reasonable to order a LAP score, additional tests are necessary for definitive diagnosis. CML is readily diagnosed by demonstrating the Philadelphia (Ph^1) chromosome in either the bone marrow (karyotypic analysis) or the peripheral blood (fluorescent in situ hybridization). Diagnosis in the other myeloid leukemias requires morphologic and cytogenetic examination of both the peripheral blood and the bone marrow.

Lymphocytosis

An absolute lymphocyte count (ALC) of more than 5,000/μL is considered absolute lymphocytosis. However, relative lymphocytosis indicates a lymphocyte percentage of more than 50% despite a normal ALC. The term "lymphocytosis," either absolute or relative, should not be used when the WBC is less than 3,000/μL. The more appropriate terminology in such cases is absolute neutropenia.

The first and most critical step in the evaluation of lymphocytosis is a peripheral blood smear evaluation to examine the morphologic features of the cells. Normal lymphocytes are usually small (slightly larger than a red cell) and have a benign-appearing round nucleus occupying almost the whole cell. However, normal lymphocytes come in many forms, and approximately 15% of the normal lymphocyte population may have abundant cytoplasm with red cytoplasmic granules. These latter forms represent either T cytotoxic ($CD3^+CD8^+$) or natural killer ($CD3^-CD16^+$) cells and are classified as large granular lymphocytes (LGL).

Lymphocytosis with "Normal-Appearing" Small Lymphocytes

When absolute lymphocytosis with "normal-appearing" small lymphocytes is found in adults, the most likely diagnosis is B-cell chronic lymphocytic leukemia (CLL). In CLL, fragile cells (smudge cells) accompany the lymphocytosis. If the patient has palpable lymphadenopathy or splenomegaly, the diagnosis of CLL becomes even more likely. However, there are other types of chronic lymphoid leukemia that are not CLL and display "normal-appearing" lymphocytosis. Therefore, the necessary subsequent step is to order lymphocyte immunophenotyping by flow cytometry to confirm clonality and accurately classify the chronic lymphoid leukemia (see Table 10). Reactive lymphocytosis usually is associated with LGL morphology (T cytotoxic cells) and not B lymphocytosis.

Lymphocytosis with LGL Morphology

The most frequent cause of LGL excess is viral infection. Therefore, if the clinical situation is consistent with a viral infection, then further investigation can be deferred until the patient recovers and the peripheral blood smear is repeated (usually in 3 months). Similarly, a mild increase in LGL, without any symptoms or cytopenia, may not require further investigation. If the increase in LGL is associated with cytopenia or symptoms, then immunophenotyping by flow cytometry is recommended to differentiate a T-cell process from a natural killer cell process. In T lymphocytosis, a reactive process can be differentiated from a clonal process by performing a T-cell receptor gene rearrangement study of the peripheral blood. A similar test is currently not available for natural killer lymphocytosis.

Lymphocytosis with "Abnormal" Morphology

More than 90% of clonal lymphocytosis is represented by CLL. The remaining 10% of cases are various B-, T-, or natural killer cell disorders (see Table 10). Some of these disorders may present without an absolute increase in the total lymphocyte or leukocyte count. Therefore, in clinically suspected cases, a peripheral blood smear and immunophenotyping by flow cytometry should be done regardless of the WBC. The immunophenotypic profile and clinical features of the variant lymphoid leukemias are summarized (see Table 10).

Monocytosis

Relative monocytosis often occurs during recovery from chemotherapy or drug-induced neutropenia. Also, the presence of absolute monocytosis in the peripheral blood is highly suggestive of a Ph[1]-negative chronic myeloid leukemia (Table 3). In particular, the possibility of chronic myelomonocytic leukemia (CMML), atypical CML, or juvenile CML should be entertained. These disorders are discussed later in the chapter. Reactive monocytosis may accompany chronic infectious, inflammatory, or granulomatous processes. Monocytosis also has been described in patients with metastatic cancer, lymphoma, and histiocytosis.

THE CHRONIC MYELOID LEUKEMIAS

These disorders represent a clonal expansion, in the peripheral blood and bone marrow, of relatively mature granulocytes or monocytes. The presence of the Ph[1] chromosome separates CML from the other subtypes (Table 3). Classification of the Ph[1]-negative entities is based on peripheral blood and bone marrow morphologic characteristics (Table 3).

Chronic Myelocytic Leukemia

Clinically, CML is characterized by left-shifted peripheral blood granulocytosis that may or may not be associated with palpable splenomegaly. Most patients present in an asymptomatic chronic phase of the disease in which antiproliferative agents, including oral hydroxyurea and subcutaneous interferon-α, easily control the leukocytosis and splenomegaly. Unfortunately, the chronic phase is transient and lasts for a median of 4 years before it transforms into the accelerated or blast phase. The only treatments that have the potential to positively alter this natural history are allogeneic bone marrow transplantation (allo-BMT) and interferon-α therapy.

PATHOGENESIS

The consistent association of CML and the Ph[1] chromosome was first recognized in 1960. The Ph[1] chromosome is a cytogenetically detectable morphologic abnormality characterized by a shorter (dwarf) chromosome 22. Later, in 1973, chromosome banding revealed that the Ph[1] chromosome constituted a reciprocal translocation of chromosome material between the long arms of chromosomes 9 and 22, t(9;22)(q34;q11). Subsequently, in the early 1980s, t(9;22) was shown to involve genetic translocations of a cellular oncogene (c-*abl*) from chromosome 9 and the *bcr* gene on chromosome 22. Investigations of the chromosome breakpoints revealed that the breakpoint on chromosome 9 occurs in a relatively large (approximately 200 kilobases, kb) variable region of the *abl* gene. In contrast, the breakpoint on chromosome 22 occurs within a much smaller 5.8-kb region designated as the major breakpoint cluster region (M*bcr*) of the *bcr* gene. As such, t(9;22) results in a fused *bcr/abl* gene.

The fused *bcr/abl* gene is oncogenic and is transcribed into a chimeric 8.5-kb messenger RNA (mRNA) (instead of the normal 6- or 7-kb mRNA from c-*abl*) translating into a tyrosine-kinase enzyme with a molecular weight of 210 kilodaltons (kd). This is different from the normal protein product (tyrosine-kinase) of c-*abl*, which has a molecular weight of 145 kd. The P210 enzyme has enhanced tyrosine-kinase activity compared with the P145 enzyme and is located in the cytoplasm (near the cell membrane) rather than the nucleus (location of P145). Recent experiments involving animal models have confirmed the pathogenetic role of the *bcr/abl* fusion gene and its product (P210) in CML. It appears that the constitutive (i.e., without stimulus) activation of the P210 enzyme initiates the oncogenic signal. The downstream events of the *bcr/abl*-induced oncogenesis are largely unknown.

LABORATORY METHODS OF DIAGNOSIS AND DISEASE MONITORING

Peripheral blood findings that are suggestive of CML include the myelocyte bulge (a disproportionate increase in myelocyte percentage) and basophilia. Although absolute monocytosis may be present, monocyte percentage is usually less than 5%. Regardless, neither this morphologic profile nor a low LAP score provides a definitive diagnosis of CML. For this, the demonstration of the 9;22 chromosome translocation is required.

Karyotypic analysis (conventional cytogenetics) reveals the Ph[1] chromosome in approximately 95% of patients with CML. This test requires analysis of cells in metaphase (dividing cells) and therefore usually necessitates bone marrow examination. Five percent of the patients have either variants of the Ph[1] chromosome or a submicroscopic translocation that is not revealed by conventional cytogenetic methods. These cases may be identified by fluorescence in situ hybridization (FISH) technology, which allows detection of t(9;22) in both metaphase and interphase cells and can be done on a wide variety of tissue types, including peripheral blood and bone marrow. The method uses DNA probes for regions at or near the chromosome region of interest, and fusion signals, detected by fluorescence, indicate translocation.

Conventional cytogenetic studies have been used to assess cytogenetic responses in patients with CML being treated with interferon-α. Cytogenetic responses have operationally been defined as complete (0% Ph[1] metaphases), major (1%-32% Ph[1] metaphases), and minor (33%-66% Ph[1] metaphases). Both randomized and nonrandomized studies have shown a survival advantage for complete or major karyotypic responders, whereas in the absence of a cytogenetic response, survival is similar to that observed with hydroxyurea therapy.

The choice of the laboratory method used to detect the 9;22 translocation in CML depends on whether the indication is for diagnosis, monitoring of treatment response, or evaluating minimal residual disease. For diagnosis, conventional cytogenetic studies are recommended because they may reveal additional cytogenetic abnormalities. If the results of cytogenetic studies do not reveal the Ph[1] chromosome, FISH should be performed to detect masked t(9;22) translocations. Currently, conventional cytogenetics is the only method with established value for following patients undergoing interferon-α therapy. Polymerase chain reaction (PCR) assays are, by far, the most sensitive methods for detecting minimal residual disease after curative treatment. However, the clinical relevance of minimal residual disease in CML has not been clarified.

PROGNOSIS

Chronic-phase disease is clearly more desirable (median survival of 4 years) than accelerated- or blast-phase disease (median survival of 6 months). Patients with chronic-phase disease are usually asymptomatic and their high leukocyte count and large spleen are easily controlled by drug therapy. The loss of disease control with drugs indicates transformation into the accelerated phase, and the blast phase is characterized by the presence of more than 30% leukemic blasts in the bone marrow. Often, patients with the blast phase of the disease are symptomatic and manifest extreme leukocytosis with circulating blasts and anemia. Bone marrow examination may reveal the acquisition of additional chromosome abnormalities, including an extra Ph[1] chromosome, trisomy 8, or isochromosome 17.

In general, the risk of blastic transformation in the first 2 years is 13%. Thereafter, the annual risk remains constant at 25%. Independent prognostic indicators of poor survival include marked splenomegaly, thrombocytosis, the presence of circulating blasts, and advanced age (Sokal's clinical prognostic criteria). The application of these criteria may identify risk groups with median survival that ranges from 2 to 6 years. The prognostic relevance of additional cytogenetic abnormalities, at diagnosis, is not clear. Finally, treatment outcome, with either allo-BMT or interferon-α, is best when therapy is instituted during the early period of chronic-phase disease (< 1 year from the diagnosis).

TREATMENT

The four major therapeutic options for CML are oral busulfan (starting dosage 4-6 mg/day), oral hydroxyurea (starting dosage 500 mg 3 times daily), subcutaneous interferon-α (starting dosage 5 million units/m^2 per day), and allo-BMT. All of these treatments cause hematologic remission in most patients with CML. The first three options are not curative, whereas allo-BMT may cure some patients. Neither busulfan nor hydroxyurea prevents blastic transformation, and thus they do not alter the natural history

Table 4
Clinical Properties of Drugs Used in Chronic Myelocytic Leukemia

	Hydroxyurea	*Interferon-α*
Drug class	Antimetabolite	Biologic response modifier
Mechanism of action	Inhibits ribonucleotide reductase	Myelosuppressive
Specificity	Affects all cell lines	Affects all cell lines
Pharmacology	Half-life $\cong$ 4 hours, renal excretion	Kidney is main site of metabolism
Starting dose	500 mg orally 3 times daily	5 million units/m^2 subcutaneously daily
Onset of action	$\cong$ 3-5 days	May take more than 1 year to achieve cytogenetic remission
Side effects observed in > 10% of patients	Oral ulcers, hyperpigmentation, nail changes	Flulike syndrome, fatigue, anorexia, weight loss, lack of ambition, alopecia
Side effects observed in < 10% of patients	Leg ulcers, diarrhea	Confusion, depression, autoimmune thyroiditis or arthritis, pruritus, myalgia
Rare side effects	Fever, liver function test abnormalities	Pruritus, hyperlipidemia, transaminasemia
Contraindications	Pregnancy, childbearing potential, breast-feeding	Anecdotal reports suggest safety during pregnancy
Cost	Annual = $1,700.00 for 500 mg 3 times daily	Annual = $40,000.00 for full dose

of the disease. This result is consistent with their inability to suppress the Ph[1]-positive clone. When the two drugs were compared head-to-head, overall survival and subsequent BMT outcome were significantly better with hydroxyurea. Furthermore, treatment with busulfan may be complicated by the development of prolonged pancytopenia, Addison disease-like syndrome, and interstitial lung disease. Therefore, we currently do not use busulfan as initial therapy for CML.

In contrast to hydroxyurea, both interferon-α and allo-BMT have the potential to prolong survival in CML because both have the ability to suppress the Ph[1]-positive clone. As such, survival benefit in patients treated with interferon-α is limited to patients who attain a complete or major karyotypic response (see page 180 for the definition of cytogenetic response). Unfortunately, only 20% to 40% of the patients treated with interferon-α are able to achieve this favorable response. Recent studies suggest that the addition of subcutaneous cytarabine (10 mg daily) may double the cytogenetic remission rates induced by interferon-α. Low-risk patients (according to Sokal's criteria) and those with early disease (< 1 year of diagnosis) have a significantly better chance of achieving a major cytogenetic response. In general, the 10-year survival rates of patients treated with interferon-α depend on the degree of treatment response and are estimated at 57% for complete hematologic responders, 68% for any cytogenetic responders, and 80% for major karyotypic responders (compared with 10% with hydroxyurea and 50%-60% with allo-BMT). The median time to achieve a cytogenetic response to interferon-α therapy

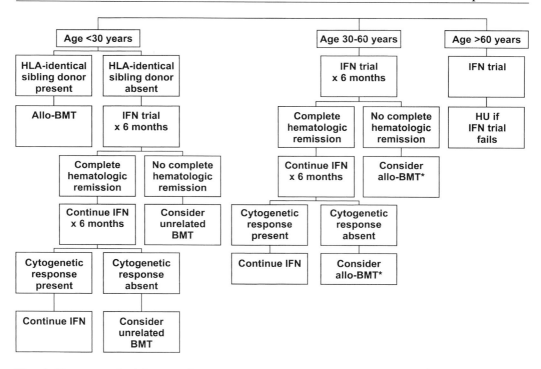

Fig. 1. Treatment decision tree in chronic myelocytic leukemia. Allo, allogeneic; BMT, bone marrow transplantation; HLA, human histocompatibility leukocyte antigen; HU, hydroxyurea; IFN, interferon-α. *HLA-identical sibling donor is preferable. If such a donor is absent, a non-sibling-related or HLA-matched unrelated donor may be considered under protocol treatment programs.

is approximately 1 year, and this causes concern regarding a possible delay in the timing of BMT. Table 4 summarizes the clinical properties of hydroxyurea and interferon-α.

Currently, the only curative therapy in CML is allo-BMT. Unfortunately, as many as a third of patients who have transplantation may die of transplant-related complications, and the survivors may experience extensive graft-versus-host disease and disease relapse. Therefore, long survival with good quality of life, rather than "cure," is the relevant goal in the treatment of CML. The outcome of allo-BMT depends on several factors, including age (age < 30 years is preferred), related versus unrelated donor (sibling donor is preferred), the degree of tissue compatibility between donor and recipient (HLA-identical match is preferred), and timing of transplant (< 1 year of diagnosis is preferred). When all these factors are favorable, the "cure" rate approaches 80% and the quality of life after transplantation is acceptable. Otherwise, long-term survival may be less than 30%, and the survivors may not have a good quality of life. In general, long-term survival with allo-BMT is superior to that with interferon-α therapy when it is applied to young patients (age < 30 years) and to those with high-risk disease. Figure 1 outlines a treatment decision tree that takes these issues into consideration. Finally, consistent with the observation that the disease-relapse rate is less in patients with graft-versus-host disease, donor lymphocyte infusions have been shown to restore remissions in patients who have relapse after allo-BMT. The role of autologous BMT in CML remains undefined.

Atypical Chronic Myelocytic Leukemia

Atypical CML is operationally defined as a Ph[1]-negative myeloid leukemia that is associated with the presence of more than 15% immature myeloid precursors (promyelocytes, myelocytes, metamyelocytes), dysgranulopoiesis, a monocyte percentage of more than 3%, and no basophilia. The dysgranulopoiesis, monocyte percentage, and lack of basophilia also characterize CMML and distinguish atypical CML and CMML from CML (Table 3). However, the distinction between atypical CML and CMML is not always clear, and a certain degree of overlap exists. In general, the percentage of myeloid precursors is less than 15% in CMML, whereas the monocyte percentage may not be increased in atypical CML (it is often increased in CMML). Atypical CML is associated with the worst prognosis among the chronic myeloid leukemias: the median survival is less than 1 year. Current therapy is ineffective, and BMT is recommended for suitable candidates.

Chronic Myelomonocytic Leukemia

CMML is currently classified under the myelodysplastic syndromes (see Chapter 11). However, certain cases of CMML may easily be categorized as atypical CML (see Table 3 for comparative features). Currently, we restrict use of the term CMML to patients with peripheral monocytosis (monocytes > 1,000/µL) that is associated with a concomitant increase in monocyte percentage and not associated with substantial left-shifted leukocytosis. The latter feature may be best described as atypical CML. The prognosis of patients with CMML is better than that of patients with atypical CML and depends on bone marrow blast percentage and the presence of anemia. Non-anemic patients with less than 5% bone marrow blasts can expect a median survival of more than 5 years and do not require specific therapy. When the bone marrow blast percentage exceeds 5%, expected survival may shorten to less than 2 years. Unfortunately, chemotherapy does not alter the natural history of the disease, and suitable candidates are often considered for BMT.

Chronic Neutrophilic Leukemia

Chronic neutrophilic leukemia (CNL) is an extremely rare disorder; fewer than 50 cases have been reported in the English literature. The characteristic clinical presentation is mature neutrophilia (> 90% PMNs) without basophilia or monocytosis. The disease should be distinguished from CML, CMML, and atypical CML. Unlike CML, the Ph[1] chromosome (or *bcr/abl* fusion) is absent and the LAP score is high. Unlike CMML, there is no peripheral blood monocytosis. Unlike atypical CML, immature neutrophil precursors and dysgranulopoiesis in the peripheral blood are absent. The disease often affects the elderly, and the presence of hepatosplenomegaly helps to distinguish CNL from leukemoid reactions. Prognosis is variable; some patients have a long chronic phase (> 5 years) and others experience transformation into acute leukemia. Various treatments, including interferon-α, busulfan, and hydroxyurea, have been used with either transient or no benefit. BMT has been successful in suitable candidates. Finally, a CNL-like syndrome has been associated with Ph[1]-positive CML with atypical chromosome 22 breakpoints (µ*bcr*), plasma cell proliferative disorders, the myelodysplastic syndrome, and chronic myeloproliferative disorders.

Table 5
The Rai Clinical Staging System in Chronic Lymphocytic Leukemia

	Stage				
	0	*I*	*II*	*III*	*IV*
Lymphocytosis (lymphocytes, $\geq$ 5,000/µL)	+	+	+	+	+
Lymphadenopathy	-	+	+/-	+/-	+/-
Splenomegaly	-	-	+	+/-	+/-
Anemia (hemoglobin, < 11 g/dL)	-	-	-	+	+/-
Thrombocytopenia (platelets, < 100,000/µL)	-	-	-	-	+
Median survival, all patients, yr	12+	8.5	6	1.5	1.5

Juvenile Myelomonocytic Leukemia

Juvenile myelomonocytic leukemia (JMML) was formerly known as juvenile CML. It usually occurs in early childhood and is characterized by hepatosplenomegaly, adenopathy, anemia, thrombocytopenia, leukocytosis, monocytosis, and cutaneous involvement. Biologic characteristics of the disease include hypersensitivity of myeloid progenitors to the in vitro exposure of granulocyte-macrophage colony-stimulating factor and abnormalities in the neurofibromatosis and *RAS* genes, whereas chromosome abnormalities are rare. Prognosis is dismal, and drug therapy has been ineffective. Allo-BMT may result in durable remission in less than a fourth of patients who have the procedure.

THE CHRONIC LYMPHOID LEUKEMIAS

These disorders represent a clonal expansion of relatively mature lymphocytes (see Table 10). Among these, the most frequent in the Western Hemisphere is chronic lymphocytic leukemia (CLL), which constitutes more than 90% of the chronic lymphoid leukemias. It is important to distinguish CLL from the other variants because of major differences in prognosis and treatment (see Table 10). The peripheral blood morphologic examination and lymphocyte immunophenotyping by flow cytometry complement each other in ensuring an accurate diagnosis (see Table 10).

Chronic Lymphocytic Leukemia

When absolute lymphocytosis with "normal-appearing" morphology is found in adults, the most likely diagnosis is B-cell CLL. However, ontogenetically mature lymphocytosis is not always either "normal-appearing" or CLL. Therefore, lymphocyte immunophenotyping by flow cytometry should be done in all cases of absolute lymphocytosis to confirm the diagnosis of CLL and exclude the possibility of other lymphoid leukemias (see Table 10). However, a bone marrow biopsy or cytogenetic study is not necessary to diagnose CLL.

CLINICAL ASPECTS AND PROGNOSIS

Clinical staging remains the most practical and reliable prognostic indicator (Table 5). Accordingly, patients presenting with lymphocytosis only are considered to have stage

Table 6
Current Indications for Treatment in Chronic Lymphocytic Leukemia

Stage III or IV disease
Stage 0, I, or II disease accompanied by one of the following:
    Bulky lymphadenopathy (> 10 cm in maximal diameter)
    Marked splenomegaly (palpable at > 6 cm below the costal margin)
    Lymphocyte doubling time of < 6 months associated with a white blood cell count
        > 50,000/μL
    A white blood cell count > 100,000/μL
    Disease-related constitutional symptoms

Table 7
Conventional Alkylator Therapy in Chronic Lymphocytic Leukemia

Schedule	Chlorambucil (oral)	Prednisone (oral)
I	4-8 mg/day	± 60 mg/day × 5 days each month
II	20 mg/m^2 every 2 weeks	± 60 mg/day × 5 days each month
III	40 mg/m^2 every 4 weeks	± 60 mg/day × 5 days each month

0 disease (low risk). Patients with stable stage 0 disease and a WBC of less than 30,000/μL have a near-normal life expectancy. Prognosis is also excellent in noncytopenic patients with lymphadenopathy (stage I) or splenomegaly (stage II) (intermediate risk). However, once anemia (stage III) or thrombocytopenia (stage IV) develops, survival is substantially compromised (high risk). Cytopenias not directly caused by decreased bone marrow reserve from leukemic infiltration do not necessarily upgrade the clinical stage. These cytopenias include anemia of chronic disease and immune thrombocytopenic purpura.

In addition to clinical staging, several laboratory factors, including cytogenetic abnormalities such as trisomy 12, which is found in 15% of patients, bone marrow infiltration pattern, and lymphocyte doubling time, have been reported to have independent prognostic value. However, their clinical impact is often not significant enough to warrant stage-independent treatment decisions. CLL is associated with hypogammaglobulinemia in 50% of cases, monoclonal gammopathy in 5%, autoimmune hemolytic anemia in 10%, and immune thrombocytopenic purpura in 2%.

TREATMENT

Not all patients with CLL require therapy. In patients with stable stage 0, I, or II disease, observation without specific therapy is at least equivalent to treatment with chlorambucil. Therefore, we do not recommend treatment for these patients. Treatment is indicated for patients with stage III and IV disease and for those with active early-stage disease (Table 6).

Until recently, oral chlorambucil alone or in combination with prednisone had been the initial treatment of choice for active CLL. It can be administered either continuously or intermittently (Table 7). The dose may be increased or decreased depending on its effect on both the disease and the hemoglobin and platelet values. In addition, patients should be given allopurinol (300 mg/day; 100 mg/day if the creatinine value is > 2 mg/dL) until the disease bulk is adequately reduced.

Table 8
NCI-WG Response Criteria in Chronic Lymphocytic Leukemia

Response	Criteria
Complete remission (CR)	No symptoms, nodes, or spleen. Lymphocyte count ≤ 4,000/µL, hemoglobin > 11 g/dL, platelet count > 100,000/µL, absolute neutrophil count > 1,500/µL, bone marrow lymphocytes < 30%
Nodular partial remission (nPR)	No symptoms, nodes, or spleen. Lymphocyte count ≤ 4,000/µL, hemoglobin > 11 g/dL, platelet count > 100,000/µL, absolute neutrophil count > 1,500/µL, bone marrow lymphocytes < 30%, persistent bone marrow nodules
Partial remission (PR)	Must fulfill 1) a ≥ 50% reduction in lymphocyte count, 2) a ≥ 50% decrease in either lymph node or spleen size, and 3) hemoglobin > 11 g/dL or platelet count > 100,000/µL or absolute neutrophil count > 1,500/µL
Overall remission (OR)	CR and PR

Abbreviation: NCI-WG, National Cancer Institute-sponsored Working Group.

Table 9
Treatment Schedule for Fludarabine or 2-Chlorodeoxyadenosine
(2-CdA) in Chronic Lymphocytic Leukemia

Agent	Dosage	Route	Frequency
Fludarabine	25 mg/m^2 per day × 5	1/2-hour intravenous infusion	Monthly × 6
2-CdA	0.1 mg/kg per day × 7	24-hour intravenous infusion	Monthly × 6
2-CdA	0.14 mg/kg per day × 5	2-hour intravenous infusion	Monthly × 6

Chlorambucil does not cure CLL but provides transient symptomatic relief and reduction of tumor bulk. According to the National Cancer Institute-sponsored Working Group (NCI-WG) on CLL response criteria (Table 8), the complete remission and overall remission rates with conventional doses of chlorambucil are less than 5% and 50%, respectively. Treatment with alkylator-based combination chemotherapy has not improved the results achieved with chlorambucil alone. Patients who respond to treatment with chlorambucil have a median survival of 3 to 4 years and median remission duration of approximately 2 years. Achievement of a complete remission, instead of partial remission, with alkylator-based chemotherapy may not be associated with improved outcome in regard to either remission duration or survival.

In the past 10 years, the purine nucleoside analogues have been shown to be effective in both previously untreated and treatment-refractory patients with CLL (Table 9). As a result, these agents have become the salvage treatment of choice in CLL. In regard to previously untreated patients, remission rates with purine nucleoside analogues appear to be superior to those achieved with chlorambucil-based chemotherapy. However, interstudy differences in patient selection and response criteria do not allow valid comparisons of efficacy and toxicity. Treatment with purine nucleoside analogues may be complicated by protracted cytopenias, opportunistic infections, and hemolytic anemia.

In a recent North American intergroup randomized trial, single-agent fludarabine was compared with chlorambucil alone or in combination with fludarabine in previously untreated patients with CLL. Complete and overall remission rates, according to the NCI-WG response criteria, were 27% and 70%, respectively, for fludarabine, 3% and 45% for chlorambucil, and 25% and 65% when the two agents were combined. Although responses were significantly more durable with fludarabine than with chlorambucil (median response duration of 32 versus 18 months, respectively), the incidence of life-threatening toxicities was significantly higher when the two drugs were combined (32%). In another randomized study of previously untreated patients which compared fludarabine with CAP (cyclophosphamide, Adriamycin [doxorubicin], prednisone), the complete remission rates were 23% and 17%, respectively, and the overall remission rates were 71% and 60%, respectively. Median response durations were 27 and 9 months for fludarabine and CAP, respectively.

Thus, in CLL, the quality and durability of treatment response are significantly better with fludarabine than with chlorambucil given in conventional doses. However, despite the use of fludarabine or 2-chlorodeoxyadenosine as front-line therapy, most patients have relapse within 3 years. Furthermore, in most patients with "true pathologic remissions," minimal residual disease is detectable with more sensitive molecular methods. Therefore, neither fludarabine nor 2-chlorodeoxyadenosine is curative in CLL, and single-agent therapy with a purine nucleoside analogue is unlikely to have an overall impact on survival.

THE ROLE OF BONE MARROW TRANSPLANTATION IN CHRONIC LYMPHOCYTIC LEUKEMIA

Both allogeneic and autologous BMT have been evaluated in the treatment of CLL. The experience is limited to fewer than 100 reported cases in each group, and most of the patients had either refractory disease or a poor prognosis at the time of transplantation. In allo-BMT, the reported rates of disease-free survival were 43% to 54% and those of treatment-related mortality were 10% to 45%. The available data suggest that the prior use of fludarabine and earlier consideration of BMT may reduce treatment-related mortality. Several studies are currently investigating the value of autologous bone marrow or peripheral blood stem cell transplantation in CLL.

FINAL COMMENTS ON THE TREATMENT OF CHRONIC LYMPHOCYTIC LEUKEMIA

There is no question that fludarabine has substantial antitumor activity in CLL. Furthermore, the quality and duration of fludarabine-induced remission may be superior to those of chlorambucil-induced remission. However, most patients treated with either fludarabine or chlorambucil have relapse in 3 years and die of their disease. Therefore, the impetus to consider allo-BMT as front-line therapy in patients younger than 60 years with treatment-requiring CLL is appreciated. At the same time, transplant-related mortality and morbidity rates remain high (25%-50%), and it is therefore reasonable to postpone the procedure until the time of relapse. In patients older than 60 years or in those without a related marrow donor, participation in clinical trials that may or may not include

Table 10
Subsets of Chronic Lymphoid Leukemia and Their
Immunophenotypic Profile and Clinical Features

Type	Clinical features
B-cell chronic lymphocytic leukemia (CLL) $CD20^+$(dim)sIg(dim)$CD5^+$ $CD23^+$	By far the most frequent. Discussed in detail in this chapter
Hairy cell leukemia (B cell) $CD20^+$(bright)sIg(bright)$CD11c^+$ (bright)$CD5^-CD25^+$(bright)$CD103^+$	Usual presentation in hairy cell leukemia is pancytopenia (monocytopenia is characteristic), splenomegaly, and recurrent mycobacterial or other opportunistic infections. Middle-aged men are mostly affected. Peripheral blood shows mononuclear cells with indented nuclei and tartrate-resistant acid phosphatase (TRAP)-positive cytoplasm. Bone marrow aspirate yields a dry tap because of reticulin fibrosis, and biopsy reveals characteristic "fried-egg" appearance (monotonous round cells with spindle-shaped nuclei separated by abundant cytoplasm). Current treatment of choice is one course of 2-chlorodeoxyadenosine (0.1 mg/kg per day continuous 24-hour infusion × 7 days or 0.14 mg/kg per day in a 2-hour infusion × 5 days). 2-Deoxycoformycin (4 mg/m^2 every 2 weeks × 12 cycles) and interferon-α (2 million units/m^2 subcutaneously 3 times a week × 1 year) are effective alternative agents
Hairy cell leukemia variant (B cell) $CD20^+$(bright)sIg(bright)$CD11c^+$ (bright)$CD5^-CD25^-CD103^-$	Hairy cell leukemia variant (HCL-V) has peripheral blood, bone marrow, and spleen morphologic features similar to those of HCL. In contrast, TRAP stain and CD25 expression are absent in HCL-V. Usual presentation is marked splenomegaly and leukocytosis. Patients with HCL-V do not respond well to treatment used in HCL
Mantle cell lymphoma (B cell) $CD20^+$(bright)sIg(bright)$CD5^+CD23^-$ $CD22^+FMC7^+$	May resemble CLL both morphologically and phenotypically. Characterized by an 11;14 chromosome translocation (involving the *bcl*-1 oncogene from chromosome 11). As a result, cyclin D (a proliferation-regulating protein) is overexpressed. The disease is morphologically similar to low-grade lymphoma but is clinically akin to aggressive intermediate-grade lymphoma. As such, its treatment is like that of intermediate-grade lymphoma (see

Table 10 continued

Type	Clinical features
	Chapter 10). Regardless, the outcome is still poor
Small cleaved cell leukemia (B cell) CD20$^+$(bright)sIg(bright)CD5$^-$CD10$^+$	Leukemic phase of low-grade follicular lymphoma. Characterized by a 14;18 chromosome translocation (involving the *bcl*-2 oncogene from chromosome 18). Treated the same way as low-grade lymphoma (see Chapter 10)
Splenic marginal zone lymphoma (B cell) CD20$^+$(bright)CD22$^+$sIg(bright), CD5$^-$CD10$^-$CD25$^-$CD103$^-$CD11c$^{+/-}$	Marginal zone lymphoma (MZL) includes three entities: splenic lymphoma with villous lymphocytes (splenic MZL), monocytoid B-cell lymphoma (nodal MZL), and mucosa-associated lymphoid tissue lymphoma (MALToma). Of these, splenic MZL may present with absolute lymphocytosis that may or may not be associated with villous lymphocytes. Usual presentation is marked splenomegaly with little lymphadenopathy. IgM monoclonal gammopathy is often detected. Treatment is deferred in asymptomatic patients. Splenectomy is the treatment of choice for cytopenia. Fludarabine has been successfully used for advanced disease
Lymphoplasmacytoid lymphoma (Waldenström's) CD20$^+$CD22$^+$sIg(bright)CD5$^-$ CD10$^-$CD25$^-$CD103$^-$CD11c$^{+/-}$	May occasionally present with peripheral lymphocytosis. The disorder is always associated with IgM monoclonal gammopathy. Treatment is similar to that of CLL
B-Prolymphocytic leukemia CD20$^+$(bright),sIg(bright), CD5$^-$CD23$^-$FMC7$^+$	Characterized by large cells with prominent nucleoli. Usual clinical presentation includes marked splenomegaly with little lymphadenopathy and high white blood cell count. The prognosis is worse than that of CLL. Some patients with CLL may undergo prolymphocytoid transformation. Conventional chemotherapy results in limited transient benefit. Purine nucleoside analogues have been shown to be effective, but the remissions are not durable. Splenectomy and splenic irradiation were reported to be successful in single case reports
T-Prolymphocytic leukemia (T-helper CLL) CD3$^+$CD7$^+$CD4$^+$CD5$^+$CD8$^{+/-}$CD25$^-$	Clinical presentation is similar to that of B-prolymphocytic leukemia, but there is frequent skin involvement. Prognosis is extremely poor, and early consideration for allogeneic bone marrow transplantation is recommended.

Table 10 continued

Type	Clinical features
	Transient responses to treatment with 2-deoxycoformycin have been reported
Hepatosplenic γ/δ T-cell lymphoma CD2$^+$(bright)CD3$^+$CD7$^+$CD16$^+$CD4$^-$ CD8$^{-/+}$CD5$^-$CD25$^-$ γ/δ receptor$^+$	Affects young adult males who present with marked hepatosplenomegaly. May be associated with isochromosome 7q, and prognosis is poor. Chemotherapy has not been effective
T-Large granular lymphocyte leukemia CD3$^+$CD8$^+$(dim)CD2$^+$(dim)CD4$^-$ CD57$^+$CD16$^+$	Neutropenia is the usual presentation. Anemia and vasculitis may develop. Most patients do not require therapy and do not have progression. Immunosuppressive therapy (prednisone 1 mg/kg orally daily, cyclophosphamide 50-100 mg orally daily, or cyclosporine 300 mg orally twice a day) is effective but is indicated only for symptomatic patients (i.e., do not treat asymptomatic neutropenia)
Adult T-cell leukemia/lymphoma (ATL) CD3$^+$(dim)CD7$^-$CD4$^+$CD25$^+$	Prevalent in Japan and the Caribbean basin. Associated with human T-cell leukemia/lymphoma virus (HTLV-1 virus) (another HTLV-1 virus-associated disease is tropical spastic paresis). ATL develops in only 5% of patients infected with HTLV-1. Opportunistic infections are prevalent in patients with ATL, and clinical presentation may be smoldering (circulating leukemic cells with normal lymphocyte count), chronic leukemic type (increased lymphocyte count with or without lymphadenopathy and skin disease), lymphoma type (lymphadenopathy without lymphocytosis), and acute type (bone marrow involvement, hepatosplenomegaly, hypercalcemia). The first two groups of patients have long survival, and the second two groups die within weeks unless treated. Latest treatment is the combination of zidovudine (AZT) and interferon
Sézary syndrome (T cell) CD3$^+$(dim)CD7$^-$CD4$^+$CD8$^-$CD25$^-$	Cutaneous lymphoma (mycosis fungoides). Erythroderma with severe pruritus with or without lymphadenopathy. Treatment depends on extent of disease. Non-erythrodermic skin disease is treated with topical nitrogen mustard, whole-body electron beam irradiation, or photochemotherapy with psoralen and ultraviolet A light (PUVA). Refractory or erythrodermic patients are treated with

Table 10 continued

Type	Clinical features
	photopheresis (extracorporeal photochemotherapy) or interferon-α. Treatment of systemic disease is palliative and may involve the use of combination chemotherapy or purine nucleoside analogues
Chronic natural killer cell lymphocytosis CD3$^-$CD20$^-$CD16$^+$CD56$^+$	Clinically similar to T-large granular lymphocyte leukemia. Treated the same way

autologous bone marrow or peripheral blood stem cell transplantation is encouraged. It is too early to comment on the value of autologous BMT, unrelated BMT, or monoclonal antibody treatment in CLL.

Treatment Summary in Chronic Lymphocytic Leukemia

Stable early-stage CLL (Rai 0, I, II) requires no therapy. Advanced-stage disease (Rai III, IV) or early-stage disease with a high tumor burden or rapid progression requires initial therapy with chlorambucil (with or without prednisone) or fludarabine. Patients in whom chlorambucil fails are offered salvage therapy with fludarabine, and vice versa. Allo-BMT is a reasonable consideration for patients younger than 60 years in whom both fludarabine and chlorambucil fail. The role of allo-BMT as part of the initial therapy in CLL remains to be defined. Various combination chemotherapy regimens are used for palliative treatment in patients who are not candidates for allo-BMT and in whom initial therapy with chlorambucil and fludarabine has failed. The role of autologous BMT and monoclonal antibody therapy is currently being investigated.

Other Chronic Lymphoid Leukemias

The laboratory and clinical features of these disorders are summarized in Table 10.

SUGGESTED READING

Cheson BD, Bennett JM, Grever M, Kay N, Keating MJ, O'Brien S, Rai KR. National Cancer Institute-sponsored Working Group guidelines for chronic lymphocytic leukemia: revised guidelines for diagnosis and treatment. *Blood* 1996; 87: 4990-4997.

Italian Cooperative Study Group on Chronic Myeloid Leukemia and Italian Group for Bone Marrow Transplantation. Monitoring treatment and survival in chronic myeloid leukemia. *J Clin Oncol* 1999; 17: 1858-1868.

Kantarjian HM, O'Brien S, Anderlini P, Talpaz M. Treatment of myelogenous leukemia: current status and investigational options. *Blood* 1996; 87: 3069-3081.

Keating MJ, O'Brien S, Kantarjian H, Plunkett W, Estey E, Koller C, Beran M, Freireich EJ. Long-term follow-up of patients with chronic lymphocytic leukemia treated with fludarabine as a single agent. *Blood* 1993; 81: 2878-2884.

Kroft SH, Finn WG, Peterson LC. The pathology of the chronic lymphoid leukaemias. *Blood Rev* 1995; 9: 234-250.

Michallet M, Archimbaud E, Bandini G, Rowlings PA, Deeg HJ, Gahrton G, Montserrat E, Rozman C, Gratwohl A, Gale RP, for the European Group for Blood and Marrow Transplantation and the International Bone Marrow Transplant Registry. HLA-identical sibling bone marrow transplantation in younger patients with chronic lymphocytic leukemia. *Ann Intern Med* 1996; 124: 311-315.

Rai KR, Sawitsky A, Cronkite EP, Chanana AD, Levy RN, Pasternack BS. Clinical staging of chronic lymphocytic leukemia. *Blood* 1975; 46: 219-234.

Saven A, Lemon RH, Kosty M, Beutler E, Piro LD. 2-Chlorodeoxyadenosine activity in patients with untreated chronic lymphocytic leukemia. *J Clin Oncol* 1995; 13: 570-574.

Shepherd PC, Ganesan TS, Galton DA. Haematological classification of the chronic myeloid leukaemias. *Baillières Clin Haematol* 1987; 1: 887-906.

Tefferi A, Litzow MR, Noel P, Dewald GW. Chronic granulocytic leukemia: recent information on pathogenesis, diagnosis, and disease monitoring. *Mayo Clin Proc* 1997; 72: 445-452.

14 Acute Leukemia

Mark R. Litzow, MD

Contents

INTRODUCTION

Acute leukemia is a malignant disorder arising in immature hematopoietic cells. Studies using X-chromosome inactivation cellular mosaicism have confirmed the clonal origin of acute leukemia and demonstrated that the leukemic process can begin in immature cells not yet committed to differentiation to a particular lineage or in more mature cells committed to develop along a particular lineage pathway (Fig. 1, Plate 16). The failure of these cells to fully differentiate and the growth advantage they demonstrate over normal cells result in cytopenias that can become life-threatening over a matter of months. Acute leukemia is broadly divided into acute myelogenous leukemia (AML) and acute lymphoblastic leukemia (ALL). This chapter reviews the etiology, classification, clinical manifestations, prognosis, and treatment of acute leukemia.

ETIOLOGY

The initial cellular events that precipitate the onset of acute leukemia are essentially unknown. Several genetic and environmental factors, however, have been associated with the development of acute leukemia. In the case of AML, an increased incidence has been noted among individuals of Eastern European Jewish extraction, in family members of patients with AML, and in association with genetic disorders such as Down's syndrome, Fanconi's anemia, Bloom syndrome, and ataxia-telangiectasia. Patients with these genetic disorders also have an increased risk for development of ALL. Environmental factors that are thought to cause DNA damage and precipitate the onset of acute

From: *Primary Hematology*
Edited by: A. Tefferi © Mayo Foundation for Medical Education and Research, Rochester, MN

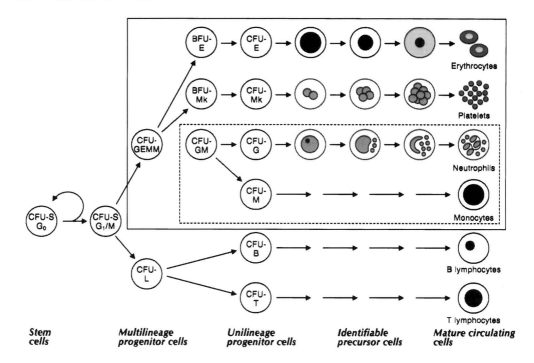

Fig. 1, Plate 16. Heterogeneity in the hematopoietic stem cell origin of acute myelogenous leukemia (AML). In some cases of AML, the disease appears restricted to stem cells committed to granulocyte/monocyte/macrophage differentiation (dotted box). In other cases of AML, the disease involves a pluripotential stem cell that is capable of differentiating to erythrocytes and megakaryocytes, in addition to granulocyte/monocyte/macrophages (red box). BFU-E, burst-forming unit–erythroid; BFU-Mk, megakaryocyte; CFU-B, colony-forming unit–B lymphocyte; CFU-E, erythroid; CFU-G, granulocyte; CFU-GEMM, granulocyte, erythroid, megakaryocyte, monocyte; CFU-GM, granulocyte macrophage; CFU-L, lymphocyte; CFU-M, monocyte; CFU-Mk, megakaryocyte; CFU-T, T lymphocyte; CFU-S G_0, stem cell, resting; CFU-S G_1/M, stem cell, cycling. (From Collins SJ. Pathobiology of human acute myeloid leukemia, in *Hematology: Basic Principles and Practice* [Hoffman R, Benz EJ Jr, Shattil SJ, Furie B, Cohen HJ, Silberstein LE, eds.], 2nd ed. Churchill Livingstone, New York, 1995, pp. 983-993. By permission of the publisher.)

leukemia include ionizing radiation, as demonstrated by the atomic bomb experience during World War II and nuclear reactor accidents such as that at Chernobyl. Exposure to benzene petroleum products and chemotherapy drugs, including alkylating agents (such as cyclophosphamide) and topoisomerase II inhibitors (such as etoposide) that are used for the treatment of other malignant or inflammatory conditions, is known to precipitate AML in some patients (Table 1). Although RNA tumor viruses (retroviruses) are known to precipitate acute leukemia in several different animal models, a clear role for the involvement of retroviruses in human acute leukemia has not been consistently demonstrated.

EPIDEMIOLOGY

AML is a relatively uncommon malignancy; approximately 11,000 new cases are diagnosed each year. The incidence increases with age, and the median age of patients

Table 1
Genetic and Environmental Associations With Acute Leukemia

Genetic predisposition	Environmental influences
Affected family member	Radiation
Down's syndrome	Benzene petroleum products
Fanconi's anemia	Alkylating chemotherapy agents
Bloom syndrome	(e.g., cyclophosphamide)
Ataxia-telangiectasia	Topoisomerase II inhibitors (e.g., etoposide)

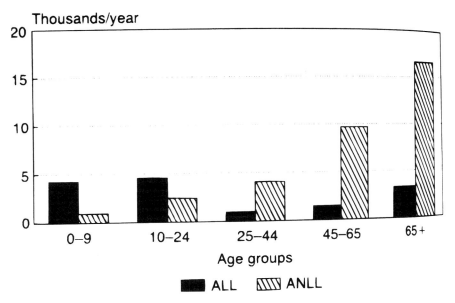

Fig. 2. Relative incidence of acute lymphoblastic leukemia (ALL) and acute myelogenous leukemia (ANLL, acute nonlymphocytic leukemia). (From Miller KB. Clinical manifestations of acute myeloid leukemia, in *Hematology: Basic Principles and Practice* [Hoffman R, Benz EJ Jr, Shattil SJ, Furie B, Cohen HJ, Silberstein LE, eds.], 2nd ed. Churchill Livingstone, New York, 1995, pp. 993-1014. By permission of the publisher.)

with newly diagnosed AML is 60 to 65 years. In adults, 90% of all acute leukemias are AML. It accounts for approximately 1.2% of all cancer deaths in the United States.

In contrast, ALL is diagnosed in 3,000 individuals per year and is the most common form of acute leukemia in children. In children, the peak incidence occurs at approximately 4 years of age. There is also a small increase in incidence in individuals older than 65 years (Fig. 2).

CLASSIFICATION OF ACUTE LEUKEMIA

Although the first documented description of a case of leukemia was made by a French surgeon, Alfred Velpeau, in 1827, it was not until early in the 20th century that the leukemias were subclassified into myelocytic and lymphocytic types. Subsequent investigators described granulocytic, erythroid, and monocytic subtypes. However, the classification scheme of the acute leukemias was not uniform until the mid-1970s, when a

Table 2
Subtypes of Acute Myelogenous Leukemia

French-American-British subtype (morphology)	Staining (MPO/ME)	Selected surface antigens
M0 Undifferentiated	-/-	Granulocytic markers CD13, CD33 (or CD14)
M1 Myeloid without maturation	+/-	CD13, CD33
M2 Myeloid with maturation	+/-	CD13, CD33
M3 Acute promyelocytic	+/-	CD13, CD33, +CD15
M4 Myelomonocytic	+/+	Granulocytic and monocytic markers
M5 Monocytic	+/+	Monocytic markers CD11b, My8, CD14
M6 Erythroleukemia	+/-	Glycophorin
M7 Megakaryoblastic	-/-	Factor VII Ag, factor VIII Ag, CD42

Abbreviations: MPO, myeloperoxidase; ME, monocyte esterase.
From Mastrianni DM, Tung NM, Tenen DG. Acute myelogenous leukemia: current treatment and future directions. *Am J Med* 1992; 92: 286-295. By permission of Excerpta Medica Inc.

group of French, American, and British (FAB) pathologists described a classification scheme based initially on morphologic features but subsequently expanded to include cytochemical stains, immunologic markers, and ultrastructural morphologic findings. They provided classification schemes for AML, ALL, and the myelodysplastic syndromes. The AMLs were initially classified into six subtypes, designated M1 to M6 (M = myeloid). Subsequent descriptions of M0 and M7 were made (Table 2). Similarly, the ALLs were classified into L1, L2, and L3 (L = lymphoid).

The FAB classification scheme has been adopted by virtually all cancer centers and cooperative oncology groups for classification of the acute leukemias. The purpose of the FAB group was to classify the acute leukemias on the basis of the similarity of the malignant cell to its normal counterparts. This classification scheme was based on the premise that most leukemic cells can be placed within the maturation sequence of a specific lineage of hematopoietic cell (Fig. 1, Plate 16). However, it did not consider some of the rare subtypes of AML, such as acute basophilic or acute eosinophilic leukemia. There are also some acute leukemias that express features of multiple lineages that are not classifiable according to the FAB criteria. These hybrid or biphenotypic leukemias are, however, rare.

The FAB classification of ALL has been less reproducible than the FAB classification of AML. Although initially widely used, it has increasingly fallen into disfavor and been replaced by an immunologic classification of ALL based on whether the cell of origin has features of B cells or T cells (Table 3).

Another limitation of the FAB classification scheme is that it did not consider clinical characteristics, cytogenetic data, or the patient's prognosis in formulating the guidelines. Incorporating this additional information has contributed to the realization that AML and ALL are not homogeneous disorders but a group of related disorders with varying clinical presentations and prognoses. Combining clinical data, morphologic findings, histochemical findings, flow cytometric data, and genetic analysis has led to the identification of syndromes of AML and ALL that have allowed clinicians to formulate more accurate prognostic information about the outcome of disease and to individualize therapy based on these characteristics (Table 4). These additional clinical and laboratory characteristics

Table 3
Immunologic Classification of Acute Lymphoblastic Leukemia

ALL subtype	Phenotypic features
Early pre-B	CD19+, CD22+, cytoplasmic (cIg), and surface (sIg)-
Pre-B	cIg+
B cell	sIg+
T cell	CD3+, CD7+, CD5+, CD2+

Abbreviation: ALL, acute lymphoblastic leukemia.
From Pui C-H. Childhood leukemias. *N Engl J Med* 1995; 332: 1618-1630. By permission of Massachusetts Medical Society.

Table 4
Acute Leukemia Syndromes

Type	Clinical findings	Morphology	Karyotype	Prognosis
Philadelphia chromosome + ALL	Older age, high leukocyte count	Pre-B	t(9;22)	Poor
Burkitt-type ALL		B-cell	t(8;14)	Good
Biphenotypic leukemia	Infants or adults, splenomegaly, high leukocyte count		t(4;11)	Poor
M4 AML with abnormal eosinophils		Myelomonocytic blasts, abnormal eosinophils	Inversion 16	Good
M3 AML	Disseminated intra-vascular coagulation, bleeding, thrombosis		t(15;17)	Good
M5 AML	Frequent skin or gum infiltration	Monocytic	t(9;11)	Poor
M2 AML	Splenomegaly, 25%; chloromas, 20%	Myeloblasts with frequent Auer rods	t(8;21)	Good
AML with normal or high platelet count		Megakaryocytes often abnormal	t(3;3) or inv (3)	Poor
Therapy-related leukemia	Occurs after use of alkylating agent		del(5), 5q-, del(7), 7q-	Poor

Abbreviations: ALL, acute lymphoblastic leukemia; AML, acute myelogenous leukemia.
Data from Koeffler HP. Syndromes of acute nonlymphocytic leukemia. *Ann Intern Med* 1987; 107: 748-758.

have been included in a new classification scheme recently proposed by the World Health Organization.

Improvements in the method of chromosome banding and identification have led to the recognition that 80% to 90% of cases of acute leukemia have an associated cytogenetic abnormality. It appears, however, that some patients with apparently normal cytogenetic patterns actually have submicroscopic abnormalities that can be detected by molecular genetic techniques. The most prominent example is in patients with a tandem duplication of a segment of the gene on the long arm of chromosome 11 (11q23), known as the ALL1 or MLL gene. Cytogenetic abnormalities can be broadly classified as translocations [exchange of genetic material between two chromosomes, such as t(9;22)], deletions of a portion or all of a chromosome [such as 5q- or del(5)], and inversions of genetic material on the same chromosome [such as inv(16)]. These chromosome abnormalities can occur as a single abnormality or as one of a series of complex abnormalities within the same cell. Cytogenetic abnormalities have emerged as one of the most powerful prognostic factors in patients with acute leukemia, and cytogenetic analysis is mandatory at diagnosis to help determine prognosis and guide therapy.

CLINICAL MANIFESTATIONS

The clinical manifestations and physical findings in patients with acute leukemia relate to decreased production of normal hematopoietic cells and invasion of other organs by leukemic cells. Most patients complain of fatigue, but this is usually of short duration (less than 2-3 months). The cell or cell lines (erythrocytes, leukocytes, or platelets) most severely affected by the leukemic process predict the patient's dominant clinical presentation. Anemia is virtually always present at diagnosis and can contribute to the patient's fatigue and cause cardiopulmonary symptoms of tachycardia and dyspnea on exertion. Normally, platelets represent the first line of defense in preventing mucocutaneous bleeding, and patients with severe thrombocytopenia present with petechiae, mucous membrane bleeding, and ecchymoses. Patients are frequently neutropenic, and fever associated with cutaneous or respiratory infections can occur. It is common for patients with undiagnosed acute leukemia to be treated with one or more courses of antibiotics and to have incomplete resolution of their symptoms before further investigation leads to the discovery of their disease. A minority of patients complain of diffuse bone tenderness in long bones, ribs, or the sternum. Such bone pain also can herald the recurrence of disease after therapy. This bone discomfort is thought to result from expansion of the intramedullary space with leukemia or invasion of the periosteum by leukemic cells.

The physical examination of patients suspected of having acute leukemia needs to be thorough to discover sites of bleeding or infection and to search for organ involvement with the disease. A digital rectal examination should, however, be avoided in patients with neutropenia, but careful inspection of the perianal area is important to exclude a rectal fissure or impending rectal abscess. Lymphadenopathy, although rare in AML, is frequent in ALL.

Up to 10% of patients can present with leukemic infiltration of the skin, which usually presents as violaceous, raised, nontender subcutaneous plaques or nodules. Known as leukemia cutis, this condition should be distinguished from Sweet's syndrome, also known as acute neutrophilic dermatosis, which is a paraneoplastic syndrome of the skin that can be associated with AML. It presents with tender red plaques and nodules that may precede the diagnosis of AML by several months or more. Gingival hyperplasia from infiltration of the gums with leukemic cells occurs most often in AML of the monocytic subtype.

Collections of leukemic blasts can occur in virtually any soft tissue organ, and these leukemic tumors have been termed chloromas, granulocytic sarcomas, or, less commonly, myeloblastomas. Common sites of involvement include the orbits, sinuses, ovaries, testes, gastrointestinal tract, and breasts. These extramedullary sites of involvement can precede the presence of leukemia in the marrow or blood by months or even years and are often initially diagnosed as lymphoma. In AML, central nervous system involvement can occur in 5% to 7% of patients and should be suspected in any patient with focal neurologic signs at diagnosis. Patients can sometimes be asymptomatic. Patients at risk with AML are those with a high blast count, increased lactate dehydrogenase value, or monocytic subtype. Whether every patient with AML should have a routine spinal tap done early in the course of the disease is controversial. However, in ALL, central nervous system involvement, although uncommon at presentation, develops in most patients unless prophylactic therapy is provided. Therefore, all patients with ALL should have an initial spinal tap done early in the course of the disease, and prophylactic therapy should be prescribed. Ideally, spinal taps should be performed when the peripheral blood differential shows no blast cells; this approach minimizes the risk that a traumatic tap could cause contamination of the cerebrospinal fluid with leukemic blast cells from the blood and lead to a misdiagnosis of central nervous system leukemia.

Patients with leukemic blast counts in the peripheral blood exceeding 50,000/μL are at high risk for leukostasis, which most commonly affects the lungs or central nervous system. Pulmonary or central nervous system hemorrhage can result. These patients should undergo emergency leukapheresis and be treated with high doses of hydroxyurea, allopurinol, and hydration with alkalinization of the urine. Definitive therapy of the disease should be initiated as soon as a diagnosis is made.

In patients with a high tumor burden, rapid lysis of the blast cells can develop with the initiation of chemotherapy. This tumor lysis syndrome is characterized by rapid onset of hyperuricemia, hyperkalemia, hyperphosphatemia, and hypocalcemia. It is important in these patients to maintain a good urine output with the initiation of therapy and also to treat them with allopurinol. This syndrome tends to be more common in patients with ALL but also can occur in AML.

An additional important complication of chemotherapy which, fortunately, occurs only rarely is necrotizing enterocolitis, also known as typhlitis. Patients with typhlitis have sudden onset of abdominal pain, fever, and abdominal distention with decreased bowel sounds. Computed tomography of the abdomen is the test of choice and usually shows thickening of the bowel wall due to edema. This disorder almost always occurs in patients with acute leukemia who have initiated chemotherapy and are neutropenic. The cause is uncertain but is probably related to occult infection. The prognosis is often poor in these patients, but some patients can be successfully managed conservatively with bowel rest, nasogastric suction, broad-spectrum antibiotics, and total parenteral nutrition. Some patients require operation if signs of perforation or peritonitis are present. The risks of operation are high.

DIAGNOSIS

In patients with acute leukemia, the complete blood cell count demonstrates varying degrees of pancytopenia. The total leukocyte count can range from less than 1.0×10^9/L to more than 200×10^9/L, but most patients have a total leukocyte count of 5 to 30×10^9/L. Most patients have circulating blast cells, which give the strongest indication of the diagnosis, but 10% of patients have no circulating blast cells. Although in patients with a high leukocyte count the laboratory can make a diagnosis by typing the peripheral blood blasts, bone marrow aspiration and biopsy are always performed to provide a comparison for subsequent bone marrow tests performed after treatment. The posterior iliac crest is the preferred site for bone marrow aspiration and biopsy because the sternal aspiration site does not allow for procurement of a biopsy sample.

Morphologically, the bone marrow typically is hypercellular with uniform replacement of the marrow cavity with immature blast forms. Normal precursors are markedly diminished in number. By definition, the diagnosis of acute leukemia requires a blast percentage of more than 30% of all nucleated cells. Although an initial Wright stain smear

Table 5
Monoclonal Antibodies Commonly Used
to Distinguish AML From ALL

AML	ALL
CD11 (anti-Mo1)	CD10 (CALLA)
CD13 (MY7)	CD2 (T11, Leu-5)
CD14 (MY4)	CD4 (T4, Leu-3)
CD15	CD5 (Leu-1)
CD33 (MY9)	CD3 (T8, Leu-2)
CD41 (platelet glycoprotein IIb/IIIa)	CD19 (anti-B4)
	CD20 (anti-B1)

Abbreviations: ALL, acute lymphoblastic leukemia; AML, acute myelogenous leukemia.

From Miller KB. Clinical manifestations of acute myeloid leukemia, in *Hematology: Basic Principles and Practice* (Hoffman R, Benz EJ Jr, Shattil SJ, Furie B, Cohen HJ, Silberstein LE, eds), 2nd ed. Churchill Livingstone, New York, 1995, pp. 993-1014. By permission of the publisher.

of the peripheral blood or marrow aspirate can give the hematologist or pathologist a high suspicion for the diagnosis of acute leukemia and offer some suggestion of the subtype, definitive diagnosis requires the use of cytochemical or immunohistochemical stains or flow cytometry with monoclonal antibodies to definitively characterize the type of acute leukemia (AML or ALL) and the specific subtype. The peripheral blood and bone marrow also should be carefully inspected for the presence of Auer rods. These are reddish rod-like filaments of aggregated lysosomes in the cytoplasm of patients with AML, most frequently of the FAB M1 or M2 subtype. Their presence is virtually pathognomonic of a diagnosis of AML.

The most important histochemical stain in the subtyping of acute leukemia is myeloperoxidase. Myeloperoxidase is a cytoplasmic enzyme that appears early in myeloid development. It is present in more than 3% of blast cells in the FAB M1 through M6 subtypes of AML (Table 2). If the peroxidase stain is positive, esterase stains then can be used to define the M1 through M5 subtypes of AML; chloracetate esterase is positive in the M1 through M3 subtypes, and nonspecific esterase is positive for the monocytic cells in the M4 and M5 subtypes. The chloracetate esterase stain is positive in the myeloid blasts of the M4 subtype (myelomonocytic). An immunohistochemical stain specific for erythrocyte precursors, such as with an antibody to glycophorin A, can be used to define the erythroblasts in the M6 subtype.

Blast cells that are negative for peroxidase, therefore, are one of the rarer subtypes of AML (M0, M7) or ALL. In these instances, the use of immunohistochemical stains with monoclonal antibodies or flow cytometry has been very beneficial to categorize these subtypes of ALL. In the past, a stain for terminal deoxynucleotidyl transferase (TdT) was thought to be specific for ALL but has subsequently been found to also be seen in some patients with AML and is now used infrequently. In the FAB M0 subtype, the presence of myeloperoxidase in the cytoplasm can be demonstrated with more sensitive monoclonal antibodies or electron microscopy. The leukocyte antigens for which monoclonal antibodies are available to diagnose AML and ALL are listed in Table 5.

Table 6
Adverse Prognostic Factors in Acute Leukemia

AML	ALL
Older age	Older age
Leukocyte count $> 100 \times 10^9$/L	Leukocyte count $\geq 50 \times 10^9$/L
Chromosome abnormalities other than t(8;21) and inv[16,t(15;17)] and normal cytogenetics	Chromosome abnormalities, including t(9;22) and t(4;11)
Antecedent hematologic disorder (e.g., myelodysplastic syndrome)	Not achieving complete remission within 4 weeks

PROGNOSIS

The acute leukemias are a heterogeneous group of disorders, and the prognosis for an individual patient can vary considerably. Table 6 outlines the major clinical adverse risk factors for AML and ALL which have been identified and are used clinically to determine prognosis.

In AML, the major adverse prognostic factors that have been identified are older age, leukocyte count more than 100×10^9/L, and chromosome abnormalities other than the favorable ones listed in Table 6. In ALL, similar prognostic factors have been identified, including older age, increased leukocyte count, and chromosome abnormalities, in particular the presence of translocations between chromosome 9 and 22 (Philadelphia chromosome) and 4 and 11. In addition, in ALL, failure to achieve complete remission within 4 weeks of initiation of therapy portends a poorer prognosis and more resistant disease. As noted in the next section on therapy, these prognostic factors are helpful in guiding therapy, particularly after achievement of remission.

THERAPY

Acute Myelogenous Leukemia

The most important chemotherapeutic agent in the treatment of AML is cytosine arabinoside (ara-C). A series of trials in the 1960s showed that a continuous infusion of ara-C over 7 days was effective for inducing complete remissions in approximately 20% of patients. Subsequent trials combining ara-C with other chemotherapeutic agents showed that a 7-day continuous infusion of ara-C (100 to 200 mg/m^2 per day) with an anthracycline antibiotic such as daunorubicin (45-60 mg/m^2 per day) by intravenous push for 3 days (known as a 3 + 7 regimen) led to complete remission rates of approximately 65%. This percentage was somewhat higher in younger patients and somewhat lower in older ones. As new anthracycline antibiotics (such as idarubicin, mitoxantrone) have been developed over the years, they have been tested in combination with ara-C and not shown to be significantly more effective than the combination of daunorubicin and ara-C. Attempts to improve the efficacy of this regimen by adding other drugs such as thioguanine or etoposide or increasing the dose of ara-C have not increased the percentage of patients entering complete remission but may play a role in prolonging the duration of remission.

Table 7
Definition of Complete Remission

Absence of circulating blasts
Bone marrow cellularity > 20% with < 5% blasts
Neutrophils ≥ 1.0×10^9/L
Platelets > 100×10^9/L
Hemoglobin concentration can be at any level

All criteria must be present for ≥ 4 weeks

A week after the initial 3 + 7 induction regimen, a repeat bone marrow aspiration and biopsy are performed. The goal of therapy at this point is to achieve marrow hypoplasia or aplasia. If residual leukemia is present in the marrow on day 14, a second course of the identical induction regimen often is given. Another marrow aspiration is then performed a week after the second course of induction therapy. If patients do not achieve marrow aplasia after the second course of induction therapy, they are thought to have refractory disease and have a poor prognosis. An alternative salvage regimen of chemotherapy combining agents such as mitoxantrone and etoposide or high doses of ara-C sometimes can lead to remission. If an HLA-identical sibling is available, a minority of these patients also can have salvage treatment with an allogeneic blood or marrow transplant.

After achievement of marrow aplasia, another 1 to 2 weeks is required for recovery of normal hematopoiesis. It is during this time that patients are pancytopenic and at risk for infection, mucositis, and bleeding. Virtually all patients require hospitalization during this time, and the total duration of hospitalization after induction therapy can be as long as 4 to 6 weeks.

After recovery of blood cell counts, patients require a second bone marrow aspiration and a biopsy to document complete remission. The hematologic and morphologic requirements for complete remission are listed in Table 7.

Once a complete remission has been achieved, post-remission therapy is required to reduce the risk of relapse of the leukemia. Randomized trials have demonstrated that even low doses of maintenance therapy with oral 6-thioguanine and subcutaneous ara-C can prolong remission compared with no post-remission therapy. In younger patients, more intensive high-dose consolidation therapy improves survival compared with lower-dose therapy. A recently published trial by a large cooperative group showed that in patients younger than 60 years, four cycles of high-dose ara-C at a dosage of 3 g/m² twice a day for 3 days led to 40% disease-free survival at 4 years compared with doses of 100 or 400 mg/m² per day by continuous infusion for 5 days. Subsequent analysis by cytogenetic subtype suggested that the main benefit of the high-dose ara-C regimen was in the group with favorable cytogenetics, including patients with inversion of chromosome 16 or those with a translocation between chromosomes 8 and 21.

Multiple large randomized trials have now also explored the role of autologous or allogeneic bone marrow transplantation compared with chemotherapy to determine which is the optimal post-remission therapy for a younger patient (< 55 years old) with AML. The results of many of these trials have now been reported in final or preliminary form. Details of the trial design have varied from one study to another in terms of the type and number of post-remission chemotherapy cycles that are given and whether attempts were made to purge or "cleanse" the autologous bone marrow of residual leukemic cells. These

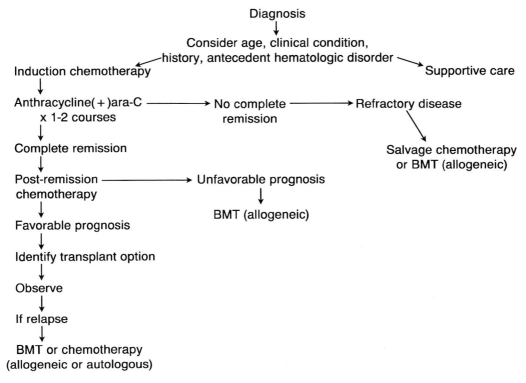

Fig. 3. Treatment options for acute myelogenous leukemia. ara-C, cytosine arabinoside; BMT, blood or marrow transplantation.

trials also demonstrated that many patients cannot complete the entire treatment program because of early relapse, excessive toxicity, or patient or physician preference to pursue an alternative form of therapy.

The results of these trials have varied somewhat but, in general, the data available have suggested equivalent or slightly improved (but generally not statistically significant) outcomes with either form of transplantation as compared with chemotherapy. It is important to bear in mind that treatment-related mortality associated with allogeneic bone marrow transplantation resulting from infection, toxicity from high-dose chemoradiotherapy, or graft-versus-host disease can reach or exceed 20%, and in autologous transplant, 10%. Therefore, many investigators now advise patients that a transplant source should be identified as soon as possible after diagnosis but that patients receive intensive consolidation chemotherapy for post-remission therapy and that transplantation be used only for relapse. These recommendations can be stratified by the patient's prognosis at diagnosis, particularly in relation to results of marrow cytogenetic analysis. Patients with good-risk cytogenetic findings can receive high-dose ara-C, given the excellent outcome in such cases. Patients with intermediate or poor-risk cytogenetic results may be considered for allogeneic bone marrow transplantation if an HLA-identical sibling is available or for autologous transplantation, depending on the preference of the patient and treating physician. The National Comprehensive Cancer Network recently published practice guidelines for the treatment of acute leukemia which incorporate these recommendations. A suggested approach is shown in Figure 3.

The described therapeutic considerations apply to all the FAB subtypes of AML except the M3 subtype, acute promyelocytic leukemia. Although this subtype makes up not more than 15% of all cases of AML, its therapy has generated intense excitement in the hematologic community because of the ability of all-*trans*-retinoic acid (ATRA) to induce complete remission in 70% to 90% of patients with AML-M3 by a unique mechanism of inducing leukemic promyelocytes to differentiate into mature cells. This therapy is the first clinically successful example of the use of differentiation therapy for a malignancy, whereas traditional approaches have relied on the cytotoxic effects of chemotherapy.

This differentiation therapy is dependent on the fact that virtually all cases of acute promyelocytic leukemia have a balanced reciprocal translocation between chromosomes 15 and 17, which results in the juxtaposition of a portion of the promyelocytic leukemia gene with a portion of the gene for retinoic acid receptor α. This fusion protein seems to play a role in preventing promyelocytes from differentiating, but pharmacologic doses of ATRA can overcome this resistance to differentiation. The malignant promyelocytes in acute promyelocytic leukemia morphologically have a hypergranular cytoplasm. Enzymes released from these granules can activate the coagulation cascade and result in disseminated intravascular coagulation, fibrinolysis, and proteolysis, which put patients at high risk for pathologic clotting and bleeding. These abnormalities can result in the death of patients from complications such as intravascular hemorrhage early in the course of the disease. Use of ATRA to induce complete remission can result in rapid resolution of the coagulopathy and lessen the number of deaths from this complication. Virtually all patients treated with ATRA alone, however, have relapse.

Additional chemotherapy given in conjunction with ATRA during induction and subsequently as post-remission therapy can significantly reduce the risk of relapse. One important complication of ATRA therapy in induction has been the "retinoic acid syndrome," which is characterized by unexplained fever, weight gain, and pulmonary infiltrates and effusions. It usually responds to discontinuation of ATRA therapy and prompt institution of dexamethasone therapy. Recently, arsenic trioxide has been found to be an effective therapy for patients with relapsed acute promyelocytic leukemia, and its role in the initial therapy of patients with this disease is being explored.

Treatment of elderly patients with AML remains problematic. The median age of patients with AML is more than 60 years, and thus half of patients with AML can be considered elderly. For multiple reasons, these elderly patients tolerate the intensive chemotherapy regimens less well than younger patients. First, most elderly patients with AML fit into poorer prognostic categories of the disease because of an antecedent myelodysplastic syndrome or the finding of poor-risk cytogenetic abnormalities at diagnosis. Second, elderly patients more frequently have comorbid conditions such as cardiopulmonary disease or renal insufficiency which make them more susceptible to complications associated with the therapy of AML, notably infections. Therefore, many elderly patients with AML are not offered intensive chemotherapy as initial treatment but are managed with supportive care with broad-spectrum oral antibiotics (such as quinolones), transfusions, and hydroxyurea to control leukocytosis. Although some elderly patients can live for several months to a year in this situation, all will die of their disease. Effective, but less toxic, therapies for the treatment of AML for this subgroup of patients are needed. For patients who are thought to be in otherwise good health, the use of a 3 + 7 regimen or intermediate doses of ara-C can produce complete remission rates of approximately 50% and 2-year disease-free survival rates of 10% to 20%. Given the improvements in supportive care of patients undergoing autologous transplantation, this therapy is being offered to an increasingly older population, and elderly patients with AML who are in otherwise good health may be candidates for autologous transplantation.

Acute Lymphoblastic Leukemia

The treatment of ALL is a triumph of the modern management of malignant disease. Current chemotherapeutic programs cure up to 70% of children with ALL, and recent programs of therapy have been directed at a risk-adapted strategy to try to reduce the intensity of therapy for good-risk patients (and, therefore, reduce toxicity) without compromising their clinical outcome and to try to modify therapy to improve the outcome of high-risk patients. Treatment with a glucocorticoid, vincristine, and asparaginase results in a complete remission in 99% of children with low-risk ALL. Included in this category are children with B-lineage ALL, aged 1 to 9 years, and with a leukocyte count less than 50×10^9/L. Post-remission therapy with 6-mercaptopurine and methotrexate for 2 to 3 years can cure more than 80% of patients with low-risk disease. The addition of an intensification phase of therapy incorporating drugs such as etoposide, ara-C, cyclophosphamide, or an anthracycline seems to bring an additional long-term survival advantage for patients in all risk groups.

Approximately 40% of children with ALL have one or more features predictive of a poorer outcome (leukocyte count more than 50×10^9/L, age older than 9 years, and T-cell immunophenotype). In these patients, the use of four or more drugs including an anthracycline seems optimal to induce complete remission, followed by a brief period of intensified treatment to eradicate residual leukemic cells. Approximately two-thirds of higher-risk patients can now be cured with this approach. Finally, there is a category of very high-risk ALL, including patients with a translocation between chromosomes 9 and 22 (Philadelphia chromosome), translocation between chromosomes 4 and 11, leukocyte count more than 200×10^9/L, and infants with rearrangement of the MLL gene on the long arm of chromosome 11. These patients should be considered for early allogeneic marrow transplantation from an HLA-matched sibling or unrelated donor because of their high risk of relapse.

Bone marrow cytogenetic abnormalities are playing an increasing role in guiding the intensity of therapy in childhood ALL. Children with hyperdiploidy (> 50 chromosomes per leukemic cell) have an excellent prognosis, and 90% of these children can be cured with antimetabolite-based treatment.

In ALL, leukemia develops in the central nervous system in most patients unless attempts are made to prevent it. Previously, it was believed that cranial irradiation was essential in all of these patients, but in low-risk children regular doses of intrathecal methotrexate can provide adequate prophylaxis. Ongoing studies are addressing whether alteration in chemotherapy regimens, including the use of high-dose intravenous methotrexate, can replace cranial irradiation because of the long-term sequelae of cranial irradiation, including brain tumors, neuropsychological deficits, and endocrine dysfunction.

Hematologists who treat adults have increasingly followed the lead of their counterparts in pediatric care and have adapted many of the successful principles used in the treatment of pediatric ALL to adults with ALL. Adults with ALL generally have a poorer prognosis than children, primarily because of higher-risk features of adult ALL compared with childhood ALL. In particular, the incidence of adults with Philadelphia chromosome-positive ALL [t(9;22)] is significantly higher than in the pediatric population. Cure rates in adult ALL are in the range of 35% with 3- to 4-year follow-up, but they also vary significantly depending on prognostic features. This poorer prognosis has meant that the role of transplantation has figured more prominently in the therapy of ALL, although randomized trials have shown a benefit for only allogeneic transplantation in patients with high-risk features. The largest randomized trial to date is being conducted by the Medical Research Council in Britain and the Eastern Cooperative Oncology Group in the United States and is exploring the role of autologous transplantation versus chemotherapy and comparing them with allogeneic transplantation from HLA-matched siblings. This trial is hoped to shed further light on the optimal therapy of adults with ALL.

SUPPORTIVE CARE

Patients with acute leukemia are subject to risks of infection and bleeding as a result of the cytopenias that accompany their disease and its treatment.

The most important risk factor for infection is an absolute neutropenia ($< 0.5 \times 10^9$ neutrophils per liter, $< 500/\mu L$). Not only the depth of the neutropenia but also its duration influences the risk of infection. Studies in the 1960s clearly documented the increased risk of infection when the neutrophil value decreases to this level. Patients with neutropenia who have fever ($> 38.5°C$ on one occasion or three or more measurements more than $38.0°C$ within 24 hours) require prompt evaluation and institution of therapy.

Aside from fever, patients may have few other signs or symptoms to pinpoint the exact source of infection, particularly once therapy of their leukemia has been initiated. However, factors other than neutropenia contribute to the risk of infection. These include disruption of normal mucosal barriers in the skin and respiratory and gastrointestinal tracts. The long-term indwelling right atrial catheters that are used for intravenous therapy and phlebotomy can be associated with both blood-borne infections and infections within the subcutaneous tunnel and exit site.

Fifteen or more years ago, the most prominent bacterial pathogens that affected patients with acute leukemia during their initial neutropenic phase were gram-negative aerobes such as *Escherichia coli* and *Pseudomonas aeruginosa*. However, in the past 10 to 15 years, gram-positive bacteria including streptococcal and staphylococcal organisms have become more frequent isolates. *Candida* and *Aspergillus* species also can be clinically significant during the initial neutropenic phase, although hepatosplenic candidiasis often manifests after recovery from neutropenia. The herpes group viruses, especially herpes simplex virus, cytomegalovirus, and varicella-zoster virus, are those most commonly associated with infection in patients with leukemia. Herpes simplex virus is by far the most common during the initial phase of therapy and contributes to the mucositis that develops in some patients.

Antibacterial antibiotic therapy of febrile neutropenia depends on the organisms cultured at the time of fever, although as many as 50% of patients with febrile neutropenia have negative cultures. All patients should receive initial empiric antibiotic therapy. The choice of an initial empiric regimen depends on the pattern of bacterial isolates and their antibiotic sensitivities that have been isolated at the center where the patient is being treated. In general, however, a third- or fourth-generation cephalosporin such as ceftazidime or, more recently, cefepime is a reasonable initial choice. Empiric vancomycin therapy in febrile patients with neutropenia should be discouraged because of emerging resistance to this antibiotic and because the most common gram-positive organism isolated is coagulase-negative staphylococcus, which has lower virulence than other bacteria. Patients with persistent fever and negative cultures in whom resolution of neutropenia does not seem to be imminent should be given empiric therapy with amphotericin B. This should be continued until resolution of the neutropenia and fever. In selected circumstances in which *Aspergillus* infection or drug-resistant *Candida* species are uncommon, fluconazole prophylaxis can be considered. Patients experiencing excessive toxicity from amphotericin B may be candidates for the newer lipid complex amphotericin preparations.

The hematopoietic growth factors granulocyte-macrophage colony-stimulating factor (Leukine) and granulocyte colony-stimulating factor (Neupogen) are both approved by the Food and Drug Administration for various supportive roles in hematologic and oncologic conditions. Multiple randomized trials have compared the use of these growth factors with placebo for shortening the duration of neutropenia and its associated complications in patients undergoing intensive chemotherapy for acute leukemia. Surprisingly, but uniformly, it has been found that these two growth factors can be given safely to patients with AML after induction chemotherapy with no increase in the incidence of relapse or progression of disease despite the fact that many AML cells have receptors for these growth factors on their cell surface. Additionally, these growth factors shorten the period of neutropenia after chemotherapy but, surprisingly, the clinical benefits in terms of reducing infections, antibiotic use, and hospitalization have been lacking in many studies in AML. In one trial, neutropenia and survival were improved and severe infections reduced, and on the basis of the study, leukine has been approved for therapy in elderly patients with AML after induction chemotherapy. Thus, although these growth factors have been shown to be safe and to shorten the duration of neutropenia, their use and clinical benefit remain controversial. In contrast, in ALL, most studies have suggested a clinical benefit for the hematopoietic growth factors in reducing morbidity and length of hospitalization.

The other potential clinical role for the hematopoietic growth factors in AML has been in initiating them before the onset of chemotherapy to transiently stimulate the growth of the leukemic cells and bring them into cell cycle in order to increase the extent of cell kill with subsequent chemotherapy, particularly ara-C. This approach has been termed "priming," and to date it remains investigational and the subject of ongoing clinical trials.

Patients with acute leukemia require frequent transfusions of erythrocytes and platelets during the course of their disease and treatment. Several studies have demonstrated that patients with acute leukemia do not have excessive bleeding until their platelet level decreases to less than 10×10^9/L. Therefore, platelet transfusions can be withheld until the platelet level decreases to this amount, unless there are intervening problems of fever (which increases platelet consumption or bleeding). Similarly, these patients will tolerate hemoglobin levels as low as 8.0 g/dL, and erythrocyte transfusions are generally unnecessary until the hemoglobin level is below this amount, but variations from this recommendation should be based on the clinical scenario. Recent studies have demonstrated that the use of leukocyte filtration devices in conjunction with erythrocyte and platelet transfusions can lessen the risk of febrile transfusion reactions and the risk of development of HLA antibodies, which can lead to subsequent platelet refractoriness. This phenomenon of alloimmunization can, if it develops, be managed with infusion of HLA-matched platelets, but it is a difficult clinical problem, and reducing the risks of its development with leukocyte filtration can be a benefit. Granulocyte transfusions are necessary only rarely with the current spectrum of antimicrobial agents available to treat infection in neutropenia. Granulocyte transfusions are considered in patients with neutropenia and overwhelming bacterial or fungal infection in whom the recovery of neutrophil number and function is not anticipated within the ensuing few days.

SUGGESTED READING

Bennett JM, Catovsky D, Daniel MT, Flandrin G, Galton DA, Gralnick HR, Sultan C. Proposed revised criteria for the classification of acute myeloid leukemia. A report of the French-American-British Cooperative Group. *Ann Intern Med* 1985; 103: 620-625.

Bloomfield CD, Herzig GP, Caligiuri MA. Acute leukemia: recent advances. *Semin Oncol* 1997; 24: 1-2.

Ganser A, Heil G. Use of hematopoietic growth factors in the treatment of acute myelogenous leukemia. *Curr Opin Hematol* 1997; 4: 191-195.

Harris NL, Jaffe ES, Diebold J, Flandrin G, Muller-Hermelink HK, Vardiman J, Lister TA, Bloomfield CD. World Health Organization classification of neoplastic diseases of the hematopoietic and lymphoid tissues: report of the Clinical Advisory Committee meeting—Airlie House, Virginia, November 1997. *J Clin Oncol* 1999; 17: 3835-3849.

Hughes WT, Armstrong D, Bodey GP, Brown AE, Edwards JE, Feld R, Pizzo P, Rolston KV, Shenep JL, Young LS. 1997 Guidelines for the use of antimicrobial agents in neutropenic patients with unexplained fever. *Clin Infect Dis* 1997; 25: 551-573.

Koeffler HP. Syndromes of acute nonlymphocytic leukemia. *Ann Intern Med* 1987; 107: 748-758.

Löwenberg B. Treatment of acute myelogenous leukaemia. *J Intern Med* 1997; 242 Suppl: 17-22.

NCCN Acute Leukemia Practice Guidelines. *Oncology* 1996; 10 Suppl: 205-221.

Pui C-H. Childhood leukemias. *N Engl J Med* 1995; 332: 1618-1630.

Strout MP, Caligiuri MA. Developments in cytogenetics and oncogenes in acute leukemia. *Curr Opin Oncol* 1997; 9: 8-17.

Tallman MS, Andersen JW, Schiffer CA, Appelbaum FR, Feusner JH, Ogden A, Shepherd L, Willman C, Bloomfield CD, Rowe JM, Wiernik PH. All-*trans*-retinoic acid in acute promyelocytic leukemia. *N Engl J Med* 1997; 337: 1021-1028.

The Trial to Reduce Alloimmunization to Platelets Study Group. Leukocyte reduction and ultraviolet B irradiation of platelets to prevent alloimmunization and refractoriness to platelet transfusions. *N Engl J Med* 1997; 337: 1861-1869.

Blood and Marrow Transplantation

Mark R. Litzow, MD

Contents

INTRODUCTION

Infusion of bone marrow for therapeutic purposes was initially attempted in the first half of the 20th century, but it was not until the development of histocompatibility testing of human leukocyte antigens (HLA) with antisera in the late 1960s that the first successful transplantation of marrow from an HLA-matched sibling was performed. Small numbers of transplantations were performed at a slowly increasing rate through the 1970s, but in the past 2 decades the procedure of blood and marrow transplantation has grown substantially in terms of numbers and types of transplants (Fig. 1).

Initially, the rationale for blood and marrow transplantation was to give patients high doses of chemotherapy or radiation therapy to eliminate their underlying disease. This treatment also destroyed the normal progenitors in their bone marrow and, thus, necessitated the infusion of a new source of normal bone marrow cells to rescue the patients from the high-dose therapy and shorten the period of cytopenias so as to lessen their risk of infection and bleeding (Fig. 2, Plate 17). This rationale is still relevant today, but new knowledge of the immune system gained from the application of transplantation over the years has demonstrated how the immune system can be harnessed to treat human malignancy.

The field of blood and marrow transplantation also has fueled advances in the field of stem cell biology. The cell of interest in transplantation, the "stem cell," has been difficult to characterize in vitro, but it is thought to be totipotent (that is, capable of giving rise to all cell subtypes in the hematopoietic system) and capable of self-renewal. A critical development in the field of transplantation was the identification of a transmembrane glycoprotein, CD34, which is expressed on both the stem cell and the immature cells committed to development along a particular lineage of cells (such as erythroid or lym-

From: *Primary Hematology*
Edited by: A. Tefferi © Mayo Foundation for Medical Education and Research, Rochester, MN

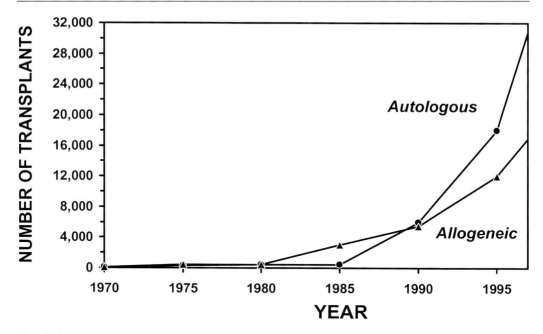

Fig. 1. Annual number of blood and marrow transplants worldwide (1970-1995). (From International Bone Marrow Transplant Registry: Autologous Blood and Marrow Transplant Registry. *1998 IBMTR/ABMTR Summary Slides: Current Status of Blood & Marrow Transplantation.* Medical College of Wisconsin, Milwaukee, 1998. By permission of the Medical College of Wisconsin.)

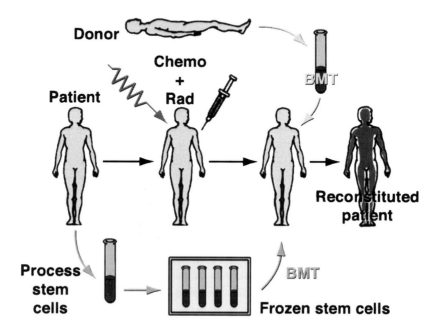

Fig. 2, Plate 17. Blood and marrow transplantation (BMT) process. Chemo, chemotherapy; rad, radiation. (Modified from Golde DW. The stem cell. *Sci Am* 1991; 265 no. 6: 86-93. By permission of the journal.)

phoid). Cells expressing CD34 are capable of reconstituting hematopoiesis in animals and humans who have received lethal doses of chemotherapy or radiation therapy. The discovery of monoclonal antibodies reacting with CD34 has led to the development of separation techniques to isolate CD34 cells and subsets of CD34 cells for clinical use.

SOURCES OF STEM CELLS

Blood and marrow cells for transplantation can be obtained from three sources: allogeneic, syngeneic, or autologous.

Sources of Blood and Marrow Cells

- Allogeneic: another human not genetically identical to the patient
- Syngeneic: an identical twin
- Autologous: the patient's own stem cells

In the allogeneic setting, cells can be obtained from a related or unrelated person who is fully or closely HLA-matched with the patient. Sources of stem cells can include the peripheral blood, bone marrow, or, more recently, umbilical cord blood, which has been found to be a rich source of hematopoietic stem cells (Fig. 3). Bone marrow is typically harvested from the posterior iliac crests while the patient is under general anesthesia.

Peripheral Blood Stem Cell Transplantation

More than 20 years ago, immature hematopoietic cells were discovered to circulate in the peripheral blood. The use of these peripheral blood stem cells (PBSCs) for transplantation was first attempted in patients who were not candidates for bone marrow transplantation because of prior damage to their bone marrow from radiation therapy or because of tumor contamination of their marrow from their underlying disease. These PBSCs were successful for promoting hematopoietic recovery after transplantation, but many apheresis procedures were necessary to collect an adequate number of these cells for transplantation.

Subsequent trials showed that stem cells could be "mobilized" from the marrow to the blood by treating the patient with a hematopoietic growth factor (such as granulocyte colony-stimulating factor [G-CSF] in a dosage of 10 μg/kg per day subcutaneously beginning 4 days before starting collections) alone or after chemotherapy. This approach increases the number of hematopoietic progenitors in the blood by 10- to 1,000-fold compared with steady-state conditions. Use of these "mobilized" PBSCs for transplantation compared with bone marrow transplantation in the autologous setting showed more rapid hematologic recovery, shorter hospitalization, lower blood product use, and lower costs. There also appears to be less risk of tumor contamination with the use of PBSCs than with bone marrow, and mobilized PBSCs have now replaced marrow as the source of stem cells of choice for autologous transplants in most transplant centers.

More recently, treatment of normal HLA-matched allogeneic donors with G-CSF for 4 days followed by a 4-hour apheresis procedure daily for 1 or 2 days resulted in collection of sufficient cells to use for transplantation. These allogeneic PBSCs also appear to result in more rapid hematopoietic recovery of the recipient, but they may result in more difficulties with chronic graft-versus-host disease (GVHD) after transplantation. Randomized trials comparing allogeneic PBSCs with bone marrow are under way.

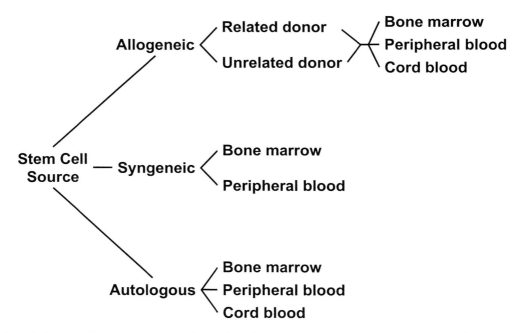

Fig. 3. Stem cell sources. (From Litzow MR. Blood and marrow transplantation, in *Transplant Surgery* [Hakim N, Danovitch GM, eds.], Springer-Verlag, Berlin [in press]. By permission of the publisher.)

Umbilical Cord Blood Transplantation

Umbilical cord blood is a rich source of hematopoietic stem cells. At delivery, a sufficient number of stem cells can be collected and cryopreserved to allow engraftment in children and small adults, although recovery of blood counts seems to be slower than with bone marrow or PBSCs. The incidence of GVHD may be lower after umbilical cord blood transplantation than after bone marrow or PBSC transplantation, and this decrease is thought to be related to the "immunologic immaturity" of umbilical cord blood. These lower rates of GVHD have suggested that greater degrees of HLA-mismatching may be clinically tolerable in umbilical cord blood transplants and, thus, give patients a greater opportunity to find a donor. After these encouraging initial results with the use of cord blood transplants, banks of these cells are being established around the world in which a large number of unrelated cord blood specimens are cryopreserved so that a patient without another allogeneic or autologous source of cells for transplantation can search for an HLA-compatible donor.

Ex Vivo Stem Cell Expansion

In the future, it will likely be possible to take a small aliquot of stem cells from bone marrow, blood, or umbilical cord blood, combine it with selected hematopoietic growth factors in an appropriate in vitro environment, and "expand" the number of immature progenitors present to a level sufficient for hematopoietic recovery after a transplantation. Early clinical trials of such stem cell expansion techniques have already been initiated. The ability to select different cell types from a stem cell source and expand them is also becoming a reality, and the ability to "engineer" a graft of stem cells for different purposes will be utilized increasingly in the future.

TECHNICAL ASPECTS

Blood and marrow transplantation should be performed in a dedicated unit by a team of experienced professionals, including representation from disciplines that encompass the wide-ranging psychosocial and physical needs of patients receiving transplants. The unit should contain special air-handling equipment with either high-efficiency particulate air (HEPA) filtration or laminar airflow to minimize patient exposure to infectious organisms. Other measures to reduce the risk of infection include thorough room cleaning, strict hand washing, diets free of fresh fruits and vegetables during the period of neutropenia, and antibiotic prophylaxis immediately before and after transplantation, including the use of absorbable or nonabsorbable antibacterial antibiotics (such as a quinolone antibiotic), antifungal (such as fluconazole), and antiviral (such as acyclovir) agents. Administration of hematopoietic growth factors (such as granulocyte-macrophage colony-stimulating factor [GM-CSF] or G-CSF) by subcutaneous injection after stem cell infusion also can accelerate hematopoietic recovery after transplantation and lessen the risk of infection. Improvements in supportive care have increased the safety of blood and marrow transplantation and allowed care of patients to be increasingly shifted to the outpatient setting, to the point that transfer of the entire transplant procedure to the outpatient setting is becoming a reality.

Pretransplantation Evaluation

Blood and marrow transplantation is a physically and psychologically demanding undertaking for patients and their caregivers, and patients must undergo a thorough evaluation of their overall health before transplantation. Representative evaluations and tests that are required before the procedure are listed in Table 1. Abnormalities in the results of these tests are not always absolute contraindications to transplantation, but they must be interpreted in light of the overall clinical situation and the patient's alternatives for treatment of the underlying disease. In the past, age limits of less than 65 years for autologous and less than 55 years for allogeneic transplants were established by most centers because of the increased toxicity of the procedure in older individuals. Improvements in supportive care, however, have increased the ability of older patients to tolerate the procedure, and more and more, a patient's functional status rather than chronologic age is being used to determine suitability for transplantation.

Related Donors

For allogeneic transplantation, donors also undergo general and serologic testing to assess their overall health and infectious risk. HLA typing by serologic and molecular techniques is essential to determine whether the patient has a donor who has inherited the same HLA-A, B, and DR phenotype. Each individual receives one HLA haplotype from each parent (three antigens from each), and the ideal donor is, therefore, a six of six match (Fig. 4 *A*, Plate 18, and Fig. 4 *B*). Although the HLA system is much more complex than these six antigen designations suggest, these HLA loci have proved to be of most importance in reducing the risks of GVHD and rejection and are still most often relied on in selecting a donor. On the basis of mendelian genetics, each individual should have a 25% chance that a sibling will be a full match. This probability is actually somewhat higher because of the genetic linkage of certain HLA types. A five of six match also seems to be acceptable for transplants, and in some centers, with the use of more intense immunosuppression, transplantations from family members with four of six or even three of

Table 1
Pretransplantation Tests

History	Cholesterol, triglyceride levels
Physical examination	ABO, Rh typing
Complete blood cell count	Urinalysis
Chemistry tests	Creatinine clearance
Human leukocyte antigen typing	Bone marrow biopsy with cytogenetic study
Hepatitis B and C tests	Electrocardiography
Human immunodeficiency virus test	Echocardiography or multiple-gated
Herpes simplex virus serology	acquisition scanning of the heart
Cytomegalovirus serology	Pulmonary function tests
Epstein-Barr virus serology	Chest radiography
Toxoplasma serology	Sinus radiography
Prothrombin time, partial	Dental evaluation
thromboplastin time test	Radiation oncology evaluation
Pregnancy test	Disease staging
Sperm or oocyte banking	

From Litzow MR. Blood and marrow transplantation, in *Transplant Surgery* (Hakim N, Danovitch GM, eds.). Springer-Verlag, Berlin (in press). By permission of the publisher.

six matches are being performed. The poorer the match, however, the higher the risk of marrow rejection or GVHD. Extended family searches occasionally identify a more distant relative who is closely HLA-matched with the recipient.

Unrelated Donors

Patients who lack a suitable family match must rely on the use of their own stem cells (if suitable) or search for an unrelated donor. Unrelated umbilical cord blood can now be used and is an appropriate option for many children and, perhaps, some adults. For most patients, an unrelated adult is the best option. In the past 10 years, large registries of volunteers who have been HLA-typed have been established and large computer databases developed so that patients and physicians can search for a histocompatible unrelated donor. The National Marrow Donor Program in the United States is the largest such registry, and it has close ties with similar registries in other countries. More than 3 million volunteers have now registered with this program, and the chances of finding a match for patients, regardless of ethnic origin, have increased substantially. Thousands of unrelated donor blood and marrow transplantations have now been performed worldwide. Results, in general, however, are somewhat inferior to those achieved with sibling donors because of the increased risk of rejection and GVHD.

Conditioning and Stem Cell Infusion

Once a patient has been selected for blood and marrow transplantation and a source of stem cells has been identified, a long-term central venous catheter with two or three lumina is placed in a central vein via a subcutaneous tunnel to facilitate infusion of stem cells, blood products, parenteral nutrition, and drugs and to allow blood removal for testing (this spares the patient repeated venipunctures). Although these catheters have been of great benefit in easing the burden of transplantation for medical personnel and patient alike, they can be sources of infection and thrombosis, which can result in the need for their removal and replacement.

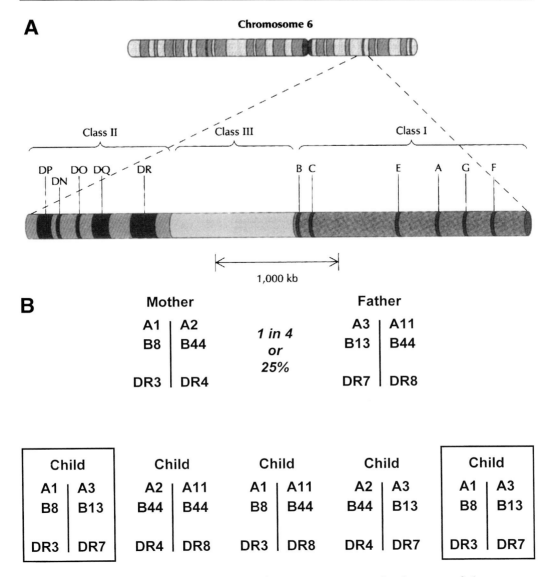

Fig. 4. *A*, **Plate 18,** The human leukocyte antigen gene system on the short arm of chromosome 6 consists of the class I region of A and B loci as well as other loci and the class II region of D loci. The class III region contains genes of the complement system. (*A* from Jagannath S, Barlogie B, Tricot G. Hematopoietic stem cell transplantation. *Hosp Pract* 1993; 28 no. 8: 79-86. By permission of the McGraw-Hill Companies, Inc. Illustration by Seward Hung.)*B*, Chances of finding an identical match among siblings.

In virtually all cases, patients undergoing blood and marrow transplantation are treated with a "conditioning" regimen before infusion of their stem cells. This conditioning regimen usually consists of high-dose chemotherapy with or without total body irradiation. The purpose of the conditioning regimen is to reduce the patient's disease burden to the lowest level possible and, in the case of allogeneic transplants, to suppress the patient's immune system to facilitate engraftment of the infused stem cells. Most of these regimens were developed empirically. The most frequently used regimens are listed in

Table 2
Examples of Frequently Used Conditioning
Regimens and Associated Diseases

Conditioning regimen	Disease
Cyclophosphamide-total body irradiation	Multiple
Busulfan-cyclophosphamide	AML, CML, genetic diseases
Carmustine (BCNU), etoposide, cytosine arabinoside, and cyclophosphamide (BEAC) or melphalan (BEAM)	Lymphoma
Melphalan-total body irradiation	Multiple myeloma
Etoposide-total body irradiation	ALL
Cyclophosphamide, thiotepa, carboplatin	Breast cancer
Cyclophosphamide-antithymocyte globulin	Aplastic anemia
Cyclophosphamide, carmustine, etoposide	Hodgkin's disease

Abbreviations: ALL, acute lymphoblastic leukemia; AML, acute myelogenous leukemia; CML, chronic myelogenous leukemia.
From Litzow MR. Blood and marrow transplantation, in *Transplant Surgery* (Hakim N, Danovitch GM, eds.). Springer-Verlag, Berlin (in press). By permission of the publisher.

Table 2. Initial successful experiments with total body irradiation in animals led to its subsequent use in humans. The Seattle group, led by Nobel laureate E. D. Thomas, M.D., later showed the benefit of a combination of total body irradiation and high-dose cyclophosphamide to cure a fraction of patients with end-stage leukemia. Subsequent studies built on this experience and substituted drugs such as busulfan for the irradiation and etoposide, melphalan, and cytosine arabinoside, among others, for the cyclophosphamide. Many of these regimens have relied on the use of alkylating agents because of their broad spectrum of antitumor activity, non–cross-resistance, and lack of significant organ toxicity at high doses. Unfortunately, few randomized trials have been performed comparing these different regimens to determine which is most efficacious in a particular disease setting.

After completion of the conditioning regimen, the patient's stem cells are infused. These can be infused directly into the recipient through the long-term central venous catheter after filtering in the operating room to remove particulate matter in the case of an ABO-compatible allogeneic marrow transplant. Frequently, additional processing is required to deplete T cells to reduce the risk of GVHD or to remove red cells in the case of an ABO-incompatible transplant. Autologous stem cells are usually cryopreserved with dimethyl sulfoxide, which stabilizes cell membranes and prevents intracellular ice crystal formation. Cryopreservation is usually done in a liquid nitrogen controlled-rate freezer, which seems to enhance long-term cell viability and is required if the stem cells are not used within 2 to 3 days of collection. Stem cells cryopreserved for 10 years or more have been shown to engraft successfully. Removal of T cells from allogeneic grafts to reduce the risk of GVHD and tumor cells from autologous grafts to reduce the risk of relapse is complicated and often controversial, and the subject is beyond the scope of this chapter. The reader is referred to other sources for discussions of this topic.

Infusion of thawed stem cells after cryopreservation can be associated with symptoms of nausea, flushing, abdominal cramps, fever and chills, hypoxia, hypertension, bradycardia, and renal insufficiency related to dimethyl sulfoxide and fragments of residual red cell membranes. Bacterial contamination of the stem cell product can cause bacteremia.

These infusion-related symptoms are usually self-limited, reversible, and rarely clinically significant, but they occasionally are severe. A CD34 cell-affinity column can be used before cryopreservation to remove accessory cells and enrich for stem cells. It significantly reduces the volume of infused cells and has been shown to lessen the incidence of toxicities.

COMPLICATIONS

Blood and marrow transplantation is a complex and intense procedure that can be associated with a myriad of complications.

Complications of Transplantation

- Regimen-related toxicity
- Toxicity due to cytopenias (infection and bleeding)
- Immune-mediated toxicity (GVHD)
- Delayed toxicity

Regimen-Related Toxicity

Regimen-related toxicity refers to complications attributed to the high-dose conditioning regimen patients receive in the initial phase of the transplantation. These toxicities are, in general, organ-specific; usually occur within the first few weeks after the procedure; and most often affect the liver, lung, heart, skin, urinary system, gastrointestinal tract, or central nervous system. Multiple organs can be affected simultaneously, and toxicity occurring initially in one organ can complicate toxicities in other organs. A syndrome of multiorgan failure also can occur after transplantation. Although these toxicities can vary in severity, they can be life-threatening and tend to be more severe in patients who enter the transplantation process with compromised organ function, poor performance status, and extensive prior therapy of the underlying disease. The affected organ systems and most frequent toxicities associated with them are listed in Table 3.

Consequences of Myelosuppression

Toxicities related to cytopenias are primarily those of infection and bleeding. Patients undergoing blood and marrow transplantation are extremely susceptible to infections of various types and for varying durations, depending on the type of transplant they receive and the complications they experience after the procedure. The type of infection correlates with the particular immune defect the patient is experiencing at the time. Figure 5 shows the spectrum of infections and time after transplantation at which they occur. Immediately after the procedure, neutropenia is the dominant immune defect, and patients are susceptible to primarily bacterial and fungal infections. Although neutropenia usually resolves within 30 days of stem cell infusion, recovery of lymphocyte function can be delayed and leave patients at risk for viral infection for prolonged periods. This protracted lymphocyte recovery is particularly prominent after allogeneic transplantation and can be significantly affected by the presence of GVHD and its treatment with immunosuppressive drugs. GVHD also affects recovery of immunoglobulin production, and patients with chronic GVHD are at risk for delayed bacterial infections.

In the early post-transplantation period, up to 40% to 50% of patients can have fever due to documented or occult bacterial infection. In the past, the predominant organisms

Table 3
Common Regimen-Related Toxicities

Site	Toxicity
Liver	Veno-occlusive disease
Lung	Diffuse alveolar damage
	Idiopathic pneumonia syndrome
Heart	Cardiomyopathy
	Arrhythmia
	Myocarditis
Skin	Acral erythema
	Alopecia
	Eruption of lymphocyte recovery
Urinary system	Hemorrhagic cystitis
	Renal insufficiency
	Radiation nephritis
Gastrointestinal system	Nausea
	Diarrhea
	Mucositis
Nervous system	Seizures
	Cerebellar toxicity
	Peripheral neuropathy

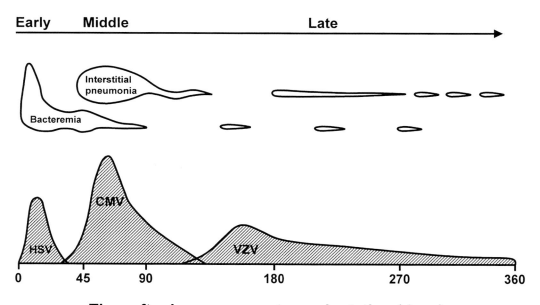

Time after bone marrow transplantation (days)

Fig. 5. Infections occurring after blood and marrow transplantation. Time is divided into early (days 0-21), middle (days 22-100), and late (days after 100). *CMV*, cytomegalovirus; *HSV*, herpes simplex virus; *VZV*, varicella zoster virus. (From Zaia JA. Infections, in *Clinical Bone Marrow Transplantation* [Blume KG, Petz LD, eds.]. Churchill Livingstone, New York, 1983, pp. 131-176. By permission of the publisher.)

were gram-negative bacilli; however, in recent years, with the use of effective prophylactic antibiotics against gram-negative organisms and the use of long-term central venous catheters, the incidence of infections with gram-positive organisms, especially *Staphylococcus epidermidis* and *Streptococcus viridans*, has significantly increased.

Once fever develops in a patient with neutropenia, a careful history and physical examination, cultures of blood and body fluids, appropriate radiographic studies, and initiation of therapy with parenterally administered broad-spectrum antibiotics are indicated. The choice of initial empiric antibiotic therapy depends on the spectrum of organisms identified at a particular institution, but frequently includes either an aminoglycoside and antipseudomonal β-lactam with or without vancomycin or, more often, monotherapy with a late-generation cephalosporin such as ceftazidime or cefipime. If no source of infection is found and fever persists for 3 or 4 days, empiric amphotericin B therapy should be initiated. Infections with *Candida* or *Aspergillus* species are the most common fungal infections after transplantation. In a randomized trial of prophylactic fluconazole versus placebo, fluconazole significantly reduced the incidence of candidal infections after allogeneic transplantation.

Post-transplantation Viral Infections

Viral infections after transplantation are predominantly due to the herpes virus family, including herpes simplex, cytomegalovirus (CMV), varicella zoster, and Epstein-Barr virus (EBV). Adenoviruses and respiratory syncytial virus also can cause significant infection. Herpes simplex virus can aggravate the chemoradiotherapy-induced mucositis patients experience early after blood and marrow transplantation, but it can be effectively prevented by prophylactic administration of acyclovir or one of the newer antiherpetic antibiotics, such as valacyclovir, in the first month after transplantation. CMV infection, especially pneumonia, was, until recently, the most dreaded viral infection after allogeneic transplantation. With the use of weekly intravenous administration of immunoglobulin from immediately before transplantation until day 100 after transplantation, as well as weekly surveillance viral blood cultures with initiation of ganciclovir therapy when the culture results are positive, the vast majority of tissue-invasive CMV infections can now be prevented. Varicella zoster infection, usually dermatomal, can occur in 25% to 50% of patients in the first year after transplantation. Cutaneous or visceral dissemination can occur in a minority of these patients. Therapy should be initiated at the first sign of infection to reduce the risk of post-herpetic neuralgia. Lymphoproliferative syndromes due to EBV infection can occur several months after transplantation, primarily in patients who have undergone allogeneic transplantation with T-cell depletion or intense immunosuppression. Infusion of small numbers of EBV-specific donor cytotoxic lymphocytes often produces remission of the syndrome.

Blood Component Transfusion After Transplantation

Virtually all patients require transfusion of red blood cells and platelets after blood and marrow transplantation. Because of patients' immunocompromised state, all cellular blood products should be irradiated (25 Gy) before administration for at least 1 year after transplantation to prevent the development of GVHD initiated by passenger T cells in the blood products. Alloimmunization to platelets is one of the most common transfusion problems after the procedure. It is caused by leukocytes in the transfused blood products which stimulate the production of HLA antibodies in the host and can lead to febrile transfusion reactions and destruction of transfused products, especially platelets, rendering random donor platelet transfusions ineffective. The development of allo-immunization can be reduced by filtration of the leukocytes before transfusion. Once alloimmunization develops, HLA-matched platelets, including those obtained by apheresis from the patient's donor, can be of benefit. Reducing the number of transfusions given also can reduce the risk of transfusion reactions, and studies now have demonstrated that withholding red cell transfusion until the hemoglobin level is less than 8 g/dL, and platelets until the platelet count is less than $10 \times 10^9/L$, is safe if the patient is otherwise stable.

Graft Failure

Failure of the blood counts to recover after transplantation, or graft failure, is, fortunately, uncommon. Although a uniform definition of graft failure does not exist, most investigators become concerned when neutrophil recovery to more than $0.5 \times 10^9/L$ has not occurred by day +30 after the procedure. Some patients have recovery subsequent to this time, but some sort of intervention often is considered. Graft failure can be primary if no increase in blood counts is achieved or secondary if a transient increase occurs followed by a subsequent decline. Mechanisms of graft failure vary depending on the type of transplant. In the autologous or syngeneic setting, considerations include an inadequate number of stem cells infused, damage to the bone marrow microenvironment inhibiting engraftment, or infections or drugs that inhibit hematopoietic recovery. In some patients, particularly in the autologous setting, partial graft failure occurs when neutrophil recovery occurs, but significant delays in red cell and platelet recovery lead to ongoing transfusion requirements.

In the allogeneic setting, graft rejection mediated by residual host T cells is one of the most frequent causes of graft failure. Allogeneic rejection can occur more frequently in patients who have transplantation for aplastic anemia or in those who have received marrow that has been depleted of T cells or has come from a mismatched donor. Rejection in these settings can be diagnosed when the number of host T cells in the peripheral blood is increased or an increase in host cells is detected in the marrow in the setting of decreased blood cell counts. Increases in host cells can be detected with cytogenetic or molecular techniques that detect sex chromosome differences in sex-mismatched transplants, donor-host HLA differences in HLA-mismatched transplants, or DNA polymorphisms in sex- and HLA-matched transplants. Graft failure frequently has a poor prognosis, and rescue cannot always be accomplished with salvage therapy. Options for treatment include infusion of additional stem cells with or without additional conditioning therapy, administration of hematopoietic growth factors, and more intensive immunosuppressive therapy.

Graft-Versus-Host Disease

GVHD is an immunologic disorder first described after blood and marrow transplantation. T lymphocytes from the donor have been established as the mediators of GVHD, and the clinical manifestations of GVHD result from T-cell recognition of foreign host antigens with subsequent activation of multiple inflammatory cytokines, including interferon-γ and tumor necrosis factor. GVHD has been divided clinically into acute and chronic forms, although there can be significant overlap between the two forms. The acute form generally occurs within the first 2 to 3 months after transplantation, whereas the chronic form usually develops after 3 months.

Table 4
Clinical Stage of Acute Graft-Versus-Host Disease According to Organ System

Stage	Skin	Liver	Intestinal tract
+	Maculopapular rash < 25% of body surface	Bilirubin 2-3 mg/100 mL	> 500 mL diarrhea/day
++	Maculopapular rash 25%-50% body surface	Bilirubin 3-6 mg/100 mL	> 1,000 mL diarrhea/day
+++	Generalized erythroderma	Bilirubin 6-15 mg/100 mL	> 1,500 mL diarrhea/day
++++	Generalized erythroderma with bullous formation and desquamation	Bilirubin > 15 mg/100 mL	Severe abdominal pain, with or without ileus

From Thomas ED, Storb R, Clift RA, Fefer A, Johnson L, Neiman PE, Lerner KG, Glucksberg H, Buckner CD. Bone-marrow transplantation (second of two parts). *N Engl J Med* 1975; 292: 895-902. By permission of the Massachusetts Medical Society.

Table 5
Overall Clinical Grading of Severity
of Acute Graft-Versus-Host Disease

Grade	Degree of organ involvement
I	+ to ++ skin rash; no gut involvement; no liver involvement; no decrease in clinical performance
II	+ to +++ skin rash; + gut involvement or + liver involvement (or both); mild decrease in clinical performance
III	++ to +++ skin rash; ++ to +++ gut involvement or ++ to ++++ liver involvement (or both); marked decrease in clinical performance
IV	Similar to grade III with ++ to ++++ organ involvement and extreme decrease in clinical performance

From Thomas ED, Storb R, Clift RA, Fefer A, Johnson L, Neiman PE, Lerner KG, Glucksberg H, Buckner CD. Bone-marrow transplantation (second of two parts). *N Engl J Med* 1975; 292: 895-902. By permission of the Massachusetts Medical Society.

ACUTE GVHD

In acute GVHD, some combination of skin, liver, and gastrointestinal tract involvement develops. The degree of involvement can be graded based on clinical severity, and an overall grade of disease is assigned based on a widely accepted grading scheme devised in the 1970s (Tables 4 and 5). Acute GVHD also can cause lymph node and thymic atrophy and hypogammaglobulinemia. In the nontransplant setting, in which acute GVHD can arise from transfusions given to immunocompromised patients, severe pancytopenia also can occur. Acute GVHD occurs in 40% to 50% of HLA-matched sibling donors and in up to 80% to 90% of mismatched family or unrelated donors. Even though the closeness of the match between donor and recipient is the most important determinant of the risk of development of acute GVHD, increasing age of donor and recipient, more intensive conditioning regimens, type of prophylaxis of GVHD, and use of a parous female donor also can increase the risk.

Prophylaxis of GVHD is essential to decrease the risk of its development and usually has consisted of pharmacologic methods of immunosuppression or T-cell depletion. The most commonly used regimen of prophylaxis is cyclosporine, 1.5 mg/kg twice daily intravenously, in the immediate peritransplantation period, followed by oral dosages of 12.5 mg/kg a day in two divided doses (adjusted according to blood level) and low-dose intravenous methotrexate given on days 1, 3, 6, and 11 after transplantation to inhibit any proliferating T cells that escape suppression by the cyclosporine. Most patients can discontinue cyclosporine use by 6 months to 2 years after transplantation if GVHD is controlled. Depletion of donor T cells by various methods can effectively prevent GVHD after transplantation, but it can lead to an increased risk of graft failure and relapse of the underlying disease. More selective T-cell depletion of subsets of T cells can lessen the risk of these adverse effects and still control GVHD. The therapy of acute GVHD depends on its severity, but it usually consists of prednisone in dosages of 1 to 2 mg/kg a day in addition to continuing cyclosporine use. Up to 75% of patients will respond to prednisone therapy. Nonresponders have a poor prognosis, but they may respond to second-line therapy, usually in the form of antithymocyte globulin, or investigational therapy.

CHRONIC GVHD

Chronic GVHD has its onset 2 to 3 months or later after transplantation. The greatest risk factor for the development of chronic GVHD is the prior occurrence of acute GVHD. Grading of chronic GVHD is not as sophisticated as that of acute GVHD and has been divided into a limited form of localized skin involvement and a nonprogressive cholestatic hepatic dysfunction or an extensive form including generalized lichenoid or scleroder- matous skin involvement, progressive hepatic dysfunction, or keratoconjunctivitis sicca, among other manifestations (Fig. 6 A, Plate 19, and Fig. 6 B, Plate 20). Patients with platelet counts less than 100×10^9/L at the time of onset and with progressive develop- ment of chronic GVHD after acute GVHD have a poorer prognosis. Chronic GVHD is associated with immunodeficiency, which can be severe and is exacerbated by the immu- nosuppressive drugs used to try to control the disease. Most patients dying of chronic GVHD succumb to infection. Therapy for chronic GVHD depends on the use of pred- nisone and cyclosporine, which are usually given in an alternating schedule of each drug every other day. Patients failing this first-line therapy have a poor prognosis, but they may respond to alternative immunosuppressive therapies.

Supportive care of patients with GVHD is essential to prevent infection and maintain function. Patients with chronic GVHD have poor splenic phagocytic function and are at risk for infection from encapsulated organisms. Penicillin prophylaxis in doses of 500 to 1,000 mg per day is effective in preventing this complication. Immunosuppressive therapy, especially with corticosteroids, requires prophylaxis for *Pneumocystis carinii* with trimethoprim-sulfamethoxazole or inhaled nebulized pentamidine. Patients with hypogammaglobulinemia may benefit from monthly intravenous infusions of gamma globulin. Good oral hygiene can lessen the risk of dental caries and oral ulcers. For patients with sclerodermatous skin changes, physical therapy and good skin care can help maintain mobility and prevent joint contractures and infections. Prolonged sun exposure should be avoided to prevent exacerbation of both cutaneous and systemic GVHD.

Delayed Complications

Although patients who survive blood and marrow transplantation and are cured of their underlying disease can go on to lead normal lives, they can be at risk for several delayed

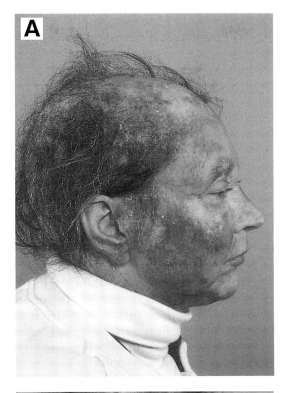

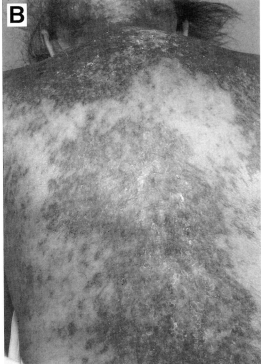

Fig. 6. *A*, **Plate 19,** Chronic graft-versus-host disease with lichenoid and sclerodermatous changes in the face and scalp with alopecia. *B*, **Plate 20,** Lichenoid hyperpigmentation of the back.

Table 6
Delayed Complications

Chronic graft-versus-host disease
Airway and pulmonary disease
Autoimmune dysfunction
Neuroendocrine dysfunction
Impaired growth
Infertility
Ophthalmologic problems
Avascular necrosis of the bone
Dental problems
Genitourinary dysfunction
Secondary malignancies
Central and peripheral nervous system
Psychosocial effects and rehabilitation

From Deeg HJ. Delayed complications,
in *On Call In . . . Bone Marrow Transplan-
tation* (Burt RK, Deeg HJ, Lothian ST,
Santos GW, eds.). Chapman & Hall, New
York, 1996, pp. 515-522. By permission of
R. G. Landes Company.

complications resulting from the conditioning regimen, complications of chronic medication use, or GVHD. These complications can, at times, have a significant impact on
their quality of life. These are too broad in scope to be discussed in detail here. These
complications are listed in Table 6.

DISEASES TREATED WITH BLOOD
AND MARROW TRANSPLANTATION

In the past 2 decades, not only the number of transplants but also the types of diseases
to which blood and marrow transplantation has been applied have increased substantially. The wider application of transplantation has been stimulated by initial successes
in leukemia and other hematologic disorders and improvements in supportive care which
have lessened the toxicity of the procedure. The most common diseases for which blood
and marrow transplantation has been used are listed in Table 7. The indications for the
procedure in the treatment of several of these diseases remain uncertain, and precisely
when a patient should have transplantation in the course of a disease remains controversial. The European Group for Blood and Marrow Transplantation recently published
guidelines for when to consider different types of stem cell sources for transplantation for
a wide variety of disorders, depending on the phase of a patient's disease (relapse or
remission).

As new therapies develop, the role that transplantation plays in particular diseases also
has to be redefined. Despite the advances in supportive care that have been made in recent
years, patients can still die of one of the many complications of BMT outlined previously,
and some patients who survive the procedure can be chronically disabled from a complication such as chronic GVHD. Mortality rates from complications vary considerably
depending on the type of transplant, the phase of the patient's disease, the extent of
pretransplantation therapy, and type of donor (matched or mismatched, related or unre-

Table 7
Diseases Treated With Blood and Marrow Transplantation

Acute leukemias
Chronic leukemias
Myelodysplastic syndromes
Agnogenic myeloid metaplasia
Hodgkin's disease
Non-Hodgkin's lymphoma
Multiple myeloma
Amyloidosis
Breast cancer
Ovarian cancer
Germ cell cancer
Sarcomas
Brain tumors
Neuroblastoma
Aplastic anemia
Autoimmune diseases
Hemoglobinopathies
Immunodeficiency states
Lysosomal and peroxisomal storage diseases

From Litzow MR. Blood and marrow transplantation, in *Transplant Surgery* (Hakim N, Danovitch GM, eds.). Springer-Verlag, Berlin (in press). By permission of the publisher.

lated). In high-risk allogeneic transplants, mortality rates from complications can be as high as 40% to 50%, whereas in good-risk patients undergoing autologous PBSC transplant-associated mortality rates can be less than 5%. All these factors must be considered in counseling a patient about the role blood and marrow transplantation plays in the treatment of their disease. The challenge for clinicians is to apply transplantation early enough in the course of the disease when the patient still has excellent functional status and few or no comorbid conditions, yet also consider the potential cure rate and outcome the patient can achieve with nontransplant therapies.

An additional challenge clinicians face is the management of patients whose disease recurs after transplantation. In general, such patients have a poor prognosis. In the past, patients with relapse after receiving an allogeneic transplant were sometimes offered a second transplant, but these transplants were associated with a high treatment-related mortality rate and disease relapse rate. A novel observation after allogeneic transplantation was that patients with GVHD had lower relapse rates than patients who did not and that relapse rates after syngeneic or T-cell–depleted transplants were even higher (Fig. 7). This phenomenon has been referred to as the graft-versus-leukemia (GVL) effect and suggests that the immune system of the donor can be used to help eradicate the patient's underlying disease. Based on these observations, a newer approach to the therapy of relapse after allogeneic blood and marrow transplantation has been leukapheresis of the donor to collect peripheral blood T cells, which are then infused into the recipient to stimulate a GVL effect. This approach has been most successful in patients with chronic myelogenous leukemia who have relapse after transplantation, but it can be beneficial for the treatment of relapse of other diseases after transplantation. Ultimately, it is hoped that a better understanding of the pathogenesis of GVHD and the mechanism of the GVL effect can help harness the GVL effect to fight the patient's disease without provoking GVHD.

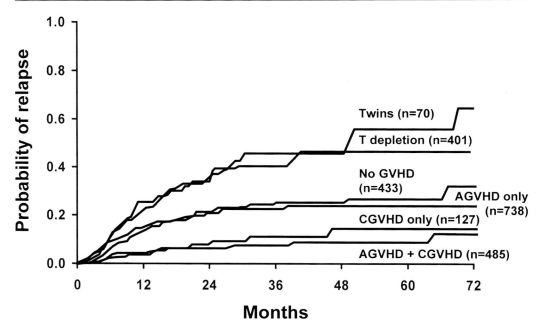

Fig. 7. Actuarial probability of relapse after bone marrow transplantation for early leukemia, according to type of graft and development of graft-versus-host disease (GVHD). AGVHD, acute GVHD; CGVHD, chronic GVHD. (From Horowitz MM, Gale RP, Sondel PM, Goldman JM, Kersey J, Kolb H-J, Rimm AA, Ringdén O, Rozman C, Speck B, Truitt RL, Zwaan FE, Bortin MM. Graft-versus-leukemia reactions after bone marrow transplantation. *Blood* 1990; 75: 555-562. By permission of the American Society of Hematology.)

FUTURE DIRECTIONS

In the future, improvements in the outcome of patients undergoing blood and marrow transplantation will depend on decreasing the toxicity of the procedure and reducing the risk of recurrence of the underlying disease after the procedure. Promising approaches include altering the conditioning regimen to target tumor cells and spare normal tissues, such as through the use of monoclonal antibodies linked to radionuclides. Another approach has been to lessen the intensity of the conditioning regimen so it is less toxic but still immuno-suppressive to allow engraftment of allogeneic cells and stimulate a GVL effect. Improved understanding of stem cell biology may allow the expansion of a small number of stem cells in vitro and lessen the toxicity of blood and marrow collections. The concept of "graft engineering" will play an increasingly prominent role in treatment strategies as our abilities to isolate and expand subsets of cells for specific purposes increase. Finally, the promise of gene therapy brings the hope that therapeutic genes can be inserted into stem cells and transplanted to correct gene defects or augment deficient functions. Blood and marrow transplantation has stimulated and will continue to stimulate new advances in immunology, stem cell biology, and the treatment of a wide variety of diseases.

SUGGESTED READING

Atkinson K. Reconstruction of the haemopoietic and immune systems after marrow transplantation. *Bone Marrow Transplant* 1990; 5: 209-226.

Bearman SI, Appelbaum FR, Buckner CD, Petersen FB, Fisher LD, Clift RA, Thomas ED. Regimen-related toxicity in patients undergoing bone marrow transplantation. *J Clin Oncol* 1988; 6: 1562-1568.

Cairo MS, Wagner JE. Placental and/or umbilical cord blood: an alternative source of hematopoietic stem cells for transplantation. *Blood* 1997; 90: 4665-4678.

Huntly BJ, Franklin IM, Pippard MJ. Unrelated bone-marrow transplantation in adults. *Blood Rev* 1996; 10: 220-230.

Lazarus HM, Vogelsang GB, Rowe JM. Prevention and treatment of acute graft-versus-host disease: the old and the new. A report from the Eastern Cooperative Oncology Group (ECOG). *Bone Marrow Transplant* 1997; 19: 577-600.

Rowe JM, Ciobanu N, Ascensao J, Stadtmauer EA, Weiner RS, Schenkein DP, McGlave P, Lazarus HM. Recommended guidelines for the management of autologous and allogeneic bone marrow transplantation. A report from the Eastern Cooperative Oncology Group. *Ann Intern Med* 1994; 120: 143-158.

Schmitz N, Gratwohl A, Goldman JM, for Accreditation Sub-Committee of the European Group for Blood and Marrow Transplantation (EBMT). Allogeneic and autologous transplantation for haematological diseases, solid tumours and immune disorders. Current practice in Europe in 1996 and proposals for an operational classification. *Bone Marrow Transplant* 1996; 17: 471-477.

Sullivan KM, Mori M, Sanders J, Siadak M, Witherspoon RP, Anasetti C, Appelbaum FR, Bensinger W, Bowden R, Buckner CD, Clark J, Crawford S, Deeg HJ, Doney K, Flowers M, Hansen J, Loughran T, Martin P, McDonald G, Pepe M, Petersen FB, Schuening F, Stewart P, Storb R. Late complications of allogeneic and autologous marrow transplantation. *Bone Marrow Transplant* 1992; 10 Suppl 1: 127-134.

Szilvassy SJ, Hoffman R. Enriched hematopoietic stem cells: basic biology and clinical utility. *Biol Blood Marrow Transplant* 1995; 1: 3-17.

To LB, Haylock DN, Simmons PJ, Juttner CA. The biology and clinical uses of blood stem cells. *Blood* 1997; 89: 2233-2258.

Wingard JR. Infections in allogeneic bone marrow transplant recipients. *Semin Oncol* 1993; 20 Suppl 6: 80-87.

IV LYMPHOID AND PLASMA CELL DISORDERS

16

Lymphadenopathy

Thomas M. Habermann, MD

Contents

INTRODUCTION

Lymphadenopathy can occur in any age group, in symptomatic or asymptomatic patients, and in a single site or multiple sites, and it is associated with innumerable disorders. Lymphadenopathy can be discovered on palpation by the patient, on physical examination by a health-care worker, or through radiologic evaluation. It may present in complex cases or be straightforward to members of the health-care team. Most importantly, patients may have underlying potentially curable malignant disorders. This review synthesizes initial general considerations, reviews issues of initial approach and subsequent directions, defines which patients and which nodes should have biopsy, and outlines a broad differential diagnosis with the use of acronyms.

INITIAL CONSIDERATIONS

Lymphadenopathy can affect all ages. The essential general considerations for the approach to the patient with lymphadenopathy include **a**ge, **l**ocation, **l**ength of time present, **a**ssociated signs and symptoms, **g**eneralized lymphadenopathy, **e**xtranodal associations, and **s**plenomegaly (acronym, ALL AGES) (Table 1).

Age is the most important factor in statistically estimating the probability of whether the lymphadenopathy is due to a benign or a malignant lesion (*1*). In young patients, the differential diagnosis should include infectious mononucleosis. Associated signs and symptoms are varied. Patients may be asymptomatic and have no other signs or symp-

From: *Primary Hematology*
Edited by: A. Tefferi © Mayo Foundation for Medical Education and Research, Rochester, MN

Table 1
General Considerations
for Lymphadenopathy

Age
Location
Length of time present

Associated signs and symptoms
Generalized lymphadenopathy
Extranodal associations
Splenomegaly

toms. Patients may present with "B" symptoms, which include fever, chills, night sweats, and weight loss. These are characteristics of lymphoproliferative disorders. Patients with Hodgkin's disease may have pain after alcohol ingestion. There may be lymphangiectatic streaking in cutaneous infections.

With regard to consistency, the nodes may be tender, warm, erythematous, or fluctuant. The nodes may be hard, fixed, rubbery, or mobile. Overall, consistency is not necessarily helpful in distinguishing a benign from a malignant lesion.

In 63% of cases, Margolis et al. (2) established a positive yield, defined as one in which the clinical diagnosis was confirmed, changed, or excluded through lymph node biopsy. Sinclair et al. (3) reported a 63% specific diagnosis rate, excluding patients with known malignancies, systemic diseases, or abnormal chest radiographs. The most critical consideration in the clinical approach to adenopathy is determining which cases are associated with benign lesions and which are associated with malignant disorders. Then, it is essential to distinguish carcinoma from lymphoma.

Global considerations in the approach to lymphadenopathy include the region involved, the differential diagnosis, and the consideration that patients present with lymphadenopathy and fever with or without splenomegaly (rdw = with or without splenomegaly). Two approaches to the differential diagnosis are the CHICAGO approach (cancer, hypersensitivity, infections, connective tissue diseases, atypical lymphoproliferative disorders, granulomatous disorders, and other unusual causes of lymphadenopathy (Table 2) and the alphabet approach (Table 3).

HISTORY

The history and physical examination are essential in the evaluation of lymphadenopathy, after which a diagnosis often can be established efficiently with a few tests. Key historic and laboratory associations may aid in establishing the diagnosis in difficult cases of lymphadenopathy. The differential diagnosis of lymphadenopathy with malabsorption includes gluten-sensitive enteropathy, Crohn's disease, amyloidosis, and Whipple's disease. Lymphadenopathy associated with arthralgias may be caused by rheumatoid arthritis, systemic lupus erythematosus, Wegener's granulomatosis, and Whipple's disease. Renal disease and lymphadenopathy may be associated with systemic lupus erythematosus, mixed connective tissue disease, amyloidosis, Whipple's disease, and Hodgkin's disease with minimal change disease. Hypogammaglobulinemia and

Table 2
Causes of Lymphadenopathy: CHICAGO[a]

Cancer

Hematologic: Lymphoma, acute and chronic leukemia, Waldenström's macroglobulinemia,
    multiple myeloma (uncommon), systemic mastocytosis
Metastatic: Breast, lung, renal cell, prostate, other cancers

Hypersensitivity

Serum sickness
Drug sensitivity: Diphenylhydantoin, carbamazepine, primidone, gold, allopurinol, indomethacin,
    sulfonamides, others
Silicone reaction
Vaccination-related
Graft-versus-host disease

Infections

Viral: Infectious mononucleosis (Epstein-Barr virus), cytomegalovirus, infectious hepatitis,
    postvaccination lymphadenitis, adenovirus, herpes zoster, human immunodeficiency virus,
    acquired immunodeficiency syndrome, human T-cell lymphotropic virus type 1
Bacterial: *Staphylococcus, Streptococcus*, cat-scratch disease, chancroid, melioidosis, tuberculosis,
    atypical mycobacteria, primary and secondary syphilis
Chlamydial: Lymphogranuloma venereum
Protozoan: Toxoplasmosis
Mycotic: Histoplasmosis, coccidioidomycosis
Rickettsial: Scrub typhus
Helminthic: Filariasis

Connective tissue diseases

Rheumatoid arthritis, systemic lupus erythematosus, dermatomyositis, mixed connective tissue
    disease, Sjögren syndrome

Atypical lymphoproliferative disorders

Angiofollicular (giant) lymph node hyperplasia (Castleman's disease), angioimmunoblastic
    lymphadenopathy with dysproteinemia, angiocentric immunoproliferative disorders,
    lymphomatoid granulomatosis, Wegener's granulomatosis

Granulomatous disorders

Tuberculosis, histoplasmosis, mycobacterial infections, cryptococcosis, silicosis, berylliosis,
    cat-scratch disease

Other unusual causes of lymphadenopathy

Inflammatory pseudotumor of lymph nodes, histiocytic necrotizing lymphadenitis (Kikuchi's
    lymphadenitis), sinus histiocytosis with massive lymphadenopathy (Rosai-Dorfman
    syndrome), vascular transformation of sinuses, progressive transformation of germinal centers

---

[a]CHICAGO, *c*ancer, *h*ypersensitivity, *i*nfections, *c*onnective tissue diseases, *a*typical lymphoproliferative
disorders, *g*ranulomatous disorders, *o*ther unusual causes of lymphadenopathy.
    From Skarin AT. Approach to the patient with suspected lymphoma, in *The Lymphomas* (Canellos GP,
Lister TA, Sklar JL, eds.). WB Saunders Company, Philadelphia, 1998, pp. 207-211. By permission of the
publisher.

lymphadenopathy may be associated with Whipple's disease and amyloidosis. Monoclonal proteins in the serum or urine may be associated with non-Hodgkin's lymphoma,
chronic lymphocytic leukemia, multiple myeloma, and amyloidosis.

Table 3
Differential Diagnosis of Lymphadenopathy[a]

A	**Acquired immune deficiency syndrome (AIDS), AIDS-related complex,** AIDS-related infectious mononucleosis-like syndrome, asbestosis, allergic bronchopulmonary aspergillosis, **adenovirus**, angioimmunoblastic lymphadenopathy, actinomycosis, agnogenic myeloid metaplasia, acanthosis nigricans, aphthous stomatitis, amyloidosis
B	**Bite-wound infection,** brucellosis, bacille Calmette-Guérin vaccine, borreliosis, bubonic plague, blastomycosis
C	**Cancer** (breast, head and neck, lung, testicular, esophageal, melanoma, prostate, retinoblastoma, nasopharyngeal, rhabomyosarcoma), cytomegalovirus, **cellulitis,** chlamydiosis, lymphogranuloma venereum, chanchroid, **chronic lymphocytic leukemia,** Castleman's disease, cold agglutinin syndrome, carinii bacterial infections, cryptococcal infections, common variable immune deficiency, Chagas' disease
D	**Drugs (diphenylhydantoin, carbamazepine, primidone, gold, indomethacin, sulfonamides, hydralazine, allopurinol), dermatopathic lymphadenopathy,** dysmyelopoietic syndrome (chronic myelomonocytic leukemia)
E	**Epstein-Barr virus,** eosinophilic granuloma, **exfoliative dermatitis,** extramedullary hematopoiesis
F	Familial Mediterranean fever, Felty syndrome, filariasis
G	**Granulomatous diseases** (such as tuberculosis, histoplasmosis, mycobacterial infections), Glander's disease
H	**Hodgkin's disease, histoplasmosis,** herpes zoster, hepatitis A, histiocytosis X, Henoch-Schönlein purpura, **human immunodeficiency virus,** human herpes virus type 6 infection, human T-cell leukemia/lymphoma, hyperthyroidism, hypersensitivity reactions (serum sickness, drugs, graft-versus-host disease)
I	**Infectious mononucleosis,** inflammatory pseudotumor, idiopathic retroperitoneal fibrosis
J	**Juvenile rheumatoid arthritis**
K	Kawasaki's disease, Kikuchi-Fujimoto syndrome (histicytic necrotizing lymphadenitis), Kaposi's sarcoma
L	**Leukemia** (acute leukemia, chronic lymphocytic leukemia, hairy cell leukemia, chronic myelogenous leukemia), large granular lymphocyte disorders, lymphomatoid granulomatosis, leishmaniasis, Lyme disease
M	**Mycobacterial infections,** melioidosis, measles, mycotic carotid aneurysm, mixed essential cryoglobulinemia, multiple myeloma, mycosis fungoides, mesenteric adenitis
N	**Non-Hodgkin's lymphomas,** necrotizing lymphadenitis, neurodermatitis
O	**Occult malignancy**
P	Posttransplantation lymphoproliferative disorders, pulmonary alveolar proteinosis, postvaccination lymphadenitis, polyarteritis nodosum, psittacosis, progressive transformation of germinal centers
Q	Q fever
R	**Rheumatologic** (systemic lupus erythematosus, rheumatoid arthritis with or without gold treatment, mixed connective tissue disease, Sjögren's syndrome), Rosai-Dorfman syndrome (sinus histiocytosis), rheumatic fever, rheumatic heart disease, relapsing fever, rubella
S	**Sarcoidosis, streptococcal,** Sjögren's syndrome, Sweet's syndrome, systemic lupus erythematosus, silicone, schistosomiasis, salmonella, syphilis, subacute bacterial endocarditis, systemic mastocytosis, sporotrichosis, Sézary's syndrome, systemic mastocytosis, storage disease (Gaucher's disease, Niemann-Pick disease, Letterer-Siwe disease)
T	**Toxoplasmosis,** tuberculosis, tularemia, toxic oil syndrome, trypanosomiasis

Table 3 continued

U	Undiagnosed disease
V	Viral-associated hemophagocytic syndrome, vascular transformation of sinuses
W	Whipple disease, Waldenström's macroglobulinemia, Wegener's granulomatosis
X	X-linked lymphoproliferative disease states
Y	*Yersinia* infection, yaws
Z	Zaharsky's disease (periadenitis mucosa necrotica recurrens)

[a]Entries in boldface are the more common causes.

PHYSICAL EXAMINATION

The size of a lymph node in conjunction with the duration that the node has been present aid in the surgical approach to the diagnosis. In one series, a lymph node size of 1.5 × 1.5 cm was the best discriminating limit for distinguishing malignant or granulomatous lymphadenopathy from other adenopathy (4). In general, lymph nodes less than 1 × 1 cm in size without other evidence of an underlying systemic disease can be observed, and lymph nodes that have been present for more than 1 month and are 1 × 1 cm or more in size without a diagnosis should be considered for biopsy if the clinical situation warrants.

SITE OF LYMPHADENOPATHY

Cervical and Axillary

The differential diagnosis of cervical lymphadenopathy includes infections and malignancy. Infectious causes include bacterial pharyngitis, dental abscesses, otitis, infectious mononucleosis, gonococcal pharyngitis, cytomegalovirus, toxoplasmosis, hepatitis, and adenovirus. The common malignancies in the cervical region include Hodgkin's disease, non-Hodgkin's lymphoma, and squamous cell carcinoma of the head and neck.

Axillary adenopathy may be caused by Hodgkin's and non-Hodgkin's lymphoma, carcinoma of the breast, and melanoma. Other characteristic causes include staphylococcal infections, streptococcal infections, cat-scratch fever, tularemia, and sporotrichosis.

A Virchow node (left supraclavicular adenopathy) heralds the presence of an abdominal or thoracic neoplasm. Common causes include breast carcinoma, non-Hodgkin's lymphoma, Hodgkin's disease, abdominal neoplasms, and bronchogenic carcinoma. Chronic fungal infections can cause supraclavicular adenopathy.

Hilar

The most common causes of hilar prominence on chest radiographs are vascular engorgement and adenopathy. On chest radiographic evaluation alone, it may be difficult to distinguish vascular enlargement from nodal enlargement. The differential diagnosis of hilar lymphadenopathy is extensive (5). Unilateral hilar adenopathy may be related to pneumonitis or neoplasia. Any pneumonia can cause unilateral hilar adenopathy, as can granulomatous pneumonitis, tuberculosis, atypical mycobacterial infections, histoplasmosis, coccidioidomycosis, *Mycoplasma* pneumonia, tularemia, psittacosis, and pertussis. Neoplastic causes include bronchogenic carcinoma, metastatic carcinoma of the breast and gastrointestinal tract, non-Hodgkin's and Hodgkin's lymphoma, and sarcoidosis (1%-3%). Bilateral hilar adenopathy may be caused by sarcoidosis, non-Hodgkin's and Hodgkin's lymphomas, metastatic carcinoma, chronic granulomatous infection, and berylliosis. Calcified hilar adenopathy may be due to tuberculosis, histoplasmosis, and silicosis (egg-shaped). The approach to evaluating hilar adenopathy includes the evaluation of previous chest radiographs, serologic tests (such as fungal and serum angiotensin-converting enzyme), cultures when appropriate, and biopsy. Mediastinoscopy is the preferred initial approach, but other approaches include a limited anterior thoracotomy or needle biopsy.

Mediastinal

The causes of mediastinal widening are varied (5). Diffuse mediastinal widening may be related to acute mediastinitis, hemorrhage, lipomatosis, or fibrosing mediastinitis. Acute mediastinitis may be bacterial and related to an entity such as esophageal rupture due to Boerhaave's syndrome, foreign body ingestion, esophageal carcinoma, penetrating or blunt chest trauma, post-esophageal dilatation, empyema, lung abscess, pericarditis, retropharyngeal abscess, or infected bronchogenic cyst. Anterior mediastinal masses may be due to thymoma, teratoma, dermoid cysts, intrathoracic goiter, Hodgkin's and non-Hodgkin's lymphoma, parathyroid masses, endodermal sinus tumors, seminoma, primary choriocarcinoma, lipoma, fibroma, hemangioma, and lymphangioma. Middle mediastinal masses may be due to non-Hodgkin's and Hodgkin's lymphoma, carcinoma of the trachea, metastatic carcinoma, granulomatous mediastinitis, bronchogenic cyst, pleuropericardial cyst, diaphragmatic hernia through the foramen of Morgagni, Castleman's disease, and vascular dilatation. Posterior mediastinal masses may be a result of neurogenic tumors, neuroenteric cysts, gastroenteric cysts, thoracic duct cysts, esophageal neoplasms and diverticula, diaphragmatic hernia through the foramen of Bochdalek, disease of the thoracic spine, and extramedullary hematopoiesis.

The initial approach to the mediastinal mass includes a history and physical examination, evaluation of previous chest radiographs, and laboratory evaluations, followed by other evaluations, which may include computed tomography with subsequent biopsy.

Inguinal

Essentially, most adults have some inguinal lymph node enlargement. Benign reactive lymphadenopathy is more common in patients who walk barefooted outdoors. Malignant causes include non-Hodgkin's lymphoma, Hodgkin's disease, malignant melanoma, squamous cell carcinoma of the penis, and squamous cell carcinoma of the vulva. Benign causes include cellulitis, syphilis, chancroid, genital herpes, and lymphogranuloma venereum.

Abdominal

Common causes of abdominal (mesenteric and retroperitoneal) lymphadenopathy include non-Hodgkin's lymphoma, metastatic adenocarcinoma, gastric adenocarcinoma, Hodgkin's disease (characteristically retroperitoneal node involvement), metastatic transitional cell carcinoma of the bladder, chronic lymphocytic leukemia, hairy cell leukemia, and tuberculosis.

The classic sign of gastric adenocarcinoma is the Sister Joseph node in the umbilical area.

Epitrochlear

Selby et al. (6), in a study of epitrochlear adenopathy, evaluated 324 patients: in 140 normal patients, no epitrochlear nodes were palpable, and 184 consecutive patients with conditions associated with adenopathy were examined. Of the 184 patients who were examined, 49 patients (27%) had epitrochlear adenopathy. The diagnoses in these 49 patients included Hodgkin's disease in 3, non-Hodgkin's lymphoma in 15, chronic lymphocytic leukemia in 4, sarcoidosis in 3, rheumatoid disorders in 9, infectious mononucleosis in 12, human immunodeficiency virus (HIV) in 1, and dermatopathic conditions in 2. Historically, epitrochlear adenopathy also has been associated with secondary syphilis, lepromatous leprosy, leishmaniasis, cytomegalovirus, rubella, glandular fever, and HIV infections.

Generalized, With or Without Fever

Common causes of malignant generalized lymphadenopathy include the hematologic malignancies of non-Hodgkin's lymphoma, Hodgkin's disease, chronic lymphocytic leukemia, and acute lymphocytic leukemia. Benign causes include infectious mononucleosis, cytomegalovirus, toxoplasmosis, tuberculosis, histoplasmosis, coccidioidomycosis, brucellosis, herpes infection, sarcoidosis, rheumatoid arthritis, systemic lupus erythematosus, HIV infections, and angioimmunoblastic lymphadenopathy.

The differential diagnosis of patients with lymphadenopathy and fever with or without splenomegaly includes the following: infectious mononucleosis, Epstein-Barr virus, cytomegalovirus, toxoplasmosis, syphilis, subacute bacterial endocarditis, histoplasmosis, sarcoidosis, salmonella, tuberculosis, acquired immunodeficiency syndrome (AIDS), Hodgkin's disease, non-Hodgkin's lymphoma, angioimmunoblastic lymphadenopathy, mixed essential cryoglobulinemia, systemic mastocytosis, chronic lymphocytic leukemia, myelofibrosis, Waldenström's macroglobulinemia, multiple myeloma, systemic lupus erythematosus, rheumatoid arthritis, Kawasaki disease, Whipple's disease, serum sickness, and Kaposi's sarcoma.

WHICH NODE TO BIOPSY?

In general, biopsy is performed on the largest node. The least helpful nodes are inguinal nodes, although if they are accessible biopsy may be useful because ancillary studies have aided significantly in the pathologic diagnosis. If multiple nodal sites are involved, then the initial biopsy should be done on the largest peripheral node outside the inguinal area, and subsequent biopsies should include mediastinal nodes and then abdominal nodes. Occasionally, multiple biopsies may be needed at the time of initial evaluation or over time. The presence or absence of symptoms in patients with adenopathy should not alter the approach because both symptomatic and asymptomatic patients may have pathologic lymphadenopathy. In a statistical analysis by Lee et al. (1), 925 patients had biopsy from 1973 to 1977, representing 0.9% of all surgical cases (Table 4). Lymphoproliferative disorders do not have an age predilection, but carcinomas have a much higher incidence in patients older than 50 years.

The region of lymph node involvement may be helpful. In patients with generalized adenopathy, it is usually best to biopsy the largest node. An alternative approach for biopsy based on sites includes, in descending order, supraclavicular, cervical, axillary, epitrochlear, and inguinal nodes.

BIOPSY OF LYMPH NODES

Biopsy of lymph nodes can be excisional (direct surgical extirpation, mediastinoscopy, or laparoscopy) or needle aspiration (core, fine-needle). In a study by Gupta et al. (7), 100 patients had concomitant fine-needle aspiration and excisional biopsy. The

Table 4
Results of Lymph Node Biopsy, by Site and Age

	Benign, %	Carcinoma, %	Lymphoma, %
Site			
All	60	28	12
Abdominal	63	33	4
Thoracic	73	26	1
Peripheral	56	29	15
Age			
All	60	28	12
< 30	79	6	15
51-80	40	44	16

From Lee et al. (*1*). By permission of Wiley-Liss, a division of John Wiley & Sons, Inc.

accuracy rates were 76.9% in reactive hyperplasia, 76.78% in tuberculous lymphadenitis, 75% in non-Hodgkin's lymphoma, and 84.6% in metastatic carcinoma. Fine-needle aspiration is simple, safe, reliable, and cost-effective, but reactive hyperplasia, Hodgkin's disease, and non-Hodgkin's lymphoma prove difficult to diagnose. In the evaluation of pancreatic and peripancreatic disorders, fine-needle aspiration biopsy is helpful for differentiating adenocarcinoma from other disorders. It is also useful in the differential diagnosis of head and neck carcinoma, thyroid lesions, malignant melanoma, relapsed lymphoproliferative disorders, or carcinomas. In patients without an established diagnosis with accessible peripheral adenopathy, excisional biopsy to ensure adequate sampling is preferred.

ATYPICAL LYMPH NODE HYPERPLASIA

The diagnosis of atypical hyperplasia occurs less with special studies, which include immunohistochemical stains, cytogenetics, and molecular genetic techniques. Schroer and Franssila (*8*) followed up 70 patients with a diagnosis of atypical hyperplasia from 1961 to 1972. A malignant lymphoproliferative disorder developed in 37% from 2 to 13 years after the diagnosis. On reexamination of the initial tissue, 19 patients had benign lesions, 10 had malignant lesions, 37 had atypical hyperplasia, and 4 had angioimmunoblastic lymphadenopathy; malignant lymphoma developed in 30% of patients with atypical hyperplasia. It is still common practice to designate a suspicious lymph node as atypical hyperplasia and request a repeat biopsy later. Malignant lymphoma has been reported to develop in 17% to 20% of patients with a nondiagnostic lymph node biopsy. With the newer immunohistochemical, cytogenetic, and genetic technologies, more accurate diagnosis is now possible (*9*). Data have not been published to confirm this impression.

KIKUCHI'S DISEASE: A RARE CAUSE OF LYMPHADENOPATHY

A rare cause of lymphadenopathy is histiocytic necrotizing lymphadenitis (Kikuchi's disease), which was first described in 1972 in Japan. The male:female ratio is 1:4. It occurs in young patients. They typically present with painless, but sometimes tender, lymphadenopathy that is unilateral in the posterior cervical region. Twenty percent of patients have generalized lymphadenopathy. This usually resolves in 3 months.

Splenomegaly is uncommon. Fever occurs in 33% of patients. Other aspects of the clinical presentation include an increased erythrocyte sedimentation rate, abnormal results of liver function tests, fatigue, arthralgias, rashes with an urticarial-like reaction, and epididymitis. The cause is unclear. Malignant transformation does not occur. Corticosteroid treatment may be indicated in some patients.

CONCLUSION

Lymphadenopathy is a simple physical finding with an extensive differential diagnosis that may present interesting challenges to the clinician. The ability to palpate peripheral lymph nodes is a skill that improves with time. Clinicians should be encouraged to consistently measure the peripheral nodes that are discovered on physical examination. A knowledge of the broad differential diagnosis, the relationships of other signs and symptoms, and key laboratory associations all aid a thoughtful and expeditious diagnosis.

REFERENCES

1. Lee Y, Terry R, Lukes RJ. Lymph node biopsy for diagnosis: a statistical study. *J Surg Oncol* 1980; 14: 53-60.
2. Margolis IB, Matteucci D, Organ CH Jr. To improve the yield of biopsy of the lymph nodes. *Surg Gynecol Obstet* 1978; 147: 376-378.
3. Sinclair S, Beckman E, Ellman L. Biopsy of enlarged, superficial lymph nodes. *JAMA* 1974; 228: 602-603.
4. Pangalis GA, Vassilakopoulos TP, Boussiotis VA, Fessas P. Clinical approach to lymphadenopathy. *Semin Oncol* 1993; 20: 570-582.
5. Fraser RG, Paré JAP. *Diagnosis of Diseases of the Chest*, 2nd ed, vol 3. WB Saunders Company, Philadelphia, 1977, pp. 1793-1870.
6. Selby CD, Marcus HS, Toghill PJ. Enlarged epitrochlear lymph nodes: an old physical sign revisited. *J R Coll Physicians Lond* 1992; 26: 159-161.
7. Gupta AK, Nayar M, Chandra M. Reliability and limitations of fine needle aspiration cytology of lymphadenopathies. An analysis of 1,261 cases. *Acta Cytol* 1991; 35: 777-783.
8. Schroer KR, Franssila KO. Atypical hyperplasia of lymph nodes: a follow-up study. *Cancer* 1979; 44: 1155-1163.
9. Knowles DM. Immunophenotypic and immunogenotypic approaches useful in distinguishing benign and malignant lymphoid proliferations. *Semin Oncol* 1993; 20: 583-610.

SUGGESTED READING

Benjamin SP, McCormack LJ, Effler DB, Groves LK. Primary tumors of the mediastinum. *Chest* 1972; 62: 297-303.
Moore RD, Weisberger AS, Bowerfind ES Jr. An evaluation of lymphadenopathy in systemic disease. *Arch Intern Med* 1957; 99: 751-759.
Skarin AT. *Approach to the patient with suspected lymphoma, in The Lymphomas* (Canellos GP, Lister TA, Sklar JL, eds). WB Saunders Company, Philadelphia, 1998, pp. 207-211.
Winterbauer RH, Belic N, Moores KD. Clinical interpretation of bilateral hilar adenopathy. *Ann Intern Med* 1973; 78: 65-71.

17

Hodgkin's Disease and Non-Hodgkin's Lymphoma

Thomas M. Habermann, MD

Contents

HODGKIN'S DISEASE

Introduction and Clinical Presentation

In the United States there are about 7,500 new cases of Hodgkin's disease (HD) per year. The age distribution is bimodal in that the peak incidences are at approximately 25 and 80 years of age. HD usually presents as a localized lymph node enlargement and progresses in an orderly manner (contiguous rather than hematogenous dissemination). However, any organ, including the bone marrow, liver, lung, pericardium, pleura, skin, bone, and the central nervous system, can be involved. Patients may present with "B" symptoms (Table 1), pruritus, jaundice, ascites, and dysphagia. The fever may have a cyclic pattern, with several days of fever alternating with afebrile periods (Pel-Ebstein fever). Some patients with HD complain of alcohol-induced pain in areas of diseased lymph nodes. Laboratory abnormalities may include cytopenias, leukocytosis, eosinophilia, abnormal liver function tests, and increased erythrocyte sedimentation rate. Paraneoplastic manifestations associated with HD include lipoid (minimal change) nephrosis, demyelinating neuropathy, and cerebellar syndromes.

More than 90% of patients with HD present with peripheral lymphadenopathy. Intrathoracic disease, common in young women with nodular sclerosing HD (Fig. 1 *A*), occurs in two-thirds of patients and is found by chest radiography or computed tomography. Occasionally, compression of the superior vena cava may result in facial swelling and distention of the veins in the neck and upper chest. Although palpable splenomegaly is an unusual finding, the spleen may be involved in up to 27% of patients undergoing staging laparotomy for clinical stage I and II disease (Table 1). However, a third of patients with clinically or radiographically enlarged spleens may not have pathologic involvement. Older patients may present with occult disease with weight loss, liver function test abnormalities, and cytopenias without lymphadenopathy.

From: *Primary Hematology*
Edited by: A. Tefferi © Mayo Foundation for Medical Education and Research, Rochester, MN

Table 1
The Cotswolds Staging System of Hodgkin's Disease

Classification	
Description	
Stage I	Involvement of a single lymph node region or a lymphoid structure (e.g., spleen, thymus, Waldeyer's ring)
Stage II	Involvement of two or more lymph node regions on the same side of the diaphragm. The "mediastinum" is considered a single site. Note that hilar nodes, internal mammary nodes, and paravertebral nodes are not part of the "mediastinum." Therefore, if the hilar nodes are involved bilaterally, it is stage II disease
Stage III	Involvement of lymph node regions or structures on both sides of the diaphragm
Stage III1	Subdiaphragmatic involvement limited to spleen, splenic hilar, celiac, or portal nodes
Stage III2	Subdiaphragmatic involvement includes para-aortic, iliac, or mesenteric nodes
Stage IV	More than one extranodal loci at any location or any involvement of the bone marrow or liver
Designations applicable to any stage of disease	
A	No "B" symptoms
B	Any "B" symptom: fever (temperature > 38°C), drenching night sweats, unexplained loss of > 10% of body weight within the preceding 6 months
X	Bulky disease: a widening of the mediastinum (by chest radiography) by more than 1/3 of the internal transverse diameter of the thorax at T5-T6, or the presence of a nodal mass with a maximal dimension of ≥ 10 cm
E	Localized, solitary involvement of extralymphatic tissue, excluding liver and bone marrow. A localized extranodal site constitutes stage IE disease. If that site accompanies a regional lymph node region or is a direct extension of a known nodal site, then it is stage IIE disease
CS	Clinical stage: based on all staging procedures, except laparotomy. Bone marrow biopsy is considered clinical staging
PS	Pathologic stage: requires laparotomy. Staging laparotomy includes splenectomy, sampling of splenic hilar nodes, liver biopsies of both lobes including a wedge biopsy, resection of suspicious nodes, and oophoropexy

Modified from Kaufman D, Longo DL. Hodgkin's disease, in *Clinical Oncology* (Abeloff MD, Armitage JO, Lichter AS, Niederhuber JE, eds.). Churchill Livingstone, New York, 1995, pp. 2075-2107. By permission of the publisher.

Pathology

The pathologic diagnosis of HD is based on the presence of Reed-Sternberg cells (Fig. 1 *B*). These are large binucleate cells with inclusion-like nucleoli (owl-eye appearance). However, Reed-Sternberg–like cells may be found in infectious mononucleosis and other viral diseases. Histologically, HD may be classified as nodular sclerosing (40%-70% of cases), mixed cellularity (20%-40%), lymphocyte-predominant, and lymphocyte-depleted (rare). However, unlike non-Hodgkin's lymphoma, the histologic features may not play an important prognostic role during the treatment of HD. The Reed-Sternberg cells in HD react with the Hodgkin's-associated markers CD15 (Leu-M1) and CD30 (ber-H2) and not with B- or T-lymphocyte markers. Recent data suggest that

B

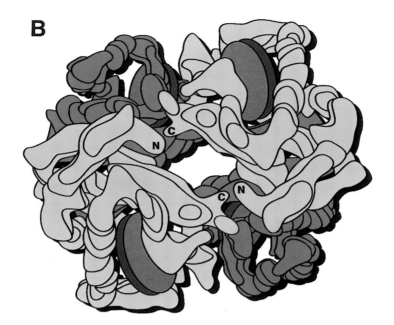

Plate 1 (from Chapter 3, Fig. 1B, p. 42.) Hemoglobin molecule. The molecule is built from four subunits: two identical α chains *(yellow)* and two identical β chains *(blue)*. "N" identifies the amino ends and "C" identifies the carboxyl ends of the two α chains. Each chain enfolds a heme group *(red disk)*.

C

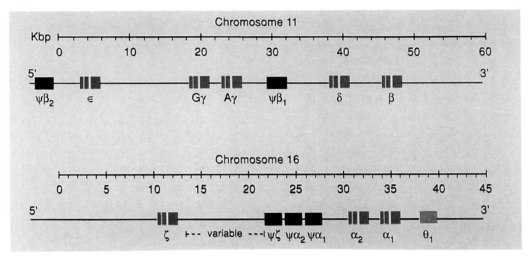

Plate 2 (from Chapter 3, Fig. 1C, p. 43.) Globin genes. (From Steinberg MH, Benz EJ Jr. Hemoglobin synthesis, structure, and function, in *Hematology: Basic Principles and Practice* [Hoffman R, Benz EJ Jr, Shattil SJ, Furie B, Cohen HJ, Silberstein LE, eds.], 2nd ed. Churchill Livingstone, New York, 1995, pp. 458–468. By permission of the publisher.)

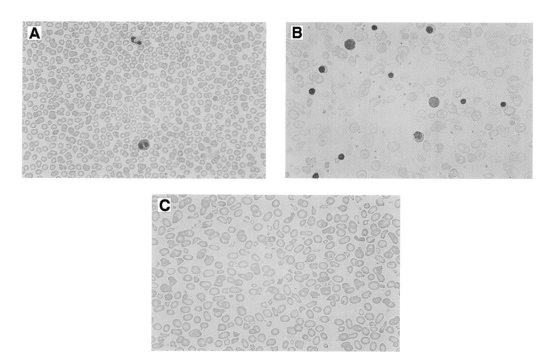

Plates 3–5 (from Chapter 3, Fig. 2, p. 48.) Peripheral smears. **(A)** Plate 3, β-Thalassemia minor: hypochromia, microcytosis, poikilocytosis, and ovalocytes. **(B)** Plate 4, β-Thalassemia major: hypochromia, polychromasia, microcytosis, anisocytosis, poikilocytosis, target cells, basophilic stippling, and nucleated red blood cells. **(C)** Plate 5, Hemoglobin H disease: marked hypochromia along with anisocytosis, poikilocytosis, basophilic stippling, polychromasia, and microcytosis.

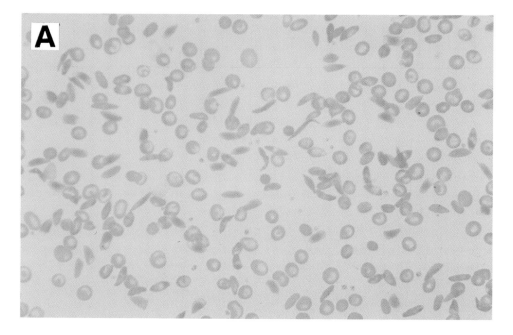

Plate 6 (from Chapter 4, Fig. 2A, p. 68.) Sickle cell disease (peripheral smear): irreversibly sickled red cell forms, other elongated forms, nucleated red blood cells (not shown), Howell-Jolly bodies, polychromasia, target cells, mild leukocytosis (not shown), and thrombocytosis.

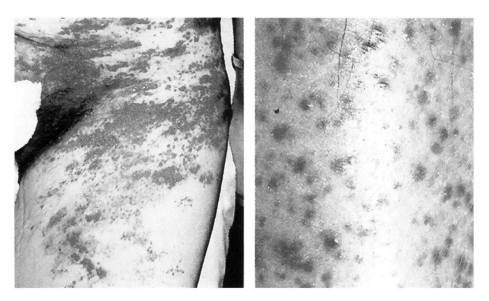

Plate 7 (from Chapter 7, Fig. 1, p. 106.) Ecchymoses (left) and petechiae (right) from severe thrombocytopenia (From Hoffbrand AV, Pettit JE. *Color Atlas of Clinical Hematology,* 2nd ed. Mosby-Wolfe, London, 1994. By permission of the publisher.)

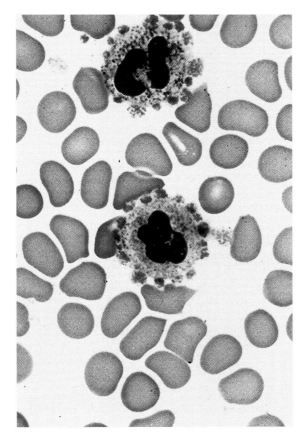

Plate 8 (from Chapter 7, Fig. 2, p. 108.) Platelet rosetting in the presence of EDTA. (From Hoffbrand AV, Pettit JE. *Color Atlas of Clinical Hematology,* 2nd ed. Mosby-Wolfe, London, 1994. By permission of the publisher.)

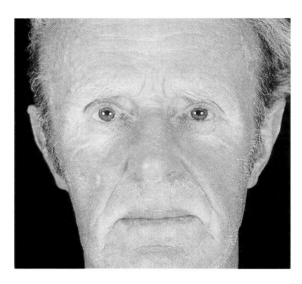

Plate 9 (from Chapter 10, Fig. 2, p. 140.) Facial plethora in a patient with polycythemia vera. Notice the ruddy skin appearance. (From Hoffbrand AV, Pettit JE. *Color Atlas of Clinical Hematology,* 2nd ed. Mosby-Wolfe, London, 1994. By permission of the publisher.)

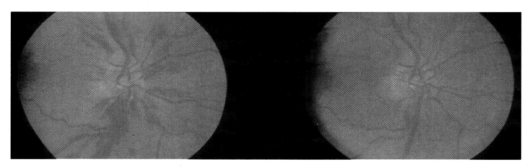

Plate 10 (from Chapter 10, Fig. 3, p. 140.) Retinal vein distention in a patient with polycythemia vera, before and after phlebotomy. Notice the thickened "sausage-shaped" appearance of the retinal veins and fundal hemorrhage. (From Hoffbrand AV, Pettit JE. *Color Atlas of Clinical Hematology,* 2nd ed. Mosby-Wolfe, London, 1994. By permission of the publisher.)

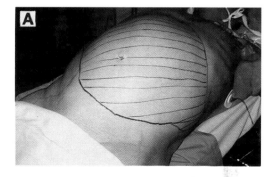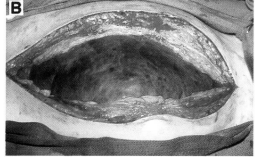

Plate 11 (from Chapter 10, Fig. 4A, p. 144), Plate 12 (from Chapter 10, Fig. 4B, p. 144.) Massive splenomegaly in a patient with myelofibrosis. (*A* from Tefferi A, Silverstein MN. Myeloproliferative diseases, in *Cecil Textbook of Medicine* [Goldman L, Bennett JC, eds], 21st ed. WB Saunders Company, Philadelphia, 2000, pp. 935–941. By permission of the publisher.)

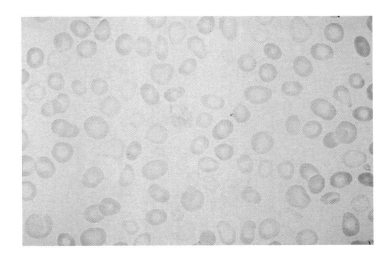

Plate 13 (from Chapter 11, Fig. 1, p. 152.) Dimorphic red cells.

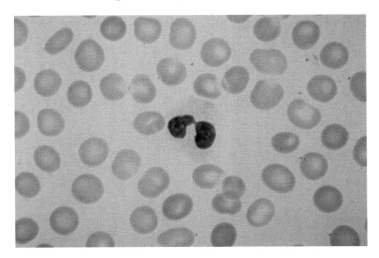

Plate 14 (from Chapter 11, Fig. 2, p. 152.) Pseudo Pelger-Huët granulocyte.

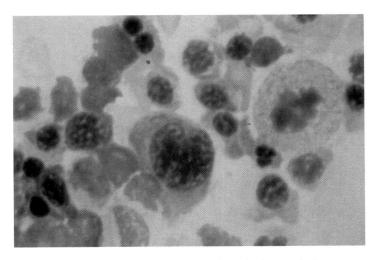

Plate 15 (from Chapter 11, Fig. 3, p. 153.) Dyserythopoiesis seen in bone marrow aspirate.

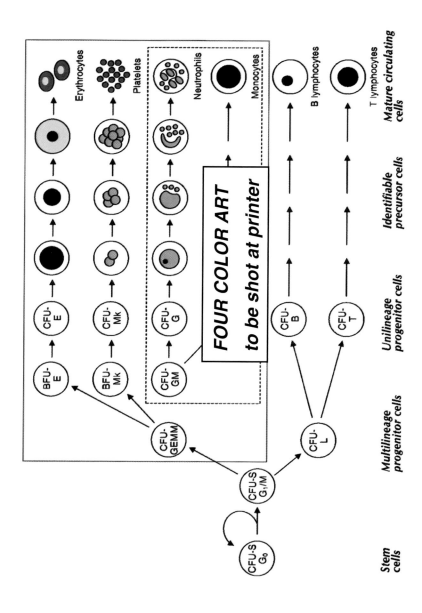

Plate 16 (from Chapter 14, Fig. 1, p. 194.) Heterogeneity in the hematopoietic stem cell origin of acute myelogenous leukemia (AML). In some cases of AML, the disease appears restricted to stem cells committed to granulocyte/monocyte/macrophage differentiation (dotted box). In other cases of AML, the disease involves a pluripotential stem cell that is capable of differentiating to erythrocytes and megakaryocytes, in addition to granulocyte/monocyte/macrophages (red box). BFU-E, burst-forming unit–erythroid; BFU-Mk, megakaryocyte; CFU-B, colony-forming unit–B lymphocyte; CFU-E, erythroid; CFU-G, granulocyte; CFU-GEMM, granulocyte, erythroid, megakaryocyte, monocyte; CFU-GM, granulocyte macrophage; CFU-L, lymphocyte; CFU-M, monocyte; CFU-Mk, megakaryocyte; CFU-T, T lymphocyte; CFU-S G_0, stem cell, resting; CFU-S G_1/M, stem cell, cycling. (From Collins SJ. Pathobiology of human acute myeloid leukemia, in *Hematology: Basic Principles and Practice* [Hoffman R, Benz EJ Jr, Shattil SJ, Furie B, Cohen HJ, Silberstein LE, eds.], 2nd ed. Churchill Livingstone, New York, 1995, pp. 983-993. By permission of the publisher.)

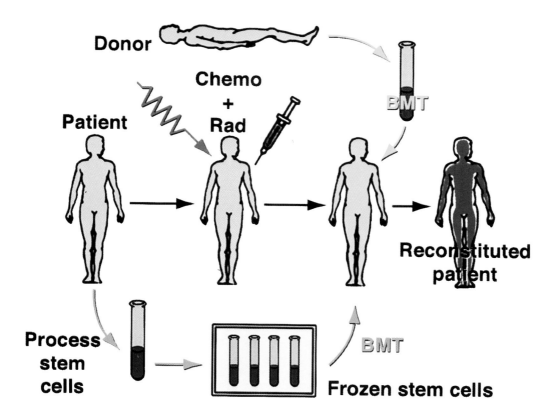

Plate 17 (from Chapter 15, Fig. 2, p. 210.) Blood and marrow transplantation (BMT) process. Chemo, chemotherapy; rad, radiation. (Modified from Golde DW. The stem cell. *Sci Am* 1991; 265 no. 6: 86–93. By permission of the journal.)

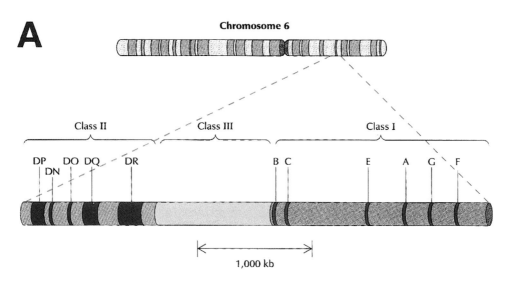

Plate 18 (from Chapter 15, Fig. 4A, p. 215.) The human leukocyte antigen gene system on the short arm of chromosome 6 consists of the class I region of A and B loci as well as other loci and the class II region of D loci. The class III region contains genes of the complement system. (A from Jagannath S, Barlogie B, Tricot G. Hematopoietic stem cell transplantation. *Hosp Pract* 1993; 28 no. 8: 79-86. By permission of the McGraw-Hill Companies, Inc. Illustration by Seward Hung.)

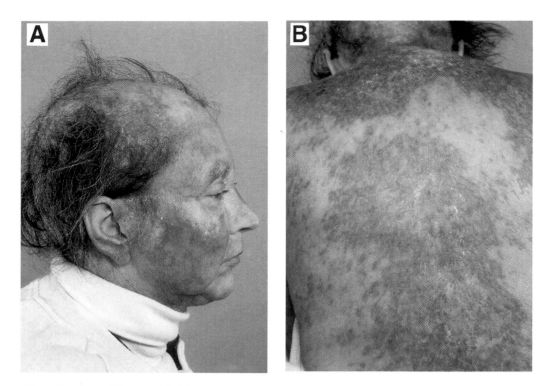

Plate 19 (from Chapter 15, Fig. 6A, p. 223.) Chronic graft-versus-host disease with lichenoid and sclerodermatous changes in the face and scalp with alopecia. **Plate 20 (from Chapter 15, Fig. 6B, p. 223),** Lichenoid hyperpigmentation of the back.

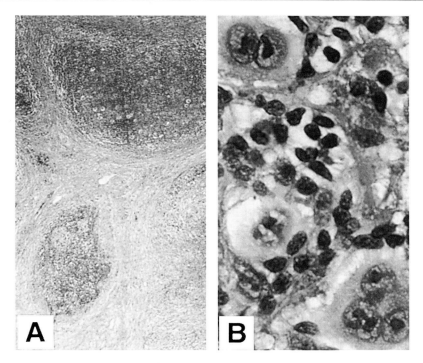

Fig. 1. Hodgkin's disease: lymph node biopsy specimens. A, Abundant bands of collagenous connective tissue separating areas of abnormal Hodgkin's tissue of the nodular sclerosing type. B, High-power view of mixed cellularity disease showing Reed-Sternberg cells surrounded by lymphocytes. (From Hoffbrand AV, Pettit JE. *Color Atlas of Clinical Hematology*, 2nd ed. Mosby-Wolfe, London, 1994. By permission of the publisher.)

lymphocyte-predominant HD is a B-cell disorder. The cause of HD is unknown. Approximately 20% to 80% of patients have Epstein-Barr virus genome in the tissue samples, but an etiologic relationship has been difficult to establish.

Staging

Disease dissemination in non-Hodgkin's lymphoma is largely hematogenous, whereas the process is often contiguous in HD. As such, disease stage is critical to the prognosis of HD and it is the principal factor in selecting treatment. The Ann Arbor staging system had been used for many years before it was modified into the currently used Cotswolds staging system (Table 1). It is important to understand that the staging system is based on "lymph node regions" and not individual lymph nodes (Fig. 2). The recommended procedures for staging are outlined below.

Recommended Procedures for Staging Hodgkin's Disease

- Obtain history of "B" symptoms (Table 1)
- Physical examination of lymph nodes, spleen, and liver
- Complete blood cell count and liver tests
- Computed tomography of chest, abdomen, and pelvis
- Bilateral bone marrow biopsy

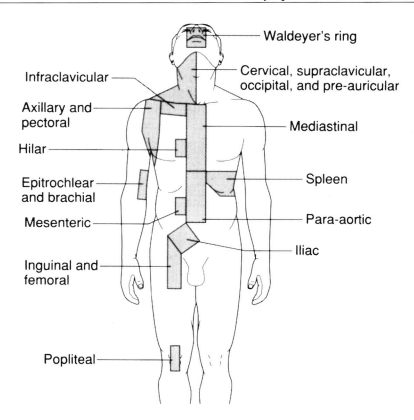

Fig. 2. Anatomical lymph node regions. (From Kaplan HS, Rosenberg SA. The treatment of Hodgkin's disease. *Med Clin North Am* 1966 Nov; 50: 1591-1610. By permission of WB Saunders Company.)

In addition to the listed tests, determination of serum calcium and creatinine values and of the erythrocyte sedimentation rate is mandatory. Increased erythrocyte sedimentation rate is associated with a poor prognosis. In addition, pretreatment gallium scanning is recommended for patients with bulky disease (especially in the mediastinum); if the tumor is gallium-avid, the response status of a residual "mass" or "scar" may be further clarified by repeat gallium scanning. Staging laparotomy and bipedal lymphangiography are not routine components of the staging procedure in HD and are now infrequently performed.

If primary radiation therapy is contemplated in patients with clinical stage I or II disease (Table 1), it might be necessary to ensure that occult subdiaphragmatic disease (especially in the spleen) is not overlooked. Therefore, these patients may require a staging laparotomy with or without lymphangiography. However, certain clinical characteristics may suggest a very low likelihood of splenic involvement (clinical stage IA in female patients, lymphocyte-predominant HD), whereas other factors (male sex, "B" symptoms, and involvement of more than two lymphatic regions, bulky disease) may suggest otherwise. Furthermore, several studies have suggested an increased rate of both fatal infections with encapsulated organisms and secondary leukemia in patients who have had splenectomy. Because we are currently inclined to use chemotherapy for patients with "B" symptoms, bulky disease, or increased erythrocyte sedimentation rate and

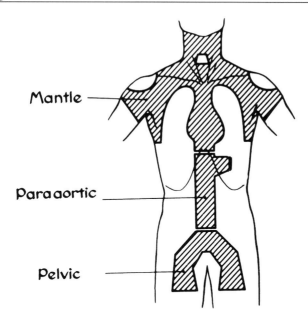

Fig. 3. Mantle, para-aortic, and pelvic irradiation fields. (From Aisenberg AC. *Malignant Lymphoma: Biology, Natural History, and Treatment.* Lea & Febiger, Philadelphia, 1991. By permission of the publisher.)

because chemotherapy is effective in most patients in whom radiation therapy fails, staging laparotomy has been used infrequently in recent years.

Treatment

Currently, the preferred treatment of non-bulky pathologic stage IA or IIA disease is radiation to an extended mantle field (mantle and para-aortic fields) (Fig. 3). The usual dose of radiation is a total of 35 to 44 Gy at the rate of 150 to 200 cGy per day for 5 days a week (4-6 weeks of therapy). The corresponding rates of freedom from progression and survival at 14 years are 93% and 83%, respectively. However, the treatment of choice for non-bulky stage IIIA2, IIIB, IVA, and IVB disease is combination chemotherapy (cure rate of about 66% with recent regimens). Although somewhat controversial, non-bulky stage IB and IIB disease also is treated with combination chemotherapy. Chemotherapy also is used in the setting of infradiaphragmatic disease, regardless of stage. The treatment of stage IIIA1 disease is controversial. Long-term remissions with radiation therapy alone are reported in 60% to 80% of patients. Regardless of stage, the presence of bulky disease requires chemotherapy, and in many cases a combination of both chemotherapy and radiation.

The MOPP (nitrogen mustard, Oncovin [vincristine], procarbazine, and prednisone) chemotherapy regimen was the standard of care until recently. However, the cure rate with MOPP was only 50%, and the therapy was associated with long-term complications, including treatment-related acute leukemia and sterility. Subsequently, regimens that were more effective (cure rates of up to 55% to 65% in advanced-stage disease on long-term follow-up) and less leukemogenic were developed (ABVD: Adriamycin [doxorubicin], bleomycin, vinblastine, dacarbazine) (Table 2). The toxicities associated with ABVD include cardiomyopathy from Adriamycin, lung injury from bleomycin, nausea

Table 2
Chemotherapy Regimens

Drug	*Side effect*
ABVD	
Doxorubicin (Adriamycin)	Dose-related cardiomyopathy
	Marrow suppression
	Alopecia
	Nausea and vomiting
	Acute nonlymphocytic leukemia
Bleomycin	Pulmonary fibrosis
	Fever, chills
	Skin pigmentation
Vinblastine (Velban)	Myelosuppression
Dacarbazine	Nausea and vomiting
CHOP	
Cyclophosphamide (Cytoxan)	Myelosuppression
	Acute nonlymphocytic leukemia and myelodysplastic syndromes (monosomy 5 and 7)
	Bladder cancer
	Cystitis
	Pulmonary fibrosis
	Alopecia
	Nausea and vomiting
Doxorubicin (Adriamycin)	Dose-related cardiomyopathy
	Marrow suppression
	Alopecia
	Nausea and vomiting
	Acute nonlymphocytic leukemia
Vincristine (Oncovin)	Peripheral neuropathy
Prednisone	Diabetes
	Aseptic necrosis
	Peptic ulcer disease
	Osteoporosis

and vomiting from dacarbazine, and infections due to neutropenia from Adriamycin and vinblastine. The risk of acute leukemia is about 7% with MOPP and about 0.7% with ABVD. A new approach being evaluated, Stanford V, intensifies the frequency of chemotherapy with weekly administration of drugs over a shorter period.

TREATMENT OF RELAPSED DISEASE

Relapse patterns are relatively predictable in HD. After radiation, relapse occurs in the first 2 years and usually involves nonirradiated sites adjacent to the treated fields. Relapse after chemotherapy occurs at sites of bulky disease. Patients who have relapse after radiation therapy have about a 66% chance of cure with salvage chemotherapy. In patients who have relapse after chemotherapy, remission with further chemotherapy depends primarily on the duration of the first complete remission. A second complete remission, with chemotherapy alone, may be possible in more than 90% of patients, with initial remissions lasting at least 12 months, whereas the rate is 29% for those with shorter durations of remission. However, when autologus bone marrow transplantation was compared with conventional chemotherapy for recurrent or refractory disease, the 3-year event-free survival rate was 53% for the transplant group and 10% for the chemotherapy group. As such, patients with HD who have relapse after modern chemotherapy are currently offered autologous stem cell or bone marrow transplantation. Patients who have relapse after transplantation may respond to palliative therapy with various chemotherapeutic agents, including single-agent vinblastine.

ADDITIONAL THERAPEUTIC ISSUES

Before treatment is started, male patients should be informed of the potential to store sperm, and female patients are advised not to become pregnant for 2 years after therapy because 75% of relapses occur during this interval. Radiotherapy is a consideration in the management of HD emergencies, including acute superior vena cava syndrome, airway obstruction, pericardial tamponade, and epidural spinal cord compression. Patients with large mediastinal masses who undergo general anesthesia may not be extubated easily, and radiation therapy may be required. Radiation therapy often results in radiation pneumonitis, which usually is associated with mild symptoms and should not be confused with HD or infection.

Complications of Therapy

Long-term complications usually occur from 5 to 20 years after therapy. The complications include hypothyroidism in patients who have received neck irradiation, pneumococcal sepsis after splenectomy, infertility, amenorrhea, cardiomyopathy due to Adriamycin or radiation therapy, radiation pneumonitis, pulmonary fibrosis, coronary artery disease, and secondary cancers. The secondary cancers include acute nonlymphocytic leukemia, myelodysplastic syndrome, non-Hodgkin's lymphoma, and solid tumors. Risk factors for development of acute leukemia include chemotherapy, age older than 40 years at diagnosis, and splenectomy. ABVD is less leukemogenic than MOPP. Patients at highest risk are those who have received multiple courses of chemotherapy. The risk for development of non-Hodgkin's lymphoma is 4% at 10 years. Radiation therapy increases the risk of solid tumors. The actuarial risk of secondary solid tumors is 13% at 15 years of follow-up and 20% at 20 years. The risk of lung and breast cancer is strongly related to radiation therapy. After 15 years of follow-up, women treated with mantle-field radiation before the age of 20 years had a 40-fold increased risk of breast cancer.

NON-HODGKIN'S LYMPHOMA

Introduction

Non-Hodgkin's lymphomas (NHLs) are malignant lymphocyte disorders that are heterogeneous in their natural history, responses to therapy, and pathologic, cytogenetic, and immunologic features. This group of diseases is responsive to treatment, but the extent, type, and duration of responses vary significantly. The precise cause of NHL is unknown. The prognosis depends on the histologic subtype, stage, clinical characteristics, and laboratory findings. It is essential to establish an accurate histologic diagnosis at the outset to ensure the most appropriate therapeutic intervention. The estimated number of new cases of NHL in the United States in 1997 was 53,600 (30,300 male and 23,300 female patients). Lymphoma represents 4% of all new cases of cancer and 4% of all deaths from cancer. The incidence has been increasing since 1957.

In the vast majority of patients with NHL, the cause of the disease is undetermined. The reported epidemiologic risk factors for NHL include human immunodeficiency virus infection, solid organ transplantation, T-cell–depleted bone marrow transplantation, Hodgkin's disease, Sjögren's syndrome, past methotrexate therapy for rheumatoid arthritis, pesticide exposure, black hair dye, red meat exposure in females, and *Helicobacter pylori* in gastric mucosa-associated lymphoid tissue lymphoma (MALToma).

Classification

The classification system has evolved. Prior classification schemes were based on pattern and cellular morphology only and were not derived from information from cytochemical, cytogenetic, or molecular genetic studies. It is not possible to compare clinical trials that use different classification systems, because not all subcategories can be translated from one classification scheme to another. The Working Formulation for Clinical Usage, which groups NHL by natural history and response to therapy, had been the most used scheme in the United States (Table 3). This and other existing schemas have been based on morphologic features only. These morphologic patterns have characteristic cytochemical, cytogenetic, and oncogene associations.

The Working Formulation broadly categorizes patients into two groups: the favorable low-grade lymphomas and the unfavorable intermediate and high-grade lymphomas. Some patients have different histologic types of the lymphoma in the same biopsy specimen or in different biopsy specimens sampled at the same time. If both follicular and diffuse areas are involved, then the lymphomas are considered follicular in the Working Formulation, but the disease has the significant characteristics of each histologic subtype, and patients are treated for the more aggressive subtype.

To recognize new entities and refine previously recognized disease categories, the International Lymphoma Study Group reported on the Revised European-American Lymphoma (REAL) classification (Table 4). The REAL classification includes established entities, classifies all follicular lymphomas into one subset, differentiates B- and T-cell disorders, includes distinct T-cell disorders, and allows identification of new entities, including mantle cell lymphoma, anaplastic large-cell lymphoma, marginal zone lymphoma, and MALToma. The REAL classification is defined by morphologic, immunologic, and genetic techniques and does not take clinical characteristics into account.

Diagnosis and Staging

For the first-time diagnosis of lymphoma, the procedure of choice is usually a surgical biopsy of the most suspicious (rapidly enlarging) lymph node if the clinical condition of the patient allows this approach. If the clinical condition of the patient is such that surgical biopsy is contraindicated or the site of disease is difficult to access, a needle biopsy may be the procedure of choice. A core needle biopsy is preferred over a fine-needle aspirate. Mediastinoscopy is a very reliable approach for mediastinal disease. Laparoscopic biopsy recently has been shown to be effective and reliable in abdominal disease. Tissue should be set aside for additional frozen-section immunohistochemical studies, possible molecular genetic studies, and possible cytogenetic studies. Staging procedures are similar to those for HD.

Prognosis

Recently, several investigators have developed a prognostic model, the International Index, based on clinical pretreatment characteristics and the relative risk of death in

Table 3
Non-Hodgkin's Lymphoma According
to the Working Formulation

Subtype	Histology
Low-grade	
A	Small lymphocytic
B	Follicular small cleaved cell
C	Follicular mixed cell
Intermediate-grade	
D	Follicular large cell
E	Diffuse small cleaved cell
F	Diffuse mixed cell
G	Diffuse large cell
High-grade	
H	Immunoblastic
I	Lymphoblastic
J	Small noncleaved cell
Miscellaneous	
	Composite malignant lymphoma
	Mycosis fungoides
	Extramedullary plasmacytoma
	Unclassified
	Other

Modified from The Non-Hodgkin's Lymphoma Pathologic
Classification Project. *Cancer* 1982; 49 no. 10: 2112-2135. By
permission of the American Cancer Society and Wiley-Liss, Inc.,
a subsidiary of John Wiley & Sons, Inc.

patients with intermediate histologic features of NHL (diffuse large cell, diffuse mixed, and immunoblastic). Clinical features that were associated with poor survival included age older than 60 years, increased lactate dehydrogenase level, poor performance status (Eastern Cooperative Oncology Group [ECOG] scale 2-4 vs. 0, 1), advanced stage (III or IV vs. I or II), and extranodal involvement at more than one site. Patients were divided into different risk groups based on the number of risk factors (Table 5).

Treatment

The paradox of NHL is that the follicular and diffuse low-grade types are associated with a long survival but are not curable, even though they are very responsive to initial oral chemotherapy. In contrast, the intermediate- and high-grade types are potentially curable but are associated with a short survival if they do not respond to therapy. Chemotherapy is the primary treatment for most types of NHL. Treatments may differ for acquired immunodeficiency syndrome (AIDS)-related lymphomas, posttransplantation lymphoproliferative disorders, and the extranodal lymphomas that involve the central nervous system, stomach, thyroid, testicle, bone, lung, reproductive organs, and skin. Indications for radiation or surgical treatment are limited and include presentation with isolated gastric, central nervous system, testicular, bowel, orbital, pulmonary, or cutaneous disease. Most recent clinical trials suggested an additional benefit of involved-field

Table 4
The Revised European-American Lymphoma (REAL) Classification

B-cell neoplasms

I   Precursor B-cell neoplasm: precursor B-lymphoblastic leukemia/lymphoma
II Peripheral B-cell neoplasms
    1. B-cell chronic lymphocytic leukemia/prolymphocytic leukemia/small
       lymphocytic lymphoma
    2. Lymphoplasmacytoid lymphoma/immunocytoma
    3. Mantle cell lymphoma
    4. Follicle center lymphoma, follicular
       Provisional cytologic grades: I (small cell), II (mixed small and large
         cell), III (large cell)
       Provisional subtype: diffuse, predominantly small cell type
    5. Marginal zone B-cell lymphoma
       Extranodal (mucosa-associated lymphoid tissue-type with or without
         monocytoid B cells)
    6. Provisional entity: splenic marginal zone lymphoma (with or without
       villous lymphocytes)
    7. Hairy cell leukemia
    8. Plasmacytoma/plasma cell myeloma
    9. Diffuse large B-cell lymphoma[a]
   10. Burkitt's lymphoma
   11. Provisional entity: high-grade B-cell lymphoma, Burkitt-like[a]

T-cell and putative natural killer-cell neoplasms

I   Precursor T-cell neoplasm: precursor T-lymphoblastic lymphoma/leukemia
II Peripheral T-cell natural killer-cell neoplasms
    1. T-cell chronic lymphocytic leukemia/prolymphocytic leukemia
    2. Large granular lymphocytic leukemia
       T-cell type
       Natural killer-cell type
    3. Mycosis fungoides/Sézary syndrome
    4. Peripheral T-cell lymphomas, unspecified[a]
       Provisional cytologic categories: medium-sized cell, mixed medium-
         sized and large cell, large cell, lymphoepithelioid cell
       Provisional subtype: hepatosplenic $\gamma\delta$ T-cell lymphoma
       Provisional subtype: subcutaneous panniculitic T-cell lymphoma
    5. Angioimmunoblastic T-cell lymphoma
    6. Angiocentric lymphoma
    7. Intestinal T-cell lymphoma (with or without associated enteropathy)
    8. Adult T-cell lymphoma/leukemia
    9. Anaplastic large cell lymphoma, CD30+, T- and null-cell types
   10. Provisional entity: anaplastic large cell lymphoma, Hodgkin-like

Hodgkin's disease

I   Lymphocyte predominance
II   Nodular sclerosis
III Mixed cellularity
IV   Lymphocyte depletion
V   Provisional entity: lymphocyte-rich classic Hodgkin's disease

[a]These categories are thought likely to include more than one disease entity.
   From Harris NL, Jaffe ES, Stein H, Banks PM, Chan JK, Cleary ML, Delsol G, De Wolf-
Peeters C, Falini B, Gatter KC. A revised European-American classification of lymphoid
neoplasms: a proposal from the International Lymphoma Study Group. *Blood* 1994; 84:
1361-1392. By permission of the American Society of Hematology.

Table 5
Risk-Group Stratification in Intermediate-Grade Lymphoma[a]

Risk group	No. of risk factors	Complete response rate, %	5-Year relapse-free survival, %	5-Year overall survival, %
Low	0 or 1	87	70	73
Low-intermediate	2	67	50	51
High-intermediate	3	55	49	43
High	4 or 5	44	40	26

[a]Poor risk factors are: 1) age older than 60 years, 2) lactate dehydrogenase value increased, 3) poor performance status (Eastern Cooperative Oncology Group 2, 3, or 4), 4) advanced disease stage (III or IV), and 5) extranodal involvement at more than one site.

radiation therapy, after a course of chemotherapy, in patients with diffuse large-cell lymphoma with clinical stage I and II disease.

Low-Grade Non-Hodgkin's Lymphoma

The low-grade NHLs are clinically differentiated as follicular lymphomas and "diffuse" low-grade lymphomas. In the REAL classification, the follicular low-grade lymphomas include follicular–small-cleaved and follicular-mixed NHLs, whereas the "diffuse" type includes small lymphocytic lymphomas, lymphoplasmacytoid lymphoma, mantle cell lymphoma, nodal marginal zone lymphoma (low-grade B-cell lymphomas of MALT), and splenic marginal zone lymphoma.

Most patients with low-grade lymphoma present with stage III or IV disease (infiltration of the bone marrow is common), and the disease is not curable. Observation has been the initial treatment of choice in asymptomatic patients with low tumor burden. Chemotherapy has not been shown to improve survival in these patients. The median survival of patients with follicular lymphoma is 5 to 8 years. Furthermore, most patients with low-grade lymphoma require therapy at a median interval of 3 years from the time of diagnosis. Spontaneous regression occurs occasionally.

Current indications for chemotherapy in low-grade NHL are the presence of disease-related symptoms, bulky disease, or peripheral blood cytopenias. Initial treatments of choice include daily oral chlorambucil or intravenous combination chemotherapy (CVP: cyclophosphamide, vincristine, and prednisone), and there is no difference in outcome. Reported overall response rates are between 57% and 80%, 5-year disease-free survival rates are 18% to 60%, and overall 5-year survival rates are 49% to 67%. The median disease-free interval is 17 months. Relapsed disease usually responds to further treatment with the same or other drugs. The duration of remission is shorter with subsequent treatments.

The first monoclonal antibody for the treatment of malignancy was approved for follicular low-grade lymphomas in 1997. Anti-CD20 (Rituxan) is administered at a dosage of 375 mg/m^2 weekly for four doses. The overall response rates were 48% (complete remission 6% and partial remission 42%) in patients who had been previously treated with two to seven previous regimens. The median time to progression was 13.7 months. Studies that combine this antibody with radioactive conjugates are now under way. The role of both autologous and allogeneic bone marrow transplantation in the treatment of low-grade lymphoma is currently unknown. Various chemotherapeutic agents, including the purine nucleoside analogs, are used as palliative therapy in patients with refractory disease. Overall, a third of patients may obtain a transient response.

One unique low-grade lymphoma is gastric MALToma. This disorder may respond to treatment for *Helicobacter pylori* infection. Short courses of double- or triple-antibiotic therapy regimens have been reported to induce remissions in about 60% of patients.

Intermediate and High-Grade Lymphomas

Anthracycline (doxorubicin)-based combination chemotherapy regimens are the hallmark of therapy, with complete remission rates of 60% to 80% and a long-term disease-free survival as predicted by the International Index (Table 5). An intergroup trial in the United States compared CHOP (cyclophosphamide, Adriamycin [doxorubicin], Oncovin [vincristine], and prednisone) with m-BACOD (methotrexate, bleomycin, Adriamycin [doxorubicin], cyclophosphamide, Oncovin [vincristine], and dexamethasone), ProMACE-CytaBOM (cyclophosphamide, doxorubicin, etoposide, prednisone, cytarabine, bleomycin, Oncovin [vincristine], methotrexate, and leucovorin), and MACOP-B (methotrexate, Adriamycin [doxorubicin], cyclophosphamide, Oncovin [vincristine], prednisone, and bleomycin). CHOP was less toxic and was as effective as the other regimens. As such, CHOP chemotherapy (Table 2) is the current initial treatment of choice in patients with intermediate- or high-grade lymphoma.

However, only 40% of patients are cured with initial chemotherapy. Fortunately, a third of patients with relapse can expect salvage with autologous bone marrow transplantation if their disease is still responsive to chemotherapy. Because of the success of this transplantation for relapse, subsequent clinical trials have compared standard treatment alone or with the incorporation of autologous bone marrow transplantation in newly diagnosed disease. So far, the additional benefit has not been realized.

Particular types of high-grade lymphoma that require a different therapeutic approach include lymphoblastic lymphoma and small noncleaved NHL. In contrast to the other lymphomas, these lymphomas have a propensity for relapse in the central nervous system. As such, intensive chemotherapy often is supplemented by central nervous system prophylaxis. One approach in treating lymphoblastic lymphoma uses CHOP and L-asparaginase in combination and central nervous system prophylaxis that includes intrathecally administered methotrexate and cranial irradiation. With this approach, almost 50% of patients may sustain a durable remission. The survival rate may reach 75% in the absence of bone marrow involvement. Similarly, up to 65% of patients with small noncleaved cell lymphoma (Burkitt-like) may achieve a lasting remission when treated with an aggressive, high-intensity, brief-duration chemotherapy program that includes cyclophosphamide, etoposide, bleomycin, vincristine, methotrexate, and doxorubicin.

SUGGESTED READING

Hodgkin's Disease

Canellos GP, Anderson JR, Propert KJ, Nissen N, Cooper MR, Henderson ES, Green MR, Gottlieb A, Peterson BA. Chemotherapy of advanced Hodgkin's disease with MOPP, ABVD, or MOPP alternating with ABVD. *N Engl J Med* 1992; 327: 1478-1484.

Leibenhaut MH, Hoppe RT, Efron B, Halpern J, Nelsen T, Rosenberg SA. Prognostic indicators of laparotomy findings in clinical stage I-II supradiaphragmatic Hodgkin's disease. *J Clin Oncol* 1989; 7: 81-91.

Linch DC, Winfield D, Goldstone AH, Moir D, Hancock B, McMillan A, Chopra R, Milligan D, Hudson GV. Dose intensification with autologous bone-marrow transplantation in relapsed and resistant Hodgkin's disease: results of a BNLI randomised trial. *Lancet* 1993; 341: 1051-1054.

Lister TA, Crowther D. Staging for Hodgkin's disease. *Semin Oncol* 1990; 17: 696-703.

Longo DL. The use of chemotherapy in the treatment of Hodgkin's disease. *Semin Oncol* 1990; 17: 716-735.

Mauch P, Tarbell N, Weinstein H, Silver B, Goffman T, Osteen R, Zajac A, Coleman CN, Canellos G, Rosenthal D. Stage IA and IIA supradiaphragmatic Hodgkin's disease: prognostic factors in surgically staged patients treated with mantle and paraaortic irradiation. *J Clin Oncol* 1988; 6: 1576-1583.

van Leeuwen FE, Klokman WJ, Hagenbeek A, Noyon R, van den Belt-Dusebout AW, van Kerkhoff EH, van Heerde P, Somers R. Second cancer risk following Hodgkin's disease: a 20-year follow-up study. *J Clin Oncol* 1994; 12: 312-325.

Non-Hodgkin's Lymphoma

Fisher RI, Gaynor ER, Dahlberg S, Oken MM, Grogan TM, Mize EM, Glick JH, Coltman CA Jr, Miller TP. Comparison of a standard regimen (CHOP) with three intensive chemotherapy regimens for advanced non-Hodgkin's lymphoma. *N Engl J Med* 1993; 328: 1002-1006.

Gianni AM, Bregni M, Siena S, Brambilla C, Di Nicola M, Lombardi F, Gandola L, Tarella C, Pileri A, Ravagnani F, Valagussa P, Bonadonna G. High-dose chemotherapy and autologous bone marrow transplantation compared with MACOP-B in aggressive B-cell lymphoma. *N Engl J Med* 1997; 336: 1290-1297.

Harris NL, Jaffe ES, Stein H, Banks PM, Chan JK, Cleary ML, Delsol G, De Wolf-Peeters C, Falini B, Gatter KC. A revised European-American classification of lymphoid neoplasms: a proposal from the International Lymphoma Study Group. *Blood* 1994; 84: 1361-1392.

Horning SJ, Rosenberg SA. The natural history of initially untreated low-grade non-Hodgkin's lymphomas. *N Engl J Med* 1984; 311: 1471-1475.

McMaster ML, Greer JP, Greco FA, Johnson DH, Wolff SN, Hainsworth JD. Effective treatment of small-noncleaved-cell lymphoma with high-intensity, brief-duration chemotherapy. *J Clin Oncol* 1991; 9: 941-946.

Miller TP, Dahlberg S, Cassady JR, Adelstein DJ, Spier CM, Grogan TM, LeBlanc M, Carlin S, Chase E, Fisher RI. Chemotherapy alone compared with chemotherapy plus radiotherapy for localized intermediate- and high-grade non-Hodgkin's lymphoma. *N Engl J Med* 1998; 339: 21-26.

Philip T, Armitage JO, Spitzer G, Chauvin F, Jagannath S, Cahn JY, Colombat P, Goldstone AH, Gorin NC, Flesh M, Laporte J-P, Maraninchi D, Pico J, Bosly A, Anderson C, Schots R, Biron P, Cabanillas F, Dicke K. High-dose therapy and autologous bone marrow transplantation after failure of conventional chemotherapy in adults with intermediate-grade or high-grade non-Hodgkin's lymphoma. *N Engl J Med* 1987; 316: 1493-1498.

The International Non-Hodgkin's Lymphoma Prognostic Factors Project. A predictive model for aggressive non-Hodgkin's lymphoma. *N Engl J Med* 1993; 329: 987-994.

The Non-Hodgkin's Lymphoma Pathologic Classification Project. National Cancer Institute sponsored study of classifications of non-Hodgkin's lymphomas: summary and description of a working formulation for clinical usage. *Cancer* 1982; 49: 2112-2135.

18 An Evaluation of Patients With Monoclonal Gammopathies

Robert A. Kyle, MD

Contents

INTRODUCTION

The monoclonal gammopathies are a group of disorders characterized by the proliferation of a single clone of plasma cells that produce a homogeneous monoclonal protein (M-protein or myeloma protein). Each M-protein consists of two heavy polypeptide chains of the same class and subclass and two light polypeptide chains of the same type. The heavy polypeptide chains are gamma (γ) in IgG, alpha (α) in IgA, mu (μ) in IgM, delta (δ) in IgD, and epsilon (ε) in IgE. Light-chain types are kappa (κ) and lambda (λ). It is extremely important to differentiate a monoclonal from a polyclonal increase in immunoglobulins because a monoclonal increase is associated with a clonal process that is malignant or potentially malignant, whereas a polyclonal increase is due to a reactive or inflammatory process.

RECOGNITION OF MONOCLONAL PROTEINS

High-resolution agarose gel electrophoresis is the best method for the detection of an M-protein. After recognition of a localized band or spike on electrophoresis, one should perform immunofixation or immunosubtraction with capillary electrophoresis to determine the presence and type of M-protein. High-resolution agarose gel electrophoresis should be performed when multiple myeloma, Waldenström's macroglobulinemia, pri-

From: *Primary Hematology*
Edited by: A. Tefferi © Mayo Foundation for Medical Education and Research, Rochester, MN

mary amyloidosis, or a related disorder is suspected. In addition, it is indicated in any patient with unexplained weakness or fatigue, anemia, increased erythrocyte sedimentation rate, unexplained back pain, osteoporosis, osteolytic lesions, fractures, hypercalcemia, Bence Jones proteinuria, renal insufficiency, or recurrent infections. Electrophoresis also should be performed in adults with unexplained sensorimotor peripheral neuropathy, carpal tunnel syndrome, refractory congestive heart failure or cardiomyopathy, nephrotic syndrome or renal insufficiency, orthostatic hypotension, or malabsorption, because these features suggest the possibility of primary amyloidosis.

An M-protein is usually visible as a discrete band on agarose gel electrophoresis or as a tall, narrow spike or peak in the g or b region or rarely in the $\alpha 2$ region of the densitometer tracing (Fig. 1). A polyclonal increase in immunoglobulins which is characterized by excess of one or more heavy-chain classes and both κ and λ light-chain types produces a broad band or a broad-based peak and is limited to the g regions (Fig. 2). Two M-proteins (biclonal gammopathy) occur in 3% to 4% of sera containing an M-protein (Fig. 3). Rarely, three M-proteins are found (triclonal gammopathy).

One must realize that a small M-protein may be present when the total protein, α, β, and γ globulin components, and quantitative immunoglobulins are all within normal limits. Bence Jones protein (monoclonal κ or λ light chain) is usually present in too low a concentration to be visible. The M-protein also may be small in cases with IgD myeloma. The electrophoretic pattern of the heavy-chain diseases (γ, α, and μ) is usually nondiagnostic. Chronic liver disease, connective tissue disorders, and chronic infection are characterized by a large, broad-based polyclonal pattern. Occasionally, lymphoproliferative disorders such as angioimmunoblastic lymphadenopathy may produce a polyclonal increase in immunoglobulins. Rarely, a polyclonal gammopathy may be present without evidence of an underlying disorder.

The type of M-protein is best determined by immunofixation. It should be performed when a sharp spike or band is found in the agarose gel or when multiple myeloma, macroglobulinemia, primary amyloidosis, solitary or extramedullary plasmacytoma, or a related disorder is suspected. It is critical for the differentiation of the monoclonal from the polyclonal increase in immunoglobulins. It is particularly helpful for the recognition and distinction of biclonal and triclonal gammopathies. Immunoelectrophoresis also may be used for the detection of an M-protein, but most laboratories do not use it. Capillary zone electrophoresis measures protein by absorbance, so protein stains are unnecessary, and no point of application is seen. Immunotyping can be performed by an immunosubtraction procedure in which the serum sample is incubated with sepharose beads coupled with anti-γ, α, μ, κ, and λ antisera. After incubation with each of the heavy- and light-chain antisera solid-phase reagents, the supernates are reanalyzed to determine which reagents removed the electrophoretic abnormality. The immunosubtraction procedure is technically less demanding and is automated, and thus it is a useful procedure for immunotyping M-proteins. IgD and IgE M-proteins must be excluded by Ouchterlony immunodiffusion, immunoelectrophoresis, or immunofixation in all patients with Bence Jones proteinemia. All patients with a monoclonal light chain in the serum (Bence Jones proteinemia) must have electrophoresis and immunofixation of a 24-hour urine specimen.

Quantitation of IgG, IgA, and IgM is best performed with a rate nephelometer. Levels of IgM may be 1,000 to 2,000 mg/dL more than the size of the M-protein in the densitometer tracing. IgG and IgA also may be spuriously increased. Consequently, the clinician must measure the M-protein by either or both techniques but must not use serum

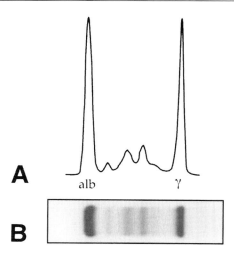

Fig. 1. *A*, Monoclonal pattern of serum protein as traced by densitometer after electrophoresis on agarose gel: tall, narrow-based peak of γ mobility. *B*, Monoclonal pattern from electrophoresis of serum on agarose gel (anode on left): dense, localized band representing monoclonal protein of γ mobility. (From Kyle RA, Katzmann JA. Immunochemical characterization of immunoglobulins, in *Manual of Clinical Laboratory Immunology* (Rose NR, de Macario EC, Folds JD, Lane HC, Nakamura RM, eds), 5th ed. ASM Press, Washington, DC, 1997, pp. 156-176. By permission of the American Society for Microbiology.)

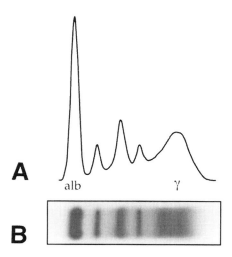

Fig. 2. *A*, Polyclonal pattern from densitometer tracing of agarose gel: broad-based peak of γ mobility. *B*, Polyclonal pattern from electrophoresis of agarose gel (anode on left). Band at right is broad and extends throughout the γ area. (From Kyle RA, Katzmann JA. Immunochemical characterization of immunoglobulins, in *Manual of Clinical Laboratory Immunology* (Rose NR, de Macario EC, Folds JD, Lane HC, Nakamura RM, eds), 5th ed. ASM Press, Washington, DC, 1997, pp. 156-176. By permission of the American Society for Microbiology.)

protein electrophoresis and then attempt to follow the patient by comparing the M-spike with nephelometric measurement at the next visit. The viscosity of serum should be measured if the patient has signs or symptoms of hyperviscosity syndrome, which is

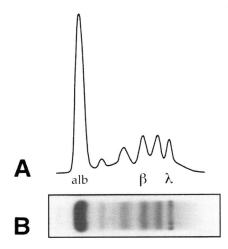

Fig. 3. *A*, Serum protein electrophoresis on agarose gel showing two γ peaks. *B*, Biclonal pattern of electrophoresis of serum on agarose gel (anode at left): two discrete γ bands. (From Kyle RA, Katzmann JA. Immunochemical characterization of immunoglobulins, in *Manual of Clinical Laboratory Immunology* (Rose NR, de Macario EC, Folds JD, Lane HC, Nakamura RM, eds), 5th ed. ASM Press, Washington, DC, 1997, pp. 156-176. By permission of the American Society for Microbiology.)

characterized by dilatation of retinal veins, flame-shaped retinal hemorrhages, blurring or loss of vision, oronasal bleeding, headaches, vertigo, nystagmus, decreased hearing, ataxia, paresthesias, diplopia, congestive heart failure, somnolence, stupor, or coma. The relationship of serum viscosity and symptoms of hyperviscosity is not precise.

Patients with a serum M-protein value more than 1.5 g/dL should have electrophoresis and immunofixation of an aliquot from a 24-hour urine collection. In addition, immunofixation of the urine should be performed initially in all patients with multiple myeloma, Waldenström's macroglobulinemia, primary amyloidosis, or heavy-chain diseases or patients in whom these entities are suspected. The amount of monoclonal light chain in the urine is a direct reflection of the tumor mass of the patient.

A classification of monoclonal gammopathies is as follows:

I. Monoclonal gammopathy of undetermined significance (MGUS)
   A. Benign (IgG, IgA, IgM, IgD)
   B. Associated with neoplasms of cell types not known to produce M-proteins
   C. Biclonal gammopathies
   D. Triclonal gammopathies
   E. Idiopathic Bence Jones proteinuria
II. Malignant monoclonal gammopathies
   A. Multiple myeloma (MM) (IgG, IgA, IgD, IgE, and free κ or λ light chains)
      1. Symptomatic multiple myeloma
      2. Smoldering multiple myeloma
      3. Plasma cell leukemia
      4. Nonsecretory myeloma
      5. Osteosclerotic myeloma (POEMS)
   B. Plasmacytoma
      1. Solitary plasmacytoma of bone
      2. Extramedullary plasmacytoma

MONOCLONAL GAMMOPATHY
OF UNDETERMINED SIGNIFICANCE (MGUS)

Monoclonal gammopathy of undetermined significance (MGUS) denotes the presence of an M-protein in persons without evidence of multiple myeloma, Waldenström's macroglobulinemia, primary amyloidosis, or other related disorders. The term "benign monoclonal gammopathy" was frequently used, but it is misleading because one does not know at the time of diagnosis whether a process producing an M-protein will remain stable and benign or will develop into symptomatic multiple myeloma or a related disorder.

MGUS is characterized by a serum M-protein spike less than 3 g/dL, fewer than 10% plasma cells in the bone marrow, or no or only small amounts of M-protein in the urine, absence of lytic bone lesions, anemia, hypercalcemia, and renal insufficiency. The proliferative rate of the plasma cells (plasma cell labeling index) is low. Most importantly, the M-protein remains stable and other abnormalities do not develop during follow-up. The finding of an M-protein is an unexpected event in the laboratory evaluation of an unrelated disorder, in investigating an increased erythrocyte sedimentation rate, or in a general health examination. It was initially considered to be benign, but it is now well established that in a proportion of patients it will evolve into multiple myeloma, macroglobulinemia, primary amyloidosis, or a related disorder.

The prevalence of MGUS is 1% in patients older than 50 years and 3% in those older than 70 years. In subjects older than 80 years, the frequency is nearly 5%, and it approaches 15% in those older than 90 years. Because of its high prevalence in the multiple fields of clinical practice in which these patients are seen, it is of particular importance to know whether the disorder will remain stable and benign or, on the contrary, progress to a symptomatic monoclonal gammopathy requiring chemotherapy.

LONG-TERM FOLLOW-UP OF M-PROTEIN

We did a long-term study of 241 patients with MGUS who were examined at the Mayo Clinic before Jan. 1, 1971. No patients were lost to follow-up. Electrophoresis and immunoelectrophoresis of serum and urine proteins were performed periodically in an effort to determine the frequency of development of multiple myeloma, primary amyloidosis, macroglobulinemia, or other disorders. The group consisted of 140 male and 101 female patients. The median age at recognition of the M-protein was 64 years. When the M-protein was detected, one-third were 70 years or older and only 4% were younger than 40 years. Hepatomegaly or splenomegaly and laboratory abnormalities, such as anemia, thrombocytopenia, increased serum creatinine value, or hypercalcemia, were the result of unrelated disorders. The initial M-protein value ranged from 0.3 to 3.2 g/dL. The median value of the M-protein was 1.7 g/dL. The heavy-chain type was IgG in 73%, IgM in 14%, IgA in 11%, and biclonal in 2%. κ Light chains were found in 62%, and the remainder were λ. The levels of uninvolved (background or normal) immunoglobulins

Table 1
Course of 241 Patients With Monoclonal
Gammopathy of Undetermined Significance

| Group | Description | At follow-up after 24-38 years | |
		No. of patients	%
1	No substantial increase of serum or urine monoclonal protein (benign)	25	10
2	Monoclonal protein ≥ 3.0 g/dL but no myeloma or related disease	26	11
3	Died of unrelated causes	127	53
4	Development of myeloma, macroglobulinemia, amyloidosis, or related disease	63	26
Total		241	100

Modified from Kyle RA. 'Benign' monoclonal gammopathy. A misnomer? *JAMA* 1984; 251: 1849-1854. By permission of the American Medical Association.

were reduced in 29% at the time of recognition of the M-protein. The percentage of bone marrow plasma cells ranged from 1% to 10% (median, 3%). Unrelated disorders such as cardiovascular or cerebrovascular disease, inflammatory disorders, connective tissue diseases, and various other conditions unrelated to the M-protein were found in three-fourths of patients.

After follow-up of 24 to 38 years, the patients were categorized into four groups (Table 1). The concentration of hemoglobin, amount of serum M-protein, type of serum heavy and light chains, decrease in uninvolved immunoglobulins, subclass of IgG heavy chain, and the number and appearance of plasma cells in the bone marrow in the group of patients with a benign or stable course did not differ substantially from those in the overall study group.

The number of living patients in whom the M-protein remained stable and who are classified as having benign disease has decreased to 25 (10%). These patients are still at risk for the development of myeloma or related disorders and continue to be followed. The M-protein disappeared in two patients. Twenty-six patients had an increase of the M-protein to 3 g/dL or more but did not require chemotherapy for myeloma or macroglo- bulinemia. Three of these patients are still living. One hundred twenty-seven patients died without developing myeloma or a related disorder. Fifty-five patients lived for 10 years or more after the serum M-protein was detected. The most frequent cause of death was cardiac disease (34%). Fifteen patients died of malignancy, but these deaths were unrelated to the M-protein.

Sixty-three patients (26%) developed myeloma, amyloidosis, macroglobulinemia, or a related disorder. The actuarially estimated cumulative incidence of these serious out- comes was 16% at 10 years and 40% at 25 years (Fig. 4). Forty-three (68%) of the 63

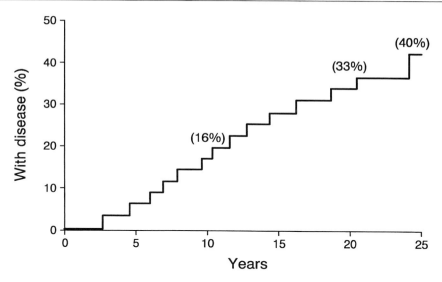

Fig. 4. Incidence of multiple myeloma, macroglobulinemia, amyloidosis, or lymphoproliferative disease after recognition of monoclonal protein. (From Kyle RA. Monoclonal gammopathy of undetermined significance [MGUS]. *Baillière's Clin Haematol* 1995; 8: 761-781. By permission of Baillière Tindall.)

Table 2
Development of Myeloma or Related Diseases in 63 Patients
With Monoclonal Gammopathy of Undetermined Significance

| Disease | No. of patients | % | Interval to diagnosis, yr | |
			Median	Range
Multiple myeloma	43	68	10.0	2-29
Amyloidosis	8	13	9.0	6-19
Macroglobulinemia	7	11	8.5	4-20
Lymphoproliferative	5	8	10.5	6-22
Total	63	100		

patients developed multiple myeloma. The interval from diagnosis of the M-protein to the diagnosis of multiple myeloma ranged from 2 to 29 years (median, 10 years). In nine of the patients, multiple myeloma was diagnosed more than 20 years after initial detection of the serum M-protein. The median duration of survival after the diagnosis of myeloma was 33 months. The development of myeloma varied from a gradual increase of the M-protein to an abrupt increase. Primary amyloidosis was found in eight patients 6 to 19 years after recognition of an M-protein. Macroglobulinemia occurred in seven patients; the median interval from recognition of the M-protein to diagnosis of macroglobulinemia was 8.5 years. In five patients, a lymphoproliferative disorder developed 6 to 22 years after recognition of the M-protein (Table 2). The risk of development of serious disease was essentially the same for IgG, IgA, and IgM M-proteins. On the basis of a proportional hazards model, the likelihood of development of myeloma, amyloidosis, or other serious disease was not influenced by age, sex, class of heavy chain, IgG subclass, type of light chain, presence of hepatomegaly, values for hemoglobin, serum M-protein spike, serum creatinine, or serum albumin, or number or appearance of the bone marrow plasma cells.

In a long-term follow-up of 430 patients with an IgM M-protein, 242 (56%) were considered to have MGUS. During a median follow-up of 7 years (1,714 patient-years), 40 (17%) of the 242 patients developed a lymphoid malignancy: macroglobulinemia (22 patients), malignant lymphoproliferative disease (9), lymphoma (6), primary amyloidosis (2), and chronic lymphocytic leukemia (1). The median duration from recognition of the IgM component to the development of these disorders ranged from 4 to 9 years.

DIFFERENTIATION OF MGUS FROM MULTIPLE MYELOMA OR MACROGLOBULINEMIA

The differentiation of MGUS from multiple myeloma may be difficult. The size of the M-protein in the serum and urine, hemoglobin value, number of bone marrow plasma cells, presence of hypercalcemia or renal insufficiency, and the presence of lytic lesions are helpful.

The presence of a serum M-protein of more than 3 g/dL usually indicates overt multiple myeloma, but some patients may have smoldering multiple myeloma and remain stable for long periods. Levels of uninvolved or background immunoglobulins may help in differentiating benign from malignant disease. In most patients with multiple myeloma or Waldenström's macroglobulinemia, the levels of normal or uninvolved immunoglobulins are reduced, but a similar reduction also may occur in MGUS. In our experience, about one-fourth of patients with MGUS had a reduction in normal or uninvolved immunoglobulins at the time of recognition of the M-protein, and yet they remained stable for many years. Thus, a reduction of uninvolved immunoglobulins is not a reliable differentiating feature.

The presence of monoclonal light chains in the serum of a patient with a monoclonal gammopathy suggests a neoplastic process. However, it is not uncommon to find patients with newly diagnosed MGUS who remain stable for many years despite the presence of a small monoclonal light chain in the urine.

Usually, the presence of more than 10% plasma cells in the bone marrow suggests multiple myeloma, but some patients with greater plasmacytosis remain stable for long intervals. Generally, the morphologic appearance of the plasma cells is of little help in differentiating malignant from benign disease. The presence of osteolytic lesions is strong evidence of multiple myeloma, but metastatic carcinoma may produce lytic lesions and be associated with an unrelated monoclonal gammopathy. The plasma cell labeling index, which measures synthesis of DNA, is useful in differentiating patients with MGUS or smoldering multiple myeloma from those with multiple myeloma. We have developed a monoclonal antibody (BU-1) reactive with 5-bromo-2-deoxyuridine (BRD-URD) in mice. Bone marrow plasma cells are exposed to BRD-URD for 1 hour. The cells synthesizing DNA incorporate BRD-URD, which is recognized by the BU-1 monoclonal antibody conjugated to a goat antimouse immunoglobulin-rhodamine complex. Binding with propidium iodide identifies the cells incorporating BRD-URD in S phase. The BU-1 monoclonal antibody does not require denaturation for its activity. Consequently, the use of fluorescent conjugated immunoglobulin antisera to κ and l identifies the population of monoclonal plasma cells. The test can be done in 4 to 5 hours. An increased plasma cell labeling index is good evidence that either multiple myeloma is present or it will soon develop. However, about 40% of patients with active multiple myeloma will have a normal plasma cell labeling index. There is also a good correlation between the peripheral blood labeling index and the bone marrow labeling index.

The presence of circulating plasma cells of the same isotype in the peripheral blood is a good marker of active disease. In a series of 57 patients with newly diagnosed smoldering multiple myeloma, 16 had progression within 12 months. Sixty-three percent of those patients who progressed had an increased number of peripheral blood plasma cells. In contrast, only 4 of 41 patients who remained stable had an increase in peripheral blood plasma cells at diagnosis.

Although β_2-microglobulin levels are important for the prognosis of multiple myeloma, they are of little value for differentiating MGUS from multiple myeloma. The presence of J chains in malignant plasma cells, increased levels of plasma cell acid phosphatase, reduced numbers of CD4 lymphocytes, increased numbers of monoclonal idiotype-bearing peripheral blood lymphocytes, an increased number of immunoglobulin-secreting cells in peripheral blood, and increased levels of interleukin-6 are all characteristic of multiple myeloma, but they are not reliable for differentiation because there is an overlap with MGUS. Fluorescence in situ hybridization (FISH) may aid in differentiation of benign from malignant disease. However, MGUS plasma cells often have abnormal findings and thus cannot be differentiated from multiple myeloma with this approach.

In summary, MGUS is usually not difficult to diagnose, and it is often an unexpected finding in the course of an unrelated process or in a routine medical examination. No single factor can differentiate patients with MGUS from those in whom a malignant plasma cell disorder will subsequently develop.

PREDICTORS OF MALIGNANT TRANSFORMATION

There is general agreement that there are no findings at the time of diagnosis of MGUS which reliably distinguish patients who will remain stable from those in whom a malignant condition will develop. As previously mentioned, the initial hemoglobin value, amount of serum and urine M-protein, and the appearance and number of bone marrow plasma cells are helpful for differentiating MGUS from myeloma; they are not useful for prediction of a subsequent malignant process.

In one report of 386 patients with a nonmyelomatous gammopathy, 51 were classified as having monoclonal gammopathy of borderline significance (MGBS) if the bone marrow plasma cell content was 10% to 30%. After a median follow-up of 70 months in the MGUS group and 53 months in the MGBS group, malignant disease developed in 23 of the 335 patients with MGUS and 19 of the 51 patients with MGBS. The relative risks of developing myeloma were 2.4 for each 1 g/dL increase of IgG, 3.5 for detectable light-chain proteinuria, 6.1 for age older than 70 years, and 13.1 for a reduction in two polyclonal immunoglobulins. The authors concluded that MGUS had a very low risk of evolution when the M-protein value was 1.5 g/dL or less, the bone marrow plasma cell value was less than 5%, polyclonal (uninvolved) immunoglobulins were not reduced, and no light-chain proteinuria was detectable. In a similar study of asymptomatic patients with stage I myeloma, disease progression occurred in 41 of 91 patients, and the median time of progression was 48 months. Hemoglobin values less than 12 g/dL, bone marrow plasmacytosis more than 25%, and an IgG spike of 3 g/dL or an IgA spike of 2.5 g/dL or greater were significant prognostic factors for progression.

The presence of peripheral blood clonal B-cell excess or the expression of serum neural cell adhesion molecule suggests multiple myeloma rather than MGUS. Bone resorption on biopsy is seen in patients with multiple myeloma but not in patients with MGUS or smoldering myeloma.

In patients whose condition evolves, myeloma usually develops after a prolonged period of stability. Thus, MGUS constitutes the pre-myeloma phase, which may persist for more than 20 years. A considerable number of patients with multiple myeloma will have had a previous MGUS. Of the 55 patients in Olmsted County, Minnesota, in whom multiple myeloma was diagnosed in recent years, 58% had a preceding MGUS, smoldering myeloma, or plasmacytoma before the diagnosis of multiple myeloma. When malignant transformation occurs, the type of M-protein is always the same as it was in the MGUS state.

ASSOCIATION OF MGUS WITH OTHER DISEASES

MGUS is often associated with other diseases, as would be expected in an elderly population. The association of two conditions depends on the frequency with which each occurs independently. Thus, appropriate epidemiologic and statistical studies and valid control populations must be used to evaluate these associations.

Lymphoproliferative Disorders

An M-protein is frequently found in lymphoma. IgM is more common than IgG or IgA. Patients with a diffuse histopathologic pattern are much more likely to have an IgM M-protein than patients with nodular lymphoma or Hodgkin's disease. Clinical response to therapy is frequently associated with a reduction in the M-protein. An M-protein is present in about 5% of patients with chronic lymphocytic leukemia. IgG and IgM are the most common types. The presence of an M-protein is not associated with a particular clinical or laboratory feature.

Other Hematologic Disorders

Monoclonal gammopathies have been reported in chronic neutrophilic leukemia, Gaucher's disease, and acquired von Willebrand's disease. There is likely some sort of an association between these entities. Monoclonal gammopathies also have been reported in a wide variety of hematologic disorders such as refractory anemia, pernicious anemia, pure red cell aplasia, idiopathic thrombocytopenic purpura, and acute leukemia. There is a lack of epidemiologic data to establish whether the incidence of an M-protein is greater in these patients than in a normal population.

Neurologic Disorders

There is an increased incidence of monoclonal gammopathies in patients with peripheral neuropathy. We found that 10% of patients with sensorimotor peripheral neuropathy of unknown cause had an associated M-protein. IgG was most common. In about half of patients with an IgM gammopathy and polyneuropathy, the IgM binds to myelin-associated glycoprotein (MAG); however, the MAG-positive peripheral neuropathies do not appear to be different clinically or in their response to therapy. Other neurologic disorders such as amyotrophic lateral sclerosis, progressive muscular atrophy, and ataxia-telangiectasia have been reported with monoclonal gammopathies, but the association may be merely coincidental.

POEMS syndrome is characterized by polyneuropathy (P), organomegaly (O), endocrinopathy (E), M-protein (M), and skin changes (S). The typical clinical feature is a chronic demyelinating polyneuropathy that is more motor than sensory. Sclerotic skeletal lesions are also typical. Cranial nerves are not involved, except for the presence of papilledema. Hepatomegaly is noted in about half of the patients, and splenomegaly and lymphadenopathy also may be present. Hyperpigmentation, hypertrichosis, angiomatous lesions, gynecomastia, and testicular atrophy may occur. IgA is common, and most patients have a l light chain. The M-component is usually less than 3 g/dL, and the bone marrow aspirate usually contains fewer than 5% plasma cells. In contrast to multiple myeloma, the hemoglobin level is normal or increased, thrombocytosis is common, and hypercalcemia and renal insufficiency rarely occur. Biopsy of an osteosclerotic lesion is generally necessary to confirm the diagnosis. Radiation of the sclerotic lesion frequently improves the peripheral neuropathy. The prognosis is better than in patients with typical myeloma.

Dermatologic Diseases

Lichen myxedematosus (scleromyxedema, papular mucinosis) is a rare disease characterized by macules and papules involving the skin and is frequently associated with a cathodal IgG λ M-protein. Pyoderma gangrenosum, necrobiotic xanthogranuloma, discoid lupus erythematosus, and diffuse plane xanthomatosis may be associated with an M-protein. Several cases of cutaneous T-cell lymphomas, such as Sézary's syndrome and mycosis fungoides, have been associated with a monoclonal gammopathy.

Immunosuppression

M-proteins have been reported in association with acquired immunodeficiency syndrome (AIDS). Monoclonal gammopathies have been reported in almost 30% of patients with a liver transplant. These M-proteins are usually small and often transient. The type of M-protein may change from time to time. Immunosuppression appears to be a major factor. Monoclonal gammopathies also have been associated with bone marrow transplantation and less frequently with solid organ transplants.

Monoclonal Gammopathies With Antibody Activity

M-proteins have shown specificity against streptolysin O, antistaphylolysin, antinuclear antibody, thyroglobulin, insulin, DNA, thyroxine, transferrin, and antibiotics. Patients have been reported with an M-protein with antiriboflavin antibody activity. This results in bright yellow coloration of the skin and hair. The M-protein may bind calcium and produce an increase in the total calcium level but without pathologic consequences, because the ionized calcium level is normal. Copper binding M-protein also has been reported. Binding of an M-protein with phosphate produces a false increase in the serum phosphorus level.

Miscellaneous

A wide variety of conditions, such as rheumatoid arthritis and its variants, polymyositis, polymyalgia rheumatica, angioneurotic edema, and chronic liver disease, have been associated with a monoclonal gammopathy. Again, it must be emphasized that a properly matched control population be used to determine the relationship of MGUS to these diseases.

MANAGEMENT OF MGUS

Because it is not possible to differentiate a patient with stable MGUS from one in whom myeloma, macroglobulinemia or a related condition develops, the clinician must continue to observe the patient. It is essential to obtain a careful history, inquiring about skeletal pain, increased fatigue, history of recurrent infections, and excessive bleeding. One must be alert for the symptoms of primary amyloidosis, such as light-headedness, change in the voice or enlargement of the tongue, weight loss, increased bruising, steatorrhea, dyspnea, edema, intermittent claudication, and paresthesias. Fever, night sweats, weight loss, blurred vision, or oronasal bleeding suggests macroglobulinemia.

The occurrence of nephrotic syndrome, renal insufficiency, congestive heart failure, sensorimotor peripheral neuropathy, carpal tunnel syndrome, or orthostatic hypotension in a patient with MGUS requires appropriate biopsies to exclude the possibility of primary amyloidosis.

If the serum M-protein value is less than 1.5 g/dL, the history and physical examination are noncontributory, and the hemoglobin, calcium, and creatinine values are normal, no additional studies are required. Serum protein electrophoresis should be repeated in 6 months, and if the results are stable, it should be done at annual intervals. In this setting, a bone marrow examination, skeletal radiographs, and a 24-hour urine specimen for immunofixation are not necessary in most instances.

If the asymptomatic patient has an M-protein value of 1.5 to 2.5 g/dL, additional studies should include nephelometry for quantitation of immunoglobulins and collection of a 24-hour urine specimen for electrophoresis and immunofixation. Serum protein electrophoretic patterns should be repeated in 3 to 6 months, and if stable, they should be repeated annually, or sooner if any symptoms or complications develop.If the serum M spike (IgG or IgA) is more than 2.5 g/dL, there is a greater likelihood of multiple myeloma, so a metastatic bone survey, including single views of the humeri and femora, should be done, in addition to quantitation of immunoglobulins with nephelometry and immunofixation of the urine. Aspiration and biopsy of the bone marrow should also be done. The plasma cell labeling index and the presence of circulating plasma cells in the peripheral blood are helpful in differential diagnosis.

If multiple myeloma is suspected, b_2-microglobulin, C-reactive protein, and lactate dehydrogenase values also should be determined. If any historical or physical features suggestive of primary amyloidosis are found, biopsy of the subcutaneous fat and bone marrow should be performed. If the results are negative and if there is clinical suspicion of amyloidosis, a rectal biopsy (including submucosa) or biopsy of an involved organ should be performed. If these studies are satisfactory, serum protein electrophoresis should be repeated in 3 to 4 months and, if stable, repeated at 6-month intervals. If the spike is still stable, electrophoresis of serum should be repeated annually.

If the serum M spike (IgM) is more than 2 g/dL, aspiration and biopsy of the bone marrow and computed tomography of the abdomen may be helpful for recognition of Waldenström's macroglobulinemia or other lymphoproliferative disorders.

A 24-hour urine specimen for electrophoresis and immunofixation should be obtained if the serum M spike is more than 1.5 g/dL. A 24-hour urine specimen also should be obtained if the serum M-protein increases or other evidence of evolving multiple myeloma, macroglobulinemia, or amyloidosis occurs.

In summary, no single factor can differentiate a patient with stable MGUS from one in whom a malignant plasma cell disorder will eventually develop. The most dependable means of follow-up is serial measurement of the M-protein in the serum and periodic reevaluation of pertinent clinical and laboratory features to determine whether myeloma, macroglobulinemia, or related disorders have developed. The patient should be told that the risk of malignancy is only 25%, and that this develops after a median of 10 years.

However, the patient and the physician also should be aware that evolution from MGUS to multiple myeloma can be abrupt and that evaluation needs to be performed promptly if untoward symptoms develop.

ACKNOWLEDGMENTS

Supported in part by Research Grant CA-62242 from the National Cancer Institute.

SUGGESTED READING

Baldini L, Guffanti A, Cesana BM, Colombi M, Chiorboli O, Damilano I, Maiolo AT. Role of different hematologic variables in defining the risk of malignant transformation in monoclonal gammopathy. *Blood* 1996; 87: 912-918.

Bladé J, López-Guillermo A, Rozman C, Cervantes F, Salgado C, Aguilar JL, Veves-Corrons JL, Montserrat E. Malignant transformation and life expectancy in monoclonal gammopathy of undetermined significance. *Br J Haematol* 1992; 81: 391-394.

Kyle RA. "Benign" monoclonal gammopathy—after 20 to 35 years of follow-up. *Mayo Clin Proc* 1993; 68: 26-36.

Kyle RA, Garton JP. The spectrum of IgM monoclonal gammopathy in 430 cases. *Mayo Clin Proc* 1987; 62: 719-731.

Kyle RA, Gertz MA. Primary systemic amyloidosis: clinical and laboratory features in 474 cases. *Semin Hematol* 1995; 32: 45-59.

Kyle RA, Greipp PR. Smoldering multiple myeloma. *N Engl J Med* 1980; 302: 1347-1349.

Kyle RA, Robinson RA, Katzmann JA. The clinical aspects of biclonal gammopathies. Review of 57 cases. *Am J Med* 1981; 71: 999-1008.

Witzig TE, Kyle RA, O'Fallon WM, Greipp PR. Detection of peripheral blood plasma cells as a predictor of disease course in patients with smouldering multiple myeloma. *Br J Haematol* 1994; 87: 266-272.

19 Multiple Myeloma and Related Disorders

Robert A. Kyle, MD

Contents

MULTIPLE MYELOMA

Multiple myeloma is characterized by the neoplastic proliferation of a single clone of plasma cells engaged in the production of a monoclonal immunoglobulin. Proliferation of the plasma cells in the bone marrow produces skeletal destruction that results in bone pain and fractures. The excessive production of the monoclonal protein (M-protein) can lead to renal failure, recurrent bacterial infections, or hyperviscosity syndrome. Anemia and hypercalcemia are other important features.

Etiology and Epidemiology

The cause of multiple myeloma is unknown. An increased risk of multiple myeloma has been reported in atomic bomb survivors and in radiologists exposed long-term to large doses of radiation. Farmers who use herbicides and insecticides may be at increased risk. Multiple myeloma has been reported in two or more first-degree relatives and in identical twins. Human herpesvirus 8 (HHV-8; Kaposi's sarcoma herpesvirus, KSHV) may play a role in the pathogenesis of multiple myeloma.

Multiple myeloma accounts for 1% of all malignant disease and slightly more than 10% of hematologic malignancies in the United States. The annual incidence of multiple myeloma is approximately 4 per 100,000. The apparent increase during the past few decades is probably related to the increased availability and use of medical facilities, especially in older persons. The incidence in blacks is twice that in whites, and rates are lower in Asian populations. It is slightly more common in men than in women. The

From: *Primary Hematology*
Edited by: A. Tefferi © Mayo Foundation for Medical Education and Research, Rochester, MN

median age at the time of diagnosis is about 65 years. Only 18% of patients are younger than 50 years and 3% are younger than 40 years.

Biologic Characteristics

Multiple myeloma is a B-cell malignancy with mature plasma cell morphology. The plasma cells are phenotypically cIg+, CD38+, PCA-1+, CD56+, and BB4 (CD138)+, and only a minority express CD10, HLA-DR, and CD20. Although still unknown, the clonogenic cell in multiple myeloma is most likely a relatively mature cell already committed to idiotypic production of immunoglobulins. There is evidence that plasma cell precursors of myeloma circulate in the peripheral blood. These circulating clonogenic pre-myeloma cells, by means of adhesion molecules, may home to the marrow, where they find an appropriate microenvironment to differentiate and further expand. CD4 T cells often are reduced in multiple myeloma. Overproduction of interleukin-1 (IL-1) and tumor necrosis factor, which have bone-resorbing activity, have been found in patients with multiple myeloma. Interleukin-6 (IL-6) is a potent plasma cell growth factor. Serum IL-6 levels correlate with disease activity and tumor mass in patients with multiple myeloma. Cytogenetic studies in multiple myeloma are difficult because of the low proliferative rate of plasma cells. Conventional cytogenetic studies show abnormal karyotypes in about 40% of patients. Hyperdiploidy occurs in about 65% of patients, whereas hypodiploidy occurs in about 10%. Fluorescence in situ hybridization (FISH) using chromosome-specific probes identifies abnormalities in up to 80% of patients. Increased expression of c-*myc*, H-*ras*, and *bcl*-2 has been found in myeloma. Approximately 15% of cases have point mutations of p53, a tumor suppressor gene. Deletions of the retinoblastoma gene (*rb*-1), p15, p16, and p18 have been reported.

Clinical Manifestations

Bone pain, particularly in the back or chest, is present at diagnosis in more than two-thirds of patients. The pain is usually aggravated by movement and, in contrast to metastatic carcinoma, does not occur at night, except with change of position. Multiple vertebral collapse may reduce the patient's height by several inches. The most common symptoms are weakness and fatigue. These are often due to anemia. Fever, when present, is usually due to an infection. An acute infection, renal failure, hypercalcemia, or amyloidosis may be the presenting feature. The most frequent physical finding is pallor. The liver is palpable in about 20% of patients and the spleen in 5%. Extramedullary plasmacytomas are uncommon and usually occur late in the course of the disease as large, purplish, subcutaneous masses.

Laboratory Findings

If multiple myeloma is suspected, the laboratory tests listed in Table 1 should be performed. A normocytic, normochromic anemia is present initially in two-thirds of patients but eventually occurs in almost all patients with multiple myeloma. Thrombocytopenia is found in approximately 15% of patients at diagnosis, whereas the leukocyte level is usually normal. Plasma cells are found in the peripheral smear in about 15% of patients. Hypercalcemia is present initially in 20% of cases, and about one-fourth have an increased serum creatinine value.

The serum protein electrophoretic pattern shows a spike or localized band in 80% of patients at diagnosis. Hypogammaglobulinemia is present in 10%, and no abnormality is seen in the remainder. An IgG M-protein is found in about 50%, IgA in 20%, light chain

Table 1
Suggested Tests for Patients in Whom
Multiple Myeloma Is Suspected

Complete history and physical examination
Complete blood cell count and differential; peripheral blood smear
Chemistry screen (including calcium and creatinine determinations)
Serum protein electrophoresis, immunofixation, quantitation of immunoglobulins
Serum viscosity if IgG value > 6 g/dL or IgA value > 5 g/dL, or symptoms of hyperviscosity are present
Routine urinalysis, 24-hour urine collection for electrophoresis and immunofixation
Bone marrow aspiration, biopsy, plasma cell labeling index, and cytogenetics
Metastatic bone survey, including single views of humeri and femurs
Peripheral blood labeling index
β_2-Microglobulin, C-reactive protein, and lactate dehydrogenase determinations

From Kyle RA. Multiple myeloma, macroglobulinemia, and the monoclonal gammopathies, in *Current Practice of Medicine* (Bone RC, ed), vol 3. Churchill Livingstone, New York, 1996, pp. 19.1-19.6. By permission of Current Medicine.

only (Bence Jones proteinemia) in almost 20%, IgD in 2%, and biclonal gammopathy in 1%. About 7% of patients have no serum M-protein at diagnosis. Immunofixation of the urine reveals an M-protein in approximately 75% of patients. The κ/λ ratio is 2:1. Ninety-eight percent of patients with multiple myeloma have an M-protein in the serum or urine at the time of diagnosis. Patients with light-chain (Bence Jones) and IgD myeloma have a higher incidence of renal failure, associated amyloidosis, smaller serum M-component, and greater light-chain excretion than those with IgG and IgA myeloma. The bone marrow usually contains more than 10% plasma cells. Bone marrow involvement may be focal, and some patients require repeat bone marrow examinations for diagnosis. Identification of a monoclonal light chain in the cytoplasm of plasma cells with immunoperoxidase or immunofluorescence is useful for differentiating myeloma from reactive plasmacytosis due to connective tissue disorder, metastatic carcinoma, liver disease, and infections.

Radiologic Findings

Conventional radiographs show abnormalities consisting of lytic lesions, osteoporosis, or fractures in 75% of patients at diagnosis. The most commonly involved sites are the vertebrae, skull, thoracic cage, pelvis, and proximal humeri and femora. Osteoblastic lesions are rare. ^{99m}Tc bone scanning is inferior to conventional radiography and is rarely helpful. Magnetic resonance imaging is particularly helpful in patients who have bone pain but no abnormalities on radiographs and in those in whom spinal cord compression is suspected.

Renal Involvement

The serum creatinine value is 2 mg/dL or more in 20% of patients at the time of diagnosis. The two major causes of renal insufficiency are myeloma kidney and hypercalcemia. Myeloma kidney is characterized by the presence of large, dense, waxy, laminated casts in the distal and collecting tubules. These casts are composed mainly of monoclonal light chains. Multinucleated giant cells surround the casts. The renal tubules dilate and atrophy, and the entire nephron becomes distorted and nonfunctional. The

Table 2
Minimal Criteria for the Diagnosis
of Multiple Myeloma[a]

Bone marrow with > 10% plasma cells *or* plasmacytoma plus one of the following:
   Monoclonal protein in serum (usually > 3 g/dL)
   Monoclonal protein in urine
   Lytic bone lesions

[a]The patient must have the usual clinical features of multiple myeloma. Connective tissue disorders, metastatic carcinoma, lymphoma, leukemia, and chronic infections must be excluded.

   From Kyle RA. Multiple myeloma and the dysproteinemias, in *Internal Medicine* (Stein JH, Daly WJ, Easton JD, Hutton JJ, Kohler PO, O'Rourke RA, Sande MA, Stein JH, Trier JS, Zvaifler NJ, eds), 2nd ed. Little, Brown and Company, Boston, 1987, pp. 1104-1108. By permission of the publisher.

extent of cast formation correlates directly with the amount of free urinary light chain and with the severity of renal failure. Dehydration contributes to acute renal failure. Hypercalcemia is a major and treatable cause of renal insufficiency. Hyperuricemia, contrast media, antibiotics, and dehydration may contribute to renal insufficiency. Amyloidosis occurs in 10% to 15% of patients and often causes nephrotic syndrome and renal insufficiency.

Neurologic Involvement

Radiculopathy is the most frequent neurologic complication and usually involves the thoracic or lumbosacral areas. Compression of the spinal cord and extradural myeloma occur in 5% of patients. Leptomeningeal involvement is uncommon but is being recognized more frequently. Peripheral neuropathy, when present, is usually due to amyloidosis. Intracranial plasmacytomas are rare.

Other Involvement

The incidence of infection is increased in multiple myeloma. Impairment of antibody response, neutropenia, treatment with glucocorticoids, and reduction of normal immunoglobulins increase the likelihood of infection.

Diagnosis

The diagnosis of multiple myeloma depends on the presence of an increased number of plasma cells in the bone marrow or plasmacytoma, an M-protein in the serum or urine, or osteolytic lesions. These features must not be related to metastatic carcinoma, lymphoma, connective tissue disorders, or chronic infections. The patient must have the usual clinical features of multiple myeloma. The minimal criteria for diagnosis are shown in Table 2.

Monoclonal gammopathy of undetermined significance (MGUS), smoldering multiple myeloma (SMM), primary amyloidosis (AL), and metastatic carcinoma are the main conditions considered in the differential diagnosis. In MGUS, the M-protein value is less than 3 g/dL, and the bone marrow contains fewer than 10% plasma cells. There are no osteolytic lesions, anemia, hypercalcemia, or renal insufficiency. SMM is characterized by the presence of an M-protein value of 3 g/dL or more and more than 10% bone marrow plasma cells but no symptoms of multiple myeloma. Hemoglobin, calcium, and creatinine levels are normal, and no lytic lesions are seen. The background or uninvolved immunoglobulins are usually decreased in multiple myeloma, but this finding is not always useful, because 30% of patients with MGUS have a reduction of uninvolved immunoglobulins. The plasma cell labeling index, which is a measure of plasma cell proliferation, is useful in differentiating MGUS and SMM from multiple myeloma. An increased labeling index strongly suggests that the patient has or soon will have symptomatic disease. However, more than a third of patients with symptomatic multiple myeloma have a normal plasma cell labeling index. Monoclonal plasma cells of the same isotype are present in the peripheral blood in up to 80% of patients with active multiple myeloma. Patients with MGUS or SMM have few or no circulating plasma cells in most instances. It is sometimes very difficult to differentiate SMM from active multiple myeloma. If there is doubt in the physician's mind, it is usually better to withhold therapy and to reevaluate the patient in 2 to 3 months.

The differentiation between AL and multiple myeloma is arbitrary, because both diseases are plasma cell proliferative disorders with different manifestations. In amyloidosis, the bone marrow plasma cell content is usually less than 20%, there are no osteolytic lesions, and the amount of Bence Jones proteinuria is modest. Obviously, there is considerable overlap between AL and multiple myeloma.

Prognostic Features

The median duration of survival in multiple myeloma is approximately 3 years, but there is a great deal of variability from one patient to another. The plasma cell labeling index and the uncorrected β_2-microglobulin level are the two most powerful prognostic factors in our experience. The presence of a low plasma cell labeling index and a low β_2-microglobulin level is associated with a median survival of almost 6 years when treated with chemotherapy. Cytogenetic abnormalities are also an important prognostic factor. The deletion of chromosome 13 and 11q abnormalities and the presence of translocations are predictors of poor outcome. The Durie-Salmon clinical staging system has been used for more than 25 years, but it is unreliable and has many shortcomings. Adverse prognostic factors are listed in Table 3.

Treatment

Although most patients with multiple myeloma have symptomatic disease at diagnosis and require therapy, some are asymptomatic and should not be treated. All symptoms, physical findings, and laboratory data must be considered. An increasing level of the M-protein in the serum or urine, development of anemia, hypercalcemia, or renal insufficiency, and the occurrence of lytic lesions or extramedullary plasmacytomas are all indications for therapy. If there is doubt about whether to begin chemotherapy, the most reasonable approach is to reevaluate the patient in 2 or 3 months and to delay therapy until progressive disease is evident.

In contrast with most hematologic malignancies, conventional chemotherapy for multiple myeloma rarely results in complete remission but in different degrees of partial response. Generally, objective response has been defined either by a 50% decrease in the serum M-protein or urinary M-protein or by a 75% reduction in the M-component synthetic rate along with clinical improvement. The point has been made that the duration of survival in patients with myeloma who achieve disease stabilization is similar whether they obtain an objective response or a partial response.

Table 3
Adverse Prognostic Factors in Multiple Myeloma

Increased β_2-microglobulin level
High plasma cell labeling index
Unfavorable cytogenetic findings
Plasmablastic morphologic features
Increased lactate dehydrogenase value
Increased thymidine kinase level
High C-reactive protein value
Hypoalbuminemia
Advanced age
Increased creatinine concentration
Hypodiploidy, low RNA content of plasma cells
Anemia, hypercalcemia, thrombocytopenia
Primary resistance to therapy with progressive disease
Rapid response to therapy and high labeling index

From Kyle RA. Multiple myeloma and other plasma cell disorders, in *Hematology: Basic Principles and Practice* (Hoffman R, Benz EJ Jr, Shattil SJ, Furie B, Cohen HJ, Silberstein LE, eds), 2nd ed. Churchill Livingstone, New York, 1995, pp. 1354-1374. By permission of the publisher.

INITIAL THERAPY

If the patient is younger than 70 years, the physician should discuss the possibility of autologous peripheral blood stem cell transplantation. Ideally, this should be done as part of a prospective study. Hematopoietic stem cells should be collected before the patient is exposed to alkylating agents.

CHEMOTHERAPY

Chemotherapy is the preferred initial treatment for overt, symptomatic multiple myeloma in persons older than 70 years or in younger patients in whom transplantation is not feasible. Melphalan and prednisone given orally produce an objective response in 50% to 60% of persons. We prefer to give melphalan in a daily dosage of 0.15 mg/kg for 7 days (8 to 10 mg/day) and 20 mg of prednisone three times a day for the same period. Melphalan should be given when the patient is fasting because food interferes with absorption. Leukocyte and platelet counts must be determined at 3-week intervals after the start of therapy, and the melphalan dosage is altered until mid-cycle cytopenia occurs. The melphalan and prednisone regimen should be repeated every 6 weeks. If the neutrophil level is less than 1.5×10^9/L or the platelet level is lower than 100×10^9/L at 6 weeks, chemotherapy should be delayed and the counts determined at weekly intervals until the pretreatment level is approached. If the neutrophil and platelet levels remain low or if the counts are unduly low at 3 weeks, the melphalan dosage in the next 7-day course should be reduced. At least three courses of melphalan and prednisone should be given before the regimen is discontinued. An objective response may not be achieved for 6 to 12 months, or longer in some patients. Furthermore, stabilization of the disease without an objective response may be beneficial for the patient.

Although the introduction of melphalan constituted an important advance in the therapy of myeloma more than a quarter century ago, the survival rate remains unsatisfactory. Thus, many chemotherapeutic agents and combinations of these drugs have been used because of the shortcomings of melphalan and prednisone. One of the best known combinations, the M2 protocol, consists of vincristine, carmustine (BCNU), melphalan, cyclophosphamide, and prednisone (VBMCP). This regimen produces an objective response in approximately 70% of patients, but the median duration of survival is not significantly different from that obtained with melphalan and prednisone. In a recent large series reported by the Medical Research Council, the ABCM regimen (Adriamycin [doxorubicin], BCNU, cyclophosphamide, and melphalan) increased both the portion of patients reaching the plateau phase and the duration of survival in comparison with melphalan alone. However, most studies have failed to show a significant survival advantage for combinations of chemotherapy over melphalan and prednisone. In fact, a meta-analysis of 18 published trials found no difference in overall duration of survival in a comparison of single and multiple alkylating agents.

Chemotherapy should be continued until the patient is in a plateau state or for at least 1 year. The plateau state is defined as having stable serum and urine M-protein levels and no evidence of progression. Continued chemotherapy may lead to the development of a myelodysplastic syndrome or acute leukemia. α_2-Interferon generally prolongs the duration of the plateau state but has a marginal benefit, if any, on overall survival. If one elects to use α_2-interferon, the dosage must be altered so that the undesirable side effects do not interfere with the patient's quality of life. The patient should be followed closely during the plateau state, and the same regimen should be reinstituted when relapse occurs, because most patients will again respond to the initial regimen.

RADIOTHERAPY

Palliative radiation in a dose of 20 to 30 Gy should be limited to patients with multiple myeloma who have disabling pain and a well-defined focal process that has not responded to chemotherapy. Analgesics in combination with chemotherapy usually control the pain. Radiation is very helpful for patients with spinal cord compression from extradural myeloma. Tumoricidal radiation is indicated for patients with solitary plasmacytoma of bone or solitary extramedullary plasmacytoma.

AUTOLOGOUS STEM CELL TRANSPLANTATION

Autologous peripheral blood stem cell transplantation has virtually replaced autologous bone marrow transplantation because there is less contamination with myeloma cells and engraftment is more rapid. Autologous stem cell transplantation is applicable for more patients than is allogeneic transplantation because the age limit extends to 70 years and a matched donor is unnecessary. However, peripheral stem cells must be collected before the patient is exposed to alkylating agents because they damage the hematopoietic stem cells. The two main challenges for autologous transplantation are that 1) the myeloma usually is not eradicated even with large doses of chemotherapy and total body radiation, and 2) infusion of autologous peripheral blood stem cells contaminated by myeloma cells or their precursors may contribute to relapse. The mortality rate from autologous transplantation is currently 1% to 2%.

Most investigators prefer to treat the patient initially with VAD (vincristine, Adriamycin [doxorubicin], dexamethasone) for 3 to 4 months to reduce the number of tumor cells in the bone marrow and peripheral blood. The patient is then given granulocyte colony-stimulating factor with or without cyclophosphamide, and the peripheral stem cells are collected. When the patient has recovered, one can proceed with transplantation in which the patient is given high-dose melphalan or a similar preparative regimen followed by infusion of the peripheral blood stem cells. The alternative is to treat the patient with alkylating agents after stem cell collection until a plateau state is reached and then maintain the patient with α_2-interferon or no therapy until early relapse. At that point, the patient is given high-dose melphalan and the previously collected peripheral blood stem cells are infused.

In a prospective trial comparing autologous bone marrow transplantation with chemotherapy, the 6-year post-diagnosis probability of overall survival was 43% in the transplant arm and 21% in the chemotherapy regimen. The difference in survival was about 15 months (42 months in the chemotherapy arm and 57 months in the transplant arm). In a nonrandomized series of 231 patients with newly diagnosed multiple myeloma, two consecutive autologous stem cell transplantations were planned. Among the 165 patients completing two transplantations, the complete response rate was 49% and the overall duration of survival was 65 months. Alternatively, the French Myeloma Group initiated a randomized study to compare single and double peripheral stem cell transplantations. Four hundred patients were randomized to receive a single autologous transplant or two autologous transplants. There was no difference in the complete response rate, event-free survival rate, or overall survival rate in the two groups when evaluated at 2 years. Additional follow-up is necessary to determine the value of double transplantation.

The role of early versus late autologous stem cell transplantation is being addressed in the current Intergroup Trial. The advantage of early transplantation is that patients are spared the inconvenience of chemotherapy, whereas delayed transplantation may be advantageous because the procedure and especially the preparative regimen may be more effective in future years. Autologous stem cell transplantation may be beneficial for patients who are refractory to primary chemotherapy. However, it is not indicated if a patient has received long-term chemotherapy and has refractory multiple myeloma. The selection of CD34+ cells is of potential value because it results in a reduction of tumor cells in the peripheral blood. It is doubtful that this translates into longer progression-free and overall survival rates.

ALLOGENEIC BONE MARROW TRANSPLANTATION

Allogeneic bone marrow transplantation has the advantages that the graft does not contain tumor cells that can subsequently lead to relapse and a graft-versus-myeloma effect. About 90% of patients with multiple myeloma cannot have allogeneic bone marrow transplantation because of their age (most are >55 years of age), lack of an HLA-matched sibling donor, and inadequate renal, pulmonary, or cardiac function. Unfortunately, the mortality rate from the procedure is approximately 25% within the first 3 months and approaches 40% overall. Complete response occurs in 40% of patients, but most will have relapse and in long-term follow-up there is no apparent survival plateau. An immunologic approach using donor lymphocytes shows promise. In one study, 8 of 13 patients with relapsed multiple myeloma after allogeneic bone marrow transplantation responded to donor leukocyte infusions. Allogeneic transplant-related mortality must be reduced. The use of T-cell-depleted peripheral blood stem cells may reduce the incidence of graft-versus-host disease and decrease transplant-related mortality.

REFRACTORY MULTIPLE MYELOMA

Patients with multiple myeloma who become refractory to initial alkylating therapy have a low response rate to subsequent chemotherapy and a short survival. The highest response rates have been reported with VAD therapy, in which vincristine and Adriamycin (doxorubicin) are given by continuous infusion for 4 days and dexamethasone, 40 mg/ day, is given on days 1 to 4, 9 to 12, and 17 to 20 of each 28-day cycle. Dexamethasone is usually given only on days 1 to 4 in even-numbered cycles because of toxicity. The major shortcomings of VAD are that vincristine and Adriamycin have to be given by a central venous catheter and that infection, myopathy, and gastrointestinal bleeding may occur from steroid toxicity. Dexamethasone can be used as a single agent in the same dosage and schedule as VAD because the steroids probably account for 80% of the benefit of VAD. Methylprednisolone, 2 g three times weekly intravenously for a minimum of 4 weeks, is helpful for refractory patients with pancytopenia. We find fewer side effects than from dexamethasone. If there is a response, the use of methylprednisolone is reduced to once or twice weekly.

We find that VBAP (vincristine, carmustine [BCNU], and Adriamycin [doxorubicin]) on day 1 and prednisone daily for 5 days every 3 to 4 weeks produces benefit in 30% of patients. If the patient's leukocyte and platelet levels are satisfactory, cyclophosphamide, 600 mg/m^2 daily intravenously for 4 days, plus prednisone, 50 mg twice a day for the same 4-day period, followed by granulocyte colony-stimulating factor, has been helpful for refractory patients with advanced disease. Use of α_2-interferon as a single agent benefits some patients, but results have been disappointing.

Management of Complications

HYPERCALCEMIA

Hypercalcemia is present in 15% to 20% of patients at diagnosis and should be suspected in the presence of anorexia, nausea, vomiting, polyuria, polydipsia, increased constipation, weakness, confusion, or stupor. If hypercalcemia is left untreated, renal insufficiency develops. Hydration, preferably with isotonic saline, plus prednisone (25 mg four times a day) is effective in most cases. If these measures fail, bisphosphonates such as pamidronate (Aredia) or etidronate (Didronel) are effective. Patients should be encouraged to be as active as possible because prolonged bed rest contributes to hypercalcemia.

RENAL INSUFFICIENCY

Reduction in renal function occurs in one-half of patients with multiple myeloma. It may develop insidiously or acutely. Hydration and prednisone or bisphosphonates are necessary if there is an accompanying hypercalcemia. Maintenance of a high urine output (3 L/day) is important for preventing renal failure in patients with Bence Jones proteinuria. Allopurinol is helpful for the treatment of hyperuricemia. Hemodialysis or peritoneal dialysis is necessary in the event of symptomatic azotemia. Plasmapheresis may be helpful in acute renal failure, but patients with severe myeloma cast formation or other irreversible changes are unlikely to benefit. Renal transplantation has been followed by prolonged survival.

SKELETAL LESIONS

Fixation of fractures or impending fractures of long bones with an intramedullary rod and methyl methacrylate has produced good results. Patients in a prospective study receiving pamidronate had fewer skeletal complications and improved quality of life when compared with those receiving placebo. Pamidronate in a dosage of 90 mg intravenously every 4 weeks is recommended for patients with multiple myeloma who have lytic lesions or osteopenia. It should be given indefinitely.

INFECTION

Prompt and appropriate therapy for bacterial infections is necessary. Pneumococcal and influenza vaccines should be given to all patients despite their suboptimal antibody response. Many infections occur within the first 2 or 3 months after diagnosis of multiple myeloma. The use of trimethoprim-sulfamethoxazole is beneficial in this setting. Prophylactic daily oral penicillin may benefit patients with recurrent streptococcal pneumonia infections. Intravenously administered gamma globulin can be used for recurrent infections but is very expensive.

OTHER COMPLICATIONS

Spinal cord compression from an extramedullary plasmacytoma should be suspected in patients with severe back pain, weakness or paresthesias of the lower extremities, or bladder or bowel dysfunction. Magnetic resonance imaging, computed tomography, or myelography must be done promptly. Dexamethasone and radiation therapy are usually helpful. Surgical decompression is rarely necessary.

Hyperviscosity is characterized by oronasal bleeding, blurred vision, paresthesias, headache, reduced cerebration, and congestive heart failure. Serum viscosity levels do not correlate well with the symptoms or clinical findings. Plasmapheresis promptly relieves the symptoms and should be done on the basis of the patient's symptoms rather than the serum viscosity level. Symptomatic anemia during the plateau phase is often benefited by the administration of erythropoietin.

VARIANT FORMS OF MULTIPLE MYELOMA

Smoldering Multiple Myeloma (SMM)

The diagnosis depends on the presence of an M-protein level more than 3 g/dL in the serum and more than 10% plasma cells in the bone marrow but no anemia, renal insufficiency, or skeletal lesions. Often a small amount of M-protein is found in the urine, and the concentration of uninvolved immunoglobulins is usually reduced. The plasma cell labeling index is low. Biologically, patients with SMM have a monoclonal gammopathy of undetermined significance (MGUS), but it is difficult to accept that diagnosis initially when the M-protein value is more than 3 g/dL and the bone marrow contains more than 10% plasma cells, because most patients with these findings have symptomatic multiple myeloma. The recognition of SMM is crucial because affected patients should not be treated unless progression occurs.

Plasma Cell Leukemia

Patients with plasma cell leukemia have more than 20% plasma cells in the peripheral blood and an absolute plasma cell count of at least 2,000/μL. It is classified as primary when it is diagnosed in the leukemic phase (60% of cases) or as secondary when there is a leukemic transformation of a previously recognized multiple myeloma (40%). Compared with patients who have secondary plasma cell leukemia, patients with primary plasma cell leukemia are younger and have a greater incidence of hepatosplenomegaly and lymphadenopathy, a higher platelet count, fewer bone lesions, a smaller serum M-component, and a longer duration of survival. Cytogenetic abnormalities are more common, and levels of serum IL-6 are higher than in patients with multiple myeloma. The response rate is higher with combination chemotherapy than with alkylating agents, but the duration of response is short. Autologous stem cell transplantation after high-dose chemotherapy is beneficial for some patients. Secondary plasma cell leukemia rarely responds to chemotherapy, because patients have already received treatment and are resistant.

Nonsecretory Myeloma

Patients with nonsecretory myeloma have no M-protein in either the serum or the urine, and this form occurs in only 2% of patients with myeloma. The diagnosis is established by identification of an M-protein in the cytoplasm of the plasma cells by immunoperoxidase or immunofluorescence. However, some cases have been reported with no M-protein in the plasma cells. The clinical picture, response to therapy, and survival in nonsecretory myeloma are similar to those in myeloma with a serum or urine M-protein except that there is less renal involvement.

IgD Myeloma

The M-protein is smaller than in IgG or IgA myelomas, and Bence Jones proteinuria of the λ type is more common. Amyloidosis and extramedullary plasmacytomas are more frequent with IgD myeloma. Survival is generally believed to be shorter than with other myeloma types, but IgD myeloma is often not diagnosed until later in its course.

Osteosclerotic Myeloma (POEMS Syndrome)

This syndrome is characterized by polyneuropathy (P), organomegaly (O), endocrin-opathy (E), M-protein (M), and skin changes (S). The major clinical finding is a chronic inflammatory-demyelinating polyneuropathy with predominantly motor disability. Sclerotic skeletal lesions are found in most cases. Except for the presence of papilledema, the cranial nerves are not involved. Hepatomegaly occurs in one-half of patients, but splenomegaly and lymphadenopathy occur in a minority. Hyperpigmentation of the skin and hypertrichosis are frequent. Gynecomastia and testicular atrophy may be present. Angiomatous lesions of the trunk are often prominent. Pulmonary hypertension has been reported in several cases. Moderate pedal edema is common and may be associated with ascites and pleural effusion. The hemoglobin level is usually normal or increased, and thrombocytosis is common. The bone marrow usually contains fewer than 5% plasma cells, and hypercalcemia and renal insufficiency rarely occur. Most patients have a λ light chain, and IgA is the most common heavy chain. Castleman's disease is frequently present. The diagnosis is confirmed by the identification of monoclonal plasma cells obtained from an osteosclerotic lesion. If the skeletal lesions are in a limited area, radiation almost always produces a substantial improvement of the neuropathy. If the patient has widespread osteosclerotic lesions, chemotherapy should be given. Autologous stem cell transplantation is another consideration.

Solitary Plasmacytoma of Bone (Solitary Myeloma)

The diagnosis depends on histologic evidence of a plasma cell tumor identical to that in multiple myeloma. Complete skeletal radiographs, bone marrow aspiration and biopsy, and immunofixation of the serum and urine should show no evidence of involvement. Occasionally, a small M-protein may be found in the serum or urine, but it usually disappears after radiation of the solitary lesion. Treatment consists of tumoricidal radiation (40-50 Gy). Overt multiple myeloma develops in approximately 55% of patients, and new solitary bone lesions or local recurrence develops in about 10%. The disease-free survival rate at 10 years ranges from 15% to 25%. Almost half of patients with solitary plasmacytoma are alive at 10 years. Magnetic resonance imaging may be helpful in identifying patients in whom multiple myeloma will develop. Progression, when present, usually occurs within 3 to 4 years.

Extramedullary Plasmacytoma

This is a plasma cell tumor that arises outside the bone marrow. It is located in the upper respiratory tract in approximately 80% of cases. The nasal cavity and sinuses, nasopharynx, and larynx are most often involved. Extramedullary plasmacytomas also may involve the gastrointestinal tract, central nervous system, urinary bladder, thyroid, breast, testes, parotid gland, or lymph nodes. There is predominance of IgA M-protein. The diagnosis depends on the finding of a plasma cell tumor in an extramedullary location in the absence of multiple myeloma after appropriate studies of the serum and urine, bone marrow examination, and radiographic studies. Treatment consists of tumoricidal radiation (40-50 Gy). Regional recurrences develop in approximately 25% of patients, but the development of typical multiple myeloma is uncommon. The patient with an apparent extramedullary plasmacytoma should be followed periodically with clinical evaluation and laboratory testing for the appearance of an M-protein in the serum or urine or other evidence of progression.

WALDENSTRÖM'S MACROGLOBULINEMIA (WM)

Macroglobulinemia is the result of an uncontrolled proliferation of lymphocytes and plasma cells which produces large amounts of IgM. It is an uncommon disease, and in our practice it is one-seventh as common as multiple myeloma. The cause is unknown, but it does occur more frequently in certain families. The median age of patients at diagnosis is about 65 years, and about 60% are male.

Clinical Manifestations

The most common presenting symptoms are weakness, fatigue, bleeding (especially oozing from the oronasal area), weight loss, and visual or neurologic disturbances. In contrast to multiple myeloma, lytic bone lesions, renal insufficiency, and amyloidosis are rare. Pallor, hepatosplenomegaly, and lymphadenopathy are often present. Fundal hemorrhages, exudates, and venous congestion with vascular segmentation ("sausage" formation) may occur. Sensorimotor peripheral neuropathy is not uncommon. Pulmonary involvement is infrequent and consists of diffuse pulmonary infiltrates, isolated masses, or pleural effusion. Small bowel and skin infiltration by lymphocytes and plasma cells is uncommon. Sudden deafness, progressive spinal muscle atrophy, and multifocal leukoencephalopathy have been reported in WM.

Laboratory Features

Moderate to severe normocytic, normochromic anemia is present in almost all patients. The increased plasma volume spuriously reduces the hemoglobin and hematocrit values. The serum electrophoretic pattern is characterized by a tall, narrow spike or dense band and is of γ mobility. Eighty percent of the IgM proteins have a κ light chain. Low-molecular-weight IgM (7S) is present and may account for a significant part of the increased IgM level. The urine contains a monoclonal light chain in 80% of patients. In contrast to multiple myeloma, the amount of light chain is usually modest. The bone marrow is often hypocellular, but the biopsy specimen is hypercellular and extensively infiltrated with lymphoid cells and plasma cells. Mast cells are frequently increased.

Diagnosis

The diagnosis is made on the basis of typical symptoms and physical findings, the presence of a monoclonal IgM protein, usually more than 3 g/dL, and lymphoplasma cell infiltration of the bone marrow. Macroglobulinemia must be differentiated from multiple myeloma, chronic lymphocytic leukemia, and MGUS of the IgM type. In some instances, the patient must be carefully observed for an indefinite period to differentiate MGUS of the IgM type from Waldenström's macroglobulinemia.

Treatment

Treatment should be withheld until the patient is symptomatic. The indications for therapy include constitutional symptoms such as weakness, fatigue, night sweats, or weight loss, anemia, hyperviscosity, or significant hepatosplenomegaly and lymphadenopathy. Chlorambucil has been a useful agent for almost 40 years. It is usually given orally in a dosage of 6 to 8 mg/day and reduced when the leukocytes or platelet counts decrease. Intermittent administration of chlorambucil and prednisone every 4 to 6 weeks is also useful. Cyclophosphamide or combinations of alkylating agents such as the M2 protocol (vincristine, BCNU, melphalan, cyclophosphamide, and prednisone) also have been useful. Patients should be treated until a plateau phase is achieved and then followed without maintenance chemotherapy. Patients must be followed closely, and chemotherapy of the same type should be reinstituted when the disease relapses.

Fludarabine or 2-chlorodeoxyadenosine has been reported to produce responses in 80% of patients. However, in a recent report, fludarabine produced objective response in only 34% of 109 patients with symptomatic Waldenström's macroglobulinemia.

Transfusion of packed red cells should be given for symptomatic anemia. Transfusion should not be given solely on the basis of the hemoglobin or hematocrit value, because the increased plasma volume produces spuriously low hemoglobin and hematocrit levels. Erythropoietin may be of benefit for patients in the plateau state who have symptomatic anemia. Symptomatic hyperviscosity should be treated with plasmapheresis. The median survival in macroglobulinemia is approximately 5 years.

HEAVY-CHAIN DISEASES

The heavy-chain diseases (HCDs) are characterized by the presence of an M-protein consisting of a portion of the immunoglobulin heavy chain in the serum or urine or both. These heavy chains are devoid of light chain and are of three major types: γ, α, and μ.

Gamma Heavy-Chain Disease (γHCD)

The abnormal protein consists of a monoclonal γ chain with significant deletions of amino acids, including the entire CH1 region and a portion of the variable region. The median age at diagnosis is approximately 60 years, but the disease has been described in patients younger than 20 years. Patients often present with a lymphoma-like illness, but the clinical findings are diverse and range from an aggressive lymphoproliferative process to an asymptomatic state. Weakness, fatigue, and fever are the most common presenting symptoms. Hepatosplenomegaly and lymphadenopathy are found in about 60% of patients. Normocytic, normochromic anemia occurs in 80%, and a Coombs-positive autoimmune hemolytic anemia has been noted in several instances. The serum protein electrophoretic pattern usually shows a broad-based band more suggestive of a polyclonal than an M-protein. The urinary heavy-chain protein concentration ranges from trace to

20 g/24 hours, but it is usually less than 1 g daily. Bence Jones proteinuria is not found. The bone marrow and lymph nodes contain an increased number of plasma cells, lymphocytes, and lymphoplasmacytoid cells.

Treatment is indicated only for symptomatic patients. The prognosis is variable, because the clinical course may range from an asymptomatic state to a rapidly progressive disease. The median duration of survival is approximately 1 year. Therapy with cyclophosphamide, vincristine, and prednisone is a reasonable choice. If there is no response, a doxorubicin-containing regimen should be tried.

Alpha Heavy-Chain Disease (αHCD)

This is the most common type of heavy-chain disease; more than 200 cases have been reported. Most patients are from the Mediterranean region or Middle East. It usually occurs in the second or third decade of life, and about 60% of patients are male. The disease most often involves the gastrointestinal tract, manifested by severe malabsorption with loss of weight, diarrhea, and steatorrhea. Infrequently, respiratory tract involvement occurs. The term "immunoproliferative small intestinal disease (IPSID)" is restricted to patients with small intestinal lesions that have the same pathologic pattern as that of αHCD. These patients do not synthesize α heavy chains.

An unimpressive broad band may appear in the α_2 or β region in half of patients, but the pattern is normal in the remainder. The diagnosis depends on the recognition of a monoclonal α heavy chain in the serum or jejunal fluid. The amount of α chain in the urine is small, and Bence Jones proteinuria is always absent. The bone marrow is also normal. Without treatment, αHCD is usually progressive and fatal. Antibiotics may produce remission in some cases. Patients who do not respond to antibiotics should be treated with combination chemotherapy consisting of cyclophosphamide, Adriamycin (doxorubicin), vincristine, and prednisone.

Mu Heavy-Chain Disease (μHCD)

This is characterized by the demonstration of a monoclonal μ-chain fragment in the serum. Most patients have an associated chronic lymphoproliferative process resembling chronic lymphocytic leukemia or lymphoma. The serum protein electrophoretic pattern contains a monoclonal spike in about 40% of cases. Hypogammaglobulinemia is frequent. Bence Jones proteinuria has been recognized in two-thirds of cases. It is usually of the κ type. There is an increase in lymphocytes, plasma cells, and lymphocytoid cells in the bone marrow. Vacuolization of the plasma cells is a clue to diagnosis of μHCD. The course of μHCD is variable; the median survival is approximately 2 years. Treatment with corticosteroids and alkylating agents has produced some benefit.

CRYOGLOBULINEMIA

Cryoglobulins are proteins that precipitate when cooled and dissolve when heated. They are designated as essential or idiopathic when they are not associated with any recognizable disease. Cryoglobulins are classified into three types: type I (monoclonal), type II (mixed), and type III (polyclonal). Type I (monoclonal) cryoglobulinemia is most commonly of the IgM or IgG class. Most patients, even with large amounts of type I cryoglobulin, are completely asymptomatic. If the cryoglobulin precipitates at a high temperature (>20°C), purpura, Raynaud's phenomenon, cyanosis, and even ulceration and sloughing of the skin may occur on exposure to the cold. Type I cryoglobulins are most commonly associated with MGUS, macroglobulinemia, or multiple myeloma.

Table 4
Immunohistochemical Identification of Amyloid

Type of amyloidosis	Congo red	κ or λ	Serum amyloid A	β₂-Microglobulin	Transthyretin (prealbumin)
Primary (AL)	+	+	–	–	–
Secondary (AA)	+	–	+	–	–
Familial Mediterranean fever (AA)	+	–	+	–	–
Dialysis (Aβ₂-M)	+	–	–	+	–
Familial (AF)	+	–	–	–	+
Senile systemic (SSA)	+	–	–	–	+

Abbreviations: AF, familial amyloidosis; β₂-M, β₂-microglobulin; SSA, serum amyloid A protein.
From Kyle RA, Gertz MA. Primary systemic amyloidosis: clinical and laboratory features in 474 cases. *Semin Hematol* 1995; 32: 45-59. By permission of W.B. Saunders Company.

Type II (mixed) cryoglobulinemia typically consists of an IgM M-protein and polyclonal IgG. In addition, monoclonal IgG or monoclonal IgA may occur with polyclonal IgM. The serum protein electrophoretic pattern is usually normal or has a polyclonal appearance. The quantity of mixed cryoglobulin is usually less than 0.2 g/dL. The most common underlying disease is hepatitis C. Vasculitis, lymphoproliferative disease, and glomerulonephritis may occur. Polyarthralgias are common. Occasionally, Raynaud's phenomenon and necrosis of the skin are present. A nephrotic syndrome may occur, but severe renal insufficiency is rare.

Early administration of corticosteroids is the most frequently used therapy. α_2-Interferon is useful, but the symptoms often recur when use of the agent is discontinued. Cyclophosphamide, chlorambucil, or azathioprine has been used. Plasmapheresis has been useful in some instances.

Type III (polyclonal) cryoglobulinemia is not associated with a monoclonal component. Type III cryoglobulins are found in many patients with infectious or inflammatory diseases.

PRIMARY AMYLOIDOSIS (AL)

Amyloid stained with Congo red produces an apple-green birefringence under polarized light. It is a fibrous protein that consists of rigid, linear, nonbranching, aggregated fibrils of 7.5 to 10 nm in width and of indefinite length. The type of amyloid cannot be differentiated by Congo red staining, organ distribution, or electron microscopy. The amyloid fibrils consist of various proteins, such as monoclonal κ or λ light chains or, rarely, heavy chains in primary amyloidosis, protein A in secondary amyloidosis (AA), transthyretin (prealbumin) in familial or senile systemic amyloidosis, or β₂-microglobulin in dialysis-associated amyloidosis. The histochemical identification of amyloid fibers is shown in Table 4.

Clinical Features

The annual incidence of AL is 0.9 per 100,000. The median age at diagnosis is 64 years, and only 1% of patients are younger than 40. Two-thirds are male. Weakness, fatigue, and weight loss are the most frequent initial symptoms. Dyspnea, pedal edema, paresthesias,

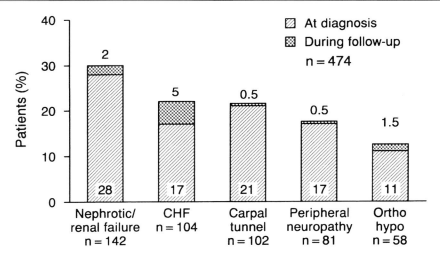

Fig. 1. Frequency of amyloid syndromes at diagnosis of primary systemic amyloidosis. CHF, congestive heart failure; Ortho hypo, orthostatic hypotension. (From Kyle RA, Gertz MA. Primary systemic amyloidosis: clinical and laboratory features in 474 cases. *Semin Hematol* 1995; 32: 45-59. By permission of W.B. Saunders Company.)

light-headedness, and syncope are frequent in patients with congestive heart failure or peripheral neuropathy. Hoarseness or change of voice and jaw claudication may occur. The liver is palpable in one-fourth of patients, but splenomegaly occurs in only 5%. Macroglossia is present in 10%. Purpura, particularly in the periorbital and facial areas, is noted in 15%. The liver is palpable in one-fourth of patients, whereas splenomegaly is present in only 5% at diagnosis.

Almost a third of patients have a nephrotic syndrome. Carpal tunnel syndrome, congestive heart failure, peripheral neuropathy, and orthostatic hypotension are other major presenting syndromes (Fig. 1). The presence of one of these syndromes and an M-protein in the serum or urine is a strong indication of AL, for which appropriate biopsy specimens must be taken for diagnosis.

Laboratory Findings

Anemia is not a prominent feature of AL and, when present, is usually due to myeloma, renal insufficiency, or gastrointestinal bleeding. Thrombocytosis (>500 platelets × 10^9/L) is present in about 10% of patients. Renal insufficiency is present in almost half of patients at diagnosis; 20% have a serum creatinine value of 2.0 mg/dL or more. The cholesterol level is increased in almost half of patients. Many of these patients have an associated nephrotic syndrome. The carotene value and the serum B_{12} levels are reduced in about 5%. An increased serum alkaline phosphatase value is not uncommon. Hyperbilirubinemia is infrequent, but when present it is an ominous sign. Factor X level is decreased in more than 10% but is rarely the cause of bleeding. The prothrombin time is increased in about 15% of patients, and the thrombin time is prolonged in 40%.

The serum protein electrophoretic pattern reveals a localized band or spike in about half of patients. When present, the median size of the spike is about 1.5 g/dL. Hypogammaglobulinemia is found in 20% of patients. A serum M-protein is present in about 70% of patients. An M-protein is found in the urine in approximately 70%. Two-thirds are λ, which is the reverse of multiple myeloma. An M-protein is found in

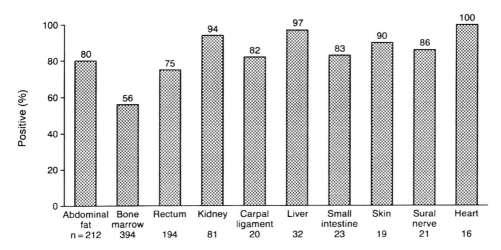

Fig. 2. Diagnosis of amyloidosis on the basis of deposits in tissues. (From Kyle RA, Gertz MA. Primary systemic amyloidosis: clinical and laboratory features in 474 cases. *Semin Hematol* 1995; 32: 45-59. By permission of W.B. Saunders Company.)

the serum or urine in almost 90% of AL patients at diagnosis. Almost half of the patients have fewer than 5% plasma cells in the bone marrow. About a fifth of patients have more than 20% plasma cells in the bone marrow, but these patients usually do not have the other features of multiple myeloma.

Congestive heart failure is present in about 20% of patients at diagnosis and develops in an additional 10% during the course of the disease. Electrocardiography frequently shows low voltage in the limb leads or characteristics consistent with anteroseptal infarction (loss of anterior forces), but there is no evidence of myocardial infarction at autopsy. Arrhythmias, including atrial fibrillation or heart block, are common. Almost three-fourths of patients have an abnormal echocardiogram. There is a relationship between the thickness of the ventricular wall and septum and the incidence and severity of congestive heart failure. Early cardiac amyloidosis is characterized by abnormal relaxation, whereas advanced involvement is consistent with constrictive cardiomyopathy. Constrictive pericarditis and hypertrophic obstructive cardiomyopathy may be difficult to differentiate from amyloid heart disease. If there is doubt, an endomyocardial biopsy is helpful.

A sensorimotor peripheral neuropathy is present in about 15% of patients at diagnosis. Autonomic dysfunction may be a prominent feature and is often manifested by orthostatic hypotension, diarrhea, and impotence. Malabsorption occurs in less than 5% of cases. Cutaneous and gastrointestinal bleeding may occur. Amyloidosis can involve the periarticular structures and produce the shoulder-pad syndrome. Involvement of the skin results in petechiae, ecchymoses, papules, plaques, nodules, alopecia, or thickening of the skin. Rarely, large amyloid deposits (amyloidomas) may cause osteolytic lesions and pathologic fractures.

Diagnosis

The diagnosis depends on the demonstration of amyloid deposits in tissues (Fig. 2) (Table 5). The possibility of amyloidosis must be considered in every patient who has an M-protein in the serum or urine and who also has nephrotic syndrome, congestive heart

Table 5
Approach to Differential Diagnosis of Amyloidosis

History
    Fatigue, weight loss, purpura, light-headedness, change in voice or tongue, jaw
        claudication, paresthesias, or dyspnea
    Family history
Physical examination
    Purpura, macroglossia, hepatomegaly, edema, neuropathy
Syndromes
    Nephrotic, congestive heart failure, carpal tunnel, peripheral neuropathy,
        orthostatic hypotension
Laboratory
    M-protein in serum or urine in 90%; bone marrow: monoclonal plasma cells
    M-protein or monoclonal plasma cells in 98%
    Echocardiogram abnormal in 75%
Diagnosis (histologic evidence needed)
    Subcutaneous fat biopsy, 80% positive
    Bone marrow, 55% positive
    Rectal biopsy, 75% positive
    Kidney, liver, sural nerve, carpal ligament biopsy, if above are negative
    If systemic amyloidosis and no monoclonal protein or monoclonal population of
        plasma cells, one must perform immunohistochemical staining with κ and λ
        antisera (AL), protein A (secondary amyloidosis) (AA), TTR (prealbumin)
        (familial or senile), and β_2-microglobulin (dialysis-associated amyloidosis)

failure, sensorimotor peripheral neuropathy, carpal tunnel syndrome, giant hepatomegaly, or idiopathic malabsorption. In 98% of patients, there is an M-protein in the serum
or urine or a monoclonal proliferation of plasma cells in the bone marrow.

The initial diagnostic procedure should be an abdominal fat aspiration, which is positive in about 80% of patients. Bone marrow aspiration and biopsy should be done to
determine the degree of plasmacytosis; amyloid stains should also be done, because they
are positive in more than half of patients. If the results of abdominal fat and bone marrow
biopsy are negative, a rectal biopsy (including submucosa) or biopsy of a suspected
involved organ, such as the kidney, liver, heart, or sural nerve, is indicated. We find that
almost 90% of patients have positive results of either subcutaneous fat or bone marrow
biopsy. Specific antisera to κ, λ, protein A, transthyretin, and β_2-microglobulin are helpful for identifying the type of systemic amyloidosis. ^{123}I-labeled purified human serum
amyloid P component is useful for detecting amyloid deposition.

Prognosis

The median duration of survival for patients with AL is approximately 13 months. Seven
percent survive for 5 or more years, and only 1% are alive at 10 years. Survival depends
mainly on the associated syndrome. In patients with congestive heart failure, the median
duration of survival is 4 to 6 months, whereas it is more than 2 years in patients with only
peripheral neuropathy. About half of deaths are due to cardiac involvement from congestive
heart failure or arrhythmias. The actual percentage of cardiac deaths is probably higher,
because some patients whose death was ascribed to "amyloidosis" very likely had a terminal cardiac arrhythmia. Infection and renal failure are other common causes of death.

Therapy

Because amyloid fibrils consist of monoclonal immunoglobulin light chains, treatment with alkylating agents that are effective against plasma cell neoplasms is warranted. A randomized placebo-controlled, double-blind trial of 55 patients with AL suggested that treatment with melphalan and prednisone was of benefit. We treated 220 patients with biopsy-proven amyloidosis in a prospective study. They were randomized to receive: 1) melphalan and prednisone, 2) colchicine, or 3) melphalan, prednisone, and colchicine. The median duration of survival after randomization was 8.5 months in the colchicine group, 18 months in the group assigned to melphalan and prednisone, and 17 months in the group treated with melphalan, prednisone, and colchicine ($P < 0.001$). Thirty-four patients (15%) survived for 5 years or longer.

Despite the results obtained with melphalan and prednisone, treatment of primary amyloidosis is still unsatisfactory. Patients with AL have had substantial clinical improvement after the administration of 4'-iodo-4'-deoxyrubicin (IDOX). This new agent appears to bind to amyloid fibrils and contributes to the resolution of amyloid deposits. Encouraging results have been reported with high-dose intravenous melphalan (200 mg/m^2) followed by autologous peripheral blood stem cell rescue. Improvement in hepatic, gastrointestinal, neurologic, renal, or cardiac involvement has been reported, along with decreased proteinuria and stable or improved performance status. The M-protein in the serum and urine and the number of bone marrow plasma cells also may decrease. Because of the short follow-up, the impact of this treatment approach on response duration and survival is to be determined.

The nephrotic syndrome should be managed with salt restriction and diuretics. If symptomatic azotemia develops, chronic renal dialysis is necessary. Patients with congestive heart failure must be treated with salt restriction and diuretics. In selected patients, cardiac transplantation appears to be beneficial. Digitalis must be used with care, because patients with amyloidosis are unusually sensitive to this drug, and heart block and arrhythmias are common. Elastic stockings or leotards may benefit orthostatic hypotension.

ACKNOWLEDGMENT

Supported in part by Research Grant CA-62242 from the National Institutes of Health.

SUGGESTED READING

Attal M, Harousseau JL, Stoppa AM, Sotto JJ, Fuzibet JG, Rossi JF, Casassus P, Maisonneuve H, Facon T, Ifrah N, Payen C, Bataille R, for the Intergroupe Français du Myélome. A prospective, randomized trial of autologous bone marrow transplantation and chemotherapy in multiple myeloma. *N Engl J Med* 1996; 335: 91-97.

Berenson JR, Lichtenstein A, Porter L, Dimopoulos MA, Bordoni R, George S, Lipton A, Keller A, Ballester O, Kovacs MJ, Blacklock HA, Bell R, Simeone J, Reitsma DJ, Heffernan M, Seaman J, Knight RD, for the Myeloma Aredia Study Group. Efficacy of pamidronate in reducing skeletal events in patients with advanced multiple myeloma. *N Engl J Med* 1996; 334: 488-493.

Falk RH, Comenzo RL, Skinner M. The systemic amyloidoses. *N Engl J Med* 1997; 337: 898-909.

Gahrton G, Tura S, Ljungman P, Bladé J, Brandt L, Cavo M, Facon T, Gratwohl A, Hagenbeek A, Jacobs P, de Laurenzi A, Van Lint M, Michallet M, Nikoskelainen J, Reiffers J, Samson D, Verdonck L, de Witte T, Volin L. Prognostic factors in allogeneic bone marrow transplantation for multiple myeloma. *J Clin Oncol* 1995; 13: 1312-1322.

Kyle RA. Multiple myeloma: review of 869 cases. *Mayo Clin Proc* 1975; 50: 29-40.

Kyle RA. "Benign" monoclonal gammopathy—after 20 to 35 years of follow-up. *Mayo Clin Proc* 1993; 68: 26-36.

Kyle RA, Garton JP. The spectrum of IgM monoclonal gammopathy in 430 cases. *Mayo Clin Proc* 1987; 62: 719-731.

Kyle RA, Gertz MA. Primary systemic amyloidosis: clinical and laboratory features in 474 cases. *Semin Hematol* 1995; 32: 45-59.

Kyle RA, Gertz MA, Greipp PR, Witzig TE, Lust JA, Lacy MQ, Therneau TM. A trial of three regimens for primary amyloidosis: colchicine alone, melphalan and prednisone, and melphalan, prednisone, and colchicine. *N Engl J Med* 1997; 336: 1202-1207.

Waldenström JG. POEMS: a multifactorial syndrome (editorial). *Haematologica* 1992; 77: 197-203.

V

THROMBOTIC AND BLEEDING DISORDERS

20 An Overview of the Hemostatic System and Interpretation of Common Screening Coagulation Tests

Rajiv K. Pruthi, MD

Contents

INTRODUCTION TO THE HEMOSTATIC SYSTEM

The coagulation system has evolved to meet two opposed functions:

1. Maintenance of fluidity
2. Formation of solid fibrin clot to prevent and stop bleeding from sites of endothelial disruption

This system, which permits rapid clotting of blood in response to a small stimulus, must be tightly controlled because inappropriate clotting of blood can obstruct vital areas of the circulation. In mammals, these requirements are met by the evolution of a highly complex coagulation cascade. This consists of multiple proteins (coagulation factors) that interact with each other and the vascular endothelium, subendothelial collagen, and circulating platelets to maintain hemostasis (Fig. 1).

The individual coagulation factors circulate in an inactive form. Thus, in order for them to participate in the coagulation cascade, they need to be activated by the action of other activated coagulation factors. This is the most important mechanism by which blood maintains its fluidity. Next, blood flow itself sweeps away excess activated clotting factors from sites of vascular injury. Finally, fluidity is maintained by the anticoagulant and fibrinolytic components of the coagulation system. The procoagulant component is crucial for clot formation to stem hemorrhage from a breach in the vasculature.

An understanding of the various components of hemostasis is essential for a rational approach to the patient with a hemostatic defect that leads to hemorrhagic or thrombotic diatheses.

From: *Primary Hematology*
Edited by: A. Tefferi © Mayo Foundation for Medical Education and Research, Rochester, MN

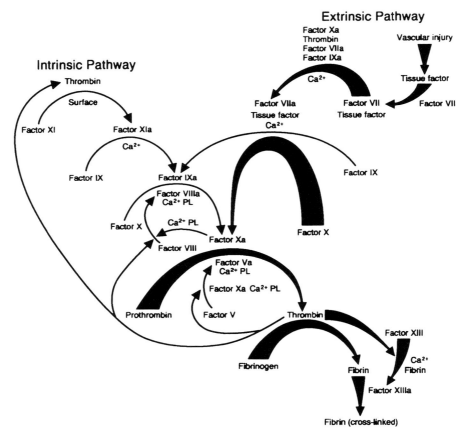

Fig. 1. Coagulation cascade. a, Activated factor; Ca²⁺, calcium; PL, phospholipid. (From Davie EW, Fujikawa K, Kisiel W. The coagulation cascade: initiation, maintenance, and regulation. *Biochemistry* 1991; 30: 10363-10370. By permission of the American Chemical Society.)

For practical purposes, three components contribute to the maintenance of hemostasis:

1. **Vascular** (endothelium and subendothelium)
2. **Platelets**
3. **Plasma coagulation factors**

Each of the three components may have one or more of the following functions:

1. Procoagulant (prothrombotic)
2. Anticoagulant
3. Fibrinolytic (breakdown of a fibrin clot)

There is an ongoing interaction among the various components of the hemostatic system; the anticoagulant component normally predominates in order to maintain blood fluidity. Vascular disruption results in the procoagulant component gaining dominance, leading to activation of procoagulant factors and ultimately to generation of thrombin. The diverse activities of thrombin make it a crucial member of the coagulation cascade. The generation of thrombin ultimately leads to the formation of fibrin clots and simultaneous activation of the anticoagulant and fibrinolytic components to prevent exuberant and disseminated clot formation.

Vascular Contribution to Hemostasis

PROCOAGULANT ACTIVITY

Endothelial cells are able to bind activated clotting factors, thus resulting in a localized and sustained effect. As shown on page 292, activation of the coagulation cascade occurs via two pathways: the intrinsic (contact) and extrinsic pathways. Endothelial cells produce an activator high-molecular-weight kininogen, which acts as a binding site for proteins involved in the intrinsic pathway.

Disruption of the endothelial layer of cells results in exposure of the subendothelial smooth muscle cells, which express tissue factor activity. This is the major stimulus for activation of the extrinsic pathway of coagulation.

ANTICOAGULANT ACTIVITY

The membrane surface of the endothelium produces heparin-like molecules that, in conjunction with antithrombin III, accelerate the breakdown of activated procoagulant proteins.

Endothelial cells synthesize an anticoagulant, thrombomodulin, that is anchored to the endothelial cell surface (see Fig. 10). Circulating thrombin binds to thrombomodulin; this binding results in a loss of the procoagulant activity of thrombin. The bound thrombin activates an anticoagulant, protein C, to activated protein C, which breaks down the activated forms of certain procoagulant cofactors (factors V and VIII).

FIBRINOLYTIC ACTIVITY

Endothelial cells express receptors for fibrinolytic proteins. This facilitates localization of the fibrinolytic activity to the site of vascular injury. An activator of factor XII, which plays a role in fibrinolysis, is also produced by the endothelium.

VASOACTIVE ROLE OF ENDOTHELIUM

Vascular relaxation, in the appropriate setting, is mediated by local release of vasoactive substances such as nitric oxide and prostacyclin. Vasoconstriction is mediated by local production and release of substances such as endothelins and thromboxane A_2. Overall, the magnitude of the contribution of these substances to hemostasis is currently being defined.

Platelets

Platelets are anucleate cells produced in the bone marrow by budding off the cytoplasm of a megakaryocyte. Once released, they circulate for approximately 7 days. There is a significant pool of platelets in the spleen which are in free interchange with the circulation and are released into the circulation when needed, as in massive hemorrhage.

The platelet membranes are rich in phospholipid and contain multiple receptors for substances that activate platelets. The cytoplasm contains numerous granules and dense bodies that contain various proteins essential for normal platelet function.

Platelets have two main functions in hemostasis:

1. Presentation of a phospholipid surface that is essential for coagulation reactions
2. Formation of a platelet plug at the site of vascular injury, which forms a framework for formation of fibrin clots

Exposure of the subendothelial tissue leads to platelet adhesion to the subendothelial collagen via the glycoprotein Ib platelet receptor. Von Willebrand factor (vWF) acts as

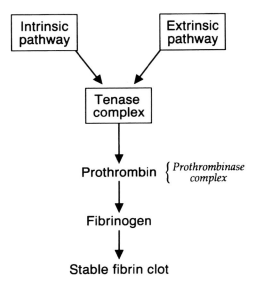

Fig. 2. Coagulation cascade: overview.

a bridge between the subendothelial connective tissue and the platelet glycoprotein Ib receptor (GpIb). Platelet activation results in activation of a second platelet receptor, glycoprotein IIb-IIIa. This is a receptor for fibrinogen, which mediates platelet aggregation. Thus, platelets are crucial for formation of the initial platelet plug.

Plasma Coagulation Cascade

A balance among the procoagulant, anticoagulant, and fibrinolytic properties of the plasma coagulation system keeps blood fluid yet initiates formation of a thrombus at the appropriate time. This chapter discusses the procoagulant functions in detail. Chapter 22, on thrombotic disorders, discusses the anticoagulant and fibrinolytic functions.

PROCOAGULANT ACTIVITY

Ultimate aims:

1. Generation of thrombin
2. Formation of a stable fibrin clot

The ultimate goal of the plasma coagulation cascade is to generate a stable fibrin clot. This occurs via two known pathways: the **extrinsic** and **intrinsic** pathways, which converge on a final common pathway. The extrinsic pathway is the dominant pathway for initiation of hemostasis, whereas the intrinsic pathway is necessary for maintenance of hemostasis. The two pathways converge and activate the final common pathway, which consists of the **tenase complex**, which subsequently activates prothrombin (in the **prothrombinase complex**). This leads to generation of thrombin, cleavage of fibrinogen to fibrin monomers, and finally stabilization of the **fibrin clot** (Fig. 2). There is simultaneous activation of the fibrinolytic and anticoagulant systems to localize clot formation.

Extrinsic Pathway (Tissue Factor Pathway)

Main components:

1. Tissue factor (TF)
2. Factor VII (FVII)

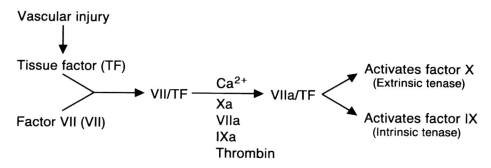

Fig. 3. Extrinsic pathway of activation of the coagulation cascade. a, Activated factor; Ca^{2+}, calcium.

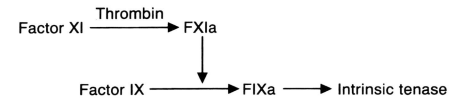

Fig. 4. Intrinsic pathway of activation of the coagulation cascade. a, Activated factor.

Ultimate aim: Activation of FVII to participate in tenase complex (Fig. 3)

Tissue factor is a procoagulant protein that, under normal circumstances, is not expressed in cells that are in direct contact with blood. It is, however, expressed in various other cells in the body, including adventitia of blood vessels, brain, and placenta. Disruption of the endothelium leads to tissue factor expression, and its contact with blood leads to formation of FVII/TF complex and activation of FVII to activated FVII (VIIa). Subsequently, the VIIa/TF complex activates factor X (extrinsic tenase complex). Factor IX is also activated in the presence of calcium. Activated factor X (Xa), thrombin (IIa), FVIIa, and FIXa also activate FVII by positive feedback activation (Fig. 1).

Intrinsic Pathway

Main components:

1. Factor XI (FXI)
2. Factor IX (FIX)
3. Factor VIII (FVIII)

Ultimate aim: Activation of factors IX and VIII to participate in the tenase complex (Fig. 4)

Factor XI (FXI) is thought to be the first component protein in the intrinsic pathway and is activated by thrombin to FXIa, which in turn activates FIX to FIXa. This participates in the tenase complex.

Tenase Complex (Fig. 5)

"Extrinsic" Tenase

Main components:

1. Factor VIIa (FVIIa)
2. Factor X (FX)
3. Tissue factor (TF)

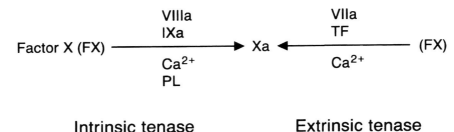

Fig. 5. Extrinsic and intrinsic tenase complexes. a, Activated factor; Ca^{2+}, calcium; PL, phospholipid; TF, tissue factor.

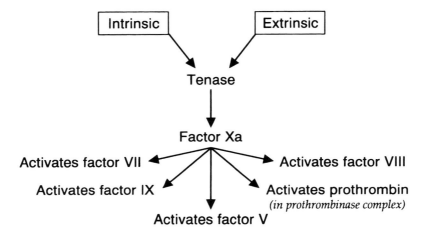

Fig. 6. Actions of activated factor X (Xa).

Ultimate aim: Generation of activated factor X (Xa)

Factor X (FX) is activated by the TF/VIIa complex in the presence of calcium. Factor Xa then participates in the prothrombinase complex that generates thrombin. The TF/VIIa complex also generates small amounts of activated factor IX (IXa).

"Intrinsic" Tenase

Main components:

1. Factor VIIIa (FVIIIa)
2. Factor IXa (FIXa)
3. Factor X (FX)

Ultimate aim: Generation of activated factor X (Xa)

Factor VIII circulates complexed with vWF. Vascular disruption and exposure of subendothelial tissue lead to vWF-mediated adhesion of platelets. Factor VIII is conveniently transported to the site of endothelial injury by vWF, where it binds to receptors on the platelet (phospholipid) membrane. Factor Xa (from the extrinsic tenase complex) activates factor VIII (FVIII) in the presence of phospholipid (platelet membrane) and calcium. Factor IXa and factor VIIIa then further activate factor X, resulting in production of activated factor X (Xa), which participates in the prothrombinase complex. Other actions of FXa are outlined in Figure 6.

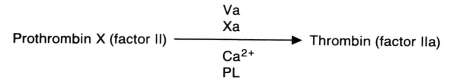

Fig. 7. Prothrombinase complex. a, Activated factor; Ca^{2+}, calcium; PL, phospholipid.

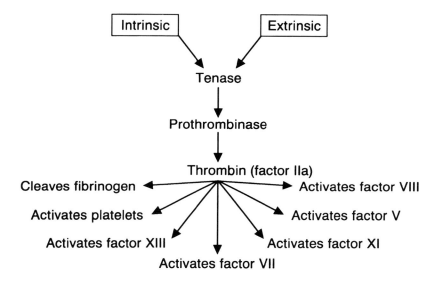

Fig. 8. Actions of thrombin (activated factor II, IIa).

Prothrombinase Complex (Fig. 7)

Main components:

1. Factor V (FV)
2. Factor X (FX)
3. Factor II (prothrombin) (FII)

Ultimate aim: Generation of thrombin (factor IIa)

Factor V is activated by factor Xa in the presence of calcium and phospholipid. It then acts as a cofactor for factor Xa, which activates prothrombin (factor II) to thrombin (IIa), in the presence of calcium and phospholipid (platelet membrane). Actions of thrombin (factor IIa) are shown in Figure 8.

Fibrin Clot Formation (Fig. 9)

Main components:

1. Thrombin
2. Fibrinogen
3. Factor XIII (FXIII)

Ultimate aim: Formation of a stable fibrin clot

Thrombin breaks down fibrinogen to fibrin monomers that cross-link to form polymers. It simultaneously activates factor XIII, which forms a stable cross-linked fibrin clot.

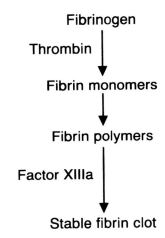

Fig. 9. Formation of fibrin clot. a, Activated factor.

ANTICOAGULANT ACTIVITY

Main components:

1. Blood flow
2. Inactivation of procoagulants by naturally occurring anticoagulants:
   a. Antithrombin (AT)
   b. Protein C (PC)
   c. Protein S (PS)

Blood flow removes activated clotting factors (procoagulants) from sites of vascular injury and transports them to the liver, where they are degraded. In addition, three known naturally occurring anticoagulants—antithrombin, protein C, and its cofactor protein S—break down (or inactivate) activated procoagulants, thus limiting excessive clot formation.

Interaction Between Vascular Endothelium and Plasma Anticoagulants

Thrombomodulin is anchored to the endothelial cell surface. Circulating thrombin, which is a procoagulant, binds to thrombomodulin (Fig. 10) and loses its procoagulant function. While bound to thrombomodulin, it activates circulating protein C to activated protein C.

Activated protein C, in conjunction with its cofactor protein S, breaks down (inactivates) two procoagulants, factor Va and factor VIIIa, curtailing their procoagulant activity and preventing spontaneous and excessive clot formation. Antithrombin, which is produced in the liver, binds to thrombin, thus inactivating it. In addition, it inactivates other clotting factors (Fig. 11). Deficiencies of the naturally occurring anticoagulants (protein C, protein S, and antithrombin) result in decreased anticoagulant activity. This results in a propensity for venous thrombosis.

FIBRINOLYTIC ACTIVITY

Plasmin is currently the only known fibrinolytic protein. Its inactive form, plasminogen, is activated by various plasminogen activators (Fig. 12). This ultimately leads to lysis of the fibrin clot, which prevents exuberant and disseminated fibrin clot formation and contributes to restoration of the vessel patency and reestablishment of vessel blood flow. This property of the fibrinolytic system is used in therapy of acute arterial (coronary

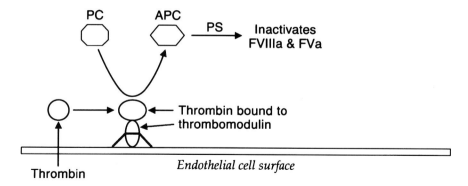

Fig. 10. Thrombomodulin, protein C, and protein S anticoagulant system. Circulating thrombin binds to thrombomodulin and activates protein C (PC) to activated PC (APC), which inactivates activated factors VIII (FVIIIa) and V (FVa). Protein S (PS) is a cofactor.

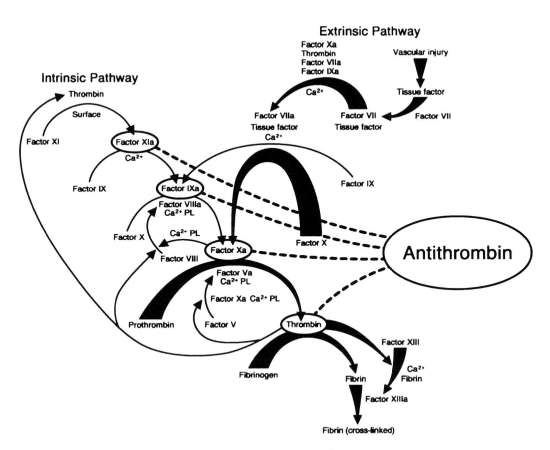

Fig. 11. Actions of antithrombin. a, Activated factor; Ca^{2+}, calcium; PL, phospholipid. (From Davie EW, Fujikawa K, Kisiel W. The coagulation cascade: initiation, maintenance, and regulation. *Biochemistry* 1991; 30: 10363-10370. By permission of the American Chemical Society.)

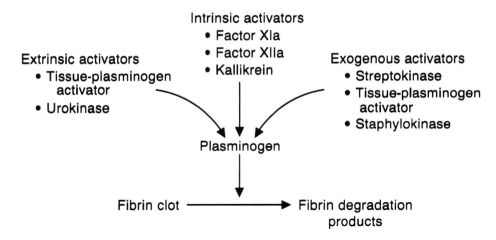

Fig. 12. Fibrinolytic system. a, Activated factor.

and peripheral) and occasional venous thrombosis. Plasminogen activator inhibitors control the rate of fibrinolysis and thus prevent bleeding complications.

INTERPRETATION OF COMMON SCREENING COAGULATION TESTS

The history and physical examination should indicate the likelihood of the presence of a bleeding diathesis. Screening tests aid in the rational application of more specific assays to establish a diagnosis.

Prothrombin Time (PT) and Activated Partial Thromboplastin Time (aPTT)

The PT and aPTT are determined to assess the function of the extrinsic and intrinsic coagulation systems (Fig. 13). For PT, a tissue factor preparation (thromboplastin) and calcium are added to patient plasma, and the time to clot formation is measured in seconds. Qualitative and quantitative abnormalities of, or inhibitors to, components of the extrinsic and final common pathways (Fig. 13) can result in prolongation of the PT. For aPTT, phospholipid extract of thromboplastin (partial thromboplastin), calcium, and an activator of factor XII (contact activator) are added to patient plasma. The time to clot formation is measured in seconds. Deficiencies or inhibitors to the clotting factors in the intrinsic or final common pathway (Fig. 13) result in a prolongation of the aPTT.

International Normalized Ratio (INR)

Differences in commercially available thromboplastins (tissue factor preparations) result in different sensitivities to the deficiencies of coagulation factors. Thus, on the basis of a patient's PT and the normal PT, the INR is calculated as follows:

$$INR = (PT \text{ of patient}/PT, \text{ mean normal})^{ISI}$$

ISI is the international sensitivity index; this is a measure of the sensitivity of the individual thromboplastin to coagulation factor deficiencies. Typically, each laboratory has a different supplier of the thromboplastin and, thus, a different ISI. The manufacturer supplies this information. Use of the calculated INR permits a more uniform monitoring

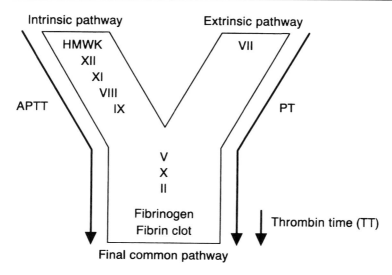

Fig. 13. Interpretation of activated partial thromboplastin time (aPTT) and prothrombin time (PT). HMWK, high-molecular-weight kininogen.

of the degree of anticoagulation in different laboratories. The INR, rather than the PT, is currently recommended for monitoring warfarin therapy.

Thrombin Time

Thrombin, when added to plasma, directly cleaves fibrinogen, resulting in fibrin formation, which subsequently stabilizes to form a stable fibrin clot. A prolonged thrombin time is indicative of a quantitative or qualitative fibrinogen abnormality or the presence of heparin. In the presence of heparin, a reptilase time should be normal.

Evaluation of a Prolonged PT and aPTT

In the laboratory, the first step in the evaluation of a prolonged clotting time (PT or aPTT) is to perform mixing studies with normal plasma. The patient's plasma is mixed with an equal volume of normal pool plasma, and the clotting assay is then repeated. Correction of the prolonged clotting time, to normal, is indicative of a clotting factor deficiency. Mixing the patient's plasma with normal plasma replenishes the deficient factor, thus correcting the clotting time.

Persistent prolongation of the clotting time indicates the presence of an inhibitor. This inhibitor could be a specific inhibitor to a clotting factor, such as a factor VIII inhibitor, or a nonspecific inhibitor, such as a lupus anticoagulant. Subsequently, assays for specific clotting factors, in the intrinsic or extrinsic pathways, lead to a diagnosis. In the absence of a coagulation factor deficiency or an inhibitor, abnormalities of fibrinogen should be considered and the thrombin time should be determined.

Bleeding Time (BT)

A test for bleeding time needs to be performed by skilled personnel. It is usually performed on the volar aspect of the forearm. A blood pressure cuff is inflated to 40 mm Hg on the upper arm, to standardize venous pressure. A controlled incision is then made, and the time required for the bleeding to cease is determined by blotting the oozing blood from the wound with a filter paper at 30-second intervals.

The test is influenced by various operator factors: the depth, direction, and location of the incision and the pressure of the inflated cuff. The time can be prolonged in patients with thrombocytopenia, fragile skin as a result of advanced age, or prolonged use of systemic or topical glucocorticoids. Platelet function defect or disorders such as vWD also can prolong the bleeding time. The utility of the bleeding time in the surgical setting has been debated. In general, although a prolonged bleeding time is a poor predictor for bleeding complications during operation, an abnormal bleeding time should prompt an investigation to rule out inherited or acquired bleeding disorders.

21 Bleeding Disorders: An Overview and Clinical Practice

Rajiv K. Pruthi, MD

Contents

HISTORY TAKING IN THE BLEEDING DISORDERS
INHERITED BLEEDING DISORDERS
ACQUIRED COAGULATION DEFECTS

HISTORY TAKING IN THE BLEEDING DISORDERS

The most important test of the hemostatic system is the patient's history of bleeding tendency. The history can be very subjective. Patients with no underlying bleeding disorder may complain of excessive bleeding problems, whereas patients who have an established bleeding disorder may not think that their bleeding tendency is anything to worry about. When possible, objective confirmation of a patient's bleeding episodes should be pursued, such as obtaining the operative report or, better yet, communicating with the surgeon of a patient who has had postoperative bleeding. A detailed history should be obtained regarding bleeding from any site (such as epistaxis or gastrointestinal). A detailed history of all surgical procedures should be obtained. Dental extraction should be inquired about separately, because most patients do not classify dental extraction as a surgical procedure.

A history of mucocutaneous bleeding with epistaxis and occasionally gastrointestinal bleeding may indicate the presence of a platelet defect or von Willebrand disease. Hemorrhage into soft tissue or joints indicates the presence of hemophilia.

INHERITED BLEEDING DISORDERS

Von Willebrand Disease

DEFINITION

Von Willebrand disease (vWD) is characterized by a quantitative or qualitative abnormality of plasma von Willebrand factor (vWF). It is the most common inherited bleeding tendency; it has a prevalence of 1% to 2% in certain populations.

BIOCHEMISTRY

vWF is produced by vascular endothelial cells and platelets. It is a large glycosylated protein of 2,813 amino acids. vWF is first synthesized as monomers, and later the C

From: *Primary Hematology*
Edited by: A. Tefferi © Mayo Foundation for Medical Education and Research, Rochester, MN

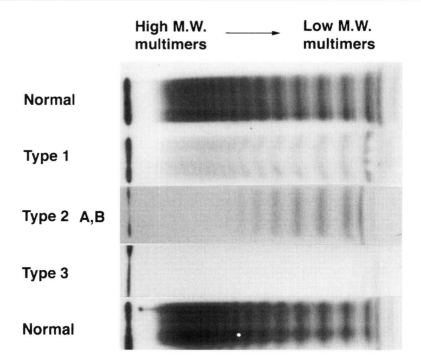

Fig. 1. Von Willebrand factor multimers. M.W., molecular weight.

termini of the monomers are linked via disulfide bonds, resulting in multimers of varying sizes (Fig. 1). These multimers are secreted into the plasma, where they circulate bound to factor VIII. vWF has a half-life of 12 to 24 hours. Endothelial cells act as a reservoir for vWF.

vWF has three main functions:

1. Adhesion of platelets to damaged vessel wall by acting as a bridge between the subendothelial connective tissue and glycoprotein receptor Ib-IX on platelets
2. Platelet-to-platelet aggregation by acting as a bridge between glycoprotein IIb/IIIa receptors on platelets
3. Carrier for factor VIII, thus transporting factor VIII to the site of platelet plug formation to facilitate formation of the fibrin clot

CLINICAL MANIFESTATIONS

Deficiency of vWF results in hemorrhagic problems. Clinical manifestations are highly variable; in mild to moderate vWD, mucocutaneous bleeding is predominant. Patients usually complain of easy bruising or epistaxis. Menorrhagia is a prominent complaint in female patients and can lead to iron deficiency. Patients can have persistent oozing after minor surgical procedures such as dental extraction or major bleed after major surgical procedures. Use of aspirin or other nonsteroidal analgesics may unmask the bleeding tendency and lead to a diagnosis of vWD.

A more severe bleeding tendency can occur in severe type 1 or type 3 disease (see below). Affected patients have a more severe bleeding tendency and may have soft tissue and intra-articular bleeds, as do patients with hemophilia.

DIAGNOSIS

Bleeding History

The patient's bleeding history is crucial for evaluation of a bleeding tendency. Obtaining a thorough personal and family history of bleeding is essential; however, absence of a history of bleeding tendency does not exclude a diagnosis of vWD. Appropriate subspecialty consultation followed by laboratory testing is recommended. The diagnosis of type 1 vWD in an individual patient may be difficult to make, and repeated testing may be necessary.

Laboratory Testing

Investigations include tests for the following:

1. Prothrombin time (PT)
2. Activated partial thromboplastin time (aPTT)
3. Bleeding time
4. vWF antigen
5. Ristocetin cofactor activity
6. vWF multimer analysis (if clinically indicated)
7. Blood group determination (ABO)

The **prothrombin time (PT)** is typically normal. vWF is a carrier for factor VIII; thus, although the **activated partial thromboplastin time (aPTT)** is typically normal, it may be prolonged if the vWF levels are low enough to result in a decreased level of factor VIII (see Fig. 13 in Chapter 20, page 301). Characteristically, the defective platelet adhesion and aggregation result in a prolonged **bleeding time**. Specific tests for vWD include assay for **vWF antigen**, formerly called factor VIII-related antigen. **Ristocetin cofactor activity**, which is a functional measurement of vWF-supported agglutination of human platelets by ristocetin, is typically decreased. Finally, assays for the multimeric forms of circulating vWF are performed; the distribution of vWF multimers is typically normal for type 1 vWD, vWF is undetectable in type 3, and higher-molecular-weight multimers are decreased in type 2.

CLASSIFICATION

1. Quantitative defects:
    Type 1 vWD: mild decrease in vWF antigen and ristocetin cofactor activity
    Type 3 vWD: severe decrease in vWF antigen and ristocetin cofactor activity
2. Qualitative defects (type 2 vWD):
    Type 2A: loss of large multimeric forms of vWF. The vWF (ristocetin cofactor) activity is lower than the vWF antigen
    Type 2B: a qualitative abnormality of vWF results in an increased affinity of the vWF receptor on the platelets to vWF. This results in a binding of vWF to platelets and increased clearance from the circulation. Thrombocytopenia is a prominent feature of this type of vWD
    Type 2N: due to defective binding of factor VIII to vWF, which results in a shortened half-life of factor VIII. This phenotype can be mistaken for mild hemophilia A because the vWF antigen and ristocetin cofactor activity are normal

CAUTIONS

Effect of hormones:

vWF levels can be increased in periods of acute stress, glucocorticoid use, estrogen use, or pregnancy. Cyclic fluctuations in endogenous estrogens, as occur during menstrual periods, may result in fluctuations in vWF levels

Effect of blood group:

vWF levels can be lower in patients with blood group O than in patients with blood groups A, B, or AB. Thus, blood group should be determined in all patients with a low vWF level

Once a diagnosis of vWD has been established, it is crucial to assess response to desamino-D-arginine vasopressin (DDAVP). This is accomplished by administration of 0.3 μg/kg of DDAVP intravenously and assaying for vWF and ristocetin cofactor activity an hour later. This test helps in assessing the response to DDAVP, which may be used in prophylaxis and management of minor bleeds.

MANAGEMENT

All patients with vWD should carry some form of identification indicating the bleeding disorder.

Management of Bleeding

Prophylaxis requires administration of appropriate products to prevent bleeding complications in anticipation of minor or major surgical procedures. Appropriate products are administered to treat an established bleeding episode. Available options include pharmacologic products (DDAVP and antifibrinolytic agents), plasma-derived products, and recombinant clotting factor concentrates.

The use of non-plasma-derived **pharmacologic products** in the management of bleeding disorders results in the elimination of transfusion-transmitted diseases. *DDAVP*, a vasopressin analog, promotes release of vWF from endothelial cells. This also results in an increase of factor VIII activity. Although the increases in vWF and factor VIII are dose-dependent, the maximal effect seems to be at a dose of 0.3 μg/kg body weight intravenously and 300 μg intranasally. The vWF levels increase to a maximum of 2 to 4 times the baseline level.

Indications for DDAVP include type 1 vWD with mild bleeding symptoms and as prophylaxis for minor surgical procedures. The patient must previously have been shown to be responsive to a test infusion of DDAVP; that is, as soon as a diagnosis of vWD is established, the patient should receive a dose of DDAVP, and the vWF antigen and ristocetin cofactor activity measured to assess the degree of increase. Patients with type 2 vWD have a qualitative defect; thus, administration of DDAVP results in release of a functionally abnormal vWF and typically provides little clinical utility for major bleeding episodes. Depending on the degree of increase in ristocetin, DDAVP could be used for management of minor bleeds.

Contraindications to the use of DDAVP include increased release of abnormal vWF, resulting in worsening thrombocytopenia in patients with type 2B vWD. Adverse effects include facial flushing, tachycardia, and hypotension. Occasionally, headache, abdominal pain, and nausea occur. Repeated use may lead to inappropriate fluid retention and hyponatremia. Repeated administration can lead to tachyphylaxis.

Antifibrinolytic agents (tranexamic acid and aminocaproic acid) bind to plasminogen, prevent its activation, and inhibit breakdown of blood clots (fibrinolysis) and can be used as an adjunct to other therapies for prophylaxis. The doses used are 15 mg /kg every 8 hours for tranexamic acid and 1 g every 6 hours for aminocaproic acid. These agents are used in combination with DDAVP to prevent bleeding before minor surgical procedures such as dental extraction. Contraindications for their use include a history of thromboembolic disease. In urinary tract bleeds, antifibrinolytics may lead to obstruction by preventing fibrinolysis of the blood clots.

Plasma-derived products are another management option. Because of the high risk of transmission of viral diseases, use of *cryoprecipitate* is not recommended. However, in emergency situations in which a vWF-rich product is not available, use of cryoprecipitate could be considered. Several commercially available *plasma-derived products* contain vWF in addition to factor VIII. Different products contain varying amounts of vWF, which affects the appropriate dose. With the current viral inactivation procedures, the risk of transfusion-transmitted disease is low. Appropriate use of clotting factor concentrates requires knowledge of the pharmacokinetics of the individual product and frequent monitoring of vWF levels to ascertain effect.

Recombinant clotting factor concentrates are free from viral contaminants and thus should make prophylaxis and therapy for vWD safe from a viral infection standpoint. Recombinant vWF concentrates are currently undergoing clinical trials and should be available in the future.

Prevention of Transfusion-Transmitted Diseases

All patients, especially patients with vWD, hemophilia, or other bleeding disorders, who have the potential to be exposed to blood products should be immunized against hepatitis A and B viruses. Vaccines against hepatitis C and human immunodeficiency virus (HIV) infections are currently not available. The use of pharmacologic agents minimizes the exposure to plasma-derived products and, hence, to viral infections. vWF factor concentrates should be used judiciously. Despite the potential for viral infections, use of plasma-derived products is safer than before, and patients should not be denied a lifesaving treatment in case of a major bleed.

CLINICALLY RELEVANT MOLECULAR GENETICS

The gene for vWF is located on the short arm of chromosome 12 and consists of 52 exons spanning 178 kb. A pseudogene located on chromosome 22 has 98% homology to exons 23-34 of the vWF gene. The disorder is transmitted in an autosomal dominant fashion, but the penetrance, that is, the expressions of vWD phenotype, varies among individuals within the same family.

Hemophilia A and B

DEFINITION

Hemophilia A and B are congenital bleeding disorders that are due to deficiencies of factors VIII (FVIII) and IX (FIX), respectively. Clinical manifestations of deficiencies of hemophilia A and B are indistinguishable.

BIOCHEMISTRY

FVIII and FIX are synthesized in the liver. FIX is produced by hepatocytes. The exact site of synthesis of FVIII in the liver is unknown; however, patients with hemophilia who undergo liver transplantation are cured of their hemophilia. Both FVIII and FIX are essential for the middle stages of blood coagulation (see Fig. 1 in Chapter 20, page 292). Activated FVIII is a cofactor for FIX, which further activates factor X in the tenase complex (see Fig. 5 in Chapter 20, page 296).

Clinical Manifestations

Patients with mild disease do not have spontaneous bleeds; they bleed only after surgery or trauma. With increasing severity, spontaneous bleeding usually occurs. Patients with hemophilia typically bleed into soft tissue and joints. They also may have easy bruising, epistaxis, and gastrointestinal hemorrhage.

Diagnosis

Bleeding History

The diagnosis of hemophilia is typically established in one of four ways:

1. In patients with a family history of hemophilia (familial), prenatal evaluation is increasingly being performed if a male fetus is thought to be at risk for hemophilia. At the appropriate gestational age, either amniocentesis or chorionic villus sampling is performed. Appropriate DNA-based techniques such as direct mutation detection or linkage analysis lead to the diagnosis in most cases.
2. Up to 30% of patients with hemophilia do not have a family history of the disease. In these cases, the disease is called sporadic hemophilia, and it reflects new mutations. Affected patients often come to attention as a result of unusually prolonged bleeding after circumcision. On occasion, the phenotype can be so mild that patients do not come to clinical attention and may escape detection altogether if they go through life without undergoing any surgery or trauma.
3. Patients who have moderate to severe disease and do not undergo circumcision at birth come to clinical attention at approximately 1 year of age when they are learning to walk and, because of multiple falls, have excessive bruising. The appropriate tests will lead to a diagnosis. On occasion, the bruises are mistaken for child abuse. Thus, one needs to ensure that patients suspected of being victims of abuse do not have an underlying bleeding disorder.
4. Occasionally, the asymptomatic patient with mild hemophilia may have a preoperative activated partial thromboplastin time that is prolonged. Further testing will lead to a diagnosis.

Laboratory Testing

The diagnosis and severity of hemophilia A and B are established by determining factor VIII and IX activity levels, respectively. Antigen levels also are measured in certain situations; however, it is the individual coagulation factor activity level that is clinically useful.

The following cautions should be noted:

1. FVIII is carried by vWF. Thus, a low FVIII activity level should lead to assays for vWF, which should be normal in hemophilia A.
2. FVIII is a labile factor. Thus, the assay for FVIII activity is best performed on a fresh plasma sample. For specimens that are frozen and sent to reference laboratories, 15% to 20% of FVIII activity can be lost as a result of freezing the sample for transportation and thawing it for the assay.
3. FIX is a vitamin K-dependent protein. Thus, depending on the FIX level, vitamin K deficiency should be ruled out when establishing a new diagnosis of hemophilia B. This is typically done by performing assays for other vitamin K-dependent proteins.
4. Children have a lower reference range than adults; thus, age should be taken into account when interpreting FIX levels.

Issues Related to Cord Blood Assays

If the sample is obtained properly, FVIII activity is accurate for establishing the diagnosis. However, neonates are all vitamin K-deficient because of an immature liver; thus, cord blood FIX activity is not reliable for evaluating hemophilia B.

CLASSIFICATION

Classification of the hemophilias is based on the coagulant activity of FVIII and FIX:

Mild: ≥ 6% to 25%
Moderate: 1% to 5%
Severe: < 1%

MANAGEMENT OF HEMOPHILIA

All patients with hemophilia should carry identification indicating their bleeding disorder. Treatment includes management of bleeding (prophylaxis and treatment of established bleeding episodes) and prevention of transfusion-transmitted disease.

HEMOPHILIA A

Management of Bleeding

Available options include pharmacologic products (DDAVP and antifibrinolytic agents), plasma-derived clotting factor concentrates, and recombinant clotting factor concentrates.

The use of non-plasma-derived **pharmacologic products** in the management of bleeding disorders results in the elimination of transfusion-transmitted diseases. *DDAVP,* a vasopressin analog, promotes release of vWF from endothelial cells to hemostatic levels. This also results in an increase of FVIII activity. Although the increases in vWF and FVIII are dose-dependent, the maximal effect seems to be at a dose of 0.3 µg/kg body weight intravenously and 300 µg intranasally. The FVIII levels increase to a maximum of 2 to 6 times the baseline level. Thus, in moderate or severe hemophilia A, the FVIII levels achieved may not be hemostatically adequate.

Indications for DDAVP include patients with mild hemophilia A in whom a trial of DDAVP has been shown to result in an increase in FVIII activity levels, treatment of mild bleeding symptoms, and as prophylaxis for minor surgical procedures.

Adverse effects include facial flushing that disappears after a few hours, occasional mild transient headache, tachycardia, and rarely, hypotension, abdominal pain, and nausea. Repeated use may lead to inappropriate fluid retention and hyponatremia.

Repeated administration can lead to tachyphylaxis. The response to the DDAVP also declines by about 30% during subsequent administrations, but a minimum 3-day interval between doses usually results in an increase to 100% response.

Antifibrinolytic agents (tranexamic acid and aminocaproic acid) bind to plasminogen, prevent its activation, and thus inhibit fibrinolysis. The doses used are 15 mg /kg every 8 hours for tranexamic acid and 1 g every 6 hours for aminocaproic acid.

These agents are used in combination with DDAVP to prevent bleeding before minor surgical procedures such as dental extraction. Contraindications for their use are a history of thromboembolic disease and upper urinary tract bleeds, in which case antifibrinolytics may lead to obstruction by preventing fibrinolysis of the blood clots.

Various **plasma-derived clotting factor concentrates** are commercially available. The FVIII content and method of viral inactivation vary. With newer techniques, the risk of viral transmission is low. The dosage of FVIII product, measured in units, varies with the indication for therapy, the baseline FVIII activity, the patient's weight, and the target FVIII activity. In general, each unit of FVIII product that is transfused leads to a 2% increase in FVIII activity. Thus, for a patient who weighs 60 kg, has a baseline FVIII activity of 5%, and has a serious bleed that requires an increase of the FVIII activity to 100% (a 95% increment in FVIII), the following formula is used:

$$(60 \times 95)/2 = 2,850 \text{ units of FVIII}$$

The post-infusion FVIII activity should be measured to assess response.

Recombinant clotting factor concentrates have the added margin of safety from viral infections. Thus, for previously untreated patients, this is likely the product of choice.

Prevention of Transfusion-Transmitted Diseases

All patients who will potentially be exposed to blood products should be vaccinated with the available hepatitis vaccines. The use of plasma-derived products should be avoided in patients who have not been exposed to these products and in those who have not been infected with the transfusion-transmitted viruses.

Pharmacologic and recombinant alternatives should be used when appropriate.

Complications of the Disease

The following complications can develop: multiple hemarthroses resulting in severe joint deformities and contractures, pseudocysts, and life-threatening bleeding problems.

Complications of Therapy

Transfusion-transmitted disease (HIV, hepatitis C, and hepatitis B) were more common before the use of high-purity clotting factor concentrates. With the increasing use of recombinant clotting factor concentrates, the infectious complications should eventually be eliminated.

The development of inhibitors to clotting factors is more common in patients with hemophilia A and is rare in patients with hemophilia B. Repeated exposure to exogenously administered FVIII results in the development of inhibitors to FVIII.

Clinically Relevant Molecular Genetics

The FVIII and FIX genes are located on the long arm of the X chromosome. Thus, the disorders are transmitted as X-linked recessive disorders, in which males are affected and females are carriers. Rarely, females may be symptomatic from low levels of the respective coagulation factors.

Because the disorder is linked to the X chromosome, female offspring of patients with hemophilia are obligate carriers of the genetic abnormality. Male offspring of patients with hemophilia are never affected, unless the hemophilic father marries a female carrier of a hemophilia defect. The mother of a hemophiliac is an obligate carrier.

FVIII protein is 2,332 amino acids long and encoded by the FVIII gene, which has 26 exons and spans 186 kb. FIX, however, is 415 amino acids long and the gene has 8 exons and spans 33.5 kb.

HEMOPHILIA B

Management of Bleeding

Available options include **pharmacologic products** (antifibrinolytics), plasma-derived clotting factor concentrates, and recombinant clotting factor concentrates.

The use of non-plasma-derived pharmacologic products in the management of bleeding disorders results in the elimination of transfusion-transmitted diseases. *Antifibrinolytic agents* (tranexamic acid and aminocaproic acid) bind to plasminogen, prevent its activation, and thus inhibit fibrinolysis. The doses used are 15 mg/kg every 8 hours for tranexamic acid and 1 g every 6 hours for aminocaproic acid.

These agents are used in combination with factor IX products for minor procedures such as tooth extraction. Contraindications for their use include a history of thromboembolic disease. In upper urinary tract bleeds, antifibrinolytics may lead to obstruction by preventing fibrinolysis of the blood clots.

Various **plasma-derived clotting factor concentrates** are commercially available. The FIX content and method of viral inactivation vary. With newer techniques, the risk of viral transmission is low. The dosage of FIX product, measured in units, varies with the indication for therapy, the baseline FIX activity, the patient's weight, and the target FIX activity. In general, each unit of FIX product that is transfused leads to a 1% increase in FIX activity. Thus, for a patient who weighs 60 kg, has a baseline FIX activity of 5%, and has a serious bleed that requires an increase of the FVIII activity to 80% (a 75% increment in FIX), the following formula is used:

$$60 \times 75 = 4{,}500 \text{ units of FIX}$$

The post-infusion FIX activity should be measured to assess response.

Recombinant clotting factor concentrates have the added margin of safety from viral infections. Thus, for previously untreated patients, this is likely the product of choice.

Prevention of Transfusion-Transmitted Diseases

All patients who will potentially be exposed to blood products should be vaccinated with the available hepatitis vaccines. The use of plasma-derived products should be avoided in patients who have not been exposed to these products and in those who have not been infected with transfusion-transmitted viruses. Pharmacologic and recombinant alternatives should be used when appropriate.

Complications of the Disease

The following complications can develop: multiple hemarthroses resulting in severe joint deformities and contractures, pseudocysts, and life-threatening bleeding problems.

Complications of Therapy

Transfusion-transmitted disease, HIV, hepatitis C, and hepatitis B were more common before the use of high-purity clotting factor concentrates. With the increasing use of recombinant clotting factor concentrates, the infectious complications should eventually be eliminated.

The development of inhibitors to clotting factors is more common in patients with hemophilia A and is rare in patients with hemophilia B.

Clinically Relevant Molecular Genetics

The FVIII and FIX genes are located on the long arm of the X chromosome. Thus, the disorders are transmitted as X-linked recessive disorders, in which males are affected and females are carriers. Rarely, females may be symptomatic from low levels of the respective coagulation factors.

Because the disorder is linked to the X chromosome, female offspring of patients with hemophilia are obligate carriers of the genetic abnormality. Male offspring are never affected, unless the hemophilic father marries a female carrier of a hemophilia defect. The mother of a hemophiliac is an obligate carrier.

FVIII protein is 2,332 amino acids long and encoded by the FVIII gene, which has 26 exons and spans 186 kb. FIX, however, is 415 amino acids long and the gene has 8 exons and spans 33.5 kb.

Hemophilia C

DEFINITION

Hemophilia C is an autosomal inherited bleeding disorder that is due to a deficiency of factor XI (FXI).

CLINICAL MANIFESTATIONS

Because of the rarity of hemophilia C, accurate classification systems have not yet been established. In general, spontaneous bleeding, although rare, even in severely deficient patients, can occur. The FXI activity levels do not accurately correlate with the severity of bleeding tendency; however, patients with an FXI activity less than 20% usually have a bleeding tendency. In selected cases, patients with a tendency to bleed may coinherit a second hemorrhagic diathesis such as vWD. The most common bleeding problems include menorrhagia and bleeding after tooth extraction, circumcision, and other surgical procedures. Soft tissue and intra-articular bleeds are uncommon.

DIAGNOSIS

Clinical History

Patients with FXI deficiency can have variable bleeding tendency. Patients with severely decreased FXI levels can have minimal or no bleeding symptoms, but patients with moderately decreased FXI levels can have fairly significant bleeding problems. Most often, the disease is diagnosed during the workup for a prolonged aPTT in an asymptomatic patient.

Laboratory Testing

Investigations include aPTT test and factor XI activity assay.

MANAGEMENT

Fresh-frozen plasma infusions are administered for bleeding episodes and in preparation for surgery. Recombinant factor XI products are undergoing clinical trials.

Inherited Platelet Disorders

These disorders include the following categories:

1. Platelet membrane glycoprotein defects
   Bernard-Soulier disease
   Glanzmann's thrombasthenia

2. Storage pool disorders
    Gray platelet syndrome
    Dense granule storage pool deficiency
    Hermansky-Pudlak syndrome
3. Defective platelet procoagulant activity
    Scott syndrome

PLATELET MEMBRANE GLYCOPROTEIN DEFECTS

Bernard-Soulier disease and Glanzmann's thrombasthenia are the best-characterized inherited platelet function disorders. These are due to defects in platelet membrane receptors which result in abnormalities in platelet adhesion and aggregation, which lead to bleeding disorders of varying severity.

BIOCHEMISTRY

Exposure of subendothelial connective tissue, as a result of vascular injury, leads to platelet adhesion to subendothelial connective tissue. vWF mediates this adhesion via a platelet glycoprotein Ib-IX receptor. Subsequent platelet activation leads to activation of a second platelet receptor, glycoprotein IIb-IIIa, that mediates platelet aggregation, resulting in formation of a platelet plug that plays an important role in the initial steps of hemostasis. Failure of the initial platelet plug formation results in a defect in the primary hemostatic response and thus leads to excessive bleeding.

CLINICAL MANIFESTATIONS

Bleeding manifestations of Bernard-Soulier disease and Glanzmann's thrombasthenia are indistinguishable. The predominant bleeding manifestations in patients with platelet defects are epistaxis, purpura, and gingival hemorrhage. Gastrointestinal and genitourinary bleeding, though rare, do occur. Soft tissue, joint, and deep visceral bleeds are uncommon. In females, menorrhagia is a prominent complaint.

The severity of bleeding is unpredictable, but it is clear that patients with either Bernard-Soulier disease or Glanzmann's thrombasthenia need prophylactic transfusions of platelets before any minor or major surgical procedures. Homozygotes are symptomatic, whereas heterozygotes are not.

DIAGNOSIS

Bleeding History

Bleeding symptoms (see below) in patients with platelet defects are characteristically mucocutaneous. Intra-articular and soft tissue hemorrhages are rare.

Laboratory Tests

Investigations include a complete blood cell count, a peripheral smear examination, bleeding time test, and platelet aggregation studies. Platelet aggregation tests are performed by exposing a patient's platelets to various agonists, such as adenosine diphosphate, collagen, epinephrine, and ristocetin, that induce platelet aggregation. The extent of aggregation is measured with a light transmission system. The major differences in laboratory results in patients with Glanzmann's thrombasthenia and Bernard-Soulier disease are shown in Table 1.

MANAGEMENT OF PLATELET FUNCTION ABNORMALITIES

All patients should carry identification indicating their bleeding disorder.

Table 1
Differences in Results of Platelet Aggregation
Studies in Patients With Bernard-Soulier
Disease and Glanzmann's Thrombasthenia

	Study			
	Adenosine diphosphate	Collagen	Arachidonic acid	Ristocetin
Bernard-Soulier	Normal	Normal	Normal	Absent
Glanzmann's thrombasthenia	Absent	Absent	Absent	Normal

Management of Bleeding

For prophylaxis, platelet transfusion and use of antifibrinolytic agents should be considered in anticipation of minor or major surgical procedures. Adequate dental hygiene is essential to prevent periodontal disease and obviate dental extractions.

The mainstay of therapy for bleeding complications consists of platelet transfusions and the use of antifibrinolytic agents, if clinically indicated. There is a risk that patients will become alloimmunized against the respective deficient glycoproteins, thus rendering the management of future transfusions more difficult.

The use of single-donor HLA-matched platelet products should be considered to reduce the overall chances of alloimmunization. Platelets from unaffected HLA-matched family members could be used.

Prevention of Transfusion-Transmitted Diseases

All patients who may potentially be exposed to blood products should be immunized against hepatitis A and B. To date, no vaccine is available to protect against hepatitis C and HIV.

Special Considerations

Iron deficiency may develop over time with persistent oozing and menstrual blood loss (in females); thus, supplementary iron replacement should be considered. Hormonal manipulations may be considered in females with menorrhagia.

ACQUIRED COAGULATION DEFECTS

Inhibitors to Plasma Coagulation Factors

INHIBITORS TO FACTOR VIII

Antibodies to plasma coagulation factor VIII (FVIII) inhibit function of FVIII. The clinical manifestations are similar to those in patients with congenital hemophilia, except that patients are usually in their sixth or seventh decade of life and both sexes are affected equally. In 50% of patients these inhibitors are idiopathic, and in the rest they are associated with connective tissue disease (such as rheumatoid arthritis or systemic lupus erythematosus), medications, or malignancies. In a subset of younger female patients, FVIII inhibitors develop during the postpartum period.

Natural History

The FVIII inhibitors disappear spontaneously in most patients in whom they develop in the postpartum period. Approximately a third of patients with spontaneously acquired inhibitors have reduction of the disease with no therapy. The remainder will respond to the use of immunosuppressive drugs. Some patients with high-titer inhibitors do not respond to immunosuppressive medication.

Diagnosis

A strong suspicion should prompt the appropriate workup. Spontaneous bleeding symptoms in an older patient should lead to screening laboratory tests (see Chapter 20, page 291). A prolonged aPTT that does not correct when the patient's plasma is mixed with normal plasma indicates the presence of an inhibitor. Subsequent assays for the appropriate individual coagulation factor should lead to the diagnosis. The titer of the inhibitor is usually determined to follow response to therapy.

Management

Actively bleeding patients are treated with high doses of FVIII products such as porcine FVIII or recombinant human FVIII. Patients who do not bleed can be managed conservatively. Activated clotting factor concentrates were used previously, but they can be associated with complications such as disseminated intravascular coagulation and thrombosis. Recently, the availability of new recombinant activated factor VII concentrates has facilitated the management of bleeding complications.

For longer-term management, aimed at reduction or elimination of the inhibitor, the use of oral glucocorticoids has resulted in remissions, failing which one could use other immunosuppressants such as cyclophosphamide or methotrexate.

Acquired von Willebrand Disease

Acquired vWD occurs in a previously normal patient without a prior history of bleeding disorders. It usually occurs in association with autoimmune disorders, myeloproliferative disorders, lymphoproliferative disorders, or dysproteinemias such as monoclonal gammopathy of undetermined significance or multiple myeloma. There are reports of acquired vWD occurring with hypothyroidism.

The diagnosis should be considered in a previously normal patient in whom bleeding problems (spontaneous or postsurgical) develop. Testing for acquired vWD is similar to that for congenital vWD. A trial of DDAVP is useful for future prophylaxis and therapy for minor bleeding. vWF-rich products are used for major surgical procedures and hemorrhages.

Acquired Platelet Dysfunction

DRUG-INDUCED PLATELET DYSFUNCTION

Aspirin

Because of its widespread use as an analgesic, and its inclusion in combinations of prescription and nonprescription analgesics, aspirin is likely the most commonly implicated drug in impairment of platelet function. In the evaluation of a patient with increased bruising, obtaining a detailed history of the use of all prescription and nonprescription drugs is crucial to eliminating drug-induced platelet dysfunction. In the appropriate clinical setting, assays for salicylate in plasma can be performed.

Thromboxane, synthesized from prostaglandin (PG) H_2, within platelets is necessary for platelet aggregation. The enzyme PGH synthetase (cyclooxygenase [COX]) is needed for generation of PG H_2. Aspirin permanently inhibits this enzyme, resulting in impaired production of thromboxane. Platelets are unable to synthesize, thus impairing more enzyme aggregation response. In effect, a single dose of aspirin results in platelet dysfunction that lasts 7 to 10 days. Thus, the use of aspirin is discontinued for 7 to 10 days before anticipated surgical procedures.

PG H synthetase, also present in the vascular endothelium, where it produces prostacyclin, is a strong inhibitor of platelet function, loss of which results in platelet dysfunction. Unlike the platelets, however, the endothelium can regenerate this enzyme.

Recently, a second form of PG H synthetase has been identified, termed PG H-synthetase-2, or COX-2. This has resulted in development of COX-2 inhibitors that have anti-inflammatory and analgesic properties, apparently without the antiplatelet effect of aspirin and nonsteroidal analgesics.

Nonsteroidal Analgesics

The mechanism of action of nonsteroidal analgesics, such as ibuprofen, is exactly that of aspirin. In contrast to aspirin, the effect on cyclooxygenase is temporary, lasting only as long as the drug is in the circulation, which is usually a few hours. Thus, nonsteroidal analgesics with a longer half-life inhibit platelet function for a longer time. It would be prudent, however, to discontinue use of the medications for at least a few days before any planned surgical procedure.

Ticlopidine and Clopidogrel

Ticlopidine and clopidogrel are specific ADP platelet receptor antagonists that prevent activation and aggregation of platelets. They are used in patients with cerebrovascular accidents and are being studied in patients with coronary artery disease. Their effects on platelets last for up to 10 days.

GpIIb/IIIa Inhibitors

GpIIb/IIIa agents are newer drugs that inhibit platelet receptors. They have shown promise in coronary artery disease.

Antibiotics

Antibiotics that share a common structure, the β-lactam ring, such as penicillin and cephalosporins, have been implicated in platelet dysfunction. Because most studies were done in critically ill patients who were taking other medications, it is difficult to ascertain the exact contribution of antibiotics to bleeding complications in patients with platelet dysfunction.

SYSTEMIC DISORDERS

Renal Failure

Renal insufficiency results in impaired platelet function. The mechanism of this impairment is multifactorial. Anemia that accompanies renal insufficiency, the presence of an as yet unidentified inhibitor, and presumably circulating toxins that are usually excreted by the kidney all impair platelet function.

Myeloproliferative Disorders

Impaired platelet function can lead to bleeding problems and, conversely, hyperaggregability can lead to thrombotic problems.

22 Thrombogenesis and Thrombotic Disorders

Rajiv K. Pruthi, MD

Contents

INTRODUCTION

Patients who have spontaneous venous or arterial thrombosis are said to be in a "hypercoagulable state" or have "thrombophilia." These terms are not clearly defined; however, persons in whom blood clots develop, either spontaneously or in high-risk situations (Table 1), likely have an underlying thrombophilia or hypercoagulable state, unlike persons who do not have development of blood clots in similar high-risk situations. Unlike the bleeding disorders, in which a global laboratory test (bleeding time, prothrombin time, or activated partial thromboplastin time) can predict a propensity to bleed, no global test can predict a propensity for development of inappropriate thrombosis. Thus, the usual approach to the patient with thrombosis consists of establishing the presence or absence of known risk factors for thrombosis (Table 1), obtaining a thorough personal and family history, and performing a physical examination. Subsequently, specific laboratory tests for inherited and acquired conditions that predispose to thrombosis may define the cause of the thrombus and aid in estimating the risk for recurrence. This information will influence the duration of anticoagulant therapy.

From: *Primary Hematology*
Edited by: A. Tefferi © Mayo Foundation for Medical Education and Research, Rochester, MN

Table 1
Risk Factors for Venous Thrombosis

Acquired	*Inherited*
Pregnancy	Strong association
Puerperium	Resistance to activated protein C
Oral contraceptives	Deficiencies of anticoagulants
Hormone replacement therapy	Antithrombin
Antiphospholipid syndromes	Protein C
Malignancy	Protein S
Trauma	Factor II 20210A
Immobilization	Dysfibrinogenemia
Orthopedic surgery of lower extremities	Thrombomodulin abnormalities
Hyperhomocystinemia	Hyperhomocystinemia
Age	Possible association
Previous thrombosis	Plasminogen deficiency
Smoking	Heparin cofactor II deficiency
Morbid obesity	
Paroxysmal nocturnal hemoglobinuria	
Myeloproliferative disorders	

OVERVIEW

Thrombi can occur within the venous and arterial vasculature. They can remain localized and be asymptomatic, produce localized symptoms, or propagate or embolize, resulting in vaso-occlusive complications at distant sites. Thrombi are composed of fibrin and blood cells (red cells, platelets, and white cells). Venous thrombi (red clot) are composed of predominantly red cells and are rich in fibrin, whereas arterial thrombi are platelet-rich (white clot) with a few strands of fibrin and usually occur in association with ruptured atherosclerotic plaques. These differences point to the disparate etiopathogenesis of the two types of thrombi.

Thrombosis occurs when there is an imbalance among the procoagulant, anticoagulant, and fibrinolytic components of hemostasis, with the procoagulant effects being more dominant than the anticoagulant and fibrinolytic effects because of abnormalities in the anticoagulant and fibrinolytic components.

The procoagulant functions of the hemostatic system were reviewed in Chapter 20. This chapter focuses on the anticoagulant and fibrinolytic properties.

ANTICOAGULANT ACTIVITIES
Vascular Endothelium

The vascular endothelium produces heparin-like molecules that, in conjunction with antithrombin, inactivate coagulation factors. Thrombomodulin is produced by the endothelium and is anchored to its surface; its anticoagulant functions are outlined below.

Plasma

The main components include 1) blood flow and 2) inactivation of procoagulants by naturally occurring anticoagulants (antithrombin, protein C, and protein S).

Blood flow removes activated clotting factors (procoagulants) from sites of vascular injury and transports them to the liver, where they are degraded. In addition, three known

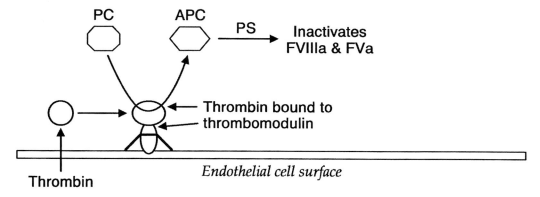

Fig. 1. Thrombomodulin, protein C (PC), and protein S (PS) anticoagulant system. Circulating thrombin binds to thrombomodulin and activates PC to activated PC (APC), which inactivates activated factors VIII and V (FVIIIa and FVa). PS is a cofactor.

naturally occurring anticoagulants (antithrombin, protein C, and protein C's cofactor protein S) break down (or inactivate) activated procoagulants, thus limiting excessive clot formation.

INTERACTION BETWEEN THE VASCULAR ENDOTHELIUM AND PLASMA ANTICOAGULANTS

Circulating thrombin, which is a procoagulant, binds to thrombomodulin, which is anchored to the endothelial cell surface (Fig. 1). Once bound, it loses its procoagulant function. In fact, while bound to thrombomodulin, it activates circulating protein C to activated protein C (APC). APC, in conjunction with its cofactor protein S, breaks down (inactivates) two procoagulants, factor Va and factor VIIIa, curtailing their procoagulant activity and preventing spontaneous and excessive clot formation (Fig. 2).

Deficiencies of the naturally occurring anticoagulants (protein C, protein S, and antithrombin) result in decreased anticoagulant activity. This results in a propensity toward venous thrombosis. It follows that if the procoagulant plasma clotting factors are in some way *resistant* to breakdown (or inactivation) by these anticoagulants, the result will be a tendency to thrombosis. In fact, factor V, which is a procoagulant, recently has been recognized to be resistant to inactivation by protein C in a subset of patients with venous thrombosis.

A discussion of thrombotic disorders traditionally has focused on congenital disorders that predispose to thrombosis. Although multiple acquired disorders predispose to thrombosis (Table 1), the interaction between congenital and acquired disorders was not emphasized until recently. Thus, in the presence of a congenital disorder that predisposes to thrombosis, the addition of an acquired risk factor compounds the risk and may lead to venous or arterial thrombosis.

CONGENITAL PREDISPOSITION FOR VENOUS THROMBOEMBOLISM

Until recently, a congenital predisposition to venous thrombosis was found in only up to 10% of patients. Since the description of the presence of APC resistance, a cause for venous thrombosis has been found in 20% to 50% of cases.

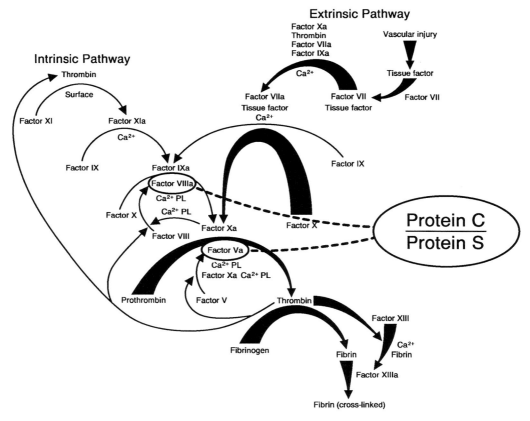

Fig. 2. Actions of protein C and protein S. a, activated factor; Ca²⁺, calcium; PL, phospholipid. (From Davie EW, Fujikawa K, Kisiel W. The coagulation cascade: initiation, maintenance, and regulation. *Biochemistry* 1991; 30: 10363-10370. By permission of the American Chemical Society.)

The most commonly recognized genetic abnormalities include the following:

1. Resistance to APC
2. Antithrombin deficiency
3. Protein C deficiency
4. Protein S deficiency
5. Prothrombin gene abnormality

Resistance to Activated Protein C (Activated Protein C Resistance, APCR)

DEFINITION

Activated factor V (Va), which is a procoagulant, is resistant to breakdown (inactivation) by APC (Fig. 1). This results in prolonged procoagulant activity of factor Va and leads to a propensity for thrombosis.

BIOCHEMISTRY

APC inactivates factor Va by cleavage at a specific amino acid (arginine) at position 506 in the factor V peptide (R506). A single-base change in the DNA results in a mutation of arginine to glutamine (R506Q). This results in a loss of the cleavage site for APC and prolonged procoagulant activity of factor Va.

Table 2
Prevalence of Inherited Coagulation Factor Abnormalities
in Patients With Venous Thromboembolism (VTE)

| | *Coagulation factor abnormality, %* | | | | |
	Protein C	*Protein S*	*Antithrombin*	*APC resistance*	*Factor II G20210A*
Healthy individuals	0.2–0.4	[a]	0.02	3–7	1–2.3
Unselected VTE[b]	3	1–2	1	20	6.2
Selected VTE[c]	1–9	1–13	0.5–7	52	18

[a]No data.
[b]Consecutive patients with VTE.
[c]Young patients, strong family history, recurrent VTE, unusual sites of VTE.
From Rosendaal FR. Risk factors for venous thrombosis: prevalence, risk, and interaction. Semin Hematol 1997; 34: 171-187. By permission of WB Saunders Company.

EPIDEMIOLOGY

APCR has a prevalence of approximately 5% to 7% in the white population. The prevalence of this abnormality is extremely low in Asian and African-American populations. Approximately 20% of consecutive patients with venous thromboembolism (VTE), and up to 50% of patients with recurrent VTE, a strong family history of VTE, or young patients with a VTE, have APCR (Table 2).

CLINICAL MANIFESTATIONS

Patients with APCR have a propensity for development of VTE, that is, deep vein thrombosis and pulmonary embolism. However, not all patients who have APCR develop VTE. Approximately 10% of patients with APCR will develop venous thrombosis during 10 years of follow-up, typically in association with other, acquired risk factors for venous thrombosis. The presence of this abnormality increases the risk of venous thrombosis in the presence of other congenital (such as antithrombin deficiency) or acquired (such as hyperhomocystinemia) risk factors.

Currently, there is no known association of APCR with arterial thrombosis.

DIAGNOSIS

An activated partial thromboplastin time (aPTT) test is performed with the patient's plasma. This is then repeated after addition of APC to the plasma. A ratio is then calculated:

$$(aPTT + APC)/aPTT$$

Because APC is an anticoagulant and curtails the procoagulant activity of factors V and VIII, the addition of APC to the patient's plasma should result in a prolongation of the aPTT. This represents the APCR ratio, which should be between 2.4 and 4.0. In the presence of APCR, the addition of APC does not result in the expected prolongation of the aPTT; it results in a lower ratio (< 2.4), which is indicative of the presence of APCR.

CAUTIONS

The APCR test is based on the aPTT; thus, an abnormally prolonged baseline aPTT precludes accurate interpretation of the APCR ratio. Common causes of a prolonged baseline aPTT include:

1. Heparin
2. Chronic oral anticoagulants
3. Lupus anticoagulant that results in prolonged aPTT
4. Clotting factor deficiencies that result in prolonged aPTT

In prolonged aPTT, one could wait until the aPTT normalizes (discontinue the use of heparin or warfarin) and then determine the APCR ratio. In a patient with lupus anticoagulant in whom the aPTT is prolonged and not likely to return to normal, a DNA test could be performed (see below). An alternative would be to mix the patient's plasma with factor V-deficient plasma, replenish the deficient clotting factors, and then perform the APCR test.

MANAGEMENT

Management of Acute Thrombosis

The presence of APCR does not affect the management of acute VTE. Standard recommended anticoagulant regimens should be followed.

Long-Term Management of Venous Thromboembolism

The presence of this abnormality predicts a significant risk of recurrent VTE, once the anticoagulation is discontinued. Thus, the presence of APCR may affect the duration of oral anticoagulation after the acute event. Patients with APCR do not need a higher-than-recommended target international normalized ratio (INR) for oral anticoagulation.

Management of Asymptomatic Family Members

Because APCR is a genetic disorder, there is a chance that family members of patients with APCR also have this abnormality. The most important aspect in the management of VTE is counseling a patient's asymptomatic family members regarding the pros and cons of testing for abnormalities that predispose to VTE. The disadvantage of testing asymptomatic family members is that they may have difficulty obtaining health and life insurance in the future. The advantages to testing include obtaining information about a patient's risk factors for VTE and thus consideration of intense thromboprophylaxis in high-risk situations, such as an orthopedic operation (Table 1).

It is essential to note that although having APCR puts one at increased risk for spontaneous VTE, currently we do not treat *asymptomatic* family members with oral anticoagulation.

Antithrombin Deficiency

DEFINITION

Antithrombin (AT, formerly called antithrombin III) is a serine protease anticoagulant. AT deficiency results in a propensity for VTE.

BIOCHEMISTRY

Thrombin is inactivated by AT when bound to it. This reaction is accelerated approximately 1,000-fold in the presence of heparin. This interaction forms the basis of the AT activity of heparin. AT also inactivates other clotting factors (Fig. 3).

EPIDEMIOLOGY

There are currently no known ethnic differences in the prevalence of AT deficiency. Its prevalences in the general population and in patients with VTE are shown in Table 2.

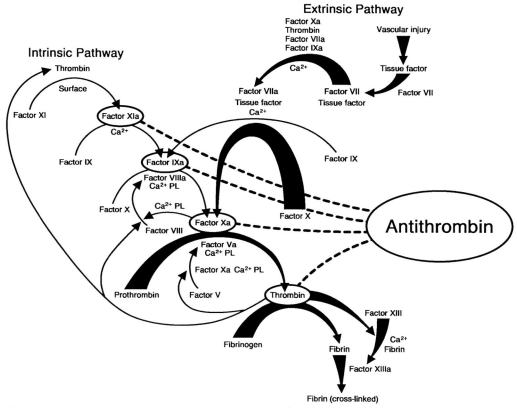

Fig. 3. Actions of antithrombin. a, activated factor; Ca^{2+}, calcium; PL, phospholipid. (From Davie EW, Fujikawa K, Kisiel W. The coagulation cascade: initiation, maintenance, and regulation. *Biochemistry* 1991; 30: 10363-10370. By permission of the American Chemical Society.)

CLINICAL MANIFESTATIONS

AT deficiency predisposes patients to VTE. The risk for venous thrombosis in AT-deficient patients is thought to be higher than the risk in patients with protein C and protein S deficiencies. Although there are occasional cases of arterial thrombosis in patients with AT deficiency, its role in the pathogenesis of arterial thrombi is unclear.

More than half of patients known to be AT deficient develop symptomatic VTE over their lifetimes and most of them will have their first VTE before 30 years of age. Approximately half of the events are spontaneous, and the rest are associated with a second (acquired) risk factor (Table 1). In patients in whom VTE does develop, the risk of recurrence is significantly increased once the anticoagulant regimen is discontinued.

CLASSIFICATION

1. Quantitative deficiency (type I)
   Decrease in both the AT activity and the antigen
2. Qualitative deficiency (type II)
   Normal AT antigen but decreased AT activity. Type II AT deficiency is a result of production of a functionally defective AT molecule

DIAGNOSIS

The AT activity assay is performed first. If it is low, then an AT antigen can be measured to further classify the deficiency state.

CAUTIONS

Neonates are born with approximately 50% the adult level of AT. Low AT levels can be due to a congenital deficiency; however, there are certain acquired causes of AT deficiency:

1. Liver disease: because AT is produced in the liver, abnormalities of liver function can lead to decreased AT levels
2. Acute thrombosis: the presence of acute thrombosis results in a decrease in circulating AT levels. Presumably this is due to its binding to thrombin that is generated during acute thrombosis.
3. Heparin therapy: this results in increased clearance of the AT
4. Nephrotic syndrome: AT is excreted in the urine in patients with nephrotic syndrome
5. L-Asparaginase therapy
6. Use of estrogen
7. Disseminated intravascular coagulation: AT is consumed in patients with this disorder
8. Postoperative patients
9. Inflammatory bowel disease and protein-losing enteropathy

AT is not a vitamin K-dependent protein, and thus warfarin use does not result in a decreased AT level. On the contrary, it results in a mild increase in the AT level through unknown mechanisms. This increase in the AT level is thought not to be significant enough to obscure a diagnosis of AT deficiency. Although a normal AT level is a reliable indicator of the absence of AT deficiency, a low AT level should be rechecked once acquired causes for decreased levels of AT are eliminated.

MANAGEMENT

Management of Acute Thrombosis

Because the main action of heparin involves its interaction with AT, AT deficiency can lead to "heparin resistance." Thus, despite therapy with large doses of intravenous unfractionated (standard) heparin, a therapeutic aPTT is difficult to achieve. One could consider replacement therapy with AT concentrate. Low-molecular-weight heparins reportedly do not prolong the aPTT. Because the doses are weight-adjusted, monitoring is not required. However, when used in patients with AT deficiency, monitoring peak and trough anti-factor Xa levels provides an indication of its therapeutic efficacy.

Long-Term Management of Venous Thromboembolism

AT deficiency increases the risk of recurrence of VTE. Thus, the duration of long-term anticoagulation needs to be modified based on the presence of this and other risk factors Indefinite anticoagulation should be considered in patients with idiopathic VTE. AT deficiency does not adversely influence the action of oral anticoagulants.

CLINICALLY RELEVANT GENETICS

The gene for AT is located on chromosome 1. Thus, it is transmitted as an autosomal dominant trait and affects both sexes equally.

Protein C Deficiency

DEFINITION

Protein C is a vitamin K-dependent serine protease anticoagulant. Its deficiency predisposes patients to VTE.

BIOCHEMISTRY

The activation and subsequent actions of protein C (PC) are outlined in Figure 1. Thrombin cleaves PC, activating it to activated PC (APC). This reaction is accelerated by the binding of thrombin to thrombomodulin. APC, in conjunction with its cofactor protein S, then inactivates factors Va and VIIIa. Quantitative and qualitative abnormalities of PC can lead to VTE disorders.

EPIDEMIOLOGY

There is no known ethnic predisposition to PC deficiency. The prevalence of PC deficiency in the general population, in consecutive patients with VTE, and in selected patients with VTE is shown in Table 2.

CLINICAL MANIFESTATIONS

Deficiency of PC leads to a propensity to develop venous thrombosis. Approximately half of patients with PC deficiency have venous thrombosis by age 40. In the large majority (about 70%) of these symptomatic patients, the initial event occurs spontaneously. The remaining patients usually have a second identifiable acquired risk factor (Table 1). The most common sites of thrombosis are the large veins of the lower extremities and the lungs. Mesenteric venous thrombosis is less common. Superficial thrombophlebitis and ischemic cerebrovascular accidents also have been reported.

The most serious clinical manifestation of PC deficiency occurs in patients with severe deficiency (< 1% PC activity). Neonates born with extremely low or undetectable PC have widespread subcutaneous thrombosis (purpura fulminans). This condition warrants immediate recognition because it can be fatal if not treated rapidly (see below).

CLASSIFICATION

1. Quantitative deficiency (type I): decrease in both PC antigen and activity
2. Qualitative deficiency: decrease in PC activity with a normal PC antigen. This occurs as a result of production of a functionally abnormal PC molecule

DIAGNOSIS

Protein C activity is measured first. If it is low, then the PC antigen could be measured to accurately classify the deficiency state.

CAUTIONS

Healthy neonates have PC levels that are 20% to 40% of adult levels. In addition to congenital causes of PC deficiency, a few acquired conditions can result in decreased PC levels:

1. Liver disease: the liver is the site of production of PC
2. Use of oral anticoagulants: PC is a vitamin K-dependent protein. Thus, oral anticoagulants decrease its activity
3. Disseminated intravascular coagulation: PC is consumed in this disorder
4. Use of heparin
5. Use of oral contraceptives
6. L-Asparaginase therapy

MANAGEMENT

Management of Acute Thrombosis

Special precautions are taken when patients with PC deficiency in whom thrombosis develops need anticoagulation. Initial therapy with heparin should be administered in the standard fashion. When oral anticoagulants are initiated, loading doses should be avoided, and heparin should be continued for at least 4 to 5 days after a therapeutic international normalized ratio (INR) is achieved.

Oral anticoagulants deplete the vitamin K-dependent proteins (factors II, VII, IX, X, protein C, and protein S). The half-lives of factor VII and PC are the shortest; thus, their levels in plasma decrease most rapidly, compared with factor II, which has the longest half-life.

If a patient has a baseline PC of approximately 50%, it will be rapidly depleted, resulting in a relative excess of circulating procoagulant (factor II), which results in coumarin-induced skin necrosis, possible extension of clots, or possibly pulmonary emboli.

Long-Term Management of Venous Thromboembolism

Recurrent VTE often occurs in patients with PC deficiency when anticoagulation is discontinued. Thus, consideration of indefinite therapy with oral anticoagulants should be considered. It is crucial to remember that PC-deficient patients will always be at risk for coumarin-induced skin necrosis each time use of their oral anticoagulant is temporarily discontinued. When this step needs to be taken in anticipation of a surgical procedure, heparin therapy should be resumed, when safe, before starting therapy with warfarin and should be continued until the INR is therapeutic and maintained for approximately 4 to 5 days. Currently, PC concentrates are not available for commercial use. When available in the future, they could be used to prevent recurrent VTE in the surgical setting.

Protein S Deficiency

DEFINITION

Protein S (PS) is a vitamin K-dependent glycoprotein. Its deficiency can predispose to VTE.

BIOCHEMISTRY

APC inactivates factors Va and VIIIa. PS acts as a cofactor (Fig. 1). Approximately 60% of PS circulates bound to C4b binding protein, and the balance circulates in free form. It is the latter form that is functional.

CLINICAL MANIFESTATIONS

VTE is the most common manifestation of PS deficiency. Approximately 50% of PS-deficient patients have a thrombotic event by age 45 years. As in PC deficiency, venous thrombosis is common, but peripheral arterial thrombosis has been reported.

CLASSIFICATION

The exact clinically useful classification of PS deficiency is debated.

1. Type I: decreased total and free PS antigen and PS activity
2. Type II: normal total and free PS antigen, but decreased PS activity
3. Type III: normal total PS antigen and decreased free PS antigen and PS activity

DIAGNOSIS

The total and free PS antigen and PS activity are assayed. The PS activity assay is difficult to perform, and if the results are low the assay should be repeated to confirm the diagnosis.

CAUTIONS

In addition to congenital deficiencies, certain acquired conditions can result in PS deficiencies:

1. Liver disease
2. Use of oral anticoagulants
3. Pregnancy
4. Use of oral contraceptives
5. Acute thrombosis
6. L-Asparaginase therapy

C4b-binding protein is an acute-phase reactant; thus, acute or chronic inflammation leads to an increase of the total PS antigen. PS activity assay is fastidious to perform; thus, abnormal results need to be interpreted with caution.

MANAGEMENT

Management of Acute Thrombosis

Patients with PS deficiency, like patients with PC deficiency, are prone to coumarin-induced skin necrosis. Thus, similar precautions should be taken, overlapping the heparin and warfarin therapy for at least 4 to 5 days when the INR is therapeutic.

Long-Term Management of Venous Thromboembolism

Patients with PS deficiency are prone to recurrent thromboembolic events once the use of warfarin is discontinued. Thus, consideration should be given to long-term anticoagulation in the right clinical setting.

Prothrombin Gene Abnormality (Factor II G20210A)

DEFINITION

A mutation in the prothrombin gene at position 20210, which results in a single-base change of a guanine to an adenine, confers an increased risk for VTE.

BIOCHEMISTRY

The mechanism for this increased risk is unclear, but it is thought that this abnormality results in an increased plasma level of thrombin (factor II).

EPIDEMIOLOGY

This mutation is present in approximately 2% of the white population. It appears to be more prevalent in the southern than the northern European population. It is rare in people of African and Asian descent. The prevalence of this abnormality in patients with venous thrombosis is shown in Table 2.

CLINICAL MANIFESTATIONS

Patients who possess this mutation have an increased propensity for development of VTE. The presence of this mutation in addition to other congenital and acquired risk factors for thrombosis likely results in an increased risk for thrombosis.

DIAGNOSIS

Although the average factor II levels in patients with II G20210A mutation is higher than in patients without this mutation, this is not a reliable indicator for the individual patient because the normal range for factor II is large. Thus, the only reliable diagnostic test is the DNA test to detect the mutation.

MANAGEMENT

Management of Acute Thrombosis

The presence of factor II G20210A does not affect management of acute thrombosis. Patients should be treated in the standard fashion with heparin followed by warfarin.

Long-Term Management of Venous Thromboembolism

The presence of this mutation may, in fact, predispose patients to recurrent VTE once the patient is not taking oral anticoagulants. Thus, knowledge of the presence of this mutation influences the duration of anticoagulation.

ACQUIRED THROMBOPHILIC DISORDERS

Antiphospholipid Antibody Syndromes (Lupus Anticoagulant, Anticardiolipin Antibody)

DEFINITION

Lupus anticoagulant and the cardiolipin antibody are considered two members of a family of antiphospholipid antibodies. The presence of these antibodies predisposes patients to venous or arterial thromboembolism.

Multisystem manifestations (outlined below) in the presence of antiphospholipid antibodies are termed the antiphospholipid antibody syndrome. Common associations of the antiphospholipid antibody syndrome include the following:

1. Venous or arterial thromboembolism
2. Obstetric
   Sequential recurrent spontaneous abortions in the late first or early second trimester
3. Hematologic
   Thrombocytopenia
   Hemolysis
4. Neurologic
   Strokes
5. Dermatologic
   Livedo reticularis
6. Cardiac
   Libman-Sacks endocarditis

BIOCHEMISTRY

Antiphospholipid Antibodies

These are IgG or IgM antibodies that interfere with in vitro phospholipid-dependent coagulation reactions. Activation of protein C and its action on factors VIIIa and Va are phospholipid-dependent; thus, interference of this reaction may lead to a prothrombotic state. Other mechnisms for the prothrombotic state include activation of platelets, interference with antithrombin activity, and interaction with other anticoagulants such as β_2-glycoprotein I.

CLINICAL MANIFESTATIONS

Antiphospholipid antibodies may be found in a significant number of patients with connective tissue disease, yet not all patients will have thrombotic complications. Antiphospholipid antibodies develop in many patients who have no underlying cause (idiopathic). Medications such as procainamide can result in formation of antiphospholipid antibodies. In children and occasionally adults, infections can lead to temporary formation of antibodies. Sites of thrombosis may be venous or arterial. Other systemic manifestations are outlined above.

DIAGNOSIS

Antiphospholipid antibodies are a heterogeneous group of antibodies that initially were thought to be directed solely against phospholipid. They are now known to be directed against proteins and protein-phospholipid complexes. The diversity of antigens against which they are directed has been recognized only recently. The currently available diagnostic tests recognize a subset of antibodies.

Lupus Anticoagulant

These antibodies are directed against phospholipid and thus interfere with phospholipid-based assays. Typically, the aPTT is prolonged, and mixing studies with normal plasma does not result in correction of the aPTT to the normal range. Additional phospholipid is added to the aPTT system in the form of platelets (platelet neutralization procedure) or exogenous phospholipid (dilute Russell viper venom time), which should result in a correction of the aPTT by 5 seconds or more.

Anticardiolipin Antibodies

Anticardiolipin antibodies (IgG and IgM) are a subset of antibodies that may be found in the antiphospholipid antibody syndrome or in asymptomatic patients. They are directed against cardiolipin and are detected by performing enzyme-linked immunosorbent assay. Although these antibodies are pathophysiologically different from lupus anticoagulants, they may be found concomitantly in patients with antiphospholipid antibody syndrome. In fact, patients may have the anticardiolipin antibody or lupus anticoagulant, both anticoagulants, or neither one and experience thromboembolic events.

CAUTIONS

A normal aPTT does *not* exclude the presence of a lupus anticoagulant.

MANAGEMENT

Routine anticoagulation in patients who have the antiphospholipid antibody and have *not* had any thromboembolic events is not routinely recommended.

Management of Acute Thrombosis

In the presence of a prolonged baseline aPTT, caused by the presence of a lupus anticoagulant, heparin levels can be monitored, because the aPTT will not be reliable for monitoring therapy with unfractionated intravenous heparin. The use of low-molecular-weight heparin obviates monitoring during the acute phase of therapy for VTE.

Long-Term Management of Venous Thromboembolism

Patients with lupus anticoagulants and anticardiolipin antibodies have an increased risk for recurrent thromboembolism. Recurrent events usually occur in the same systemic vascular distribution as the original event, that is, a venous event usually follows a venous event and an arterial event usually follows an arterial event. Thus, the seriousness of the initial event and the presence of other risk factors for thromboembolism dictate the duration of anticoagulation.

Intravascular Coagulation and Fibrinolysis
(Disseminated Intravascular Coagulation)

DEFINITION

Intravascular coagulation and fibrinolysis (ICF), or disseminated intravascular coagulation (DIC) as it is commonly referred to, is a complex disorder that occurs in defined clinical situations. A hallmark of the disorder is diffuse intravascular coagulation resulting in consumption of plasma procoagulants and anticoagulants and activation of the fibrinolytic system resulting in both thrombotic and hemorrhagic complications.

ETIOLOGY

The cause of ICF is varied and multisystemic:

1. Malignancy
   Disseminated malignancy
   Acute leukemia, especially promyelocytic leukemia
2. Infection
   Gram-negative sepsis
   Other overwhelming infections (viral and bacterial)
3. Obstetric
   Amniotic fluid embolism
   Abruptio placentae
   Eclampsia
   Retained dead fetus
4. Transfusion-related complications
   Hemolytic transfusion reactions
5. Burns
6. Crush injury/trauma
7. Hepatocellular disorders
   Acute hepatocellular injury
   Chronic liver disease

PATHOPHYSIOLOGY

The initiating event in ICF can range from release of procoagulant proteins from malignant cells to activation of the coagulation system by endotoxin. Whatever the stimulus, excess thrombin is generated. This leads to simultaneous activation of the coagulation and fibrinolytic systems (Fig. 4).

Thrombin cleaves fibrinogen to generate fibrin monomers, which, in the normal course of events, are stabilized by factor XIII, forming a stable fibrin clot. Activation of the fibrinolytic system leads to generation of plasmin, which cleaves fibrinogen into degradation products X, Y, D, and E. The fibrin degradation products also form complexes with platelets, resulting in platelet dysfunction. The fibrin degradation products can form complexes with fibrin monomers before stabilization by factor XIII, resulting in soluble fibrin monomers and unstable fibrin clots. The excess plasmin also breaks down the stable fibrin clots to fibrin degradation products (D-dimers). Thus, there is ongoing intravascular thrombosis and simultaneous fibrinolysis, resulting in consumption of coagulation factors, thrombocytopenia, and bleeding.

DIAGNOSIS

Both the clinical and the laboratory findings need to be considered when establishing a diagnosis of ICF. In the appropriate clinical setting in a patient who is bleeding and has

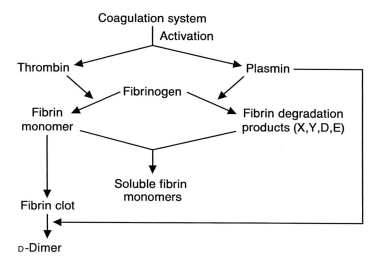

Fig. 4. Pathophysiology of intravascular coagulation and fibrinolysis. (Modified from Bick RL. Disseminated intravascular coagulation: pathophysiological mechanisms and manifestations. *Semin Thromb Hemostas* 1998; 24: 3-18. By permission of Thieme Medical Publishers.)

evidence of thrombosis, ICF should be considered. Laboratory findings include thrombocytopenia, prolonged clotting times (prothrombin time, aPTT), low fibrinogen level, increased D-dimer value, and the presence of circulating soluble fibrin monomer complexes. Specific procoagulant factors and anticoagulant activity levels are decreased, reflecting ongoing consumption.

THERAPY

Treatment of ICF is directed toward supportive care of the patient and replenishment of the coagulant and anticoagulant factors with plasma, cryoprecipitate, and platelet concentrates while the underlying cause is diagnosed and appropriately treated.

DISORDERS THAT MAY BE INHERITED OR ACQUIRED
Hyperhomocystinemia

DEFINITION

Homocysteine is a sulphur-containing amino acid that is formed during the metabolism of methionine. Although it is not a part of the coagulation system, increased levels of homocysteine have been implicated in venous thrombosis.

BIOCHEMISTRY

Homocysteine is formed during metabolism of methionine. It is further "recycled" via the remethylation cycle to generate methionine (Fig. 5). This consists of enzymatic remethylation to methionine, for which vitamin B_{12} is a cofactor. The methyl group donor is generated from 5,10-methylenetetrahydrofolate, which requires folic acid and the enzyme 5,10-methylenetetrahydrofolate reductase.

Homocysteine enters the transsulfuration pathway to generate cysteine or if an excess of homocysteine overwhelms the remethylation pathway. Abnormalities in the remethylation or transsulfuration pathway can lead to accumulation of homocysteine.

The exact mechanism by which homocystinemia leads to venous thrombosis is being studied; however, among other actions it has been shown to alter the antithrombotic

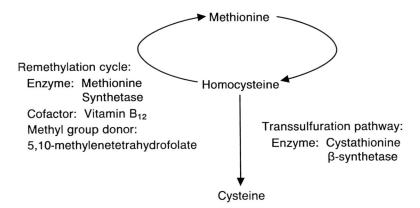

Fig. 5. Homocysteine metabolism.

properties of the endothelium by inhibiting the expression of thrombomodulin and thus affecting the anticoagulant actions of protein C.

CLINICAL MANIFESTATIONS

The presence of hyperhomocystinemia increases the risk for thrombosis and adds to the risk of thrombosis in the presence of other risk factors (Table 1).

DIAGNOSIS

Fasting homocysteine levels can be assayed in specialized laboratories.

ETIOLOGY

Plasma levels of homocysteine are increased in nutritional deficiencies of vitamin B_{12}, folic acid, vitamin B_6, renal insufficiency, and hypothyroidism.

GENETIC DEFECTS

Cystathionine β-synthetase is an essential enzyme for the transsulfuration pathway. Severe (homozygous) deficiency of this enzyme leads to severe hyperhomocystinemia with premature atherothrombotic complications. Other clinical manifestations include mental retardation, ectopia lentis, skeletal deformities, and premature atherosclerosis.

Milder (heterozygous) deficiency of cystathionine β-synthetase results in milder clinical manifestations.

Homozygous deficiency of 5,10-methylenetetrahydrofolate reductase (remethylation pathway) results in marked hyperhomocystinemia and resulting atherothrombosis. A variant of 5,10-methylenetetrahydrofolate reductase, called the thermolabile variant, is due to a mutation, C677T, which results in a substitution of valine to alanine. When present in the homozygous state, this leads to an exaggerated increase in plasma homocysteine levels when the patient is deficient in vitamins B_{12} and B_6 and folic acid. This may lead to an increased risk for VTE.

CAUTIONS

Fasting homocysteine levels may be normal, and a methionine-loaded test may need to be performed to unmask homocystinemia.

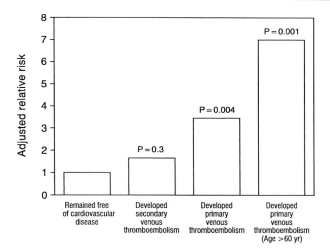

Fig. 6. Adjusted relative risk for future venous thromboembolism among apparently healthy men with factor V Leiden mutation. (From Price DT, Ridker PM. Factor V Leiden mutation and the risks for thromboembolic disease: a clinical perspective. *Ann Intern Med* 1997; 127: 895-909. By permission of the American College of Physicians.)

MANAGEMENT

Management of Acute Thrombosis

Treatment of acute thrombosis should not be affected by the presence of increased plasma homocysteine levels. Standard anticoagulation therapy with heparin and warfarin should be used.

Long-Term Management of Venous Thromboembolism

The presence of homocystinemia likely increases the risk for recurrent VTE. Thus, acquired causes of hyperhomocystinemia should be pursued, with replenishment of the appropriate vitamin as indicated.

INTERACTION OF ACQUIRED AND INHERITED RISK FACTORS FOR VENOUS THROMBOEMBOLISM

Inherited risk factors for venous thrombosis, such as the presence of activated protein C resistance (APCR), are prevalent among the general population (Table 2). Yet not all patients with these abnormalities develop venous thrombosis. Figure 6 demonstrates the relative risk for development of VTE in a group of men known to have the mutation responsible for APCR, factor V Leiden.

The combination of an inherited risk factor for VTE and an acquired risk factor results in a marked increase in the risk for VTE (Figs. 7 and 8). Thus, venous thrombosis is a multifactorial disorder with defined inherited and acquired risk factors that, if combined, result in an increased relative risk for thromboembolism.

MANAGEMENT OF VENOUS THROMBOSIS

The majority (approximately 85%) of deep vein thrombosis occurs in proximal veins (popliteal and femoral), and the remainder occurs in the distal (calf) veins. Venous

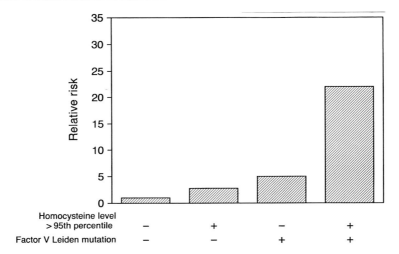

Fig. 7. Interrelationships of factor V Leiden mutation and hyperhomocystinemia. (From Price DT, Ridker PM. Factor V Leiden mutation and the risks for thromboembolic disease: a clinical perspective. *Ann Intern Med* 1997; 127: 895-909. By permission of the American College of Physicians.)

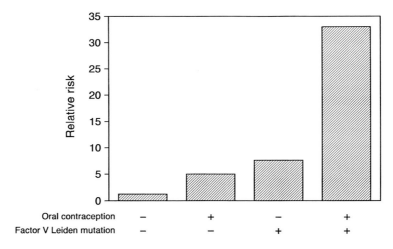

Fig. 8. Interrelationships of factor V Leiden mutation and use of oral contraceptives. (From Price DT, Ridker PM. Factor V Leiden mutation and the risks for thromboembolic disease: a clinical perspective. *Ann Intern Med* 1997; 127: 895-909. By permission of the American College of Physicians.)

ultrasound examination is reliable for accurately diagnosing proximal venous thrombosis, but it is less reliable for calf vein thrombosis. Thus, a negative ultrasound examination of the calf veins in a patient with suspected calf vein thrombus should prompt a repeat ultrasound in 1 week to detect progression of the calf vein into more proximal veins. Alternatives such as venography are more accurate, but the potential side effects and cost preclude its routine use in the diagnosis of venous thrombosis. Initial management of venous thrombosis consists of objectively establishing its presence. Clinical diagnosis of venous thrombosis is notoriously inaccurate; thus, a clinical impression of venous thrombosis should be confirmed with objective radiologic investigations.

Unless there are contraindications to anticoagulation (active hemorrhage, recent neurosurgery, or severe thrombocytopenia), therapy with intravenous unfractionated heparin (UFH) should be initiated as soon as the diagnosis is established. Recent randomized trials suggest that subcutaneous therapy with low-molecular-weight heparin on an outpatient basis in selected patients is as safe and likely more cost-effective than intravenous heparin. For hemodynamically significant pulmonary embolism, thrombolytic therapy or pulmonary thrombectomy may be indicated.

Intravenous UFH is currently the standard therapy for venous thrombosis. Given its large size and nonspecific protein binding, a bolus of 5,000 units of UFH is initially administered, followed by a continuous infusion of approximately 1,200 units per hour. Therapy with UFH is monitored with the aPTT. The aPTT should be checked 4 to 6 hours after initiation and each change in dose of UFH. The dose of heparin infusion is adjusted to achieve a therapeutic aPTT of 1.5 times control. Extension of the thrombus and the recurrence rate of venous thrombosis are increased in patients not achieving a therapeutic aPTT within 24 hours of initiation of heparin. Oral anticoagulant therapy can be initiated on the second day of therapy with heparin and is monitored with the international normalized ratio (INR). The heparin therapy can be discontinued when the INR is therapeutic for at least 2 days, which typically takes 5 to 7 days, and this interval ensures that the antithrombotic effect of oral anticoagulant (reduction of prothrombin) has occurred.

The aim of oral anticoagulation after initial therapy with heparin is to decrease the risk of recurrence of the venous thrombosis. Given the inconvenience of long-term administration of intravenous or subcutaneous heparin, oral anticoagulation is the method of choice. There appears to be no benefit to giving large "loading" doses of oral anticoagulants in the initial management of venous thrombosis. A dose of 5 mg daily with appropriate changes based on the INR is a reasonable approach. The target INR is typically between 2 and 3. The duration of anticoagulation varies with the clinical situation and is tempered by the presence or absence of risk factors (temporary or permanent). With isolated distal (calf vein) thrombosis, short-term therapy (6 to 8 weeks) may be reasonable. For patients with proximal venous thrombosis, in the absence of persistent risk factors, up to 6 months of oral anticoagulation may be appropriate. For patients with permanent (genetic or acquired) risk factors, consideration should be given to indefinite anticoagulation.

VI MISCELLANEOUS TOPICS IN HEMATOLOGY

23

Transfusion Medicine: Practical Issues

S. Breanndan Moore, MD

Contents

INTRODUCTION

The name change from "blood bank" to "transfusion medicine" has been implemented in many institutions (especially those that are hospital-based) to reflect the broadening scope of activities now included in the repertoire of such entities. Twenty-five years ago, blood banks recruited blood donors, collected and separated their blood into a handful of components, and performed a few simple tests on patients and donors, such as ABO/Rh typing, red cell crossmatching, and Coombs (antiglobulin) testing. Collected blood also was tested for hepatitis B surface antigen and for evidence of syphilis exposure. Currently, departments of transfusion medicine collect blood and other products from a much broader spectrum of donors, fractionate it into many more components, test each donation for a broad range of potentially transmissible agents, and perform many more direct services for patients such as therapeutic apheresis, intraoperative blood salvage, and histocompatibility testing and matching for bone marrow, stem cells, and solid organ transplants. In addition, many establishments are already involved in the manipulation of stem cell populations, and some are beginning to extend those manipulations to include gene transfection and gene therapy. To avail of these services for one's patients, it behooves the clinician to investigate the "repertoire" of his or her hospital's transfusion medicine department and, if it does not collect blood, the range of services provided by the institution's chief blood supplier.

TRANSFUSION MEDICINE SERVICES

Therapeutic Apheresis

In many settings, this service is provided by the "blood bank." Therapeutic apheresis is divided into two main categories: cytapheresis (removal of cells) and plasmapheresis (removal of plasma). Indications for cytapheresis include treatment of the blast-crisis phase of chronic myelogenous leukemia, in which extremely increased counts of peripheral white

From: *Primary Hematology*
Edited by: A. Tefferi © Mayo Foundation for Medical Education and Research, Rochester, MN

blood cells are associated with so-called white cell infarcts of the brain. One to two exchanges during about 2 hours usually promptly reduce the peripheral leukocyte count by about 50%, thereby reducing the risks while medications such as hydroxyurea begin to take effect. Similarly, cytapheresis can dramatically halve the greatly elevated platelet count in patients with essential thrombocytosis or polycythemia vera. Photopheresis, a form of cytapheresis, uses psoralens and ultraviolet light to extracorporeally treat white cells of patients with mycosis fungoides or Sézary syndrome.

Therapeutic plasma exchange is indicated for several neurologic disorders such as acute Guillain-Barré syndrome, myasthenia gravis, and chronic inflammatory demyelinating polyradiculoneuropathy. The role that plasma exchange plays varies with the disease and its particular stage or rate of progression. Plasma exchange also is used in the treatment of thrombotic thrombocytopenic purpura, in which it is associated with dramatic responses in many cases. Plasma exchange also has been used with considerably less success in cases of platelet alloimmunization with refractoriness. However, it has been very effective in the treatment of rapidly progressive glomerulonephritis, Goodpasture's syndrome, and hyperviscosity syndromes associated with ultrahigh immunoglobulin levels in myeloma and related disorders.

Intraoperative Blood Salvage

The ability to collect, process, and reinfuse a patient's own red blood cells during operation was revolutionized by the development of devices which could process a unit of blood (approximately 450 mL) in a few minutes. This method of blood conservation is particularly useful when blood loss is potentially copious, such as during cardiac and liver operations. We and others have used this method with success in liver transplantation. This method is contraindicated in cases of known or suspected bacterial contamination of the operative site (such as bowel operation) or in cases in which malignant cells are likely to be shed into the blood being aspirated for processing. In a recent year at our institution, 17% of all red cell units transfused were operatively salvaged. This represents a considerable reduction in allogeneic red cell requirements and in donor exposures. In some elective orthopedic procedures, 86% of patients received solely autologous blood (preoperative and intraoperative collection).

Transfusion of Blood Products

Frequently Used Transfusion Products

• **Packed red cells**: Donor blood is collected by an aseptic method in which citrate is used as an anticoagulant and adenine as a preservative. The whole blood is then centrifuged and the plasma separated. Blood is stored at 4° to 6°C for up to 42 days.

• **Platelets**: Slow centrifugation allows separation of platelets, providing a unit of platelets from 1 donor unit of blood. Transfusion of 1 unit results in an increase in platelets of 5,000 to 10,000/μL. Usually, 4 to 6 units are required for a session of platelet transfusion. Currently, platelets can be stored for 5 days.

• **Fresh frozen plasma**: This is rapidly frozen plasma separated from fresh blood and stored at less than −30°C. The frozen plasma from 1 donation of whole blood is about 200 mL.

• **Cryoprecipitate**: A bag of cryoprecipitate contains a few milliliters (10 to 20 mL) of cold insoluble material remaining after slow thawing (at 4°C) of a bag of single-donor fresh frozen plasma, and each bag contains 80 to 100 units of factor VIII

---

and 150 to 250 mg of fibrinogen. It also contains adequate levels of von Willebrand factor and factor XIII.

• **Factor VIII concentrates**: These are prepared from plasma (cryoprecipitation followed by further purification by precipitating agents) pooled from thousands of donors.

• **Recombinant factor VIII:** This is prepared by DNA methods and not from donor plasma. Therefore, it is not associated with a risk of viral transmission.

RED BLOOD CELLS

The indications for this product are well established, but the "transfusion trigger" hemoglobin has undergone considerable change in recent years. It is now generally accepted that most patients tolerate a hemoglobin level of 7 to 8 g/dL quite well unless certain other factors are at play. These factors include the rate at which anemia developed (chronic anemia is tolerated much better than acute blood loss) and the age, cardiac, cerebrovascular, and pulmonary status of the patient. Each case must be evaluated individually, but current institutional transfusion audits tend to set the unquestioned hemoglobin "trigger" at 7 to 8 g/dL. In other words, transfusions at hemoglobin levels higher than this are evaluated for appropriateness. In the average 70-kg recipient who is hemodynamically stable, 1 unit of red blood cells increases the hemoglobin value by approximately 1 g/dL. Smaller or larger patients have inversely proportionate changes. Red blood cells can be modified to fit certain clinical needs. Leuko-reduced red blood cells (that is, $< 5 \times 10^6$ white blood cells/unit) reduce the incidence of alloimmunization in patients likely to receive multiple transfusions, such as those with hematologic malignancies. They also reduce the incidence of febrile reactions, and a preponderance of data indicate that they can be considered highly unlikely to transmit cytomegalovirus (i.e., are generally considered to be "cytomegalovirus-safe").

Red blood cells can be frozen in glycerol for long-term storage (up to 10 years). This method is extremely costly and somewhat unwieldy because each unit must be individually thawed and "deglycerolized" before it can be safely transfused. This thawing process takes about 1 hour and so is unsuitable for rapid or emergency use. The freeze/thaw process usually is reserved for units that have some particular medical value (such as negative for a high-frequency antigen or autologous units). Once a unit is thawed and washed clear of glycerol, it must be infused within 24 hours. Similarly, unfrozen RBC units can be mechanically washed to remove most of the plasma elements. Again, post-wash outdating is 24 hours. Such washing sometimes is used to prevent repeated severe allergic reactions. It also can be used to reduce IgA protein levels to acceptable levels (< 0.5 mg/dL) for patients who have anti-IgA and a history of anaphylactic transfusion reactions (see below).

Before transfusion of red blood cells, certain tests should have been completed. Naturally, no blood product should be made available for possible selection for a patient until all the standard donor tests have been completed and the results found acceptable. By mandate of the Food and Drug Administration, these tests must include the following:

• ABO/Rh typing and antibody screen
• Anti-HIV-I and II (human immunodeficiency virus)
• Anti-HCV (hepatitis C virus)
• Anti-HBc (hepatitis B core antigen)
• HBsAg (hepatitis B surface antigen)

- p24 Ag (p24 antigen)
- Anti-HTLV-I and II (human T-cell leukemia virus)
- Rapid plasma reagin (or similar test for syphilis)

In addition, under certain circumstances other tests may be considered reasonable, such as anti-cytomegalovirus or anti-*Trypanosoma cruzi* in certain geographic regions.

Hemolytic Transfusion Reaction

During red cell transfusion from a donor to a recipient, the major danger is hemolysis of donor red cells in the recipient, resulting in a potentially fatal *hemolytic transfusion reaction*. For this to be avoided, compatibility between donor red cell antigens and the plasma antibodies of the recipient must be ensured. Antibodies to red cell antigens may occur either naturally or after sensitization (because of previous blood transfusion or pregnancy). The red cell antigens responsible for hemolytic transfusion reactions are several and are classified into different red cell antigen systems (the "blood group systems"). These antigen systems differ in their immunogenic potential, and two of the most clinically important systems are the "*ABO antigen system*" and the "*Rh (rhesus) antigen system*." Examples of other clinically important antigen systems include Kell, Duffy, and Kidd, whereas Lewis system antibodies are extremely unlikely to cause hemolytic transfusion reactions.

ABO System

Approximately 85% of fatal hemolytic transfusion reactions involve ABO incompatibility. *Most of these events are due to clerical error.* The ABO system consists of three allelic genes at one genetic locus: A, B, and O. The A and B genes (which are codominant alleles), but not the O gene, produce specific enzymes responsible for the addition of single carbohydrate residues to a basic red cell surface glycoprotein called the H antigen, thus transforming it to an A or B antigen. This results in the red cell expression of the A, B, or H antigen, depending on the ABO gene constituency of the individual.

Accordingly, AA genes express A red cell antigens, BB genes express B antigens, and OO genes express H antigens. Similarly, AB genes express AB antigens, AO genes express A antigens, and BO genes express B antigens. Therefore, individuals can express the A, B, AB, or H antigens. *Accordingly, the ABO system consists of four blood groups: A, B, AB, and O.*

Humans have naturally occurring (without known stimulation by foreign red cells) plasma antibodies against the A (if they lack the A antigen) and B (if they lack the B antigen) antigens but not the H antigen. *Therefore, a person with blood group A has anti-B antibodies, blood group B has anti-A antibodies, blood group AB has no antibodies, and blood group O has both anti-A and anti-B antibodies.* The antibodies against the ABO antigens are usually IgM antibodies capable of fixing complement and causing intravascular hemolysis. Persons with blood type O usually also have IgG anti-A and anti-B, and type O mothers may have babies who have ABO hemolytic disease of the newborn. Most other red cell antibodies are formed only after stimulation by foreign red cells.

The most frequent blood group is O (in 79% of Native Americans, 49% of blacks, 45% of whites). The next most frequent blood group is A, and the least frequent is AB (in <1% of Native Americans and about 5% of the rest).

Rh System

The Rh system consists of allelic genes at three closely linked loci: Cc, Dd, and Ee. C, D, E expression results in the formation of the corresponding antigens C, D, and E. These antigens are absent in persons expressing c, d, and e who express the corresponding c and e antigens. The Rh genes are inherited in sets such as cde, CDe, and cDE. *The D antigen is the most immunogenic.* Antibodies to the Rh antigens do not occur naturally. However, they usually develop as a result of previous antigen exposure through blood transfusions or pregnancy. Anti-D has been responsible for most of the rhesus clinical problems, and a simple subdivision of subjects into Rh-D-positive and Rh-D-negative was sufficient for clinical purposes. Anti-D antibodies are of the IgG subclass and capable of transplacental passage. Prevention of pregnancy-related formation of anti-D has greatly decreased the problems caused by this antibody in both pregnancy and transfusion settings.

Type and Crossmatch

When red cell transfusion is contemplated, a small sample of blood is collected from the recipient to determine his or her blood group (*typing*) and to determine the donor blood product most suitable for the recipient (*crossmatching*). *ABO typing* is done by checking the recipient's red cells for agglutination by serum from type B and type A persons containing anti-A and anti-B antibodies, respectively. The results are confirmed by checking the ability of the recipient's serum to agglutinate known type A or B cells. *Rh typing* is performed by reacting the recipient's cells with anti-D serum, which should cause, in an Rh-positive person, agglutination in the presence of albumin.

After recipient typing for the ABO and Rh systems, red cells from the donor unit are tested against the recipient's serum to detect agglutination, which indicates incompatibility (crossmatching). Futhermore, the recipient's serum is screened for red cell antibodies. During this procedure, control red cells (not belonging to either the donor or the recipient) containing optimal combinations of desirable antigens are mixed with the recipient's serum to detect possible incompatibility. This procedure allows the avoidance of transfusions of red cells expressing the incompatible antigens.

The testing on the patient should include ABO/Rh typing, red blood cell antibody screen (and identification if positive), and crossmatching (see above for details). The crossmatching traditionally has been performed by reacting recipient serum against donor red blood cells in test tubes using different methods designed to detect various types of antibodies that might cause clinical hemolysis. The recent development of highly sensitive antibody screening methods has resulted in acceptance by the Food and Drug Administration of so-called computer crossmatching, whereby the computer checks that the patient and donor have been validly ABO/Rh typed, that the patient has a negative antibody screen and no history of previous antibodies, and that the blood units in question have been properly tested for all designated pathogens as well as ABO/Rh.

Full serologic crossmatching takes about 90 minutes from time of acquisition of a patient's blood sample to completion of the serologic compatibility testing. An abbreviated crossmatching (so-called first phase) can take about 45 minutes, but this may be less sensitive. In an emergency, when there is insufficient time for proper testing, type O Rh-negative units can be transfused with about 99% assurance that hemolytic reactions will not occur.

Computer crossmatching takes about 5 minutes when the patient's blood has already been determined to be negative for antibodies.

PLATELETS

The national trend in recent years has been an overall slight reduction in red cell transfusions, but the use of platelets continues to increase. Indications for platelets include thrombocytopenia and clinical settings associated with dysfunctional platelets. Although the consensus is that platelet transfusions should be used to maintain a circulating level of at least 10×10^9/L, there are several exceptions to this "trigger." These include chronic idiopathic thrombocytopenic purpura, in which patients often compensate and maintain hemostasis with a platelet count less than this level. In fact, platelet transfusions are usually contraindicated in these cases because they can initiate increased destruction of platelets (including the patient's own), resulting in a rebound worsening of the thrombocytopenia. For patients with hematologic malignancies complicated by fever, sepsis, hypertension, or headache, a level of 20×10^9/L should be maintained. Similarly, a level of 50×10^9/L should be attained before operation and 100×10^9/L before neurosurgical procedures. For patients who are actively bleeding, the target level should be that at which the patient seems to maintain normal hemostasis (that is, does not bleed). Although several clinical factors influence responses to platelets, one expects each unit of platelet concentrate (from 1 unit of donated whole blood) to increase the peripheral count (1 hour after transfusion) by approximately 7.5×10^9/L. The factors recognized as causes of refractoriness to platelets (that is, unexpectedly low increments) include the following:

- Sepsis or fever
- Splenomegaly
- Bleeding
- Diffuse intravascular coagulation
- Recent bone marrow transplantation
- Alloimmunization to HLA
- Inadequate "dose"
- Certain antimicrobial agents

Only one of these—alloimmunization—is an indication for HLA-matched platelets obtained by apheresis. Platelets obtained by apheresis are more expensive and are not intrinsically superior to random platelet concentrate except when HLA matching is necessary. Alloimmunization can be assessed by various lymphocytotoxicity and solid-phase techniques, and it is strongly recommended that this testing be performed before embarking on a course of expensive HLA-matched platelets in order to establish a rational basis for the use of this product.

Platelets are obtained from two sources:

1. From donations of whole blood, from which the platelets are separated from the other elements and stored for up to 5 days at room temperature on a special agitating device to maintain airflow and gas exchange across the plastic of the bag. Each of these units of platelet concentrate contains about 5.5×10^{10} platelets.
2. From apheresis donors whose donation is collected solely to give about 3×10^{11} platelets per unit. This method is largely used to acquire platelets from donors with HLA phenotypes required to circumvent the HLA antibodies that develop in some patients as a result of multiple transfusion exposures.

FRESH FROZEN PLASMA

A consensus conference called by the National Institutes of Health about 5 years ago concluded that there were very few real indications for fresh frozen plasma and these were related to the rapid reversal of warfarin-based therapy (usually for emergency operations) and its use in the treatment of thrombotic thrombocytopenic purpura as a replacement fluid during plasma exchange. It is also indicated for treatment of patients who have a coagulant factor deficiency for which there is no specific factor concentrate available. Fresh frozen plasma should not be used as a simple volume replacement or for its protein content. Crystalloid solutions are generally less expensive and equally good for volume replacement, and normal serum albumin (5%) is preferable for short-term protein replacement. Solvent-detergent–treated fresh frozen plasma (so-called SD plasma) has been approved by the Food and Drug Administration for clinical use. Such treatment destroys lipid-enveloped viruses such as HIV, hepatitis B virus (HB), and HCV but not hepatitis A virus or parvovirus B19. It must be remembered that SD plasma is made from pools of several hundred donors.

CRYOPRECIPITATE

Cryoprecipitate is prepared from fresh frozen plasma that is slowly thawed at 0°C. Fresh frozen plasma contains a high concentration of factor VIII, factor XIII, and fibrinogen. It is now used mostly for liver transplantation and in the preparation of cryoprecipitated fibrinogen (so-called fibrin glue). Fibrin glue is applied topically to decrease bleeding from raw surfaces or as a biologic glue to hold severed nerve ends or small middle ear bones in apposition until they heal. Commercially prepared fibrin glue is not approved by the Food and Drug Administration.

ADVERSE REACTIONS TO TRANSFUSIONS
Pathogen Transmission

Like any medication, blood transfusions may have adverse reactions. Because of the acquired immunodeficiency syndrome (AIDS) epidemic and because of its transmissibility by blood, AIDS is probably the most widely feared adverse reaction among the general population. In fact, less than 1% of AIDS cases overall have been caused by blood transfusion—and virtually all of those cases preceded the introduction of a test for HIV antibodies now routinely performed on each donated unit. As that particular risk was being addressed, many other improvements in the safety of blood were concomitantly introduced, including much more intrusive donor questions and more donor education about lifestyle risk factors. New tests were also introduced for HCV and HTLV-I and II. Although all tests can have false-negative results and donors may be in a "window period" when donating, the overall safety of blood transfusions today is considerably better than at any time in the past. The so-called window period refers to the phenomenon whereby a donor has been exposed to a pathogen (such as HIV or HCV) and is actually incubating the virus but has not yet produced an antibody to a level that would make it detectable by current testing technology. The window period for each pathogen keeps shrinking as tests with greater sensitivity are developed and introduced to replace their less sensitive predecessors. The national figures for the risk of pathogen transmission by transfusions (per unit) are today estimated to be less than (based on data published in 1996) the following:

HIV	1:500,000-1:1.5 million
HBV	1:65,000
HCV	1:103,000
HTLV-I/II	1:650,000

These risks are actually getting smaller each year as new-generation (more sensitive) tests are replacing older versions. These figures should be put into some perspective for patients by pointing out that the odds of death/person per year are 1:5,000 for anyone who drives an automobile in the United States. If they were always logical, patients should fear more the drive to the hospital than the blood transfusion when they get there. Caution and care in the use of transfusions are wise and responsible. However, illogical or hysterical fears should not prevent physicians and patients from using this resource appropriately. Patients have died unnecessarily because an illogical and exaggerated fear of transfusions prevented them from receiving lifesaving transfusions.

Hemolytic Reactions

Although antibodies to red blood cell antigens other than those in the ABO system can and do cause hemolytic reactions, they are rarely fatal. Most such antibodies are detected before transfusion, and antigen-negative blood can be provided. Likewise, delayed (7 to 10 days after transfusion) hemolytic reactions occur (approximately 1:4,000 transfusions) as a result of the anamnestic increase in titer of an antibody that was not detectable (because of low titer) before transfusion. These reactions are sometimes missed clinically and can cause fever, rigors, and unexplained decrease in hemoglobin level accompanied by an increase in the level of indirect bilirubin. These are usually mild reactions.

However, there is one feature of modern medical practice that actually increases the risks of hemolytic reactions, that is, the practice of same-day admissions for operation. One should be aware that a sample for antibody screening must be sent to the laboratory at least 12 hours (preferably 24) before the expected time of operation for antibodies to be detected, their specificities identified, and antigen-negative red cells located and prepared. Otherwise, a blood sample may be sent to the laboratory just as the patient enters the operating room. The surgeon may then find that the patient is already bleeding just as the laboratory detects a positive screening result, which necessitates several hours of complex laboratory work to identify the specificity of the antibody.

The most devastating hemolytic reactions are, of course, ABO mismatches. The vast majority of these reactions are caused by simple clerical errors of identification of blood samples or of the patient at transfusion. Fully one-third of transfusion-related fatalities are caused by such errors. Therefore, transfusion medicine laboratories have to be fanatical about complete and correct identification of samples for testing of patients for transfusion. Any error in this chain of evidence, however small, can be and sometimes is fatal. About 24 patients die each year in the United States as a result of ABO-mismatched transfusions, and about 90% of those deaths are clearly due to such simple clerical errors. Hemolytic reactions are divided as follows:

Immediate: Caused by preexisting red blood cell antibody in the recipient; manifests within minutes to hours of beginning the transfusion
Delayed: Caused by anamnestic (recall) antibody undetected at time of transfusion; classically manifests 1 to 3 weeks after transfusion

Immediate reactions can present as a catastrophic reaction within minutes to hours. The patient may present with acute disseminated intravascular coagulation and passage of bright red urine (hemoglobinuria), fever, rigors, chest pain, and cardiovascular collapse. The patient (if conscious) may express a feeling of impending doom, and about 20% of such patients indeed die. The cause is usually the presence of a complement-fixing recipient antibody to donor red blood cell antigens, causing intravascular lysis. The most common example of such catastrophes is an ABO mismatch. Antibodies that do not fix complement in vivo tend to give rise to less dramatic hemolysis with extravascular lysis at a rate of about 1 unit destroyed in 24 hours (that is, about 1 g/dL decrease in hemoglobin level in a 70-kg patient). Patients generally complain of fever, rigors, tiredness, or weakness, and they may notice jaundice or dark urine (urobilinogen). Laboratory tests for a hemolytic episode-include pretransfusion and posttransfusion antibody screening, posttransfusion direct antiglobulin testing, and visual inspection of plasma and urine, possibly followed by tests for plasma-free hemoglobin and haptoglobin and urine-free hemoglobin. A complete blood cell count will reveal an unexpectedly low hemoglobin level, and results of tests for indirect bilirubin and lactate dehydrogenase generally are increased. One of the most important things a clinician can do is to alert the laboratory to his or her suspicion because specialized testing may be performed to confirm the presence of a hemolyzing antibody.

Febrile Nonhemolytic Reactions

These occur in about 3% to 5% of transfusions and are particularly likely in patients who have had multiple pregnancies or multiple transfusions. They often are caused by antibodies to white blood cell antigens. Simple filtration of the product (red blood cells or platelets) with modern blood filters provides 3 to 4 log reduction (that is, 99.99%) of white blood cells. Reduction to this level almost always prevents reactions caused by this mechanism. Another mechanism at play in some cases is the accumulation of cytokines (such as tumor necrosis factor-α, interleukin-1β, interleukin-6) derived from "contaminating" white blood cells in the product during storage. This is especially true for platelets. Again, prestorage filtration (as opposed to bedside filtration) removes the white blood cells that are the source of these cytokines. Filtration adds another expense to the cost of the transfusion, but for some patients this may be cost-effective because it eliminates their febrile transfusion reactions and the resultant delays and laboratory investigation.

Allergic Reactions

SIMPLE ALLERGIC

Hives and localized urticarial wheals, for example, complicate approximately 3% of transfusions. These are usually caused by recipient antibodies (IgE) directed to plasma protein to which the patient has been previously exposed by pregnancy or transfusion. Premedication with antihistamines usually prevents such further reactions.

ANAPHYLACTOID/ANAPHYLACTIC

These are very rare but devastating reactions that classically occur after infusion of a few milliliters of blood. In affected patients, widespread hives, urticaria, upper airway obstruction and laryngeal edema, hypotension, a feeling of impending doom, loss of consciousness, and cardiovascular collapse that is sometimes fatal develop very rapidly. An unknown proportion of these reactions are caused by antibodies to IgA that arise in patients who congenitally lack IgA or a portion of the molecule and respond to transfusion, pregnancy, or even immunization by forming the antibody. These patients require IgA-deficient products to prevent recurrence, such as washed red blood cells or platelets or plasma from IgA-deficient donors.

BLOOD DONATION

Availability of resuscitation crystalloid or colloid solutions has eased somewhat the burden on blood donors. However, to date, actual blood donations have not been superseded by synthetic products for red blood cells, platelets, granulocytes, and most plasma proteins. Only about 4% of the general population who are eligible actually donate. This puts a very heavy burden on clinicians to use great care and caution in the utilization of this precious, altruistically derived resource. Unnecessary or wasteful use of blood products is harmful to patients and threatens the lives of future patients if donations are inadequate to meet their legitimate needs.

The donors are routinely tested for a list of pathogens at each donation (as indicated above) but, even more important, are also subjected to a detailed questionnaire about a broad range of activities that might put them in a higher risk group for exposure to pathogens. These questions are quite specific and intrusively intimate. Donors whose responses are unsatisfactory or whose honest responses indicate a risk factor are deferred (permanently in some cases), depending on the risk in question. For example, deferral is permanent for persons who use intravenous drugs (ever), and deferral is about a month for a recent flu episode.

Patients may donate blood for their own use in some elective circumstances. The demand for this type of donation (autologous) has diminished as the safety of the regular (allogeneic) supply has increased. Occasionally patients may demand that their friends or relatives be used as their donors. This action is based on their assumption that such chosen or directed donors are naturally going to be safer than the anonymous blood bank donors. In reality, the anonymous donors are probably safer because the extreme pressure on family or friends to donate for a particular patient may lead to less than completely honest responses to intimate questions. Directed donors lose anonymity also. If recipients have any adverse reactions (trivial or serious) that they attribute (correctly or not) to the blood from a particular donor, they tend to blame the donor and may even consider a lawsuit against the donor. People who are requested to act as directed donors should be aware of the unfortunate position in which they may find themselves—all as a result of their altruism.

Summary Points

- In an asymptomatic patient, red cell transfusion may not be necessary when the hemoglobin level is more than 8 g/dL.

- One unit of a red cell product increases the hemoglobin value by approximately 1 g/dL.

- Clerical error is the major cause of hemolytic transfusion reactions.

- In asymptomatic patients with chronic thrombocytopenia, platelet transfusions are best avoided.

- The "transformation trigger" platelet count in nonbleeding patients receiving chemotherapy is 10,000/µL.

- The risk of HIV transmission in a transfusion unit is less than 1:500,000 to 1:1.5 million.

SUGGESTED READING

AuBuchon JP, Kruskall MS. Transfusion safety: realigning efforts with risks. *Transfusion* 1997; 37: 1211-1216.

Lumadue JA, Ness PM. Current approaches to red blood cell transfusion. *Semin Hematol* 1996; 33: 277-289.

Moore SB. Blood component therapy, in *Clinical Laboratory Medicine* (McClatchey KD, ed). Williams & Wilkins, Baltimore, 1994, pp. 1725-1748.

Moore SB. Hypotensive reactions: are they a new phenomenon? Are they related solely to transfusion of platelets? Does filtration of components play a role? *Transfusion* 1996; 36: 852-853.

Practice guidelines for blood component therapy: A report by the American Society of Anesthesiologists Task Force on Blood Component Therapy. *Anesthesiology* 1996; 84: 732-747.

Rossi EC, Simon TL, Moss GS, Gould SA (eds). *Principles of Transfusion Medicine*, 2nd ed. Williams & Wilkins, Baltimore, 1996.

24 Hereditary Hemochromatosis: A Disease for All Physicians

Virgil F. Fairbanks, MD

Contents

PREVALENCE

Numerous studies conducted during the past 15 years leave no doubt that the gene for hereditary hemochromatosis (HH) is the commonest deleterious gene in persons of European ancestry. The highest prevalence of the hemochromatosis mutation is in the region around the North Sea and the European littoral of the North Atlantic and among people whose ancestors were from this region: Iceland, Sweden, Norway, Denmark, the Netherlands, Germany, France (especially the Brittany Peninsula), Ireland, Scotland, England, Spain, and northern Portugal. The same high prevalence also has been in people of Canada, the states of New York, Minnesota, Missouri, Utah, and California, and in Australia, New Zealand, and the Caucasian people of South Africa. Approximately 10% to 15% of the members of these populations are heterozygous for the major HH mutation; 2% to 5% are homozygous and at risk of clinical disease. The prevalence of HH is slightly lower in persons of northern Italian ancestry and in Alabama. HH is much less common in persons of eastern and southern European origin, and it is rare in those of Middle Eastern, Ashkenazic or Sephardic Jewish, African, Asian, Native American, or Polynesian origin. Few studies have been done, as yet, of the prevalence of HH in Latin American countries. It is easily estimated that more than 1,000,000 persons in the United States are homozygous for the hemochromatosis gene. So far as we know, among genetic disorders, only essential hypertension has a higher prevalence in North America.

From: *Primary Hematology*
Edited by: A. Tefferi © Mayo Foundation for Medical Education and Research, Rochester, MN

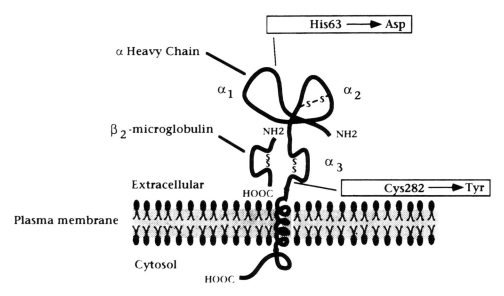

Fig. 1. The HFE protein that is affected by the hemochromatosis mutations. It is a class I MHC-like transmembrane protein that is structurally similar to components of immunoglobulins and intimately associated with β_2-microglobulin. The major hemochromatosis mutation 845A corresponds to substitution of tyrosine (Y) for cysteine (C) at amino acid position 282, which disrupts a normally present disulfide bridge. The lesser hemochromatosis mutation of C to G at nucleotide 187 corresponds to substitution of aspartic acid (D) for histidine (H) at amino acid position 63, presumably causing a less severe structural change in the HFE protein. (From Feder JN, Gnirke A, Thomas W, Tsuchihashi Z, Ruddy DA, Basava A, Dormishian F, Domingo R Jr, Ellis MC, Fullan A, Hinton LM, Jones NL, Kimmel BE, Kronmal GS, Lauer P, Lee VK, Loeb DB, Mapa FA, McClelland E, Meyer NC, Mintier GA, Moeller N, Moore T, Morikang E, Prass CE, Quintana L, Starnes SM, Schatzman RC, Brunke KJ, Dryana DT, Risch NJ, Bacon BR, Wolff RK. A novel MHC class I-like gene is mutated in patients with hereditary haemochromatosis. Nat Genet 1996; 13: 399-408. By permission of Nature America.)

GENETICS

In people of European ancestry, hemochromatosis is HLA-linked. The hemochromatosis gene is on the short end of chromosome 6, approximately 6 Mbp (6 million nucleotide base pairs) telomeric to the major histocompatibility (MHC) complex. It consists of a sequence of 1,029 base pairs, arranged in 7 exons, of which 6 are encoded in a protein that contains 343 amino acids. This has now been designated the *HFE* (for hemochromatosis) gene.

On the basis of the *HFE* gene nucleotide sequence, the protein is similar to MHC class I molecules, including a signal sequence, a peptide-binding region, an immunoglobulin-like domain, a transmembrane region, and a small cytoplasmic portion (Fig. 1). The extracellular portion of the molecule, as in other MHC class I proteins, has three domains, designated $\alpha1$, $\alpha2$, and $\alpha3$. Each of these contains several β-pleated sheets. The $\alpha3$ domain is closely associated with β_2-microglobulin, which is encoded by a gene on chromosome 15. This protein, now designated HFE, appears to be expressed in nearly all cell lines that have been tested.

HFE protein is present within the cell membranes of most cells of the body, where it interacts with transferrin receptor to regulate the formation of the iron-transferrin-trans-

Table 1
Terminology for HFE Gene and Its Known Mutations

Nucleotide notation	Amino acid notation	Simplified	Comment
187C/187C	C282C/C282C	w/w	Homozygous normal
845A/845A	C282Y/C282Y	y/y	Homozygous for severe mutation, high risk of severe HH
187G/187G	H63D/H63D	d/d	Homozygous for minor mutation, slight risk of HH
187C/845A	C282C/C282Y	w/y	Heterozygote, no risk of HH
187C/187G	C282C/H63D	w/d	Heterozygote, no risk of HH
845A/187G	C282Y/H63D	y/d	Compound ("double") heterozygote, slight risk of HH

Abbreviation: HH, hereditary hemochromatosis.

ferrin receptor complex that initiates the intake of iron by the cell. Mutations of the HFE protein impair this regulatory function, and the cellular uptake of iron is then unimpeded. Iron absorption by duodenal mucosal cells is also normally regulated by the interaction of HFE protein with transferrin receptor within the Golgi zone of enterocytes of the crypts of Lieberkuhn. Mutations of the HFE protein, which impair this regulatory mechanism, result in increased iron absorption by the mucosal cells.

Several mutations of the *HFE* gene have now been described. At least two of these are significant in the cause of HH: at nucleotide (nt) 845 G → T and at nt 187 C → G. These correspond to amino acid substitutions 282 Cys → Tyr (abbreviated C282Y) and 63 His → Asp (abbreviated H63D), respectively. The cysteinyl normally present at amino acid position 282 is involved in a disulfide bridge; replacement by tyrosinyl at this position would significantly alter the quaternary structure of the protein and thus its function.

Because chromosomes and genes come in pairs, six genotypes can be defined for combinations of the normal gene and the two mutant alleles, when taken two at a time. Table 1 shows the six genotypes and their designations. The most logical system of nomenclature is based on the DNA nucleotide change, in which the common normal ("wild-type") gene is designated 187C; however, this designation has not been widely adopted. The least logical, but the most widely adopted, designation is based on the amino acid change postulated for the HFE protein, for the wild-type gene, C282C (meaning no change), C representing amino acid cysteine (C) at position 282; for the more severe mutant gene, C282Y, indicating a change of cysteine to tyrosine (Y) at amino acid position 282; for the less severe mutant gene, H63D, indicating a change of histidine (H) to aspartic acid (D) at position 63. The United Kingdom Haemochromatosis Consortium uses a still different, although similar, notational system. For the sake of simplicity, I have adopted the symbols w (for the common, wild-type gene), y (for the severe mutation, 845A or C282Y), and d for the less severe mutant gene (187G or H63D).

One cannot have the wild-type gene (187C, C282C, or w) on both chromosomes and also have a mutant gene. Nor can one have the severe mutation (845A, C282Y, or y) on both chromosomes and also have either the wild-type gene or less severe mutation (187G, H63D, or d) on one of the two chromosomes. The presence of either the wild-type gene or one of the two mutations on a chromosome excludes the presence of any other on that chromosome. In genetic parlance, these genes are alleles. An exception to this principle

Table 2
Approximate Prevalence of the *HFE* Genotypes
in Caucasians of the United States and Northwestern Europe

Genotype	Population frequency, %	Estimated no. of Americans with this genotype[a]
Homozygotes		
w/w	59.6	131,120,000
y/y	0.4	880,000
d/d	1.0	2,200,000
Heterozygotes		
y/w	9.0	19,800,000
y/d	2.0	4,400,000
w/d	28.0	61,600,000

[a]Assumes that Americans of northwestern Europe ancestry represent approximately 220,000,000 and that the prevalence of the HFE mutations in other ethnic groups is low and so has not been included in these calculations. The observed frequency of d/d homozygotes is less than predicted from allele frequency.

is theoretically possible as a result of meiotic crossing over. To date, one recombination of these genes has been reported in which both mutations are on one chromosome.

Numerous studies that have been conducted throughout the United States and Europe indicate that the prevalence of these six HFE genotypes in Caucasians of predominantly North European ancestry is about as shown in Table 2. Approximately two of every five Caucasian Americans have one or both of the HFE gene mutations, and more than a million are at risk of serious clinical disease from iron overload. In view of the extraordinarily high prevalence rates for these mutant genes, hemochromatosis is clearly the most common, serious, single-gene genetic disorder among Caucasians of North America and Europe (essential hypertension is more common, but appears to be polygenic). Homozygous HH (y/y) is 10 times more common in this population than is cystic fibrosis (the next most common serious hereditary disorder among Caucasians). In comparison with nongenetic malignant disorders, it is approximately 100 times more common than multiple myeloma, and it is also 100 times more common than polycythemia vera.

In most series, approximately 83% of cases of clinically severe HH have been found to be homozygous for the 845A mutation (i.e., are of genotype y/y). Another 7% of cases are compound heterozygotes for both the 845A and 187G mutations (i.e., are of genotype y/d). Lower frequencies of the y/y genotype have been reported in Italian cases of HH and in cases of HH studied in Birmingham, Alabama. Although 1% of the Caucasian population are homozygous for the 187G mutation (i.e., are of d/d genotype), the clinical features of HH develop in few of them. However, of the approximately 50 known homozygotes of genotype d/d, approximately a third have significant iron overload, some with features of HH. Therefore, when DNA tests are performed to detect the HH mutation, tests should be made for both *HFE* gene mutations (845A and 187G).

Clearly, the molecular genetics of hemochromatosis has only begun to be revealed. Tests for mutation 845A and 187G account for 90% of cases of homozygous hemochromatosis. What of the other 10% of cases? Do they represent diagnostic errors, or iron overloading that is not of genetic basis, or are there other mutations of this gene that also may cause hemochromatosis? The answers to these questions still need to be resolved. Furthermore, the molecular genetics of non-HLA-linked African hemochromatosis has yet to be eluci-dated. A strain of mice that lack β_2-microglobulin have iron overload that closely resembles human HH. Absence of the HFE α3 domain–β_2-microglobulin complex on the cell surface apparently results in loss of ability to prevent absorption of iron. However, analogous mutation of the β_2-microglobulin gene has not been found in humans with HH.

Many studies have shown that the African-American gene pool is at least 30% to 35% European in origin. Indeed, mitochrondrial DNA studies suggest that more than 40% of the African-American gene pool is European in origin. During the past 300 years, con-siderable mixing of the gene pool has occurred. For the purpose of this chapter, the African-American gene pool is assumed to be one-third European, predominantly north-ern European or British. It is, then, easily estimated that the frequency of HH homozy-gotes in African-Americans is approximately $(1/3)^2$, or 1/9 that in Caucasian Americans. Because African-Americans are approximately 1/10 of the population of the United States, one may predict that HH due to the HLA-linked hemochromatosis gene must occur once in an African-American for every 90 cases in Caucasian Americans. The fact that hemochromatosis experts very rarely find HH in African-Americans is consistent with this prediction.

Another form of HH that is *not* linked to the HLA locus on chromosome 6 is common in black people of central and southern Africa, where the gene frequency appears to be as high as the gene frequency of HLA-linked HH in Europeans. This non–HLA-linked HH is also a cause of serious morbidity and death in sub-Saharan Africa. It is unknown whether there is a significant frequency of non–HLA-linked HH in African-Americans whose ancestry is believed to derive predominantly from western Africa. However, in the absence of this information, it would be imprudent to assume that HH is rare in African-Americans.

The prevalence of HH in Asian people is unknown, but it is believed to be rare.

CLINICAL FEATURES

HH is a disorder that causes considerable morbidity and mortality and that cannot be diagnosed early on the basis of clinical symptoms or signs. The symptoms, signs, and laboratory findings in hemochromatosis are shown in Tables 3 and 4 and in Figure 2.

Of persons who are homozygous for the major HH mutation, 845A/845A (y/y), approx-imately half develop symptoms or signs of severe iron overload. Of the half who are without symptoms or signs, half (or 25% of all homozygotes) have significant iron overload, but approximately one-fourth of all homozygotes appear not to accumulate excess iron. It is not clear why some homozygotes develop severe iron overload with clinical manifestations and some do not. Other factors, such as alcohol abuse or viral hepatitis, may be contributory. Less marked iron overload and less severe clinical manifestations may occur in some persons who are compound heterozygotes, of y/d genotype, or d/d homozy-gotes. However, most such persons do not develop clinically significant disease.

The most common early manifestations of HH are no symptoms, no signs, and no abnormalities on routine physical or laboratory tests. When symptoms do appear, they are nonspecific. They are often erroneously attributed to stress, anxiety, depression, or psy-choneurosis. These symptoms include fatigue, which may be overwhelming, abdominal pains, arthralgias, impotence (in males) and amenorrhea (in females), extrasystoles, and "solitary" atrial fibrillation. Nearly every organ system is involved in hemochromatosis. Accordingly, patients may be seen initially for symptoms or signs by general practi-tioners, gynecologists, urologists, psychiatrists, neurologists, endocrinologists, gastro-

Table 3
Clinical Problems Associated With Hemochromatosis
and the Medical Specialties in Which They May Be Noted

Clinical problems	Specialty
Impotence, loss of libido (males)	Urology, psychiatry
Infertility (males, females)	Endocrinology
Premature menopause	Internal medicine
Hypopituitarism, hypogonadism	Family practice
Thyroid disease: hypothyroidism	Gynecology
Diabetes mellitus	Endocrinology
Liver disease, unexplained increase of liver enzymes, especially aspartate aminotransferase	Gastroenterology, internal medicine
Hepatomegaly	Family practice
Portal hypertension	Gastroenterology
Hepatic cirrhosis	Gastroenterology
Esophageal varices	Gastroenterology
Hepatic failure	Gastroenterology
Ascites	Gastroenterology
Hepatocellular carcinoma	Gastroenterology
Skin pigmentation: gray or bronze	Dermatology
Porphyria cutanea tarda	Internal medicine
Telangiectasia	Family practice
Koilonychia	Dermatology
Caput medusae	Gastroenterology
Arrhythmias: supraventricular, ventricular	Cardiology
Cardiomegaly, cardiomyopathy, hypertrophic or dilated type	Internal medicine, family practice
Congestive heart failure	Pulmonary
Pleural effusion	Thoracic surgery
Arthropathy: 2nd or 3rd metacarpophalangeal joints	Rheumatology
Knees: with or without chondrocalcinosis	Orthopedics
Hip	Internal medicine
Pseudogout	Rheumatology
Seronegative rheumatoid arthritis	Rheumatology
Unusual color or excised cartilage or synovium	Rheumatology
Iron-loading anemias	Hematology
β-thalassemia minor	Internal medicine
Sideroblastic anemia	Hematology
Liver biopsy specimen	Pathology
Hepatic cirrhosis without hepatitis	Pathology
Hepatocellular carcinoma	Pathology
Synovium with brown or gray hue	Pathology
Systemic infection (e.g., from *vibrio vulnificus*)	Infectious disease
Alcoholics with increased liver iron	All specialties, gastroenterology
Increased percentage saturation of transferrin or serum ferritin	All specialties

Table 4

Clinical and Laboratory Features of Hemochromatosis

Symptoms[a]	Signs[a]	Laboratory findings
Fatigue (often severe)	Tachycardia or irregular pulse	Increased serum transaminases, especially aspartate aminotransferase
Pain and swelling of joints	Hepatomegaly	
Impotence	Splenomegaly	Hyperglycemia
Amenorrhea	Spider telangiectasias	Complete blood cell count: normal or
Cold intolerance	Cardiomegaly	macrocytosis targets
Dry hair	Pleural effusion	Thrombocytopenia
Sluggishness	Ascites	Serum iron ↑
Shortness of breath	Caput medusae	Total iron-binding capacity normal or ↓
Palpitations	Joint deformity:	% saturation > 55
Polydipsia, polyposia,	2nd, 3rd	Ferritin > 400 µg/L
polyuria	metacarpophalangeal,	Thyroxine ↓
Weight loss	hip, knee	Thyroid-stimulating hormone ↑
Tarry stools	Koilonychia	Gonadotropins ↓
Swelling of abdomen	Hyperpigmentation	Chest radiograph: pleural effusion,
	Testicular atrophy	cardiomegaly
	Hair loss (males)	Electrocardiogram: arrhythmia (any kind)
		Echocardiogram: normal or restrictive cardiomyopathy

[a]All of these must be viewed as late symptoms and signs. Under optimal circumstances, the diagnosis is made when there are no symptoms, no abnormalities on physical examination, and only increases in serum iron concentration, percentage transferrin saturation, and serum ferritin concentration.

enterologists, or cardiologists. HH usually does not affect the hematopoietic system. Hematologists may become involved because there may be thrombocytopenia as an expression of liver disease, or because they are asked to evaluate splenomegaly. Because hematologists commonly deal with the converse of iron overload (i.e., iron deficiency) and because they so often have patients with iron overload that is due to chronic anemia, this other disorder of iron metabolism also attracts the interest of many hematologists.

This disease "for all physicians," which masquerades in the guise of other conditions, often leads clinicians astray. A particular danger for specialists is focusing on the organ, or organ system, of one's specialty and failing to recognize that one is dealing with a polysystem disease. Some erroneously believe that HH is rare and claim they have never seen a patient with HH. But they are of this opinion because they have not looked for it. (*Chi non cerca nulla trova*, he who doesn't look doesn't find.) In view of the ratio of clinicians to the population of the United States, it may be predicted that, on average, there are 5 persons who are homozygous for HH among the average clinician's patients. This statistic means, of course, that during their careers most clinicians will have a few patients with HH, a few clinicians will have many, and a few will have no patients with HH.

It is critical that the diagnosis be made early, particularly in the presymptomatic phase, because many of the complications of HH are irreversible, and once hepatic cirrhosis develops, there is a 30% probability that highly malignant hepatocellular carcinoma will develop. Early diagnosis permits effective treatment, reduces morbidity, and dramatically extends longevity. However, early diagnosis requires universal screening of all persons age 20 years or older. Until clinicians routinely screen all persons for HH, there

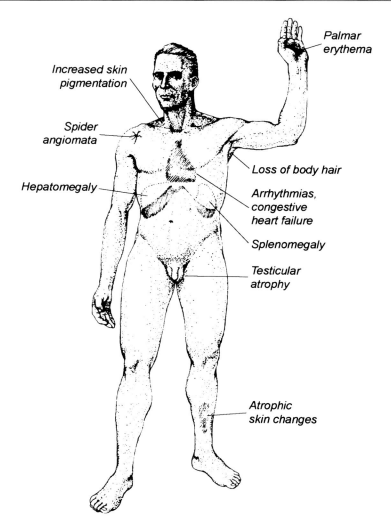

Fig. 2. Hemochromatosis is a multisystem disease that mimics many other disorders. (From Fairbanks VF, Fahey JL, Beutler E. Clinical Disorders of Iron Metabolism, 2nd ed revised and expanded. Grune & Stratton, New York, 1971. By permission of Harcourt Brace Jovanovich.)

will continue to be excessive morbidity and death and malpractice litigation as a result of making a diagnosis too late for effective intervention.

SCREENING

Three studies have analyzed the cost-effectiveness of routine screening for HH, using serum iron and transferrin saturation as the screening test. All three studies concluded that routine screening for HH would be highly cost-effective. The estimates of cost per year of life saved ranged from $850 to $2,500 (including all costs for additional tests, physicians' office visits, liver biopsy when indicated, histopathologic evaluation, and measurement of liver iron content). Even in an era of increasing cost consciousness and efforts to reduce the costs of medical care, universal screening for HH would be a bargain. Tables 5 and 6 compare the cost-effectiveness of HH screening with that for other screening procedures that have been widely advocated.

Table 5
Screening Programs: Cost-Effectiveness Comparisons

Screening program	Estimated cost per year of life gained, $[a]
Hemochromatosis	850–6,000
Cancer of the breast	600,000–6,000,000
Cancer of the colon	30,000–60,000
Cancer of the uterine cervix	15,000–30,000
Ovarian cancer	15,000–30,000
Hypertension	12,200–42,600
Human immunodeficiency virus in surgeons (to avoid transmission of the virus from infected surgeons to patients)	458,000

[a]Each of these cost estimates includes both indirect and direct costs (e.g., follow-up testing, physician office visits, biopsies when appropriate). The cost estimates vary depending on charges made for these tests in different medical centers; therefore, these can be considered only approximate.

Table 6
Approximate Costs of Initial Screening Tests per Case
Detected, Comparison With Accepted Screening Tests[a]

Screening program	Cost, $
Hemochromatosis	5,000
Cancer of the breast	70,000
Cancer of the colon	100,000
Sickle cell anemia	3,000
Phenylketonuria	30,000
Congenital adrenal hyperplasia	24,000
Congenital hypothyroidism	8,000
Galactosemia	140,000

[a]Comparison is made with mammography for detection of cancer of the breast in women after age 50, screening for colon cancer beginning at age 40, as specified by the American Cancer Society; other disorders listed are detected by neonatal screening on dried blood spots.

Because patients with untreated HH have an average shortening of survival of approximately 10 years, the estimate of cost-effectiveness includes this gain in survival. Early diagnosis and treatment would significantly reduce health care costs for society and for third-party payers.

None of the cost-effectiveness studies of screening for HH have considered the health care costs of an alternative approach that was universally used until recently: not diagnosing HH until signs of organ damage are present, as exemplified in the traditional criteria of cutaneous hyperpigmentation, hepatic cirrhosis, and diabetes mellitus. Today, the medical care costs of a diagnosis made too late include those for the treatment of arthritis, cardiac arrhythmias, heart failure, diabetes, pituitary insufficiency, hypothyroidism, esophageal varices, hepatocellular carcinoma, and hepatic failure. Some patients with late-stage hemochromatosis have been subjected to liver transplantation; for some, heart transplantation has been considered. The costs of organ transplants may exceed $200,000, and for patients with late-stage HH who require liver transplantation, long-term survival is poor. For patients with HH who have required liver transplantation, median survival is 3 years, whereas median survival is more than 7 years in those who had transplantation for other causes of liver failure. A further potential cost of a diagnosis made too late is the cost of malpractice litigation, and this also is a cost of medical care, because the cost of malpractice insurance is reflected in higher health care insurance premiums. However, the medical care costs that result from a diagnosis made too late are so variable from case to case that we have no formula by which to incorporate them in a cost-benefit analysis.

The cost estimates for screening for the early diagnosis of HH include the assumption that the initial screening be done by the least expensive method. Studies at Mayo Clinic indicated that this can be accomplished by incorporation of the serum iron and total iron-binding capacity (TIBC) assay in the conventional "serum chemistry group"; the incremental cost is approximately $1.50 per specimen. Screening for hemochromatosis would be cost-effective only if the initial screening test cost less than $8.00. Currently at Mayo Clinic, the serum iron and TIBC assays must be ordered separately from the other tests in the serum chemistry group, thereby increasing the cost of these assays 5- to 15-fold. This much greater cost, which results from separate ordering of serum iron and TIBC testing, is difficult to justify when demands for control of the costs of medical care are increasing.

The cost of HH screening would not be significantly less were it targeted at only white Americans. Indeed, concerns about racially determined inequities and who decides and how one decides whether a patient is, for example, 90% Caucasian or 20% Caucasian, would almost certainly make population-targeted screening socially and economically unacceptable.

Although the rationale for universal screening for HH is unassailable, concerns have been expressed about the psychological effect of the diagnosis of HH and the effect on insurability of persons so diagnosed. These concerns led to the recommendation that universal screening not be implemented until these concerns have been more adequately addressed.

Recommended Screening and Follow-Up Tests

The initial screening test should be a fasting, morning measurement of *serum iron (SI) and total iron-binding capacity (TIBC)*. From results of these assays is calculated the transferrin saturation (Tsat):

$$\text{Tsat } (\%) = 100 \times \text{SI/TIBC}$$

If the Tsat is more than 50%, additional studies are indicated. It must first be ascertained whether the patient is receiving (or recently received) iron either orally or parenterally. Often, this is not known to the physician, because the patient may have assumed that this information is not important or that a multiple vitamin-mineral supplement does not contain enough iron to matter. However, many over-the-counter supplements contain 18 mg or more of iron, and this is more than enough to increase the serum iron substantially and increase the Tsat to more than 60%. If the patient is a young woman, it is necessary to ascertain whether she is taking contraceptive medication, which may also increase SI and Tsat markedly. The patient must also be evaluated for other parenchymal liver disease, such as viral hepatitis or steatohepatitis, both of which may cause an increase in transferrin saturation with or without an increase in serum ferritin concentration. These conditions also may cause an increase in serum transaminases. The serum iron and TIBC assay must be repeated while the patient is fasting in the morning and after at least several days of abstention from iron medication or contraceptives. At the same time, the serum ferritin assay should be performed to evaluate the increase, if any, in total body iron content.

A presumptive diagnosis of HH is made when, in both the initial and follow-up blood specimens, Tsat is more than 50% (either sex) and the serum ferritin concentration is more than 200 µg/L in female patients or more than 300 µg/L in male patients. An increase in both serum iron and Tsat is characteristic of hemochromatosis and should be considered the hallmark of this disease. Very early, the serum iron and Tsat are increased, but the ferritin concentration is normal. As iron progressively accumulates, the serum ferritin concentration steadily increases. In advanced cases, the serum ferritin concentration often exceeds 1,000 µg/L and may exceed 3,000 µg/L. It is a poor practice to wait for these very high values of serum ferritin concentration to develop because, by then, much organ damage may be done, and this may be irreversible.

Increases in Tsat and the serum ferritin concentration are an indication for liver biopsy to ascertain the degree of iron overload and whether cirrhosis is present. The biopsy specimen should be stained with hematoxylin-eosin and Perls' iron stain, and a portion should be submitted for chemical iron assay. From the chemical iron assay and the patient's age, a very useful criterion for hemochromatosis can be derived, the hepatic iron index (HII), by this calculation:

$$\text{HII} = \text{hepatic iron concentration: µmol per gram of liver,}$$
$$\text{dry weight/patient's age (years)}$$

An HII more than 1.9 indicates HH with significant iron overload.

Not every patient consents to liver biopsy. For those who refuse this diagnostic test, the physician should note this choice in the medical record and then proceed to treat with at least weekly phlebotomies until the serum ferritin concentration is less than 20 µg/L.

Because HH is a disorder with autosomal recessive inheritance, other family members must also be screened for hemochromatosis. In affected families, on average, one-fourth of the sibship (including the ascertained case) will be homozygous for hemochromatosis. However, among the siblings of an ascertained (index) case, on average approximately one in seven also will be homozygous for HH. Parents and children of homozygotes are not usually affected. In view of the high prevalence of the gene in the Caucasian population, homozygotes often marry heterozygotes. Consequently, in about 10% of families, the disease appears in two or more generations. All first-degree relatives (parents, siblings, and children) must undergo serum iron and TIBC testing and have the transferrin saturation calculated, and further testing as indicated by the results of these tests.

A direct DNA analysis for the HH-associated mutations at nucleotides 845 and 187 is now available in a small number of laboratories, including the molecular genetics laboratory of Mayo Clinic and Mayo Medical Laboratories. This test is expected to identify approximately 90% of persons who have, or are at risk for development of, clinically severe hemochromatosis. Early diagnosis of homozygotes by DNA typing (y/y, 845A/845A, or C282Y/C282Y) may obviate liver biopsy in some cases. Homozygotes who are asymptomatic, do not have either hepatomegaly or splenomegaly, who have normal blood glucose and normal serum ALT transaminase, and whose serum ferritin is more than 300 µg/L but less than 1,000 µg/L are quite unlikely to have sufficient hepatocellular injury to cause cirrhosis. It is reasonable to diagnose HH in such cases without liver biopsy and to begin phlebotomy therapy.

Conventional HLA typing has no value in testing for hemochromatosis. It is too expensive and it is nondiagnostic, irrespective of the HLA types that may be demonstrated.

TREATMENT

The proper treatment of HH is phlebotomy, with the removal of 500 mL of blood once or twice weekly, until the serum ferritin concentration is 20 µg/L. This may require 50 to 150 phlebotomies over 1 to 2 years. If the diagnosis is made early enough, fewer phlebotomies may be required. As a rule, removal of 500 mL of blood removes 200 to 250 mg of iron; thus, removal of 1 g of iron requires four or five phlebotomies. Patients with severe iron overload may have 20 to 40 g of iron in their tissues which must be mobilized by phlebotomy. After the excess iron has been removed, it is usually necessary to remove 2 to 6 half-liters of blood every year, depending on the serum ferritin concentration, to avoid reaccumulation of iron.

Treatment of specific organ dysfunction also may be required, such as for cardiac arrhythmias or failure, diabetes mellitus, or arthritis, and hormonal replacement therapy may be needed for estrogen, androgen, and thyroxine deficiency, as warranted.

All consumption of ethanol should be forbidden.

No attempt at dietary restriction of iron intake is appropriate. A well-balanced diet is proper, with moderate meat intake. The ingestion or handling of uncooked marine seafood should be avoided. Patients with HH should not eat raw oysters. A marine bacterium, *Vibrio vulnificus*, proliferates explosively in an iron-abundant environment and may cause death from septicemia in patients with HH who handle or eat uncooked seafood.

Iron chelation therapy is not appropriate. It is too inconvenient, too costly, and too inefficient. If an effective oral iron chelator becomes available in the future (none are presently on the horizon), it may be useful as maintenance therapy after completion of the initial course of phlebotomy; it will not be appropriate for initial treatment.

PROGNOSIS

If the diagnosis is made early enough and treatment has been sufficiently aggressive to deplete the iron overload, survival is not different from that of the rest of the population. Adverse prognostic factors are cirrhosis of the liver and diabetes mellitus. These are not usually reversible, and hepatocellular carcinoma ultimately develops in 30% of those with cirrhosis, but hardly ever in those who have been adequately treated before the development of cirrhosis. Cardiac and hepatic function improve after removal of iron. Arthritis, diabetes, and hormonal insufficiencies (pituitary hypogonadism and hypothyroidism) generally do not improve; replacement therapy must be continued indefinitely.

THE ROLE OF LIVER TRANSPLANTATION

The need for liver transplantation in HH is evidence of failure to make the diagnosis and provide treatment in a timely manner. Liver transplantation is extremely costly, and the morbidity is high even if the procedure is successful. The median survival after liver transplantation for late-stage HH is 3 years, which is much poorer than results after liver transplantation for other causes of liver failure, in which median survival is more than 7 years.

OTHER CAUSES OF IRON OVERLOAD

There are many other causes of iron overloading which may lead to severe tissue injury. Hematologists are familiar with acquired iron overload that is the result of transfusion therapy of severe chronic anemias such as thalassemia major. Treatment of these requires iron chelation therapy with desferrioxamine, usually by subcutaneous infusion with a battery-operated pump for 12 to 16 hours daily at least 6 days per week, indefinitely. A hoped-for and long-awaited alternative in the form of orally administered iron chelating agents is still not available. The L1 bubble burst a few years ago: "deferiprone" is highly toxic but not very effective. We will have to wait for something better to be developed and, until then, continue to use desferrioxamine.

Hemochromatosis With β-Thalassemia Trait

A few such cases have been described. We recently did DNA analysis of one such case and proved that the patient was homozygous for HH (845A) and had β-thalassemia trait. Other investigators have now made similar observations.

Hereditary Sideroblastic Anemia

This X-chromosome–linked disorder has now been shown to be due to mutation of the δ-aminolevulinic acid synthase gene. It is characterized by hypochromic, microcytic erythrocytes and elliptocytes or ovalocytes in a dimorphic blood picture, iron overloading, predominantly male inheritance pattern, and ringed sideroblasts in bone marrow aspirates, on Perls' stain. Untreated, many of these patients develop all the features of HH. They should be treated with phlebotomy. It is often possible to increase the blood hemoglobin concentration sufficiently to permit phlebotomy therapy by administration of pyridoxine, at least 100 mg/day, and folic acid, 1 mg/day.

Iatrogenic Iron Overload

Iron overload from oral or parenteral iron therapy given to nonanemic persons has been reported in only a few cases. The overload was a result of iron given either orally or parenterally because of a misdiagnosis of iron deficiency. These cases are rare because the time required for oral iron overload to develop is long, about 25 years. We recently studied such a patient, who responded well to phlebotomy therapy. DNA study showed that she was homozygous normal at the *HFE* gene.

Congenital Atransferrinemia

To our knowledge, there is only one known case in the Western Hemisphere (a Mayo Clinic case), and only nine have been reported worldwide. They are characterized by hypochromic, microcytic anemia, very high serum ferritin concentration, extremely low serum iron concentration, and TIBC near 0. If patients are untreated, or inadequately treated, all the features of tissue injury develop as in HH. In addition, they have high susceptibility to bacterial infections. We have successfully treated our patient with monthly infusions of normal plasma, preceded by 500-mL phlebotomy. She requires replacement estrogen and progesterone; she is a young woman whose principal problem is osteoporosis as a result of hypothalamic, hypopituitary hypogonadism.

Porphyria Cutanea Tarda

This disorder is associated with mild-to-moderate iron overload, and it is ameliorated by phlebotomy therapy. Some studies have shown an increased frequency of the 845A and 187G mutations of the *HFE* gene in patients with porphyria cutanea tarda.

Congenital Dyserythropoietic Anemia Type II

This condition, characterized by moderate-to-severe anemia, is associated with iron loading that may result in severe complications of hemochromatosis, including heart failure. Treatment with phlebotomy or with desferrioxamine is appropriate.

SUGGESTED READING

Balan V, Baldus W, Fairbanks V, Michels V, Burritt M, Klee G. Screening for hemochromatosis: a cost-effectiveness study based on 12,258 patients. *Gastroenterology* 1994; 107: 453-459.

Barton JC, Edwards CQ, Bertoli LF, Shroyer TW, Hudson SL. Iron overload in African Americans. *Am J Med* 1995; 99: 616-623.

Beutler E, Gelbart T, West C, Lee P, Adams M, Blackstone R, Pockros P, Kosty M, Venditti CP, Phatak PD, Seese NK, Chorney KA, Ten Elshof AE, Gerhard GS, Chorney M. Mutation analysis in hereditary hemochromatosis. *Blood Cells Mol Dis* 1996; 22: 187-194.

Burke W, Thomson E, Khoury MJ, McDonnell SM, Press N, Adams PC, Barton JC, Beutler E, Brittenham G, Buchanan A, Clayton EW, Cogswell ME, Meslin EM, Motulsky AG, Powell LW, Sigal E, Wilfond BS, Collins FS. Hereditary hemochromatosis: gene discovery and its implications for population-based screening. *JAMA* 1998; 280: 172-178.

Cogswell ME, McDonnell SM, Khoury MJ, Franks AL, Burke W, Brittenham G. Iron overload, public health, and genetics: evaluating the evidence for hemochromatosis screening. *Ann Intern Med* 1998; 129: 971-979.

Feder JN, Gnirke A, Thomas W, Tsuchihashi Z, Ruddy DA, Basava A, Dormishian F, Domingo R Jr, Ellis MC, Fullan A, Hinton LM, Jones NL, Kimmel BE, Kronmal GS, Lauer P, Lee VK, Loeb DB, Mapa FA, McClelland E, Meyer NC, Mintier GA, Moeller N, Moore T, Morikang E, Prass CE, Quintana L, Starnes SM, Schatzman RC, Brunke KJ, Dryana DT, Risch NJ, Bacon BR, Wolff RK. A novel MHC class I-like gene is mutated in patients with hereditary haemochromatosis. *Nat Genet* 1996; 13: 399-408.

Feder JN, Penny DM, Irrinki A, Lee VK, Lebron JA, Watson N, Tsuchihashi Z, Sigal E, Bjorkman PJ, Schatzman RC. The hemochromatosis gene product complexes with the transferrin receptor and lowers its affinity for ligand binding. *Proc Natl Acad Sci U S A* 1998; 95: 1472-1477.

Gordeuk V, Mukiibi J, Hasstedt SJ, Samowitz W, Edwards CQ, West G, Ndambire S, Emmanual J, Nkanza N, Chapanduka Z, Randall M, Boone P, Romano P, Martell RW, Yamashita T, Effler P, Brittenham G. Iron overload in Africa. Interaction between a gene and dietary iron content. *N Engl J Med* 1992; 326: 95-100.

Guyader D, Jacquelinet C, Moirand R, Turlin B, Mendler MH, Chaperon J, David V, Brissot P, Adams P, Deugnier Y. Noninvasive prediction of fibrosis in C282Y homozygous hemochromatosis. *Gastroenterology* 1998; 115: 929-936.

Merryweather-Clarke AT, Pointon JJ, Shearman JD, Robson KJ. Global prevalence of putative haemochromatosis mutations. *J Med Genet* 1997; 34: 275-278.

Niederau C, Fischer R, Sonnenberg A, Stremmel W, Trampisch HJ, Strohmeyer G. Survival and causes of death in cirrhotic and in noncirrhotic patients with primary hemochromatosis. *N Engl J Med* 1985; 313: 1256-1262.

Olynyk JK, Cullen DJ, Aquilia S, Rossi E, Summerville L, Powell LW. A population-based study of the clinical expression of the hemochromatosis gene. *N Engl J Med* 1999; 341: 718-724.

Roberts AG, Whatley SD, Morgan RR, Worwood M, Elder GH. Increased frequency of the haemochromatosis Cys282Tyr mutation in sporadic porphyria cutanea tarda. *Lancet* 1997; 349: 321-323.

Waheed A, Parkkila S, Saarnio J, Fleming RE, Zhou XY, Tomatsu S, Britton RS, Bacon BR, Sly WS. Association of HFE protein with transferrin receptor in crypt enterocytes of human duodenum. *Proc Natl Acad Sci U S A* 1999; 96: 1579-1584.

25 Hematologic Manifestations of HIV Disease

Zelalem Temesgen, MD

Contents

INTRODUCTION

Infection with the human immunodeficiency virus (HIV) has been associated with abnormalities of the various components of hematopoiesis. In general, these abnormalities may be a consequence of HIV infection itself, an adverse effect of therapies directed against HIV infection or its associated conditions, or involvement of the bone marrow by HIV-related opportunistic infections and neoplasms.

This chapter provides a general discussion of specific hematologic abnormalities associated with HIV disease, including their pathogenesis and therapy. The discussion is directed toward primary care physicians and, as such, is not intended to be an exhaustive coverage of the subject matter.

ANEMIA

Anemia is a very common complication in HIV infection. Its prevalence increases with the stage of HIV disease. The causes of HIV-related anemia are diverse and include HIV infection itself, medications, and conditions that involve the bone marrow directly, such as opportunistic infections and neoplasms.

HIV Infection as a Direct Cause of Anemia

Some studies suggest that HIV infection itself or cytokines generated by HIV infection lead to suppression of the hematopoietic progenitor cell, resulting in decreased production of erythrocytes. Other studies have implicated soluble factors in the serum of

From: *Primary Hematology*
Edited by: A. Tefferi © Mayo Foundation for Medical Education and Research, Rochester, MN

Table 1
Myelosuppressive Drugs Commonly Used
in HIV Infection That Cause Anemia

Zidovudine (ZDV, AZT)	Antineoplastics
Trimethoprim-sulfamethoxazole	Doxorubicin (Adriamycin)
Dapsone	Cyclophosphamide
Sulfadiazine	Methotrexate
Pyrimethamine	Vinblastine
Pentamidine	Interferon-α
Ganciclovir	
Cidofovir	
Amphotericin B	
5-Flucytosine	

HIV-infected patients with inhibitory effects on hematopoiesis. Still others suggest that a relative deficiency in the hormone erythropoietin may play a role.

Drug-Induced Anemia

Several drugs used to treat HIV infection or to treat or prevent HIV-related opportunistic infections and neoplasms cause anemia (Table 1). Zidovudine (ZDV, AZT), a nucleoside analog antiretroviral agent, is probably the most common cause of anemia in HIV-infected patients. Anemia due to zidovudine is accompanied by macrocytosis (mean erythrocyte corpuscular volume, > 100 femtoliters). Patients with early-stage disease seem to have a lower incidence of zidovudine-induced severe anemia than patients with advanced disease.

Anemia Caused by Conditions That Directly Involve the Bone Marrow

Various HIV-related infections and neoplasms can infiltrate the bone marrow and cause hematologic abnormalities (Table 2). Two such infections, *Mycobacterium avium* complex (MAC) disease and parvovirus B19 infection, are discussed below.

MYCOBACTERIUM AVIUM COMPLEX (MAC)

MAC refers to a group of related species of mycobacterium that are the cause of one of the most common systemic bacterial infections in patients with advanced HIV disease. MAC infection is characterized by nonspecific symptoms such as fever, night sweats, fatigue, weight loss, and anorexia. High-grade bacteremia and other laboratory abnormalities, including anemia, accompany these symptoms. Stains and cultures of biopsy specimens from bone marrow demonstrate the organisms. Anemia tends to be relatively worse than neutropenia or thrombocytopenia.

PARVOVIRUS B19

Parvovirus B19 is a small DNA virus that is the cause of a common childhood exanthem, erythema infectiosum, also known as fifth disease. Parvovirus B19 infects, replicates in, and causes lysis of erythroid progenitor cells. It has been associated with transient aplastic crisis in patients with various underlying hematologic disorders, such as sickle cell disease. Parvovirus B19 also causes pure red cell aplasia in HIV-infected persons. Parvovirus B19 infection can be diagnosed by demonstration of the virus in

Table 2
HIV-Related Conditions That Can Directly Involve
the Bone Marrow

Infections	Neoplasms
Mycobacteria	Non-Hodgkin's lymphoma
Mycobacterium avium complex (MAC)	Hodgkin's disease
Mycobacterium tuberculosis (TB)	Kaposi's sarcoma
Fungi	
Histoplasma capsulatum	
Coccidioides immitis	
Cryptococcus neoformans	
Pneumocystis carinii	
Virus	
Parvovirus B19	
Cytomegalovirus	

the blood and bone marrow with molecular and immunologic techniques (such as polymerase chain reaction and hybridization assays). Examination of the bone marrow shows characteristic giant pronormoblasts. Anemia due to parvovirus B19 infection can be successfully treated with intravenous immunoglobulin infusions. Relapse can occur, requiring repeat treatment.

Treatment of Anemia in HIV Infection

The treatment of HIV-related anemia depends to a large extent on the underlying cause or diagnosis. However, there is a loss of the normal compensatory erythropoietin response to anemia regardless of the cause. The normal compensatory erythropoietin response is an attempt to correct the anemia by increasing the production of erythropoietin. The administration of recombinant erythropoietin is effective for treating HIV-related anemia caused by various conditions. This beneficial effect of erythropoietin occurs in patients with endogenous erythropoietin levels less than 500 IU/L.

GRANULOCYTOPENIA

HIV-associated granulocytopenia can be a consequence of HIV infection itself, an adverse effect of medications used to treat HIV or its associated conditions, or a complication of opportunistic infections and neoplasms that directly infiltrate the bone marrow. As has been noted in other disease states, the risk of infection increases with the decline of granulocyte counts. A recent retrospective analysis showed that HIV-infected patients with absolute granulocyte counts less than 500×10^6 L have a significantly higher risk of hospitalization for bacterial infections. However, some studies suggest that infectious episodes in neutropenic HIV-infected patients are fewer than in patients with hematologic malignancies.

HIV as a Cause of Granulocytopenia

Some investigators have suggested decreased colony growth of the progenitor cell leading to impaired granulopoiesis as the mechanism that accounts for granulocytopenia in some patients. Others postulate an autoimmune mechanism involving antigranulocyte antibodies. Neither of these hypotheses has been proved or validated.

Drug-Induced Granulocytopenia

This is the most common form of granulocytopenia seen in clinical practice. Various drugs used to treat HIV or HIV-related opportunistic infections and neoplasms are known to cause granulocytopenia (Table 1). Zidovudine is probably the most common drug causing granulocytopenia in HIV disease.

Impaired Neutrophil Function

In addition to granulocytopenia, patients with HIV infection may have abnormalities in the function of their granulocytes. The abnormalities that have been detected include defects in chemotaxis, superoxide anion production, bacterial killing capability, and phagocytosis. Although these defects in neutrophil function may account, in part, for the increased susceptibility of HIV-infected patients to bacterial and fungal infections, such a clear clinical correlation has not been established.

Treatment of HIV-Associated Granulocytopenia

The causes of granulocytopenia in HIV infection are diverse, and treatment may need to address the underlying disease process or the causative drug. In this regard, steps that may need to be taken include discontinuation of use of the offending drug and treatment of the opportunistic infection or neoplasm that infiltrated the bone marrow. In addition, myeloid growth factors—granulocyte colony-stimulating factor (G-CSF) and granulocyte-monocyte colony-stimulating factor (GM-CSF)—have been found to increase the granulocyte count and correct some neutrophil functional abnormalities. This effect permits continued use of critical first-line drugs to treat either HIV or its associated conditions. Unfortunately, GM-CSF has been associated with up-regulation of HIV replication, leading to increases in HIV RNA and P24 levels. This up-regulation has not been noted with the use of G-CSF.

THROMBOCYTOPENIA

Thrombocytopenia is also frequently noted in association with HIV disease and can be caused by reduced bone marrow production or destruction of platelets. The destruction of platelets can be mediated by immune or nonimmune mechanisms.

HIV as a Direct Cause of Thrombocytopenia

HIV can directly infect megakaryocytes. HIV RNA and proteins have been detected in megakaryocytes. The presence of HIV in these cells may lead to decreased production of platelets and expose altered antigens that may subsequently become targets of antiplatelet antibodies.

HIV-Associated Immune Thrombocytopenic Purpura (HIV-ITP)

Immune thrombocytopenic purpura (ITP) is a major cause of thrombocytopenia in HIV disease. The pathogenesis is thought to be increased reticuloendothelial clearance of platelets coated with antibody or circulating immune complexes. Examination of the bone marrow shows an increased number of megakaryocytes as a manifestation of a compensatory increase in platelet production. However, this compensatory increase in platelet production is not of sufficient magnitude to correct the thrombocytopenia in the peripheral blood. Although the potential for bleeding exists, clinical bleeding is unlikely until the platelet count decreases to less than 20,000/dL.

Treatment of HIV-ITP

Many patients with HIV-ITP do not require treatment. Therapy is reserved for those with clinically significant symptoms such as bleeding. Zidovudine has successfully been used to treat HIV-ITP. The mechanism of action is thought to be related to its antiviral effect. Other antiretroviral agents, including currently used combination treatment regimens, are expected to have a similar beneficial effect on HIV-ITP, but reports addressing this issue have been limited.

Other treatments have been used to treat HIV-ITP with varying degrees of success. These include interferon-α high-dose intravenous immunoglobulin infusion, corticosteroids, danazol, anti-Rh immunoglobulin, and splenectomy.

Other Causes of Thrombocytopenia in HIV Infection

As discussed in the sections on anemia and neutropenia, infections or neoplasms that infiltrate the bone marrow and myelosuppressive medications used to treat HIV and its associated conditions can cause thrombocytopenia (Tables 1 and 2).

CONCLUSION

Various hematologic abnormalities occur in the course of HIV infection. The causes of these abnormalities are diverse. Clinicians caring for patients with HIV should be knowledgeable about these conditions, address the underlying problem, and institute proper treatment, including, when appropriate, the use of hematopoietic growth factors.

SUGGESTED READING

Ballem PJ, Belzberg A, Devine DV, Lyster D, Spruston B, Chambers H, Doubroff P, Mikulash K. Kinetic studies of the mechanism of thrombocytopenia in patients with human immunodeficiency virus infection. *N Engl J Med* 1992; 327: 1779-1784.

Doweiko JP, Groopman JE. Hematologic complications of human immunodeficiency virus infection, in *AIDS: Etiology, Diagnosis, Treatment and Prevention* (DeVita VT Jr, Hellman S, Rosenberg SA, eds). Lippincott-Raven, Philadelphia, 1997, pp. 617-628.

Ellis M, Gupta S, Galant S, Hakim S, VandeVen C, Toy C, Cairo MS. Impaired neutrophil function in patients with AIDS or AIDS-related complex: a comprehensive evaluation. *J Infect Dis* 1988; 158: 1268-1276.

Fischl M, Galpin JE, Levine JD, Groopman JE, Henry DH, Kennedy P, Miles S, Robbins W, Starrett B, Zalusky R, Abels RI, Tsai HC, Rudnick SA. Recombinant human erythropoietin for patients with AIDS treated with zidovudine. *N Engl J Med* 1990; 322: 1488-1493.

Folks TM, Kessler SW, Orenstein JM, Justement JS, Jaffe ES, Fauci AS. Infection and replication of HIV-1 in purified progenitor cells of normal human bone marrow. *Science* 1988; 242: 919-922.

Frickhofen N, Abkowitz JL, Safford M, Berry JM, Antunez-de-Mayolo J, Astrow A, Cohen R, Halperin I, King L, Mintzer D, Cohen B, Young NS. Persistent B19 parvovirus infection in patients infected with human immunodeficiency virus type 1 (HIV-1): a treatable cause of anemia in AIDS. *Ann Intern Med* 1990; 113: 926-933.

Frumkin LR, Dale DC. The role of colony stimulating factors in HIV disease. *The AIDS Reader* 1996; 6: 185-193.

Jacobson MA, Liu RC, Davies D, Cohen PT. Human immunodeficiency virus disease-related neutropenia and the risk of hospitalization for bacterial infection. *Arch Intern Med* 1997; 157: 1825-1831.

Kaplan LD, Kahn JO, Crowe S, Northfelt D, Neville P, Grossberg H, Abrams DI, Tracey J, Mills J, Volberding PA. Clinical and virologic effects of recombinant human granulocyte-macrophage colony-stimulating factor in patients receiving chemotherapy for human immunodeficiency virus-associated non-Hodgkin's lymphoma: results of a randomized trial. *J Clin Oncol* 1991; 9: 929-940.

Mitsuyasu RT. Clinical uses of hematopoietic growth hormones in HIV-related illnesses. *AIDS Clin Rev* 1993/1994; 189-212.

Ratner L. Human immunodeficiency virus-associated autoimmune thrombocytopenic purpura: a review. *Am J Med* 1989; 86: 194-198.

Richman DD, Fischl MA, Grieco MH, Gottlieb MS, Volberding PA, Laskin OL, Leedom JM, Groopman JE, Mildvan D, Hirsch MS, Jackson GG, Durack DT, Nusinoff-Lehrman S, and the AZT Collaborative Working Group. The toxicity of azidothymidine (AZT) in the treatment of patients with AIDS and AIDS-related complex. A double-blind, placebo-controlled trial. *N Engl J Med* 1987; 317: 192-197.

The Swiss Group for Clinical Studies on the Acquired Immunodeficiency Syndrome (AIDS). Zidovudine for the treatment of thrombocytopenia associated with human immunodeficiency virus (HIV). A prospective study. *Ann Intern Med* 1988; 109: 718-721.

Zucker-Franklin D, Cao Y. Megakaryocytes of human immunodeficiency virus-infected individuals express viral RNA. *Proc Natl Acad Sci USA* 1989; 86: 5595-5599.

26 Hematopoietic Growth Factors in Clinical Practice

Pierre Noël, MD

Contents

ERYTHROPOIETIN

Erythropoietin (EPO) is a glycoprotein produced in the peritubular cells of the kidney. A heme-containing protein senses oxygen need and triggers the production of EPO and its release in the bloodstream. EPO interacts with receptor-bearing cells in the bone marrow, where physiologic oxygen demands are translated into increased red cell production. Under normal conditions, the plasma EPO level is maintained between 10 and 20 U/L.

Recombinant human EPO has been approved in the United States for the treatment of anemia caused by chronic renal insufficiency, cancer, or cancer therapy and of patients infected with the human immunodeficiency virus (HIV) who are undergoing zidovudine therapy. EPO is also approved for patients undergoing operation.

Clinical Uses of Recombinant EPO

ANEMIA OF RENAL FAILURE

Anemia related to chronic renal failure is partly due to EPO deficiency. Recombinant EPO is indicated in the treatment of anemia in patients with chronic renal failure, including patients undergoing dialysis. Nondialysis patients with symptomatic anemia considered for therapy should have a hematocrit value less than 30%.

Before initiation of therapy, the transferrin saturation should be at least 20% and the ferritin value at least 100 ng/mL. The subcutaneous route of administration is more efficacious, permitting patients to reduce their dose of erythropoietin by 30% to 50%.

From: *Primary Hematology*
Edited by: A. Tefferi © Mayo Foundation for Medical Education and Research, Rochester, MN

The recommended starting dosage of EPO is 50 to 100 U/kg three times a week. The anticipated increase in hematocrit is 0.11%/day for a dosage of 50 U/kg three times a week and 0.18%/day for a dosage of 100 U/kg three times a week. By the end of 2 months of treatment, most patients are transfusion-independent. When the hematocrit reaches 36%, a maintenance dose of EPO should be initiated. The median maintenance dose is 75 U/kg three times a week for patients undergoing dialysis and 75 to 150 U/kg a week for patients with chronic renal failure not undergoing dialysis.

The only significant toxicities include iron deficiency, hypertension, and seizures. Blood pressure increases are noted in 35% of previously hypertensive patients and in 44% of previously normotensive patients.

ANEMIA IN HIV INFECTION

Relative to their degree of anemia, patients with AIDS have inappropriately low endogenous EPO levels. While taking zidovudine, their EPO levels usually increase but still remain disproportionately depressed.

Before EPO is considered, other treatable causes of anemia need to be excluded. Evaluation of iron stores and iron replacement, if necessary, should be initiated before beginning EPO therapy.

Patients with AIDS receiving zidovudine whose EPO level is more than 500 U/L do not respond to EPO at a dosage of 100 U/kg three times a week. Only when EPO levels are less than 500 U/L do patients benefit from EPO.

EPO therapy should be started at a dosage of 100 U/kg three times a week subcutaneously. If the reticulocyte count has not improved at 10 days, the dosage of EPO should be doubled; if it has not improved at a dosage of 300 U/kg three times a week, discontinuing the EPO therapy should be considered.

Cost and benefit analyses are needed. In patients requiring less than 4 to 6 units of transfused red cells a month, EPO is an expensive option.

CANCER PATIENTS RECEIVING CHEMOTHERAPY

Many patients with cancer are anemic; in some cases, this anemia is caused by the production of cytokines, such as tumor necrosis factor, which inhibit erythropoiesis. Chemotherapy, particularly with platinum analogs, worsens the anemia. Cisplatin blunts the production of EPO in response to anemia.

Patients who have an EPO level more than 200 U/L are unlikely to respond to EPO. Patients who are transfusion-dependent at the onset of EPO treatment are less likely to respond than patients who have never had transfusion. Approximately 30% of patients will not respond to EPO.

In both myeloma and other malignancies with marrow infiltration, EPO improves erythropoiesis and decreases the transfusion requirement. The recommended starting dosage is 150 U/kg three times a week.

ANEMIA OF CHRONIC DISEASE

Increased tumor necrosis factor is found in the serum of 50% of anemic patients with rheumatoid arthritis. EPO improves erythropoiesis in a subset of anemic patients with rheumatoid arthritis. EPO also can be used to facilitate autologous collection of blood in this patient population.

MYELODYSPLASTIC SYNDROMES

Patients with myelodysplastic syndromes have an increased EPO level. The rationale for treating them with pharmacologic doses of EPO is to overcome the defective proliferation and maturation of erythroid precursors. With treatment, the hemoglobin level increases to more than 15 g/L or the transfusion is no longer required in 16% of patients with myelodysplastic syndromes.

The response is better in refractory anemia and refractory anemia with excess blasts than in refractory anemia with ringed sideroblasts. No response occurs in patients with refractory anemia with ringed sideroblasts whose EPO level is more than 200 U/L or in transfusion-dependent patients with this disorder.

AUTOLOGOUS TRANSFUSION

The administration of EPO increases the amount of blood donated by patients by about 40%. EPO therapy given preoperatively reduces the need for red blood cell transfusions and provides a method to increase the number of autologous units collected.

The patients who benefit the most from EPO therapy are those whose initial hematocrit value is 33% to 39% and whose surgical blood losses are anticipated to be 1,000 to 3,000 mL. The most cost-effective regimen may be 4 weekly subcutaneous doses of erythropoietin, starting at 100 U/kg, with increases up to 600 U/kg, if necessary, to produce evidence of reticulocyte response.

GRANULOCYTE COLONY-STIMULATING FACTOR

Granulocyte colony-stimulating factor (G-CSF) is a glycoprotein produced by monocytes, fibroblasts, and endothelial cells. It reduces the time required for maturation of neutrophils and prolongs their lifespan in circulation. In addition, G-CSF is an activator of neutrophil function. G-CSF has minimal direct in vivo effect on other hematopoietic cell types.

Side effects of G-CSF include bone pain, increases in leukocyte alkaline phosphatase and lactic acid dehydrogenase values, exacerbation of dermatologic conditions such as psoriasis, and, with chronic therapy, splenomegaly and hair loss. G-CSF should not be used 24 hours before or after cytotoxic chemotherapy.

The recommended starting dosage of G-CSF is 5 µg/kg per day either subcutaneously or by short intravenous infusion. Use of G-CSF should be discontinued once marrow recovery has occurred and the neutrophil count has reached 10,000/µL. When used for peripheral blood progenitor collection, G-CSF is often given at a dosage of 10 µg/kg per day.

Clinical Uses of G-CSF

AFTER CHEMOTHERAPY FOR CANCER

G-CSF was approved for clinical use to reduce the incidence of infection in patients with nonmyeloid malignancies receiving myelosuppressive chemotherapy; this approval was based predominantly on the results of a phase III trial in patients with small-cell lung cancer receiving cyclophosphamide, doxorubicin, and etoposide. This regimen caused profound and sustained myelosuppression. This trial demonstrated shortening of the duration of neutropenia, decreased length of stay in the hospital, and decrease in the number of days of intravenous antibiotic use.

In 1996, a panel convened by the American Society of Clinical Oncology concluded that treatment with G-CSF or granulocyte-macrophage colony-stimulating factor

(GM-CSF) is unnecessary in patients with neutropenia of less than a week in duration but that it may benefit patients with prolonged neutropenia.

In a trial of G-CSF in patients with severe chemotherapy-induced afebrile neutropenia of short duration, G-CSF shortened the time of neutrophil recovery, but it had no impact on the incidence of hospitalization, the length of stay in the hospital, the number of days of treatment with parenteral antibiotics, or the number of culture-positive infections.

In children with established febrile neutropenia, a randomized trial comparing G-CSF with placebo failed to show benefit in terms of number of proven infections. The G-CSF group had a more rapid neutrophil recovery, shorter hospital stay, and fewer median days of antibiotic treatment.

The greatest benefits of G-CSF after chemotherapy occur after the use of chemotherapy regimens commonly associated with a high risk for development of neutropenic fever. The use of G-CSF reduces the incidence of neutropenic fever by 25% to 30% when the overall incidence of the event approaches 50% to 60%.

In elderly patients with acute myeloid leukemia undergoing chemotherapy, G-CSF shortens the period of neutropenia. G-CSF does not increase the leukemic relapse rate in this setting. There is controversy regarding any improvement in remission rate or survival when G-CSF is used after chemotherapy for acute myeloid leukemia.

AFTER AUTOLOGOUS AND ALLOGENEIC STEM CELL TRANSPLANTATION

Patients undergoing autologous transplantation for lymphoid malignancies or solid tumors have a more rapid recovery of their neutrophil count and a reduction in the days of febrile neutropenia when G-CSF is used after stem cell infusion. There is no difference in survival between patients treated with G-CSF and those given placebo.

In a randomized trial of G-CSF versus placebo conducted in patients with myeloid and nonmyeloid malignancies who were undergoing allogeneic transplantation, the number of days of severe neutropenia was significantly reduced. The role of G-CSF after transplantation in myeloid malignancies remains controversial.

PERIPHERAL BLOOD PROGENITOR COLLECTION

G-CSF increases the yield of mononuclear and early stem cells (CD34+) that are harvested during a peripheral blood progenitor collection. G-CSF-stimulated progenitor cells reduce the duration of neutropenia significantly compared with nonstimulated progenitor cells.

CHRONIC NEUTROPENIAS

Patients with severe congenital neutropenia, cyclic neutropenia, and idiopathic neutropenia benefit from G-CSF therapy. G-CSF increases their neutrophil count, and the incidence of infections is decreased. The Severe Chronic Neutropenia International Registry demonstrated that the median dosage of G-CSF required for each one of these groups is, respectively, 11.5, 3, and 1.4 µg/kg per day. Leukemic transformation occurs in 9% of patients with severe congenital neutropenia. Leukemic transformation does not occur in cyclic neutropenia or in idiopathic neutropenia.

MYELODYSPLASTIC SYNDROMES

G-CSF increases the neutrophil count in most patients with myelodysplastic syndromes. Occasional patients have an increase in their reticulocyte and platelet counts, and some patients experience a worsening of their thrombocytopenia. G-CSF is not used prophylactically in the management of myelodysplastic syndromes.

HIV INFECTION

G-CSF increases the neutrophil count of patients with HIV, and it also increases the neutrophil count of patients treated with zidovudine. G-CSF does not increase the level of HIV antigens. Currently, G-CSF is not approved in the United States for the treatment of neutropenia associated with HIV. In clinical practice, G-CSF is frequently used for patients with severe neutropenia that cannot be managed by adjustments of their myelosuppressive drugs. In patients with HIV, a starting dosage of G-CSF of 0.5 to 2 µg/kg per day is suggested.

GRANULOCYTE-MACROPHAGE COLONY-STIMULATING FACTOR

Granulocyte-macrophage colony-stimulating factor (GM-CSF) is a glycoprotein that stimulates the proliferation and maturation of granulocytes and eosinophils. At high doses, GM-CSF has potent monocyte/macrophage potentiating activity.

The toxic effects of GM-CSF consist of arthralgias, myalgias, fever, pleuropericarditis, and a first-dose effect. They are more pronounced after intravenous bolus than with subcutaneous administration. The first-dose effect consists of respiratory distress, hypoxia, flushing, hypotension, and syncope after the first administration of GM-CSF in a particular cycle. These effects resolve with symptomatic treatment and usually do not recur with subsequent doses in the same cycle of treatment. This syndrome may recur with the first dose of each cycle that a patient receives. The first-dose effect is thought to be due to sequestration of neutrophils in the pulmonary microcirculation. The usual dosage of GM-CSF is 250 µg/kg per day intravenously or subcutaneously.

Clinical Uses of GM-CSF

ACUTE MYELOID LEUKEMIA INDUCTION IN PATIENTS OLDER THAN 55 YEARS

GM-CSF shortens the time for neutrophil recovery after induction chemotherapy, but it does not shorten erythroid or megakaryocytic recovery. GM-CSF reduces the incidence of severe infections and deaths related to infection. GM-CSF has no significant impact on complete remission rate or survival.

MOBILIZATION AND ENGRAFTMENT OF PERIPHERAL BLOOD PROGENITOR CELLS

Compared with nonmobilized progenitor cell collection, GM-CSF used for progenitor cell mobilization increases the yield of progenitor cells collected. GM-CSF shortens the time to neutrophil, platelet, and red cell recovery and decreases the length of stay in the hospital.

AUTOLOGOUS PROGENITOR CELL TRANSPLANTATION

In patients with lymphoid malignancies, GM-CSF administered after progenitor cell infusion is associated with a more rapid neutrophil recovery and a shorter hospital stay. Similar results have been reported in patients with solid tumors undergoing transplantation.

ALLOGENEIC PROGENITOR CELL TRANSPLANTATION

GM-CSF administered after allogeneic progenitor cell infusion is associated with more rapid neutrophil recovery, fewer infections, a shortened hospital stay, and a lower incidence of grade 3 or 4 mucositis. GM-CSF does not increase the incidence or frequency of graft-versus-host disease or the incidence of disease relapse.

BONE MARROW TRANSPLANT FAILURE OR ENGRAFTMENT DELAY

Patients with autologous or allogeneic graft failure derive a survival advantage from being treated with GM-CSF. The probability of survival is increased if the graft is autologous, if the transplant was done for a nonleukemic malignancy, and if total body irradiation was not part of the conditioning regimen.

MYELODYSPLASTIC SYNDROMES

A dose-dependent increase in the absolute neutrophil count occurs in 80% of patients. Reticulocytes increase in 20%, but this change usually does not translate into an increase in hematocrit. Platelets increase in 6%, but thrombocytopenia occurs in 6%.

Leukemic transformation has been described in patients with an excess of 14% blasts treated with GM-CSF. Splenomegaly may increase with GM-CSF therapy. GM-CSF is currently being used in patients with febrile neutropenia, but the prophylactic use of GM-CSF is not recommended.

HIV INFECTION

GM-CSF may augment HIV replication. It also has been shown to augment the antiretroviral agent zidovudine by increasing intracellular concentration of the biologically active triphosphate form.

GM-CSF increases the neutrophil count of patients with HIV and of patients treated with myelosuppressive drugs.

INTERLEUKIN-11

Interleukin-11 (IL-11) is produced by various stromal cells, including fibroblasts, epithelial cells, and osteoblasts. IL-11 is indicated for the prevention of severe thrombocytopenia and the reduction of platelet transfusion needs after myelosuppressive chemotherapy in patients with nonmyeloid malignancies. IL-11 is not indicated after myeloablative chemotherapy.

IL-11 protects small intestine cells after combined radiation and chemotherapy, reduces experimental mucositis, and ameliorates injury in models of inflammatory bowel disease. The mechanisms by which IL-11 protects the mucosa are unclear. The ability of IL-11 to inhibit macrophage production of tumor necrosis factor, IL-1, and IL-12 may prevent epithelial apoptosis.

IL-11 at a dose of 50 μg/kg was administered to patients who had severe thrombocytopenia after chemotherapy; it was given at the time of their next cycle of the same chemotherapy without dose reduction. Approximately 20% of patients avoided platelet transfusions compared with a placebo group.

A randomized, double-blind, placebo-controlled phase II study in patients undergoing autologous bone marrow transplantation after myeloablative chemotherapy failed to show improvement in the time to platelet engraftment or the incidence of platelet transfusions.

Side effects with IL-11 include fluid retention, dilutional anemia, and transient atrial arrhythmias. The atrial arrhythmias occur in 10% of patients. Papilledema has been reported in 1.5% of patients and the development of antibodies to IL-11, in 1%.

The recommended dose of IL-11 in adults is 50 mg/kg given once daily subcutaneously. The IL-11 therapy is usually continued until the platelet count reaches 50,000/μL.

Therapy with IL-11 can be initiated 6 to 24 hours after chemotherapy and should be discontinued at least 2 days before the start of the next cycle of chemotherapy.

STEM CELL FACTOR

Stem cell factor (SCF) is an early-acting hematopoietic cytokine that supports the proliferation and survival of pluripotent progenitor cells and increases their receptivity to lineage commitment and differentiation in response to lineage-specific cytokines.

In addition to hematopoietic progenitor cells, the receptor for SCF is expressed in mast cells, melanocytes, neurons, and germ cells. The Food and Drug Administration is currently considering approval of SCF for noninvestigational clinical use.

SCF has little clinical cytokine activity as an isolated molecule at low doses. However, in combination with other growth factors, SCF synergistically increases the size and number of hematopoietic progenitor cells.

G-CSF in combination with SCF has been used as a peripheral blood progenitor mobilizing agent. In clinical trials, the yield of mononuclear cells is doubled compared with G-CSF used as a single agent.

Toxic effects consist of allergic-type reactions. Virtually all patients have a pruritic wheal-and-flare response at the injection site. In phase I trials, 25% of patients have anaphylactic-like reactions. These reactions are believed to be mast-cell–mediated and dose-related, occurring primarily in patients who received more than 25 μg/kg per day of SCF. When patients are premedicated with antihistamines and β-agonists, SCF is well tolerated.

SUGGESTED READING

Aboulafia DM. Use of hematopoietic hormones for bone marrow defects in AIDS. *Oncology (Huntingt)* 1997; 11: 1827-1834.

Ganser A, Hoelzer D. Clinical use of hematopoietic growth factors in the myelodysplastic syndromes. *Semin Hematol* 1996; 33: 186-195.

Glaspy J. Clinical applications of stem cell factor. *Curr Opin Hematol* 1996; 3: 223-229.

Goodnough LT, Monk TG, Andriole GL. Erythropoietin therapy. *N Engl J Med* 1997; 336: 933-938.

Hartmann LC, Tschetter LK, Habermann TM, Ebbert LP, Johnson PS, Mailliard JA, Levitt R, Suman VJ, Witzig TE, Wieand HS, Miller LL, Moertel CG. Granulocyte colony-stimulating factor in severe chemotherapy-induced afebrile neutropenia. *N Engl J Med* 1997; 336: 1776-1780.

Isaacs C, Robert NJ, Bailey FA, Schuster MW, Overmoyer B, Graham M, Cai B, Beach KJ, Loewy JW, Kaye JA. Randomized placebo-controlled study of recombinant human interleukin-11 to prevent chemotherapy-induced thrombocytopenia in patients with breast cancer receiving dose-intensive cyclophosphamide and doxorubicin. *J Clin Oncol* 1997; 15: 3368-3377.

Means RT Jr. Erythropoietin in the treatment of anemia in chronic infectious, inflammatory, and malignant diseases. *Curr Opin Hematol* 1995; 2: 210-213.

Mitchell PL, Morland B, Stevens MC, Dick G, Easlea D, Meyer LC, Pinkerton CR. Granulocyte colony-stimulating factor in established febrile neutropenia: a randomized study of pediatric patients. *J Clin Oncol* 1997; 15: 1163-1170.

Sheffield R, Sullivan SD, Saltiel E, Nishimura L. Cost comparison of recombinant human erythropoietin and blood transfusion in cancer chemotherapy-induced anemia. *Ann Pharmacother* 1997; 31: 15-22.

Tepler I, Elias L, Smith JW II, Hussein M, Rosen G, Chang AY, Moore JO, Gordon MS, Kuca B, Beach KJ, Loewy JW, Garnick MB, Kaye JA. A randomized placebo-controlled trial of recombinant human interleukin-11 in cancer patients with severe thrombocytopenia due to chemotherapy. *Blood* 1996; 87: 3607-3614.

Vose JM, Armitage JO. Clinical applications of hematopoietic growth factors. *J Clin Oncol* 1995; 13: 1023-1035.

27 A Primer of Chemotherapy

Alex A. Adjei, MD, PhD

Contents

INTRODUCTION

The word *chemotherapy*, derived from *chemical* and *therapy*, refers to the use of chemical agents to destroy organisms (bacteria, parasites, viruses) or to destroy tissue (cancer). The use of this term has become increasingly synonymous with the chemical therapy of cancer. In cancer therapy, a strict definition of chemotherapy considers only the use of cytotoxic agents. Thus, chemotherapy is differentiated from hormonal therapy (estrogens, progestins, androgens and their antagonists), biologic therapy (cytokines and growth factors), immunologic therapy (vaccines, antibodies), and genetic therapy of cancer. This chapter focuses on clinically useful and promising cytotoxic agents.

BRIEF HISTORY

The concept of treating cancer with drugs goes back more than 500 years, when preparations of mercury, silver, and zinc were used. The first documented case of cancer chemotherapy was by Lissauer in 1865. He gave Fowler's solution (potassium arsenite) to a patient with leukemia, and the patient had "beneficial effects." The modern era of chemotherapy started when the war gas sulfur mustard was used in patients in 1931, first topically and then by direct intratumoral injection; but this agent was thought to be too toxic for human use. The second-generation mustard, nitrogen mustard, subsequently

From: *Primary Hematology*
Edited by: A. Tefferi © Mayo Foundation for Medical Education and Research, Rochester, MN

was tested by Gilman and colleagues, first in mice and then in a patient with lympho-sarcoma, in 1942. Gilman and Philips published a review of the use of nitrogen mustard in the treatment of human cancer, in 1946. One of the first nitrogen mustards found to be clinically active at that time, mechlorethamine, is still used in cancer therapy.

PRINCIPLES OF CHEMOTHERAPY

Adjuvant chemotherapy refers to the use of chemotherapy postoperatively in a patient with cancer who may be possibly cured but is at significant risk for recurrence and death from micrometastatic disease. The therapies used typically have been shown in random-ized trials to delay tumor recurrence and prolong survival. Adjuvant therapy is of proven benefit in treating breast cancer, colorectal cancer, and osteosarcoma.

Neoadjuvant chemotherapy is used to debulk tumors before definitive operation. Can-cers of the head and neck, esophagus, lung, and breast, osteosarcomas, and soft tissue sarcomas are the usual candidates. This approach can improve the probability of com-plete resection, reduce the morbidity of operation, and serve as a prognostic indicator.

The objective of cancer chemotherapy is to reduce the tumor cell population to zero. Most drugs have been developed empirically by testing large numbers of chemicals on rapidly growing transplantable rodent tumors and, recently, human tumor xenografts. This approach predominantly has identified DNA-active drugs. These agents are used in cycles of intensive therapy, used as frequently as allowed by the tolerance of dose-limiting tissues. The aim is to ablate tumor cells through the multiplicative effect of fractional cell kill. Current cancer chemotherapy regimens are guided by several paradigms.

The *fractional cell kill hypothesis* states that a constant fraction of tumor cells will be killed per cycle of constant drug dosing, regardless of total body burden. For example, if a drug kills 99% of tumor cells per cycle of treatment, the tumor burden of 10^{11} cells will be reduced to approximately 10 cells after five cycles of therapy [(10^{11} cells) $\times$ $(0.01)^6 < 10$]. This hypothesis has been validated in rapidly proliferating homogeneous rodent tumors, but it is unclear how applicable this concept is in biologically heteroge-neous human solid tumors.

The concept that neoplastic tumors have a "steep" *dose-response curve*, with a linear relationship between dose of drug administered and efficacy, underlies the administra-tion of chemotherapy. Thus, the highest possible dose of drugs is administered at the shortest possible intervals. Even a modest dose reduction may lead to substantial reduc-tions in tumor cell kill. This concept has led to the idea of dose intensity, defined as the amount of drug delivered per week of therapy. A more dose-intense regimen is expected to yield superior responses. This concept has not been consistently proved in clinical studies.

The *Goldie-Coldman hypothesis* states that a tumor undergoes a spontaneous mutation of about 1 cell in 105 cells per gene. The minimal detectable tumor size in humans is 1 g (109 cells). Such a tumor may contain 104 resistant clones to a given drug. Resistance to two drugs, however, should occur in 1 cell of 1,010 cells (1 resistant clone per 10 g of tumor). It therefore follows that multidrug therapy is significantly more effective than single-agent therapy. As with the other paradigms of cancer chemotherapy, this hypoth-esis was generated retrospectively. Combination therapy was known to be more effective than single-agent therapy before this hypothesis was generated.

In addition to overcoming tumor resistance, combination therapy is important for limiting drug toxicity, because several agents with nonoverlapping toxicities can be used.

Table 1
Some Known Mechanisms of Drug Resistance

Mechanism	Drugs
Decreased influx (alteration in transport protein)	Methotrexate, nucleoside analogues
Increase in drug efflux (P-glycoprotein amplification)	Natural products Vinca alkaloids, taxoids Anthracyclines Epipodophyllotoxins
MRP overexpression	Similar to MDR
Increased drug detoxification (increased glutathione levels, glutathione S-transferase overexpression)	Alkylating agents, platinum compounds
Increased DNA repair (O^6-alkyl guanine alkyltransferase overexpression)	Triazenes, nitrosoureas
Alterations in target enzymes	Methotrexate, 5-fluorouracil, topoisomerase inhibitors
Defective apoptosis (overexpression of anti-apoptosis genes, e.g., *bcl*-2), inactivation of pro-apoptotic genes, e.g., p53	Most cytotoxic drugs

Abbreviations: MDR, multidrug resistance; MRP, multidrug resistance protein.

One of the first curative regimens for a solid tumor (testicular cancer) was comprised of bleomycin, vinblastine, and cisplatin—three agents with different mechanisms of action and non-overlapping toxicities.

Drug resistance, either present at initial treatment or developing at relapse, inevitably occurs in all but a few cancers and is the reason for incurability of most nonoperable cancers. Such resistance probably results from random, spontaneous accumulations of somatic mutations by tumor cells. Clinical resistance emerges by positive selection for resistance clones. Important resistance mechanisms to chemotherapy agents are outlined in Table 1. In a particular tumor type, multiple mechanisms may occur.

ANTIMETABOLITES

The antimetabolites are structural analogues of naturally occurring compounds which interfere with the production of nucleic acids by two major mechanisms. Some agents inhibit the production of deoxyribonucleoside triphosphates, which are immediate precursors of DNA in its synthetic pathway. Other agents are similar enough in structure to the normal nucleosides to be used as fraudulent nucleotides in DNA synthesis, leading to chain termination of the elongating DNA strand.

Antifolates

The importance of folates in tumor growth was demonstrated in 1948, when Farber and colleagues demonstrated that remissions were induced in children with leukemia who were treated with the folate antagonist aminopterin (4-amino-folic acid). Subsequently,

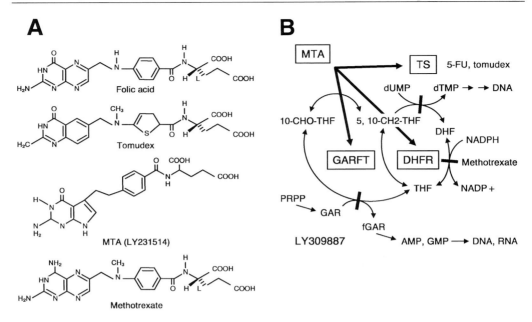

Fig. 1. *A*, The structures of folic acid and antifolate drugs. *B*, Target enzymes for antifolate and related drugs. Multitargeted antifolate (MTA) is a novel agent undergoing broad clinical trials. AMP, adenosine monophosphate; 10-CHO-THF, formyl tetrahydrofolate; DHF, dihydrofolate; DHFR, dihydrofolate dehydrogenase; dTMP, deoxythymidylate; dUMP, deoxyuridine monophosphate; fGAR, formyl glycinamide ribonucleotide; 5-FU, 5-fluorouracil; GAR, glycinamide ribonucleotide; GARFT, glycinamide ribonucleotide formyl-transferase; GMP, guanosine monophosphate; NADP, nicotinamide adenine dinucleotide phosphate; NADPH, reduced form of NADP; PRPP, phosphoribosylpyrophosphate; THF, tetrahydrofolate; TS, thymidylate synthase. (From Adjei AA. A review of the pharmacology and clinical activity of new chemotherapy agents for the treatment of colorectal cancer. *Br J Clin Pharmacol* 1999; 48: 265-277. By permission of Blackwell Science.)

another folate analogue, methotrexate (4-amino-10-methyl-folic acid), was found to have similar effectiveness, but it was less toxic. All classic antifolate drugs are transported into cells by the reduced folic acid carrier and are extensively anabolized to the more active polyglutamated form by folylpolyglutamyl synthase. This results in products containing up to 12 glutamic acid residues. Cellular retention is increased because of this extensive polyglutamation. The structures of folic acid and its antagonists are shown in Figure 1.

METHOTREXATE

Methotrexate is the most widely used antifolate in cancer chemotherapy. Its mechanism of cytotoxicity is through 1) inhibition of dihydrofolate reductase, resulting in depletion of reduced folates, which are the one-carbon donor for several metabolic processes; 2) inhibition of de novo purine and thymidylate synthesis by methotrexate and its dihydrofolate polyglutamates; and 3) formation of DNA strand breaks, which occurs through depletion of thymidylate and purine nucleotides and by incorporation of deoxyuridine triphosphate into DNA. The major resistance mechanisms described for methotrexate are listed in Table 1.

Methotrexate is administered orally, intravenously, or intrathecally. The major route of elimination is through the kidneys. Renal excretion is inhibited by nonsteroidal anti-inflammatory agents, penicillin, cephalosporins, and probenecid. In the setting of impaired renal function, the dose of methotrexate should be reduced in proportion to the creatinine clearance. The drug accumulates in third-space fluid collections, such as ascites, leading to increased toxicity. Such fluid collections should be drained before methotrexate therapy is started. The major toxic effects of methotrexate are myelosuppression, mucositis, nephrotoxicity, acute and chronic hepatotoxicity, pneumonitis, and neurotoxicity (high-dose therapy). Hypersensitivity reactions rarely occur. Methotrexate is used clinically in leukemia, lymphoma, breast cancer, head and neck cancer, osteogenic sarcoma, and choriocarcinoma. Standard and high-dose regimens with leucovorin rescue are used.

SPECIFIC THYMIDYLATE SYNTHASE INHIBITORS

Thymidine monophosphate (TMP) is anabolized in cells to the triphosphate, which is essential for DNA synthesis and repair. An enzyme critical to the de novo synthesis of TMP is thymidylate synthase. The substrate for thymidylate synthase is deoxyuridine monophosphate, which is converted to TMP. The carbon donor for this reaction is the folate cofactor, 5,10-methylenetetrahydrofolate (CH2FH4) (Fig. 1). Various heterocyclic folate analogues are potent thymidylate synthase inhibitors. The first such inhibitor to be evaluated clinically was CB3717, which was active in several preclinical tumor models but exhibited life-threatening nephrotoxicity in early clinical testing. Several second-generation agents are currently in different stages of clinical development.

Tomudex (ZD-1694)

Tomudex (N-[5-(N-[3,4-dihydro-2-methyl-4-oxoquinazolin-6-ylmethyl]-N-methyl-amino)-2-th enoyl]-L-glutamic acid) is the first specific thymidylate synthase inhibitor to be approved for clinical use. This is a water-soluble second-generation quinazoline analogue of folic acid which is transported into cells by the reduced folate carrier and is extensively anabolized to the more active (600-fold more cytotoxic) polyglutamated forms. Cellular retention is increased because of the extensive polyglutamation. Tomudex is administered as a single intravenous infusion every 3 weeks. Toxic effects are myelosuppression, mucositis, increased hepatic transaminase value, asthenia, and alopecia. This agent is currently used for the treatment of metastatic colorectal cancer.

PYRIMIDINE ANALOGUES

The pyrimidine antagonists comprise nucleic acid bases and their pro-drugs, which inhibit thymidylate synthase, and nucleoside analogues, which become incorporated into the elongating DNA strand and inhibit DNA synthesis.

5-Fluorouracil (5-FU)

5-FU was rationally synthesized in 1957 by Heidelberger, who had observed that rat hepatoma cells used uracil more efficiently than normal rat intestinal mucosa, a suggestion that uracil metabolism might represent a target for cancer chemotherapy. The predominant mechanisms of 5-FU cytotoxicity are the inhibition of thymidylate synthase by fluorodeoxyuridine monophosphate (FdUMP), the 5-FU anabolite, and the incorporation of fluorouridine triphosphate (FUTP) into RNA, resulting in alterations in RNA processing. Some of the documented mechanisms of resistance of 5-FU are shown in Table 1. The drug is administered intravenously on various schedules. Common toxic effects of 5-FU are myelosuppression (bolus schedules), mucositis, ocular toxicity (blepharitis, conjunctivitis), plantar-palmar erythrodysesthesia, also known as hand-foot syndrome (continuous infusion schedules), and cardiac and neurologic symptoms.

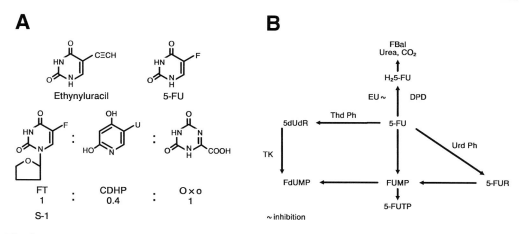

Fig. 2. The structures of fluorouracil (5-FU) and its modulators. Ethynyluracil and chlorodihydropyrimidine (CDHP) are inhibitors of dihydropyrimidine dehydrogenase (DPD). Oxonic acid (Oxo) is an inhibitor of pyrimidine phosphoribosyl transferase. Ftorafur (FT) is an oral pro-drug of 5-FU in clinical trials. S-1 comprises FT, CDHP and Oxo in the molar ratio shown. This agent is in clinical trials. *B*, The metabolism of 5-FU with key enzymes. 5dUdR, 5-deoxyuridine; EU, ethynyluracil; FBal, fluorobeta alanine; FdUMP, fluorodeoxyuridine monophosphate; FUMP, fluorouridine monophosphate; 5-FUR, 5-fluorouridine; 5-FUTP, 5'-fluorouridine triphosphate; Thd Ph, thymidine phosphorylase; Urd Ph, uridine phosphorylase; TK, thymidine kinase. (From Adjei AA. A review of the pharmacology and clinical activity of new chemotherapy agents for the treatment of colorectal cancer. *Br J Clin Pharmacol* 1999; 48: 265-277. By permission of Blackwell Science.)

Eighty-five percent of administered 5-FU is eliminated through catabolism (Fig. 2). The initial rate-limiting enzyme in this pathway is dihydropyrimidine dehydrogenase (DPD), which is abundant in the gastrointestinal tract, liver, and peripheral blood mononuclear cells. An inherited variability in the activity of this enzyme has been described, and it is thought to explain the wide interpatient variability in 5-FU pharmacokinetics, toxicity, and oral bioavailability. The exact proportion of the population with DPD deficiency is unknown. In these individuals, standard doses of 5-FU cause profound myelosuppression, mucositis, alopecia, neurologic toxicity, coma, and sometimes death. The combination of 5-FU or its pro-drugs with inhibitors of DPD has produced several novel oral agents being tested currently for clinical use (Fig. 2).

Several important interactions between 5-FU and other agents have been described. Leucovorin provides reduced folates to enhance the inhibition of thymidylate synthase. Thymidine and uridine can antagonize the host toxic effects of 5-FU, but they may abrogate antitumor efficacy. Methotrexate pretreatment increases the formation of 5-FU nucleotides. 5-FU is used for gastrointestinal malignancies and for esophageal, head and neck, and breast cancers.

Capecitabine (Xeloda)

Pyrimidine nucleoside phosphorylase (thymidine phosphorylase) catalyses the formation of pyrimidine bases from nucleosides. Levels of this enzyme are significantly higher in several tumor tissues than in normal tissue. Recently, pyrimidine nucleoside phosphorylase was shown to be a tumor-associated angiogenic factor, identified as platelet-derived endothelial cell growth factor, whose expression has correlated with poor clinical outcome. 5'-Deoxyfluorouridine, which is a substrate for this enzyme, was synthesized in an attempt to increase the efficacy of 5-FU by increasing intratumoral delivery

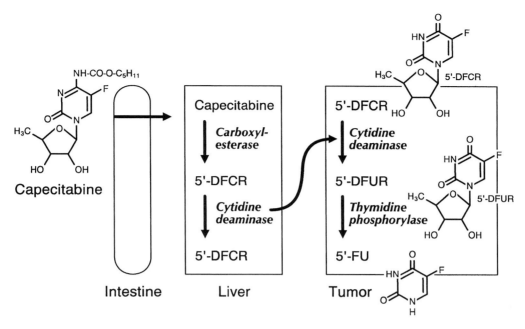

Fig. 3. The metabolic activation of capecitabine. 5'-DFCR, 5'-deoxy-5-fluorocytidine; 5'-FU, 5'-fluorouracil; 5'-DFUR, 5'-deoxy-5-fluorouridine. (From Adjei AA. A review of the pharmacology and clinical activity of new chemotherapy agents for the treatment of colorectal cancer. *Br J Clin Pharmacol* 1999; 48: 265-277. By permission of Blackwell Science.)

of the drug. In subsequent human testing, response rates similar to those achieved by 5-FU in colorectal carcinoma (30%–35%) could be obtained only after protracted venous infusion, up to 3 months in one study. Unfortunately, an alternative trial of oral administration was limited by diarrhea, presumably due to the release of 5-FU in the gastrointestinal tract through the activity of intestinal pyrimidine nucleoside phosphorylase.

Capecitabine has been developed to circumvent the problem of gastrointestinal toxicity from oral 5'-deoxyfluorouridine. This oral pro-drug of 5-FU is absorbed through the gastrointestinal mucosa as an intact molecule. It is sequentially activated by carboxylesterase, cytidine deaminase, and pyrimidine nucleoside phosphorylase (Fig. 3), leading to the intratumoral release of 5-FU. The drug is administered orally in two divided doses daily for 14 days with 1 week off. Major toxic effects are diarrhea, which is dose-limiting, palmar-plantar erythrodysesthesia, and stomatitis. These are typical of protracted infusion of 5-FU. The antitumor activity of capecitabine has been demonstrated in breast cancer, for which it has been approved.

Cytosine Arabinoside (Ara-C)

Ara-C was isolated from the Caribbean sponge *Cryptothethya crypta*. The ribose moiety of cytosine has been substituted with an arabinose group in this agent (Fig. 4). It is a standard agent in the treatment of acute myelogenous leukemia, but it has minimal activity against solid tumors. Ara-C is transported intracellularly via the facilitated diffusion nucleoside transport system and anabolized intracellularly to ara-CTP, the active anabolite. Two inactivating enzymes, cytidine deaminase and deoxycytidine monophosphate (dCMP) deaminase, can form inactive metabolites from either ara-C or ara-CMP. This can affect the amount of intracellular ara-CTP and is critical for the drug's activity.

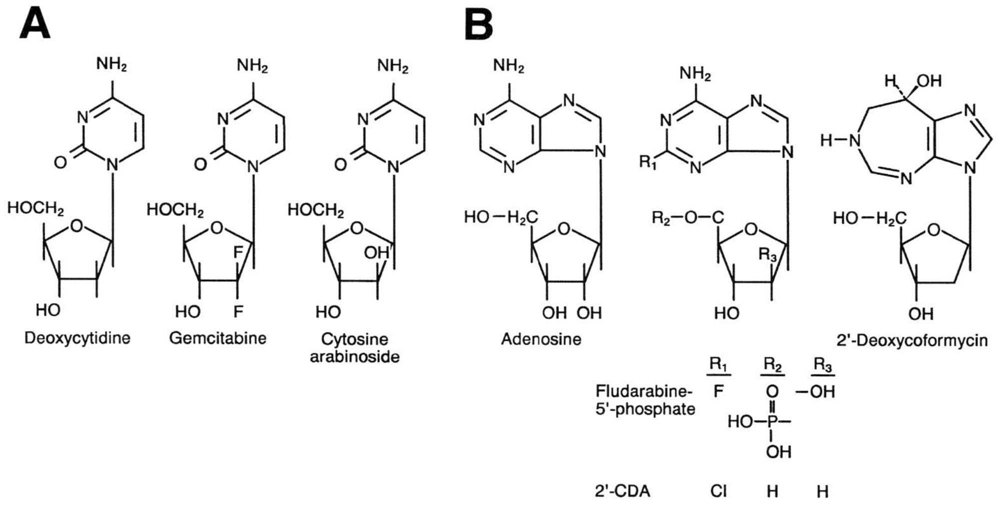

A

B

Fig. 4. The structures of clinically useful nucleoside analogues.

Ara-CTP inhibits DNA polymerase alpha and beta, leading to inhibition of DNA synthesis and repair. It is also incorporated into DNA, leading to chain termination.

Some of the resistance mechanisms described for ara-C are shown in Table 1. The presence of high concentrations of cytidine deaminase in liver and gastrointestinal epithelium prevents the oral use of ara-C, whose plasma half-life is a short 7 to 20 minutes. The drug is therefore administered on an every 8- to 12-hour schedule for 5 to 7 days or as a continuous infusion. Ara-C achieves cerebrospinal fluid levels of 20% to 40% of serum levels and is given intrathecally to treat meningeal leukemia and carcinomatosis. It can be given on a high-dose schedule of 2 to 3 g/m^2 every 12 hours for 6 days. In regular doses, the major toxic effects are myelosuppression and gastrointestinal effects. Intrahepatic cholestasis and rare pancreatitis occur. In high-dose therapy, the toxic effects are more severe. In addition, cerebral and cerebellar dysfunction, pulmonary toxicity, conjunctivitis, and a cutaneous reaction with plaques or nodules (neutrophilic eccrine hydradenitis) occur.

Gemcitabine

Gemcitabine (2',2'-difluorodeoxycytidine, dFdC, Gemzar) is a fluorinated analogue of deoxycytidine (Fig. 4). Gemcitabine has major differences in activity and clinical effects compared with those of other deoxycytidine analogues, such as cytosine arabinoside. The drug was initially synthesized as an antiviral agent, but it was not evaluated further because of toxicity. Gemcitabine is a pro-drug, transported into cells via the facilitated diffusion nucleoside transport carrier and phosphorylated sequentially to the triphosphate form. The rate-limiting enzyme in the phosphorylation is deoxycytidine kinase. In comparison with cytosine arabinoside, gemcitabine is a better substrate for the nucleoside transporter of tumor cells and has greater affinity for deoxycytidine kinase.

The principal cytotoxic metabolite of gemcitabine is 2',2'-difluorodeoxycytidine triphosphate (dFdCTP). It directly competes with deoxycytidine triphosphate (dCTP) for incorporation into the elongating DNA strand. Incorporation of dFdCTP results in termination of DNA chain elongation and inhibition of DNA synthesis. Critical to the cytotoxic effect is the prolonged intracellular retention of dFdCTP that is related to its

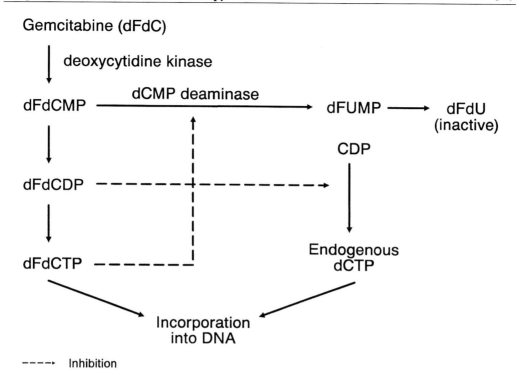

Fig. 5. The metabolic activation of gemcitabine-CDP, cytidine diphosphate; dCMP, deoxycytidine monophosphate; dCTP, deoxycytidine triphosphate; dFdCDP, 2',2'-difluorodeoxycytidine diphosphate; dFdCMP, 2',2'-difluorodeoxycytidine monophosphate; dFdCTP, 2',2'-difluorodeoxycytidine triphosphate; dFdU, 2',2'-difluorodeoxyuridine; dFUMP, 2',2'-difluorodeoxyuridine monophosphate.

self-potentiation through various mechanisms. Because dFdCTP inhibits ribonucleotide reductase for phosphorylation, competing endogenous deoxyribonucleotide pools (including dCTP) are reduced. In addition, dFdCTP inhibits its own catabolizing enzyme, deoxycitidine monophosphate deaminase, an enzyme that converts 2'2'-difluorodeoxycytidine monophosphate (dFdCMP) to 2',2'-difluorodeoxyuridine monophosphate (dFUMP), which is then metabolized to 2',2'-difluorodeoxyuridine (dFdU), an inactive catabolite. The metabolic pathway of gemcitabine is summarized in Figure 5. The solid tumor selectivity of gemcitabine, in contrast to other nucleoside analogues, is related to the prolonged intracellular retention of dFdCTP.

The side effects of gemcitabine include a flu-like syndrome, fever, hypotension, myelotoxicity, and liver toxicity. Other toxic reactions are nausea and vomiting, mild hematuria, dyspnea, edema, rash, and somnolence. Most patients (> 85% to 90%) do not experience hair loss or mucositis. Gemcitabine is administered intravenously and exhibits striking schedule-dependent toxicity. The maximal tolerated dose (MTD) of the drug given weekly for 3 weeks every 4 weeks ranges from 790 to 2,400 mg/m^2. The MTD on an every-other-week schedule exceeds 3,000 mg/m^2, whereas the MTDs for schedules of twice a week and 5 days a week every 4 weeks are 65 mg/m^2 and 12 mg/m^2, respectively. Gemcitabine is active in pancreatic, ovarian, lung, breast, bladder, and head and neck cancer. It is now approved for use in the treatment of metastatic pancreatic carcinoma and non-small cell lung cancer in the United States.

PURINE ANALOGUES

Until recently, the two major drugs in this category were the thiopurines 6-mercaptopurine (6-MP) and 6-thioguanine (6-TG), which are analogues of hypoxanthine and guanine, respectively. These drugs were synthesized almost 50 years ago and continue to be used in the therapy of the acute leukemias. 6-MP is used for maintenance therapy of acute lymphocytic leukemia and 6-TG is used for acute myelogenous leukemia. Both drugs require conversion to either the monophosphate or triphosphate anabolite before exerting their cytotoxic effects. These agents inhibit de novo purine synthesis and, in nucleotide form, can be incorporated into DNA or RNA, resulting in inhibition of DNA synthesis and RNA processing, respectively. These drugs are sometimes said to be self-limiting because their incorporation into DNA can be decreased when total DNA synthesis is inhibited by purine starvation. Thus, in some systems, these agents are less cytotoxic at high concentrations than they are at lower concentrations.

Resistance to the thiopurines is mediated through decrease in the activating enzyme hypoxanthine-guanine phosphoribosyltransferase and increase in catabolic enzymes. The primary cytotoxic mechanism of these drugs can be different because a lack of cross-resistance has been demonstrated in several systems. Both drugs have a variable oral bioavailability of 20% to 50%. Enhanced 6-MP toxicity may result from the concomitant administration of allopurinol (a xanthine oxidase inhibitor), and the dose of 6-MP must be reduced by 25% to 50%. 6-TG is not a substrate for xanthine oxidase, and this drug interaction does not occur. The thiopurines are eliminated by several metabolic alterations. At high doses, 20% to 40% of 6-MP is eliminated through the kidneys, and dose reduction is required for renal dysfunction. Myelosuppression and gastrointestinal effects are the major toxic effects of these drugs. Hepatotoxicity is more common with 6-MP. Thiopurine methyltransferase (TPMT) is an important inactivating enzyme for these agents. Genetic polymorphisms have been described for this enzyme. Significant functional deficiency may occur in approximately 0.4% of the population. In these individuals, standard doses of these agents can be fatal.

High activity of the enzyme is found in approximately 10% of the population. In these individuals, standard doses of these drugs may be ineffective. Another drug substrate for this enzyme which is subject to all the given caveats is azathioprine. At the Mayo Clinic, the TPMT phenotype of patients is routinely obtained before therapy with the thiopurines.

Deoxycoformycin (dCF, Pentostatin)

Adenosine deaminase (ADA) is a key enzyme in purine salvage which converts adenosine to inosine. It is widely distributed in mammalian tissues and plasma. In 1972, Giblett et al. observed that children with congenital ADA deficiency were lymphopenic and both T- and B-cell immunodeficient. They postulated that an inhibitor of ADA might be useful in the therapy of lymphoproliferative disorders. dCF (Fig. 4) is an adenosine analogue isolated from *Streptomyces antibioticus*. It is a potent inhibitor of ADA and has an inhibitory constant of 2.5 pM. Cytotoxicity appears to be related to accumulation of dATP, which inhibits ribonucleotide reductase, accumulation of deoxyadenosine, which inhibits S-adenosylhomocysteine hydrolase, and incorporation of nucleotide metabolites of dCF into DNA. dCF is administered by intravenous infusion and has activity in hairy cell leukemia, cutaneous T-cell lymphoma, chronic lymphocytic leukemia, and T-cell acute lymphocytic leukemia. Toxic effects are myelosuppression, nausea, vomiting, acute renal failure, neurotoxicity (lethargy, seizures), and reversible hepatic dysfunction.

2-Chloro-2'-Deoxyadenosine (2-CdA, Cladribine)

2-CdA is an analogue of deoxyadenosine with a 2-chloro group on the adenine ring. This chloride substituent makes 2-CdA resistant to adenosine deaminase and it induces a lymphopenic state similar to what occurs in ADA deficiency. It is transported by the nucleoside transport system into cells and phosphorylated to the active 5'-triphosphate anabolite. This triphosphate species causes chain termination after incorporation into DNA. It also inhibits DNA polymerase alpha. Inhibition of ribonucleotide reductase has also been documented. 2-CdA has been given as a 7-day continuous infusion, but the drug has been shown to be 100% bioavailable when given subcutaneously. Levels in cerebrospinal fluid reach 25% of systemic levels. The drug is excreted through renal tubular secretion, and it should be administered with care in patients with renal dysfunction.

2-CdA has major activity in indolent lymphoid malignancies such as hairy cell leukemia, chronic lymphocytic leukemia, low-grade non-Hodgkin's lymphoma, and cutaneous T-cell lymphoma. Myelosuppression occurs with 2-CdA. Cumulative thrombocytopenia is dose-limiting after repeated courses. Fever, most frequently related to lysis of hairy cell leukemia cells, occurs. Infection related to central venous catheters is common. 2-CdA is immunosuppressive and affects both T and B lymphocytes equally. Restoration of T-cell function occurs between 6 and 12 months after 2-CdA therapy, compared with 2 years or more for resolution of B-cell lymphopenia. No gastrointestinal, renal, hepatic, cardiac, neurologic, or pulmonary toxic effects have been observed after standard doses of 2-CdA. Alopecia does not occur.

Fludarabine Phosphate (2-Fluoro-Ara AMP)

Fludarabine is unique among the nucleoside analogues in having modifications in both the base and the sugar portions of the molecule. The parent compound is insoluble; the drug is therefore formulated as the monophosphate. After administration, it is rapidly dephosphorylated to 2-F-ara-A, which enters cells by the facilitated diffusion nucleoside transport system and undergoes phosphorylation to the active triphosphate form. This active form is incorporated into 3' termini of DNA, in contrast to ara-C, which is incorporated into 5' termini. 2-F-ara-A is also incorporated into RNA. It inhibits ribonucleotide reductase, DNA polymerase alpha, DNA ligase 1, DNA primase, and RNA primer formation. Fludarabine has significant clinical activity against chronic lymphocytic leukemia, including the refractory type and low-grade lymphomas. Myelosuppression is the most common dose-limiting toxicity. Gastrointestinal toxicity is frequent, as is mild increase of hepatic transaminases. Reversible somnolence and fatigue occur. Lymphopenia has been associated with frequent infections. Neurotoxicity occurred with the high doses given initially in early clinical trials, but it is rare with current doses and schedules.

ALKYLATING AGENTS

These compounds were the first chemotherapeutic agents to be used for cancer treatment. They share a common mechanism of action. These agents attack negatively charged, electron-rich, nucleophilic sites of DNA. They add alkyl groups to oxygen, nitrogen, phosphorus, and sulfur atoms. The favorite sites of alkylation are N-7 guanine, N-3 cytosine, O-6 and N-1 guanine, O-4 thymidine, and N-1,3,7 adenine. Alkylating agents are cytotoxic in all phases of the cell cycle. Described mechanisms of resistance for these agents are shown in Table 1. Common toxic effects of alkylating agents include nausea and vomiting of varying severity, alopecia, and myelosuppression. All of these agents are considered carcinogenic and can lead to the development of secondary malignancies. However, their carcinogenic potential is variable. Melphalan appears to be more carcinogenic than cyclophosphamide. Most secondary malignancies are acute leukemias. The alkylating agents differ in chemical reactivity and clinical uses. They are classified as *nitrogen mustards* (mechlorethamine, chlorambucil, melphalan, cyclophosphamide, ifosfamide), *ethylenimines (aziridines)* (thiotepa, hexamethylmelamine, mitomycin C), *triazines* (dacarbazine, procarbazine), *nitrosoureas* (CCNU, BCNU, methyl-CCNU, streptozotocin), and *alkane sulfonates* (busulfan).

Cyclophosphamide

Cyclophosphamide (CTX) is a pro-drug that is converted to the 4-hydroxy form by the hepatic microsomal oxidase system. 4-Hydroxycyclophosphamide reenters the circulation and is converted by tumor and peripheral tissues to acrolein and phosphoramide mustard. Phosphoramide mustard is thought to be the main cytotoxic product. CTX is used orally and intravenously. The active metabolites are eliminated mainly through the kidneys. Renal failure results in prolonged levels but not in increased toxicity. Toxicities peculiar to CTX include hemorrhagic cystitis, which is related to damage from acrolein in urine. Late sequelae from this toxicity include bladder fibrosis and contractures as well as transitional cell carcinomas. Bladder toxicity may be avoided by hydration (3-4 liters/day) with frequent voiding for 24 hours after drug administration. Thiol-producing agents such as *N*-acetylcysteine and sodium-2-mercaptoethane sulfonate (MESNA) are also effective. CTX also can cause syndrome of inappropriate secretion of antidiuretic hormone and cardiac toxic effects after high-dose therapy. This agent has activity in various solid tumors, including breast, ovary, and lung cancers, and lymphomas and leukemias.

Ifosfamide

Ifosfamide is a congener of CTX which has a lower affinity for the activating enzymes. A fourfold increase in dosage is required to achieve antitumor effects equivalent to those of CTX. Hemorrhagic cystitis is more common with ifosfamide, and uroprotection with MESNA is standard. Central nervous system toxic effects such as lethargy, somnolence, confusion and seizures occur. This drug is used clinically in the treatment of sarcomas, lung cancer, and testicular cancer.

Mechlorethamine

This agent is currently used solely for the treatment of Hodgkin's lymphoma and was the first alkylating agent introduced for clinical use. It possesses all the properties of alkylating agents and is considered a potent teratogen and carcinogen.

Chlorambucil

This is the alkylating agent of choice in chronic lymphocytic leukemia. It is completely absorbed after oral administration, reaching peak plasma levels approximately 60 minutes after an oral dose. It is extensively metabolized in the liver. In addition to the usual toxic effects of the alkylating agents, chlorambucil can cause pulmonary fibrosis.

Melphalan

This phenylalanine derivative of nitrogen mustard was rationally synthesized to target melanoma, which actively takes up phenylalanine for the synthesis of tyrosine and melanin. It was, however, found to be ineffective in melanoma and is principally used to treat multiple myeloma. The activity of this agent is impaired by tamoxifen, doxorubicin, aminophylline, and indomethacin. This agent is more carcinogenic than cyclophosphamide and causes sterility and amenorrhea.

Procarbazine

This agent was discovered in a search for monoamine oxidase inhibitors and possesses some of the properties of this class of agents. Hypertensive crises have occurred when used with sympathomimetics, tricyclic antidepressants, or foods containing high levels of tyramine such as red wines, bananas, yogurt, ripe cheese, and dark beer (ales). It can cause a disulfiram-like reaction of sweating, flushing, headache, nausea, and vomiting when taken with alcohol. Hypersensitivity reactions including a maculopapular rash and pulmonary infiltrates are relatively common. Peripheral neuropathy is uncommon. Although the drug is highly toxic to the reproductive organs, teratogenic effects have not been reported after administration in all trimesters of pregnancy. Procarbazine is thought to be the principal carcinogen in the MOPP regimen for Hodgkin's disease. This agent is also used extensively in gliomas.

Dacarbazine (DTIC)

This agent was synthesized as an analogue of 5-aminoimidazole-4-carboxamide (AICAR), an intermediate in de novo purine synthesis. However, the imidazole nucleus was thought to be unnecessary for the activity of DTIC. This agent is activated by the hepatic microsomal mixed-function oxidase system. Activation may be increased by phenytoin and barbiturates, which can induce these enzymes. The active species, however, remains unknown. This is one of the most emetogenic of all antineoplastic agents. Acute fatal hepatotoxicity has been reported. Myelosuppression is moderate and non-dose limiting. This drug is administered intravenously and has activity in melanoma, Hodgkin's disease, and soft tissue sarcomas.

Nitrosoureas

These agents are used principally for the therapy of gliomas. Prolonged use can lead to cumulative bone marrow toxicity and aplastic anemia. Nadir blood counts typically occur 4 to 6 weeks after administration. Mild reversible hepatotoxicity occurs. Pneumonitis is dose-related and is common after cumulative doses of 1,200 mg/m^2. Streptozocin is a naturally occurring antibiotic used principally to treat islet cell tumors of the pancreas. Renal toxicity is manifested as proteinuria and azotemia. In patients with creatinine clearance less than 25 mL/min, drug doses should be reduced by 50% to 75%. This drug causes hypoglycemia. Myelosuppression is uncommon. The pharmacology of other alkylating agents in the ethylenimine and alkylsulfonate class is summarized in Table 2.

PLATINUM AGENTS

Rosenberg and coworkers observed in 1965 that a current delivered between platinum electrodes inhibited the growth of *Escherichia coli*. These inhibitory effects were found to be due to the formation of inorganic platinum-containing moieties in the presence of ammonium and chloride ions. Cisplatin (*cis*-diamminedichloroplatinum II, CDDP) was the most active of these platinum complexes in experimental tumor systems and was introduced into clinical practice in the early 1970s. Cisplatin has a broad spectrum of

Table 2
Pharmacology of Ethylenimines and Alkylsulfonates

Drug	Principal route of administration	Pharmacologic characteristics	Toxicity
Ethylenimines			
Thiotepa	Intravenous, intravesical	Absorption from bladder can cause myelo suppression. Indications: bladder cancer, breast cancer	Anorexia, nausea, vomiting, bone marrow depression
Hexamethyl-melamine	Oral	Rapid demethylation by cytochrome P-450 to its active form. Used in ovarian cancer	Nausea and vomiting, neurotoxicity, bone marrow depression
Mitomycin-C	Intravenous	Appears to be a substitute for P-glycoprotein activity in carcinomas of breast and lung, head and neck sarcomas, upper gastrointestinal cancer	Cumulative bone marrow depression, pulmonary, renal, nausea, vomiting, vesicant
Alkylsulfonates			
Busulfan	Oral	Enters cells by diffusion. Used for chronic myelogenous leukemia as preparative regimen for bone marrow transplantation	Pulmonary, bone marrow, amenorrhea, impotence, sterility, hepatic veno-occlusive disease

activity against epithelial cancers and has become the foundation of curative regimens in testicular and ovarian cancers. It also demonstrates significant activity against cancers of the lung, head and neck, esophagus, bladder, cervix, and endometrium. However, toxicities of cisplatin are substantial. Carboplatin (cis-diammine-1,1- cyclobutane-dicarboxylatoplatinum II, CBDCA), an analogue of cisplatin, was introduced into clinical trials in 1981 to help circumvent some of the toxicities of cisplatin. Both cisplatin and carboplatin are platinum(II) complexes with two ammonia groups in the cis position. Cisplatin has two chloride "leaving" groups, and carboplatin possesses a cyclobutane moiety (Fig. 6).

The pharmacologic behavior of cisplatin is determined largely by an initial aquation reaction in which the chloride groups are replaced by water molecules. This reaction is driven by the high concentration of water and low concentration of chloride in tissues. The aquated platinum complex can then react with various macromolecules. In intact DNA, cisplatin seems to bind preferentially to the N-7 position of guanine and adenine. This may be due to the high nucleophilicity at this position. The cytotoxicity of cisplatin correlates closely with platinum DNA interstrand cross-links and to the formation of intrastrand bifunctional N-7 adducts. Carboplatin has a mechanism of action similar to that of cisplatin, but requires 10 times higher drug concentrations and 7.5 times longer incubation time than cisplatin to induce the same degree of DNA damage. Some of the resistance mechanisms to the platinum agents are shown in Table 1.

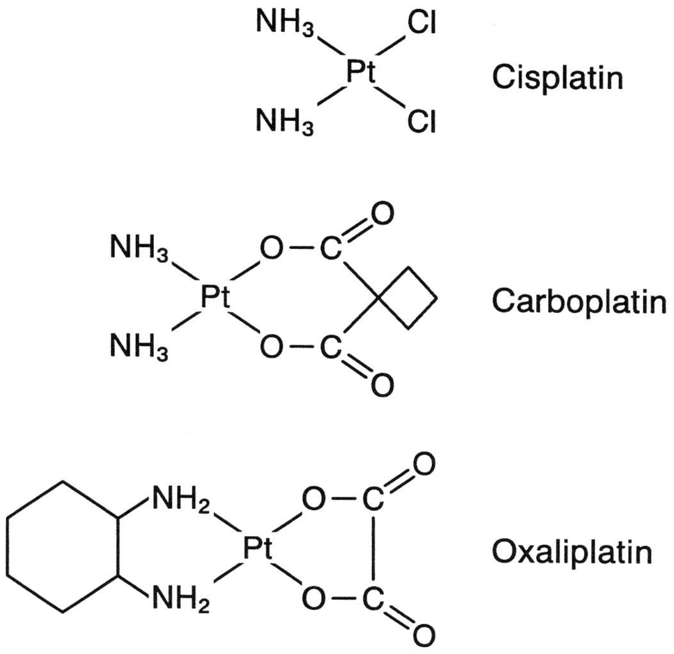

NH₃ ... Cl — Cisplatin
NH₃ ... Cl (Pt)

Cisplatin

Carboplatin

Oxaliplatin

Fig. 6. Structures of clinically useful platinum analogues.

About 25% of the cisplatin dose is eliminated from the body during the first 24 hours, and renal clearance is responsible for more than 90%. Unlike cisplatin, carboplatin is not significantly secreted by renal tubules, and thus renal clearance is similar to the glomerular filtration rate (GFR). The area under the drug concentration-time curve (AUC) is the ratio of the amount of a drug that reaches the systemic circulation and the clearance of the drug. The AUC of a drug, therefore, typically correlates with its toxicity and clinical efficacy. Carboplatin has relatively simple pharmacokinetics, with GFR accounting for almost all drug elimination. The remainder of the drug binds to body proteins. The clearance of carboplatin is, thus, linearly related to the GFR, so that GFR is related to the AUC of this drug. A formula (Calvert formula) has been derived to calculate the dose of carboplatin necessary to achieve a particular AUC. This formula has been validated prospectively and has been shown to predict AUCs with a margin of error of about 15%:

$$\text{Dose (mg)} = \text{target AUC (mg/mL} \times \text{min)} \times (\text{GFR [mL/min]} + 25)$$

In the original study, GFR was measured by the [51]CrEDTA method. Estimation of GFR by creatinine clearance, which is more convenient, is now widely used, although this simplified approach has not been validated prospectively. Target AUC values of 5 and 7 mg/mL × min are recommended for single-agent carboplatin in previously treated and untreated patients, respectively. These doses have been shown to lead to acceptable thrombocytopenia (platelet nadirs of about 30% of the pretreatment value) and efficacy.

Immediate (< 24 hours after treatment) or delayed (> 24 hours after treatment) nausea and vomiting are the most common side effects of cisplatin-based chemotherapy. In contrast to cisplatin, carboplatin-related nausea and vomiting are much less severe and frequent. Nephrotoxicity was dose-limiting for cisplatin in early clinical trials, with effects ranging from reversible azotemia to irreversible renal failure requiring dialysis.

Hydration with normal saline, hypertonic saline infusion, and mannitol, or furosemide-induced diuresis, has been used to effectively decrease this toxicity. The mechanism of cisplatin-induced nephrotoxicity is believed to be similar to its tumor cytotoxicity (i.e., formation of highly reactive aquated platinum species that cross-link DNA). This aquation reaction is dependent on ambient chloride concentrations. Hydration and diuresis can reduce the urinary concentration of cisplatin, whereas forced chlorouresis provides high chloride levels in the kidneys, thus minimizing the aquation of cisplatin in renal tubules.

In the presence of preexisting renal insufficiency, cisplatin should not be used if the GFR is less than 30 mL/min. Full-dose cisplatin can be used if the GFR is more than 50 mL/min. Dosage adjustment is required for a GFR between 30 and 50 mL/min. Dose reduction should be proportional to the reduction in GFR (normal GFR is assumed to be 100 mL/min). Thus, at a GFR of 40 mL/min, 40% of the full dose of cisplatin should be given.

Thiol-containing compounds have also been used to reduce cumulative renal toxicity. The most promising agent to date is amifostine, WR-2721, S-2 (3-amino-propylamino)-ethylphosphorothioic acid. It is a pro-drug that is preferentially taken up and metabolized by normal cells. The active thiol moiety acts as a nucleophile, which can inactivate carbonium ions generated by alkylating agents and prevent DNA damage. In various trials, pretreatment with amifostine conferred protection against cisplatin-induced nephrotoxicity without compromising antitumor efficacy. Reduction in other cisplatin-related toxicities, including myelosuppression and neurotoxicity, was noted as well.

Renal impairment is rare with the administration of carboplatin except at very high doses. There seems to be no significant cumulative damage after long-term follow-up, as seen in a series of treated patients with germ cell tumors. Because it is excreted primarily as an unchanged drug in the kidneys, carboplatin is not directly toxic to the renal tubules. However, the presence of renal impairment will significantly increase its plasma level, leading to other systemic toxicities. Dosage according to the desired AUC is then modified according to the Calvert formula.

Neuropathy is now the major dose-limiting toxicity of cisplatin. This includes peripheral sensory neuropathy, which is the most common, hearing loss, autonomic neuropathy, Lhermitte's sign (electric shock-like sensation transmitted down the spine on neck flexion), seizures, and encephalopathy. It is dose-dependent and occurs in about 85% of patients with a cumulative dose of more than 300 mg/m². In 30% to 50% of cases, this is irreversible. Neuropathy is additive when cisplatin is administered with other neurotoxic agents, including paclitaxel and docetaxel. Neurotoxicity is infrequent as a result of carboplatin treatment. Peripheral neuropathies develop in about 3% of patients. Myelosuppression, in particular thrombocytopenia, is the dose-limiting toxicity of carboplatin. This is cumulative. Platelet count nadirs can be delayed up to 21 days after treatment with carboplatin.

ANTITUBULIN AGENTS

Microtubules are eukaryotic cell components that perform important functions, including regulation of cell morphology, signal transmission, intracellular transport, formation of the mitotic spindle during cell division, cellular motility, and anchorage of receptors in the cell membrane. Microtubules are assembled from tubulin, which is a 100-kDa protein comprising two subunits, α and β, of 50 kDa each. Structurally, microtubules are a collection of 13 protofilaments arranged longitudinally to form hollow cylinders, which are in equilibrium with free tubulin. The equilibrium shift between microtubule assembly and disassembly is controlled by various factors, such as free guanidine triphosphate, calcium ions, temperature, and proteins (including microtubule-associated proteins), and can also be modified by drugs.

The antitubulin agents comprise two broad classes of compounds. The first and older class prevents polymerization of tubulin dimers and inhibits microtubule formation. This class comprises the vinca alkaloids (vincristine, vinblastine, vindesine, vinorelbine). The second class comprises the taxoids, which enhance both the rate and the extent of micro-tubule assembly in vitro and inhibit the disassembly of microtubules, thereby leading to bundles of microtubules in cells. These agents bind to specific sites on tubulin. The antitubulin agents are metabolized mainly in the liver and are excreted in stool. Dose modification is imperative in patients with hepatic dysfunction, especially in those with obstructive liver disease.

Vinca Alkaloids

These natural alkaloids were originally extracted from the periwinkle plant *Cath-aranthus rosea.* Vindesine is a synthetic alkaloid. Vincristine has activity in acute lymphocytic leukemia, Hodgkin's and non-Hodgkin's lymphoma, Wilms' tumor, sar-comas, and neuroblastoma. This drug is a potent vesicant. It causes syndrome of inap-propriate secretion of antidiuretic hormone. Peripheral neurotoxicity is dose-limiting. Vinblastine is used clinically for testicular germ cell tumors, Hodgkin's disease, and lung cancer. It is a potent vesicant. Myelosuppression is dose-limiting. Neurotoxicity is very rare. Alopecia and mucositis are common. Vinorelbine (3',4'-didehydro-4'-deoxy-C'-nor-vincaleukoblastine, Navelbine) is a semisynthetic vinca alkaloid that differs from other vinca alkaloids by substitutions on the catharanthine rather than the vindoline ring of the vinca alkaloid molecule (Fig. 7). Unlike other vinca alkaloids, vinorelbine acts primarily on nonaxonal microtubules, with specific binding to the microtubules of the mitotic spindle. This is thought to be the reason for the minimal neurotoxicity with this agent. In preclinical studies, vinorelbine inhibited mitotic spindle microtubules at a concentration of 2 μmol/L. However, axonal microtubule depolymerization occurred only at a concentration of 40 μmol/L. Vincristine and vin-blastine also inhibit mitotic microtubular formation at the same concentration as vinorelbine. However, they produce axonal microtubular depolymerization at lower concentrations (vincristine, 5 μmol/L; vinblastine, 30 μmol/L).

Neutropenia is the major dose-limiting toxicity of vinorelbine. The drug is fairly well tolerated overall. Although 20% to 25% of patients have some symptoms of peripheral neuropathy, grade 3 or 4 neuropathy is rare, occurs in fewer than 5% of patients, and is usually reversible. Other toxicities (usually mild) include fatigue, nausea, vomiting, constipation, diarrhea, alopecia, phlebitis, and injection site reactions. As with other vinca alkaloids, dose reductions are not needed in renal failure. Although the use of vinorelbine in patients with hepatic dysfunction has not been studied, dose adjustments in the range of 50% are recommended for patients with mild hepatic dysfunction (total bilirubin, > 2.0 mg/dL). For patients with total bilirubin exceeding 3.0 mg/dL, a 75% dose adjustment is recommended.

Taxoids

The taxoids are a new class of anticancer drugs that include paclitaxel (5β,20-epoxy-1,2α,4,7β,10β,13α-hexahydroxytax-11-en-9-one 4,10-diacetate 2-ben-zoate 13-ester with [2R,3S]-N-benzoyl-3-phenylisoserine; Taxol) and docetaxel

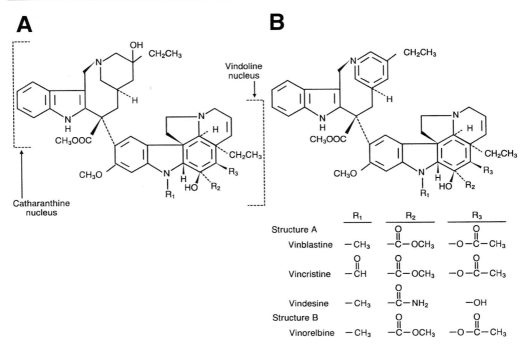

Fig. 7. Structures of the vinca alkaloids.

(5β,20-epoxy-1,2α,4,7β,10β,13α-hexahydroxytax-11-en-9-one 4-acetate 2-benzoate, trihydrate 13-ester with [2R,3S]-N-carboxy-3-phenylisoserine, N-*tert*-butyl ester; Taxotere). Paclitaxel was discovered during the screening of more than 30,000 natural products by the National Cancer Institute in the 1960s. A crude extract from the bark of the Pacific yew (*Taxus brevifolia*) had cytotoxic activity against many tumors. Paclitaxel was determined to be the active constituent of this extract in 1971. Horwitz later described the unique mechanism of action of paclitaxel. Despite initial problems of solubility and unexpected toxic effects, several clinical trials were begun in the 1980s. Paclitaxel is now approved in the United States for use in the treatment of ovarian, breast, and non-small cell lung cancer. In 1986, a semisynthetic taxoid was prepared through use of a precursor, 10-deacetyl baccatin III, obtained from the needles of the European yew (*Taxus baccata*). The active constituent of this extract is docetaxel, which has two chemical modifications of paclitaxel's structure (Fig. 8). Docetaxel has been approved for the treatment of breast cancer. The taxoids, however, have a broad spectrum of activity in other solid tumors, including small cell lung cancer and bladder, esophageal, cervical, and head and neck cancers.

Both drugs have similar mechanisms of action, as already described. The stable, abnormal microtubules formed with taxoid therapy lead to cell cycle arrest in the G_2 and M phases of the cell cycle, because the cells are unable to form normal mitotic spindles and divide. Mechanistically, docetaxel differs from paclitaxel by being twice as potent an inhibitor of microtubule depolymerization and promoter of tubulin assembly. Docetaxel binds to tubulin with a 1.9-fold higher affinity than paclitaxel. This difference may explain why, in comparative studies, docetaxel is 1.3- to 12-fold more cytotoxic in vitro than paclitaxel. In addition to its effect on microtubules, paclitaxel has other properties that may contribute to its cytotoxicity. Recent investigations have suggested that

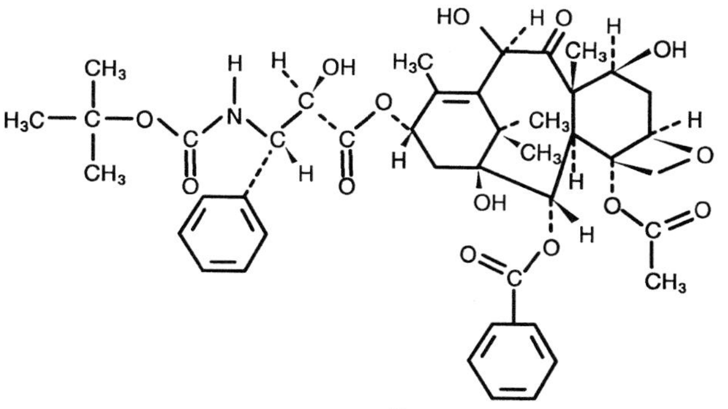

Fig. 8. The taxoids.

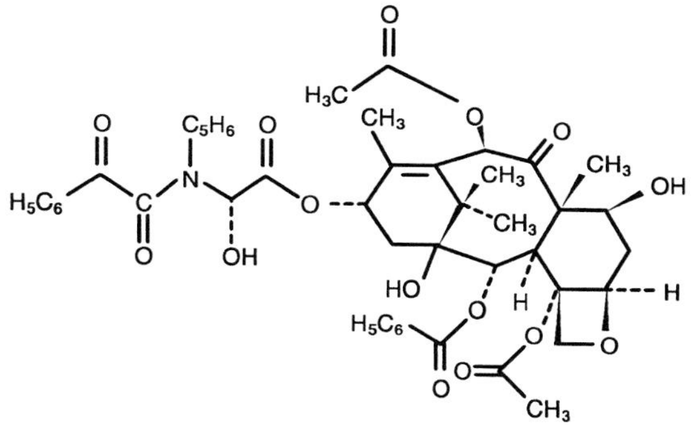

paclitaxel may have significant antiangiogenic activity. Noncytotoxic doses of the drug inhibit the angiogenic response induced by tumor cell supernatant in mice experiments. In vitro experiments also showed inhibition of endothelial cell proliferation, motility, and invasiveness in a dose-dependent manner. Paclitaxel also inhibits the production of matrix metalloproteinases, which are enzymes that degrade matrix and thereby contribute to tumor invasiveness. Further, paclitaxel induces the expression of the gene for tumor necrosis factor-α. However, it is not clear what relevance these effects have in the clinical activity of the drug.

Major toxic effects of the taxoids are neutropenia, mucositis, thrombocytopenia, peripheral neuropathy, alopecia, and myalgias. The dose-limiting toxicity of both paclitaxel and docetaxel is usually neutropenia, which tends to be reversible and noncumulative. Severe acute hypersensitivity reactions occurred in 20% to 30% of patients treated with paclitaxel in early phase 1 trials. These included hypotension, dyspnea, flushing angioedema, and an erythematous rash. Hypersensitivity is related to the polyoxyethylated castor oil (Cremophor) vehicle in which the water-insoluble drug is dissolved. Because the reactions with paclitaxel resembled those with iodinated contrast dye, a similar schedule of premedication was adopted. This consisted of dexamethasone (20 mg administered 12 and 6 hours before chemotherapy), as well as cimetidine (300 mg) and diphenhydramine (50 mg), both given intravenously preceding administration of paclitaxel. The incidence of hypersensitivity reactions was reduced to less than 5%. The need for routine use of dexamethasone 6 and 12 hours before paclitaxel administration recently has been questioned. Some investigators have used a single dose of dexamethasone, 16 to 20 mg, given intravenously 30 minutes before paclitaxel infusion, and no increase has been found in the incidence of hypersensitivity reactions. Anaphylactic reactions are rare with premedication. Neurotoxicity, which has been better characterized for paclitaxel, occurs with both agents. It is a result of the toxicity of these drugs to nerve cell bodies or axons. Peripheral neuropathy follows a "stocking and glove" distribution, tends to be symmetrical, and is mainly sensory. Motor abnormalities have been described in a minority of patients. Paclitaxel-induced neurotoxicity can be dose-limiting and tends to occur more frequently in patients with preexisting neuropathy. It is reversible, dose-dependent, and related to cumulative dose. Neuropathy is also more frequent in patients receiving paclitaxel in combination with other neurotoxic agents, such as cisplatin.

The most striking, unusual toxicity noted with docetaxel is a fluid retention syndrome characterized by both peripheral and generalized edema. Pleural effusion, ascites, pericardial effusion, and increased capillary fragility also can occur. The incidence was 30% to 50% in patients receiving 75 to 100 mg/m^2 of docetaxel every 3 weeks, and it rapidly increased at cumulative doses of more than 400 mg/m^2. This toxicity has been decreased by premedication with oral dexamethasone, 4 to 8 mg given twice daily 48 to 72 hours before and after docetaxel administration. With this schedule, the median cumulative dose to onset of fluid retention is about 700 mg/m^2. When fluid retention occurs, it is treated with diuretics, dose reduction, or discontinuation of treatment, and it is slowly reversible. Because hypersensitivity reactions appear to be less frequent with docetaxel and patients receive dexamethasone routinely to minimize fluid retention, premedication with histamine antagonists, as with paclitaxel administration, is unnecessary.

The dosage of the taxoids in hepatic dysfunction has not been well studied, but in patients with significant liver dysfunction (total bilirubin > 3 mg/dL), the dose needs to be reduced by at least 50%. Because renal clearance of the drug is less than 10%, dose modifications are not necessary in renal failure. The mechanisms of inherent or acquired resistance to the taxoids have not been fully elucidated (Table 1).

TOPOISOMERASE INHIBITORS

Topoisomerases are enzymes that uncoil DNA before replication. There are two classes of topoisomerases: topoisomerase I and topoisomerase II. Topoisomerase II inhibitors, such as the anthracyclines and epipodophyllotoxins, have been widely used in chemotherapy. Camptothecin, a plant alkaloid derived from the tree *Camptotheca acuminata*, was the first mammalian topoisomerase I inhibitor to be identified and showed impressive activity in several clinical studies. However, during phase 1 trials in the early 1970s, severe and unpredictable toxicity, including hemorrhagic cystitis, myelosuppression, nausea, and vomiting, halted its further development. The water insolubility of camptothecin was thought to contribute to its unpredictable toxicity. Irinotecan (7-ethyl-10-[4-(1-piperidino)-1-piperidino]carbonyloxycamptothecin; CPT-11; Camptosar) and topotecan ([S]-dimethylaminomethyl-10-hydroxycamptothecin; Hycamtin) are topoisomerase I inhibitors that are semisynthetic, water-soluble analogues of camptothecin. The structure of the parent compound with the substitutions for topotecan and irinotecan is shown in Figure 9. The analogues have greater in vivo and in vitro activity and less severe and more predictable toxicity than camptothecin. Both have shown activity in a wide variety of solid tumors. Irinotecan and topotecan were recently approved in the United States for use in recurrent colon cancer and recurrent ovarian cancer, respectively.

The cytotoxicity of irinotecan and topotecan depends on the inhibition of the eukaryotic nuclear enzyme DNA topoisomerase I. This enzyme, which is critical for DNA

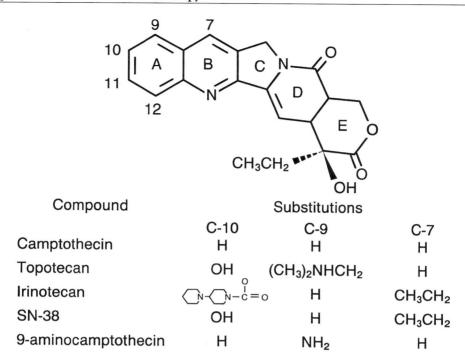

Compound	Substitutions		
	C-10	C-9	C-7
Camptothecin	H	H	H
Topotecan	OH	(CH₃)₂NHCH₂	H
Irinotecan	⟨N⟩-⟨N⟩-C=O	H	CH₃CH₂
SN-38	OH	H	CH₃CH₂
9-aminocamptothecin	H	NH₂	H

Fig. 9. Structure of the camptothecin molecule and the clinically useful derivatives. (From Adjei AA. A review of the pharmacology and clinical activity of new chemotherapy agents for the treatment of colorectal cancer. *Br J Clin Pharmacol* 1999; 48: 265-277. By permission of Blackwell Science.)

replication and transcription, causes transient breaks in a single strand of DNA by forming a transient DNA-enzyme "cleavable complex." These breaks release the torsional strain caused by strand separation required for synthesis of a new strand of DNA or RNA. The camptothecins target this DNA-topoisomerase I complex, preventing the reannealing of the nicked DNA strand (Fig. 10). This inhibition results in intracellular accumulation of drug-stabilized topoisomerase I-DNA cleavable complexes, arrest of DNA replication, and subsequent cell death.

Irinotecan is a water-soluble pro-drug that is rapidly hydrolyzed to its active form, 7-ethyl-10-hydroxycamptothecin (SN-38), primarily by hepatic microsomal carboxylesterases. The topoisomerase I inhibition of irinotecan is accounted for by the intracellular concentrations of SN-38, which are about 3,000 times more potent than the parent drug. SN-38 is inactivated by glucuronidation to SN-38G, a reaction catalyzed by the 1A1 isoform of hepatic uridine diphosphate glucuronyltransferase (UGT1A1). Genetic variations in the activity of this enzyme exist. This leads to variations in the inactivation of SN-38. Studies suggest that patients with low UGT1A1 levels, such as those with Gilbert's syndrome, may be at high risk for irinotecan toxicity. An intact lactone ring in camptothecin and related compounds, including irinotecan and topotecan, enhances antineoplastic activity. The lactone functional group undergoes a pH-dependent hydrolytic ring opening to the relatively inactive hydroxy acid form, with the closed ring form predominating at low pH.

The major dose-limiting toxicity of both irinotecan and topotecan is neutropenia. The incidence of grade 4 neutropenia with irinotecan is approximately 6%. This neutropenia

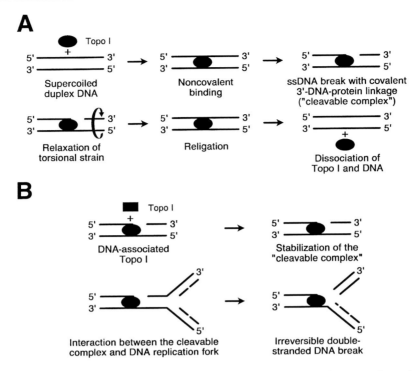

Fig. 10. *A*, Catalytic cycle of DNA topoisomerase I. *B*, Mechanism of action of topoisomerase I inhibitors.

is reversible, lasts mostly for less than 5 days, and is usually asymptomatic. Nonhematologic toxicity is generally mild with topotecan. In contrast, irinotecan has significant nonhematologic toxicity, including diarrhea, nausea and vomiting, abdominal cramps, and flushing. Diarrhea is a dose-limiting toxicity of irinotecan. Early-onset diarrhea, during or within 30 minutes after irinotecan infusion, is due to a cholinergic response and is easily controlled with anticholinergic therapy, such as atropine, 0.5 to 1.0 mg intravenously. Late-onset diarrhea, 5 to 10 days after drug administration, is believed to be related to biliary excretion of SN-38. Early recognition and prolonged administration of loperamide are effective for late-onset diarrhea, having decreased the incidence of grade 4 diarrhea from 20%-30% to 5%-10% in different studies. The appearance of concomitant severe neutropenia and diarrhea has been fatal in a few cases.

Topotecan is associated with severe, grade 4, neutropenia in more than 80% of patients. Grade 4 thrombocytopenia has been noted in 26% of patients and severe anemia (< 8 g/dL) in 40% of patients. Nonhematologic toxic reactions are mainly nausea, vomiting, diarrhea, constipation, alopecia, fatigue, and abdominal pain. The dosage of irinotecan in renal and hepatic failure is unclear. However, because the drug is metabolized in the liver, dose adjustments are probably necessary in patients with hepatic dysfunction. At physiologic pH, the closed-ring lactone species of topotecan (active form) is predominant over the open-ring hydroxy acid species (less potent form). Pharmacokinetic studies indicate that dose adjustment is not necessary in patients with liver impairment but is required in patients with moderate renal impairment (creatinine clearance, 20 to 39 mL/min). Patients with mild renal impairment (creatinine clearance, 40 to 59 mL/min) also do not need dose adjustment.

Topoisomerase II-Directed Agents

DNA topoisomerase II (topo II) is a homodimeric nuclear enzyme that cleaves both DNA strands. An enzyme subunit becomes covalently linked to the 5' phosphoryl end at the site of each DNA strand break. This allows strand passage during replication and segregation of chromosomal DNA and is therefore critical for cell division. In addition, topo II can catalyze the unknotting of knotted DNA and the decatenation of intertwined DNA molecules. Topo II inhibitors trap a key reaction intermediate, "the cleavable complex," leading by an unknown mechanism to DNA fragmentation and cell death.

Epipodophyllotoxins

This class of natural compounds isolated from the mandrake plant comprises etoposide (VP-16) and teniposide (VM-26). These agents were initially thought to interfere with microtubule assembly, but in recent years their mechanism of cytotoxicity has been found to be due to targeting of topo II. Approximately 30% to 45% of these agents is recovered as unchanged drug in the urine. In patients with impaired renal function, dose modification is required. As with all natural products, expression of the multidrug resistance phenotype with increased p170 protein expression results in efflux of drug from neoplastic cells with subsequent resistance. Alteration in topo II activity with decreased topo II levels or mutated topo II with decreased drug binding has also been described as a mechanism of cytotoxicity. Myelosuppression is dose-limiting for these agents. Mucositis, alopecia, and rare hypersensitivity reactions occur. Etoposide is used clinically for the treatment of leukemias, non-Hodgkin's lymphomas, and testicular, lung, and upper gastrointestinal tract cancers. Teniposide is used in the treatment of childhood acute lymphocytic leukemia and neuroblastoma.

Anthracyclines and Anthracenediones

The anthracyclines doxorubicin (Adriamycin) and daunorubicin (daunomycin) are antibiotics isolated from various species of *Streptomyces*. Both drugs have a characteristic four-ring structure that is linked, via a glycosidic bond, to an amino sugar, daunosamine. They differ only by the presence of either a hydroxyl or hydrogen at position 14. Idarubicin, which is 4-demethoxy-daunorubicin, has a structural alteration that makes the drug more lipophilic and alters the metabolism to yield a longer bioactive half-life. In addition to inhibiting topo II, these agents stack between paired bases in DNA to form tight DNA-drug complexes that contribute to their cytotoxicity. These agents also generate free radicals and may inhibit DNA helicase. Thus, they possess multiple mechanisms of cytotoxicity. Renal clearance for these agents is minor. They are metabolized significantly in the liver, and drug doses should be modified in the setting of hepatic dysfunction (bilirubin, > 3 mg/dL). The initial metabolic step involves reduction to doxorubicinol and daunorubicinol, which are active cytotoxic agents themselves. Described resistance mechanisms for these agents include increased drug efflux mediated by p170 protein, alterations in topo II, and increased levels of glutathione-dependent detoxification enzymes. The anthracyclines are extreme vesicants.

Other toxicities are myelosuppression and mucositis (which are dose-limiting), alopecia, radiation sensitization (radiation recall), and cardiotoxicity, which can be acute or chronic and is the most significant sequela of treatment. The acute cardiac toxicity occurs in the week after drug administration and manifests as electrocardiographic changes of tachycardia, ectopy, and ST-T wave changes. Dysrhythmias typically resolve within a few hours, whereas ST-T wave changes may last for up to 2 weeks. This syndrome occurs in approximately 11% of patients. The chronic toxicity manifests as cardiomyopathy, which typically presents as severe, rapidly progressive congestive heart failure. Antecedent symptoms are rare, and the condition develops late, up to 6 months after the last dose of drug. This toxicity is cumulative and dose-dependent, and the risk is considerable after a cumulative dose of 500 mg/m^2 of doxorubicin. The dose limit for daunorubicin is 900 mg/m^2. Mediastinal irradiation and potentially cardiotoxic chemotherapy agents such as cyclophosphamide, mitomycin-C, and paclitaxel increase the risk of cardiotoxicity after doxorubicin dosing. In patients receiving mediastinal radiation or alkylating agents, the total cumulative dose of doxorubicin should probably be limited to 400 mg/m^2.

The mechanism underlying cardiotoxicity appears to be the generation of oxygen-derived free radicals that react with myocardial cells. Also, lipid peroxidation of myocardial cells by the anthracyclines has been implicated. This mechanism appears to be the more relevant one, because the only agent shown to be clinically effective in preventing anthracycline cardiotoxicity is dexrazoxane (Zinecard, ICRF-187). This agent is hydrolyzed intracellularly to an open ring form that is a potent chelator of iron and copper. Anthracycline-induced lipid peroxidation has been shown to require iron. Dexrazoxane is currently approved for use in patients with anthracycline-sensitive tumors who have exceeded maximal safe doses of these agents. Toxicities of this agent include myelosuppression, mild reversible hepatotoxicity, and anemia. Doxorubicin is used clinically in the treatment of breast, ovarian, thyroid, and lung cancers and soft tissue sarcomas. Daunorubicin is used in the treatment of leukemias (acute lymphocytic and acute myeloid). In an attempt to identify agents with a broader spectrum of activity and less cardiac toxicity than doxorubicin, a large number of analogues have been tested. Two that have been approved for clinical use are idarubicin and epirubicin. Both agents have a mechanism of cytotoxicity and resistance similar to that of doxorubicin. Idarubicin has marked activity in acute myeloid leukemia and is used solely for this indication. Epirubicin is used widely in Europe for breast cancer. These agents possess lesser cardiac toxicity.

Mitoxantrone (dihydroanthracenedione) is a planar tetracyclic compound that, unlike the anthracyclines, lacks a glycosidic substituent. This agent inhibits topo II but possesses significantly reduced potential for free radical formation and lipid peroxidation in membranes and cardiac tissue. These findings may explain its diminished ability to cause cardiac toxicity. The potential for causing extravasation injury, alopecia, and nausea and vomiting is also markedly reduced. This agent, however, has a much narrower spectrum of activity compared with doxorubicin. Its clinical use is confined to breast cancer, leukemias, lymphomas, and prostate cancer.

MISCELLANEOUS AGENTS

Bleomycin

The bleomycins are water-soluble glycopeptide antibiotics isolated from cultures of *Streptomyces verticillus.* These compounds differ only in their terminal amine moieties. Bleomycin refers to the commercial preparation, which is composed of 70% bleomycin A2 and 30% bleomycin B2. The primary action of bleomycin is to produce single-strand and double-strand DNA breaks. The A2 peptide has DNA-binding and iron-binding regions at opposite ends of the molecule. An oxidized iron-bleomycin complex catalyzes the reduction of oxygen to superoxide or hydroxyl radicals, which cause DNA damage. Cells are more sensitive to the drug in the G2 phase of the cell cycle.

Bleomycin can be administered subcutaneously, intravenously, or intramuscularly, and there are no differences in response rates. It can be administered into the pleural or peritoneal space to control malignant effusions. The drug is mainly excreted in urine (40%–75% in the first 24 hours). Dose modification is required in patients with compromised renal function. Bleomycin resistance has been explained by increased degradation through bleomycin hydrolase, enhanced DNA repair, and decreased drug activity. Bleomycin is essentially devoid of myelosuppressive activity. Hypersensitivity reactions and Raynaud's phenomenon occur. Dermatologic toxicity is manifested as erythema, induration, desquamation, and hyperpigmentation. Pulmonary toxicity is the most significant adverse effect. The syndrome presents with dyspnea, tachypnea, and a nonproductive cough. Fine rales may be heard in the lungs, and chest radiographs may show patchy infiltrates, nodules, and diffuse interstitial fibrosis. The frequency of pulmonary toxicity is about 10%. This is relatively constant at lower doses but increases markedly above a cumulative dose of 400 units of bleomycin. Older age (more than 70 years), prior thoracic radiotherapy, renal insufficiency, and exposure to high oxygen tensions increase the risk of pulmonary toxicity. Bleomycin is used in combination protocols to treat squamous cell carcinomas of the skin, genitalia, and head and neck. It is part of the curative therapy for testicular carcinomas and has activity against Hodgkin's and non-Hodgkin's lymphomas, for which it is no longer used clinically.

Mitotane (o,p'-DDD)

1,1-Dichloro-2(o-chlorophenyl)-2-(p-chlorophenyl)ethane is used only in the palliative treatment of adrenocortical carcinoma. Its use followed the observation that the insecticide DDD, an analogue of DDT, produced necrosis of the adrenal cortex in dogs. The isomer o,p'-DDD is the principal cytotoxic agent. This agent acts directly on the adrenal gland, but the biochemical mechanism of cytotoxicity is unknown. The drug is administered orally and is 40% bioavailable. Like DDT, a significant amount of the drug is stored in body fat, and on discontinuing therapy the drug disappears slowly from the serum over a period of months. The major toxic effects are gastrointestinal. Central nervous system side effects such as ataxia, somnolence, lethargy, and visual disturbances occur. This drug is metabolized in the liver, and caution should be used in patients with hepatic dysfunction.

NOVEL AGENTS

With advances in molecular and cell biology, numerous anticancer agents are in clinical testing. Some of these agents are new drugs directed against known targets. The most exciting research, however, is with drugs that are directed against novel targets. A partial list of these drugs is given in Table 3.

New Drugs, Old Targets

This class includes oral 5-FU pro-drugs. Eniluracil (776C85) is an inhibitor of DPD. The combination of 5-FU and eniluracil makes 5-FU orally bioavailable. UFT is a combination of ftorafur (FT), an oral pro-drug of 5-FU, and uracil, which is the natural substrate for DPD. S-1 is an oral formulation of ftorafur and its modulators in a molar ratio of 1.0:1.0:0.4. Oxonic acid is a potent inhibitor of gastrointestinal pyrimidine phosphoribosyl transferase (PPRT), and 5-chlorodihydropyrimidine is a DPD inhibitor (Fig. 2). Gastrointestinal toxic effects can be dose-limiting when 5-FU is administered

Table 3
Examples of Cancer Chemotherapy Agents Directed Against Novel Targets

Target	Agent	Stage of development[a]
Angiogenesis	Endogenous	
Proliferating endothelial cells	Angiostatin	Preclinical
	Endostatin	Preclinical
	Thrombospondin-I	Preclinical
	Platelet factor-4	Preclinical
	Fragment of prolactin	Preclinical
	Methoxyestradiol	Preclinical
	Synthetic	
	CAI	Phase 2
	TNP-470	Phase 3
	Thalidomide	Phase 2
	α-Interferon	Phase 2
	Interleukin-12	Phase 1
	COL-3	Phase 1
Intercellular matrix		
Matrix metalloproteinase (MMP) inhibitors		
MMP–2,9	BAY 12-9566	Phase 3
MMP–2,3,3	AG 3340	Phase 2/3
MMP–2,3,9,11	CGS 27023A	Phase 2
MMP–1,2,3,7,9	MARIMASTAT	Phase 3
Signal transduction		
Farnesyl transferase inhibitors	R115777	Phase 2
SCH66336	Phase 2	
L744832	Phase 1	
Protein kinase C	Bryostatin-I	Phase 2
UCN-01	Phase 2	
CGP-41251	Phase 2	
Cyclin-dependent kinases		
cdkl/cdk2	Flavopiridol	Phase 2
Growth factor receptors		
Platelet-derived growth factor	SU101	Phase 2

[a]Phase 1, small studies to evaluate toxicity and determine the dose for future studies; phase 2, small trials to determine efficacy; phase 3, large trials comparing new therapy with best available treatment.

as a prolonged infusion. Diarrhea is a major toxic effect with chronic dosing schedules of 5-FU plus eniluracil and UFT plus leucovorin. PPRT activates 5-FU to 5-FU monophosphate and consequently 5-FU triphosphate (5-FUTP), which is incorporated into RNA. The incorporation of 5-FUTP into RNA is thought to primarily mediate the gastrointestinal toxicity of 5-FU. Theoretically, S-1 should have antitumor activity similar to that of 5-FU plus eniluracil, or UFT, but less toxicity. A multitargeted antifolate (MTA) that targets thymidylate synthase (TS), dihydrofolate reductase (DHFR), and glycinamide ribonucleotide (GAR) formyltransferase (Fig. 1) is in phase 3 trials. DNA topoisomerase I and II inhibitors (rebeccamycin), DNA alkylating agents, and minor groove binders (bizelesin) are being tested. The platinum compound oxaliplatin (Fig. 6) has significant activity in colon, lung, and ovarian cancers and is in phase 3 trials.

Novel Targets

With the exception of the antitubulin agents, all current chemotherapeutic agents target DNA, either directly (alkylating agents) or indirectly (antimetabolites). Currently, agents directed against novel targets are available for clinical testing. The most important targets can be classified as *signals, vessels,* and *connective tissue.*

SIGNALS

Cell proliferation and differentiation are regulated by a myriad of hormones, growth factors, and cytokines. These effector molecules interact with cellular receptors and communicate with the nucleus through intracellular signaling pathways. In cancer cells, key components of these pathways are subverted by oncogenes through overexpression or mutation, leading to unregulated cell signaling and cellular proliferation. The components of these dysregulated signaling pathways represent potential targets for new anti-cancer therapies. Agents currently in clinical trials target cell cycle regulation, growth factors, and intracellular second messengers. The farnesyltransferase inhibitors are a prototype of this class of agents. Ras is a membrane-localized guanine nucleotide-binding protein that functions as a molecular switch linking receptor and nonreceptor tyrosine kinase activation to downstream cytoplasmic and nuclear events. Three mammalian *ras* proto-oncogenes have been identified, encoding three related and highly conserved proteins. Activating mutations in these ras proteins result in constitutive signaling that stimulates cell proliferation and tumorigenesis. Mutated oncogenic *ras* has been identified in 30% of all human tumors, with the highest prevalence in pancreatic (90%) and colon (50%) cancers. Posttranslational modification of the ras protein is required for membrane localization and is essential for ras function. This reaction is catalyzed by the enzyme protein farnesyltransferase. Thus, this enzyme is an appropriate biochemical target for the development of inhibitors of ras-mediated cellular transformation. Three farnesyltransferase inhibitors recently have been introduced into clinical trials. Initial results indicate that these agents are tolerable and safe. Efficacy data are awaited with interest.

VESSELS

Angiogenesis, or new blood vessel formation, is important in tumor growth and metastasis. Without new vessel formation, a tumor nodule is unable to grow. It is clear from previous experience that targeting tumor cells is problematic because of the development of drug resistance. Interestingly, normal host tissues do not develop any resistance to the cytotoxic effects of drugs. Because new capillary formation stimulated by tumor cells develops from normal host tissue, targeting blood vessels may provide a more effective method of treating tumors. Several agents that target new blood vessel formation are currently in clinical trials.

CONNECTIVE TISSUE

The extracellular matrix that supports tumor cells and their vasculature is critical for tumor growth and metastasis, analogous to blood vessel formation. Enzymes called matrix metalloproteinases are able to break down the intercellular matrix and allow tumors to grow and metastasize. These proteinases contain a zinc atom in a highly conserved active site and are responsible for the turnover and remodeling of extracellular matrix proteins. To date, 14 matrix metalloproteinases are known. Currently, several agents target the matrix metalloproteinases and are in different stages of clinical testing. These agents are complementary to the angiogenesis inhibitors and target elements other than the tumor itself, preventing growth and metastasis by "starving" the tumor.

ACKNOWLEDGMENT

Supported by Grant CA77112 from the National Cancer Institute.

SUGGESTED READING

Chabner BA, Longo DL (eds). *Cancer Chemotherapy and Biotherapy: Principles and Practice*, 2nd ed. Lippincott-Raven, Philadelphia, 1996.

Farber S, Diamond LK, Mercer RD, Sylvester RF Jr, Wolff JA. Temporary remissions in acute leukemia in children produced by folic acid antagonist, 4-aminopteroyl-glutamic acid (aminopterin). *N Engl J Med* 1948; 238: 787-793.

Folkman J. Fighting cancer by attacking its blood supply. *Sci Am* Sept 1996; 275: 150-154.

Gilman A, Philips FS. The biological actions and therapeutic applications of β-chloroethyl amines and sulfides. *Science* 1946: 103: 409-415.

Goldie JH, Coldman AJ. A mathematic model for relating the drug sensitivity of tumors to their spontaneous mutation rate. *Cancer Treat Rep* 1979; 63: 1727-1733.

Perry MC (ed). *The Chemotherapy Source Book*, 2nd ed. Williams & Wilkins, Baltimore, 1996.

Pratt WB, Ruddon RW, Ensminger WD, Maybaum J. *The Anticancer Drugs*, 2nd ed. Oxford University Press, New York, 1994.

Rajkumar SV, Adjei AA. A review of the pharmacology and clinical activity of new chemotherapeutic agents in lung cancer. *Cancer Treat Rev* 1998; 24: 35-53.

Saltiel AR. Signal transduction pathways as drug targets. *Sci Am Sci Med* 1995; 2: 58-67.

Teicher BA (ed). *Cancer Therapeutics: Experimental and Clinical Agents*. Humana Press, Totowa, NJ, 1997.

28 An Approach to Porphyria

Lawrence A. Solberg, Jr., MD, PhD

Contents

WHO SHOULD BE EVALUATED FOR PORPHYRIA?

Patients with porphyria may have cutaneous or neurologic symptoms or both. Cutaneous signs include vesiculobullous skin eruptions, crusted ulcers, scarring, and hyperpigmentation in sun-exposed areas. Fragile skin also develops. Patients with neuropathic porphyrias often have episodic attacks of abdominal pain with variable or no symptoms between attacks. Some may have chronic abdominal pain with a few acute attacks or long periods of remission punctuated by acute attacks. The acute attacks usually last for several days. Most attacks start after pubescence. Hypertension, hyponatremia from vomiting, and seizures can occur.

CLASSIFYING THE SYMPTOMS OF A PATIENT WITH POSSIBLE PORPHYRIA

The physician should first classify a patient's symptoms into one of three groups: cutaneous only, neurologic only, or neurologic and cutaneous.

Inherited, fully expressed porphyrias are easily diagnosed when appropriate tests on blood, urine, and stool are conducted during acute symptoms due to the porphyria. In many cases patients have symptoms, such as chronic pain and abnormal patterns of porphyrin excretion, but do not have true inherited porphyria. The most common such circumstance is increased urinary excretion of coproporphyrins in patients who have chronic pain. Making an incorrect diagnosis of porphyria in these patients is not helpful, although sometimes both patient and physician are relieved to have an apparent diagnosis.

From: *Primary Hematology*
Edited by: A. Tefferi © Mayo Foundation for Medical Education and Research, Rochester, MN

Table 1
Porphyrias Producing Cutaneous Manifestations Only

Porphyria	Characteristics
Porphyria cutanea tarda	Most prevalent cutaneous porphyria in North America. Most cases are acquired; there are some familial forms. Usually, first signs are in adults with liver disease
Erythropoietic protoporphyria	Often first diagnosed in adults. Skin involvement (pain, pruritus, and erythema) is acutely related to sun exposure
Congenital erythropoietic porphyria	Rare, autosomal recessive. Usually presents dramatically in children
Hepatoerythropoietic porphyria	Rare; basically a severe, inherited form of porphyria cutanea tarda. Presents dramatically in children

Cutaneous Manifestations Only

Specific forms of porphyria that must be considered when only cutaneous manifestations are present are listed in Table 1.

Neurologic Manifestations Only

Acute intermittent porphyria (AIP) is the most common form of neuropathic porphyria in North America. AIP does not cause cutaneous manifestations. There is only one other, extremely rare, form of acute neuropathic porphyria that never involves the skin, and thus mimics AIP. This is aminolevulinic acid dehydratase deficiency porphyria.

The clinician should be careful before classifying a patient as having neurologic symptoms only. Two inherited types of neuropathic porphyria can also produce dermatologic disease, which may be mild. History is important here.

Neurologic and Cutaneous Manifestations

Hereditary coproporphyria and variegate porphyria are two forms of neuropathic porphyria in which sun-sensitive skin damage can occur. These conditions are less prevalent in North America than porphyria cutanea tarda (PCT) or AIP.

Hereditary coproporphyria is particularly important to discuss because the most common form of secondary porphyrinuria (i.e., increased excretion of a porphyrin in the urine) that is not due to a true porphyria disorder is increased 24-hour excretion of coproporphyrin in the urine. This usually raises concern about an underlying porphyria.

TESTING FOR PORPHYRIA

As mentioned, but worth reinforcing, true attacks of cutaneous or neuropathic porphyria are readily diagnosed if appropriate samples of urine, stool, and blood are collected at the optimal time. The samples need to be processed and transported correctly and then analyzed by a reference laboratory. Some caveats about collecting samples of urine, stool, and blood for evaluating porphyria are summarized in Table 2.

Table 2
Principles of Specimen Collection for Evaluating Porphyria

Specimen	Principles

Urine
  24-hour urine for quantitative porphyrins
For the initial evaluation of a neuropathic
  porphyria, the clinician should be certain
  that the preporphyrins porphobilinogen
  (PBG) and aminolevulinic acid (ALA) are
  also measured. (Mayo Medical Labora-
  tories measures PBG automatically with
  urinary porphyrins, but the ALA excretion
  needs to be ordered separately)
	Timing: This must be collected during
	  acute symptoms. If symptoms are chronic,
	  the sample should be collected when the
	  patient says he or she is having symptoms
	  being attributed to the suspected porphyria.
	  The reference laboratory should be capable
	  of reporting levels of the various intermedi-
	  ates of uroporphyrinogen II metabolism
	  (e.g., heptacarboxyl porphyrins, hex-a).
	  A full 24-hour collection is necessary.
	  The specimen should be protected from
	  light and 5 g sodium carbonate used
	  as a preservative.

Stool
  Porphyrins, feces
	Timing: This can be collected during or
	  between attacks. The reference laboratory
	  should be capable of reporting the various
	  metabolites of uroporphyrinogen and also
	  various dicarboxyl porphyrins such as proto-
	  porphyrins. Patients should discontinue use
	  of all medications, if possible, for 1 week.
	  Patients should avoid eating any red meat
	  for 3 days before collection. The collection
	  should be for 24 hours and transported frozen
	  on dry ice. The adequacy of stool collections
	  can be determined from the 24-hour weight,
	  which is typically not less than 10 g and not
	  more than 100 g

Blood and plasma
  Several tests are possible, including
  measurements of plasma porphyrins,
  red cell protoporphyrins, red cell
  enzymes, such as uroporphyrinogen
  decarboxylase, coproporphyrinogen
  oxidase, porphobilinogen deaminase
  (I-uroporphyrinogen-synthase), and
  aminolevulinic acid dehydratase
	Check carefully with the reference laboratory
	  for transport conditions. Enzymatic activities
	  can degrade during transit. Critical tests
	  on red cell enzymes should be confirmed
	  with two separate studies.

Molecular studies	Molecular genetic testing is not routinely
	  available, but specific DNA mutations have
	  been identified in various families. The clini-
	  cian can search the literature, find a report
	  by a research laboratory on the enzyme of
	  interest, and contact the investigator

Cutaneous Manifestations Only

If an adult patient has cutaneous signs only, the goal of testing is to determine whether the patient has PCT or erythropoietic protoporphyria. If the patient is a child, congenital erythropoietic porphyria and hepatoerythropoietic porphyria need to be considered.

SUSPECTED PORPHYRIA CUTANEA TARDA

For suspected PCT, initial testing should include a plasma porphyrin measurement, a 24-hour quantitative urine porphyrin analysis (which should include measurement of the preporphyrin porphobilinogen), and measurement of the red cell enzyme uroporphyrinogen decarboxylase.

Patients with PCT have increased total plasma porphyrin levels. These can be used to monitor treatment with phlebotomies. The patients also have a unique pattern of abnormal uroporphyrin excretion in the urine with abnormally increased quantities of uroporphyrins having 7 (thus the name heptacarboxylporphyrin), 6 (hexa-), 5 (penta-), and 4 (tetra-) uroporphyrins. The uroporphyrin that has 4 carboxylate groups is called coproporphyrin. PCT is not a neuropathic porphyria, and thus porphobilinogen excretion is always normal in these patients. PCT can be diagnosed if a patient has cutaneous signs and the typical increase in plasma porphyrin and urinary uroporphyrins as described.

In a patient with typical, fully expressed, acquired PCT, 24-hour fecal porphyrin testing is not needed to make a diagnosis. If done, however, findings will support the diagnosis. One looks for abnormally increased levels of a unique porphyrin metabolite called isocoproporphyrin in the stool. Isocoproporphyrin is made from uroporphyrinogen I isomers that are increased in PCT. During normal porphyrin synthesis, the active intracellular metabolites are isomer iii forms of octa-, hepta-, hexa-, penta-, and tetrauroporphyrinogen. These are in equilibrium with a small fraction of isomer I forms of the molecules. In PCT, both isomer II and I forms accumulate and enzymatic action on coproporphyrinogen I leads to isocoproporphyrin.

The clinician who makes a diagnosis of PCT should recall that there are rare familial forms of PCT. The history is the most important tool for determining whether familial PCT exists.

One test on red cells which can be useful to obtain additional evidence for familial PCT is to measure the red cell enzyme activity of uroporphyrinogen decarboxylase. Uroporphyrinogen decarboxylase is an enzyme that repetitively decarboxylates uroporphyrinogen III, which has 8 carboxylate groups, to those intermediates having 7, 6, 5, or 4 carboxylate groups. In familial or acquired PCT, this enzymatic activity is decreased and there is a buildup and increased excretion in urine and stool of the intermediates.

Some patients with familial PCT have low levels of uroporphyrinogen decarboxylase, and this red cell enzyme test can be used to screen family members who may be afflicted. There have been rare families, however, in which low red cell enzyme uroporphyrinogen decarboxylase was not expressed, although this enzymatic activity was abnormal in the liver. Thus, ultimately, family history and measurement of abnormal patterns of porphyrin excretion in the urine or stool are the principal means of detecting familial PCT.

SUSPECTED ERYTHROHEPATIC PROTOPORPHYRIA

Erythrohepatic protoporphyria (EPP) produces sun-related skin changes that can be first expressed in adults. Over time, some patients with EPP may accumulate enough protoporphyrin in the liver that severe liver disease develops. The clinician should think of EPP when initial testing for PCT does not show evidence for PCT although the patient does have a definite sun-related skin disorder.

If EPP is suspected, the clinician should order total and fractionated red cell protoporphyrin testing (which should include free and zinc-bound protoporphyrin), a 24-hour urine test for quantitative porphyrins and porphobilinogen, and a 24-hour fecal collection for porphyrins.

In EPP, iron is not inserted effectively into protoporphyrin IX, which accumulates in red cells as free protoporphyrin (i.e., with no iron or zinc-bound). Protoporphyrins are too water-insoluble to be excreted in the urine, and thus the hallmark of EPP is a marked increase in stool excretion of protoporphyrins. In EPP there is no dominant excretion of coproporphyrins in the urine or stool, unlike hereditary coproporphyria, in which both urine and stool levels are typically increased. EPP is not a neuropathic porphyria, and 24-hour excretion of porphobilinogen (PBG) therefore will not be increased. If it is markedly increased in the urine of a patient suspected of having EPP, variegate porphyria should be considered.

Suspected Congenital Erythropoietic Protoporphyria (CEP) and Hepatoerythropoietic Porphyria (HEP)

These forms of porphyria are rare; fewer than 300 cases of both combined have been reported. Patients invariably present to those caring for young children, such as pediatricians or family practitioners. Major sun-related skin damage should trigger an investigation. CEP and HEP are inherited as autosomal recessive disorders, so a family history is most useful.

If the clinician suspects CEP or HEP, a 24-hour quantitative urinalysis should be ordered, as well as measurement of total and fractionated red cell protoporphyrins and the red cell enzymes uroporphyrinogen decarboxylase and uroporphyrinogen III cosynthase. Patients with CEP have an abnormal enzyme, uroporphyrinogen III cosynthase, which is necessary for forming the normal uroporphyrinogen III isomer. HEP is an inherited, severe deficiency of uroporphyrinogen decarboxylase in which the pattern of partially decarboxylated porphyrins accumulating in urine and stool is the same as in adult acquired PCT.

Neurologic Manifestations Only

Suspected Acute Intermittent Porphyria and Aminolevulinic Acid Dehydratase Deficiency Porphyria

Acute intermittent porphyria (AIP) is the most common form of neuropathic porphyria in North America. AIP differs from other neuropathic porphyrias (hereditary coproporphyria and variegate porphyria) because it does not produce any skin-related damage. Only one other, extremely rare, form of acute neuropathic porphyria never involves the skin and thus mimics AIP. This is aminolevulinic acid dehydratase deficiency porphyria.

If AIP is suspected, a 24-hour quantitative urine study for porphobilinogen, aminolevulinic acid, and urinary porphyrins should be ordered. *It is very important that the urine collection be done during an attack of suspected porphyria or during active chronic symptoms suspected to be from porphyria.* I also recommend measurement of the red cell enzyme porphobilinogen deaminase (also known as uroporphyrinogen-1-synthase) and the red cell enzyme aminolevulinic acid dehydratase with the first round of testing for AIP. Mayo Medical Laboratories automatically combines measurement of the enzyme aminolevulinic acid with uroporphyrinogen-1-synthase, which is a useful combination.

During an acute attack of AIP, the 24-hour porphobilinogen excretion is always increased markedly (3- to 20-fold). There are no significant increases of uroporphyrins in the urine and no increase in excretion of coproporphyrins or protoporphyrin in the stool of patients with AIP. The red blood cell enzyme uroporphyrinogen-1-synthase is reduced by at least 50% in most patients with active AIP. This enzyme activity can be used to screen family members for this autosomal dominant porphyria. In a patient with aminolevulinic acid dehydratase deficiency, symptoms are identical to those of AIP, the 24-hour urinary excretion of aminolevulinic acid is increased, the excretion of PBG is usually not increased, the aminolevulinic acid dehydratase red blood cell enzyme activity is low, and urinary porphyrin excretion shows increased levels of coproporphyrin III.

Neurologic and Cutaneous Manifestations

VARIEGATE PORPHYRIA (VP) AND HEREDITARY COPROPORPHYRIA (HC)

VP and HC are different inherited forms of porphyria, but they are discussed together here because their cutaneous and neurologic symptoms overlap. VP is autosomal dominant and common in South Africa. VP has more severe or prominent skin damage than HC. HC is more prevalent in North America.

The clinician who suspects VP or HC should order quantitative tests of urinary porphyrins and porphobilinogen on a 24-hour specimen. *This urine collection should be made when the patient is experiencing active neurologic symptoms being attributed to the porphyria. If necessary, the clinician should counsel the patient to be ready to collect urine whenever the patient is having the symptom complex being attributed to porphyria.* A 24-hour fecal porphyrin analysis should also be ordered. At the time of initial studies, I also recommend measurements of the red cell enzyme activities for coproporphyrinogen oxidase, uroporphyrinogen-1-synthase, and aminolevulinic acid dehydratase.

If the patient has HC, there will be an unequivocal increase of PBG during an attack. *This finding is so important that no neuropathic porphyria should be diagnosed unless one has found evidence of abnormally increased excretion of PBG or, as mentioned, rarely, of aminolevulinic acid.* Coproporphyrin excretion in the urine and stool will also be increased. In HC, the abnormally increased PBG excretion can return to normal between attacks, but the increased stool coproporphyrin characteristically remains so. The stool protoporphyrins may be increased somewhat but are not as dominant as the coproporphyrin. Patients with HC typically have a 50% reduction in the activity of the red cell enzyme coproporphyrinogen oxidase. This is the enzyme that decarboxylates coproporphyrinogen III to protoporphyrin.

As in uroporphyrinogen decarboxylase, there are families who inherit genetic lesions that are not expressed in red cells—so once again, the constellation of clinical signs, increased PBG excretion, and increased coproporphyrin excretion in stool and urine allow HC to be diagnosed. In a family with HC and low coproporphyrinogen oxidase levels, this enzyme can be used to screen family members.

If the patient has VP, the PBG will be unequivocally increased during an attack. There may be some minor increases in uroporphyrin excretion in urine, but the cardinal finding in VP is a markedly increased fecal excretion of protoporphyrin in the stool. This pattern occurs because the deficient enzyme in VP is protoporphyrinogen oxidase, which leads to a buildup of non-oxidized protoporphyrins that are not water-soluble and therefore are primarily excreted in bile and stool. For screening families, 24-hour stool collections can be used to identify asymptomatic individuals with markedly increased protoporphyrin excretion.

COMMON DIAGNOSTIC PROBLEMS

Secondary Coproporphyrinuria:
The Most Common Condition Confusing Clinicians

Confusion in testing patients for possible neuropathic porphyrias starts when patients with chronic pain are found to have an abnormal increased excretion of coproporphyrin. Typically, all the other uroporphyrin and PBG values are normal.

In most instances, these patients are excreting more coproporphyrins in the urine because of one or both of two underlying processes. First, they may have ingested a substance, handled by the liver, or may have a hemolytic process that has secondarily stimulated porphyrin metabolism. Second, they may have a relative decrease in the ability of their hepatocytes to transport coproporphyrins from the hepatocyte into the biliary tract system, again because of an acquired situation or because they have Dubin-Johnson-like syndrome.

If a patient has increased urinary coproporphyrins but the urinary excretion of PBG is normal during pain, a neuropathic porphyria, (i.e., AIP, HC, or VP) is not present. Additional evidence against neuropathic porphyrias includes normal fecal porphyrins, which is major evidence against VP or HC, and normal red cell enzymes for coproporphyrinogen oxidase, porphobilinogen deaminase, or aminolevulinic acid dehydratase.

Acquired factors and Dubin-Johnson syndrome can impede the transport of coproporphyrin into bile from hepatocytes. The hepatocyte-bile transport route is particularly efficient at excreting coproporphyrin I isomers. If biliary excretion of coproporphyrin I is decreased, more is excreted in the urine. Normally 20% to 45% of total urinary porphyrins are coproporphyrin I isomers. Coproporphyrin I values more than 60% of total urinary coproporphyrins suggest Dubin-Johnson syndrome. Clinicians can order the measurement of coproporphyrin isomers I and III in the urine for patients who have increased excretion of total urinary porphyrins but no evidence of a neuropathic porphyria.

Traits for Porphyrias

Patients being evaluated for porphyria often have marginally low values for enzymes such as coproporphyrinogen oxidase or porphobilinogen deaminase even though they are never found to have increases of porphobilinogen associated with symptoms attributed to a possible neuropathic porphyria.

These patients have a possible trait for HC or AIP, or this condition can occur for any porphyria. Patients who have such traits should not be told they have active neuropathic porphyria. Generally, persons with traits for HC, or other porphyrias, do not have any symptoms during their life. However, I do recommend to patients with traits (e.g., low values of coproporphyrinogen oxidase, but no proven attacks of acute porphyria) that they avoid factors that might precipitate attacks of full-blown neuropathic porphyria such as exposure to drugs like phenobarbital or to prolonged fasting. Modern low-dose estrogen oral contraceptives can be used in patients with these traits.

Pseudoporphyria or Intoxication Porphyria

Patients with pseudoporphyria have skin lesions identical to those of PCT triggered by exposure to a drug. Typically tests of urine and stool do not confirm the diagnosis of PCT or any porphyria disorder, although if enough testing is done, some evidence of abnormal porphyrin excretion can be identified. Nonsteroidal anti-inflammatory agents such as naproxen have been implicated in several case reports. Skin biopsy specimens resemble those found in cutaneous porphyria.

Some, but not all, of these patients have inherited traits for porphyria, and under certain conditions there is a transient disturbance of porphyrin metabolism with the transient accumulation of enough photosensitizing porphyrins to produce sun photosensitivity. These patients are asymptomatic if precipitating drugs are avoided.

Many agents such as lead, heavy metals, halogenated aromatic hydrocarbons, and drugs can alter porphyrin metabolism. If urine, blood, and stool samples are collected during active disturbances, the findings are various. Typically, red cell zinc-bound proto-porphyrins may be increased, and PBG or aminolevulinic acid in the urine (e.g., with lead) can be increased. Porphyrin excretion in urine and stool also can be increased. It is critical to remove patients from environments that produce heavy chemical exposure to determine whether their test results return to normal. Unfortunately, many acquired causes of increased coproporphyrin excretion (e.g., alcohol) can have a persisting influ-ence on porphyrin excretion for months. Daniell et al. (1) published an excellent review of this area.

SUMMARY

Patients with sun-sensitive skin blistering or pain and erythema may have cutaneous porphyria. Patients with acute unexplained or chronic abdominal pain or neuropathy may have a neuropathic porphyria. The clinician should first classify the patient as having cutaneous only, neuropathic only, or cutaneous and neuropathic porphyria. Targeted tests of urine, stool, and blood should then be done. It is critical to collect urine during acute attacks or when a patient agrees he or she is having symptoms being attributed to the porphyria. Test specimens must be obtained, transported, and analyzed effectively. Fully expressed inherited or acquired porphyrias are easy to diagnose. If making a diag-nosis is difficult, a secondary porphyrinuria, pseudoporphyria, intoxication porphyria, or a trait for a porphyria may be present. In these cases, consultation may be warranted.

REFERENCE

1. Daniell WE, Stockbridge HL, Labbé RF, Woods JS, Anderson KE, Bissell DM, Bloomer JR, Ellefson RD, Moore MR, Pierach CA, Schreiber WE, Tefferi A, Franklin GM. Environmental chemical expo-sures and disturbances of heme synthesis. *Environ Health Perspec* 1997; 105 Suppl 1: 37-53.

SUGGESTED READING

Kappas A, Sassa S, Galbraith RA, Nordmann Y. The porphyrias, in *The Metabolic Basis of Inherited Disease*, 6th ed. (Scriver CR, Beaudet AL, Sly WS, Valle D, eds). McGraw-Hill, New York, 1989, pp. 1305-1365.

29

Ethical Issues in the Care of Patients With Hematologic Diseases

C. Christopher Hook, MD

Contents

INTRODUCTION

Medicine is inherently an area of ethical concern because medicine is, first and foremost, a relationship. Although our knowledge and science have contributed greatly to the practice of medicine in general, and hematology specifically, they do not fully define the healing relationship between caregiver and patient. If this were not true, then medicine would be only a profession that has existed for a few decades. In reality, medicine is an art that has been practiced for at least the past 2,400 years. In medicine, understanding the underlying healing relationship is critical because even when our knowledge is inadequate, we can still provide our presence, our support, and our comfort to our patients. We are genuinely healers in this capacity. In fact, it is in the humbling times when we no longer have additional types of chemotherapy or other interventions to offer that we may be our best at being what the patient requires, because it is in those times that *we* are the therapy.

This chapter explores some of the fundamental ethical concerns that develop in the care of patients with hematologic diseases.

FOUNDATIONAL PRINCIPLES

Throughout its long history, Western medicine has been guided by different oaths and codes, the most well known of which is the Hippocratic Oath. Recently, individuals working in the field of medical ethics have tried to identify specific principles to help frame many of the concerns about the physician-patient relationship. Beauchamp and Childress *(1)* stated that most of the concerns of medical ethics may be understood in the framework of four major principles: 1) autonomy, 2) beneficence, 3) nonmaleficence, and 4) justice. Although additions have been made to these four principles, they do provide a reasonable framework from which to derive many other significant issues. For the purposes of this chapter, the first three of these principles are reviewed.

From: *Primary Hematology*
Edited by: A. Tefferi © Mayo Foundation for Medical Education and Research, Rochester, MN

Autonomy

Autonomy derives from two Greek words: *autos* ("self") and *nomes* ("rule"). The principle of autonomy is the articulation that all individuals have the right to determine their individual values and goals and, within certain limitations, to govern the conduct of their lives. Fundamentally, autonomy also may be understood as a respect for persons, that is, the need to recognize the value of each individual and the circumstances unique to his or her life, including the individual's beliefs and the choices that result from those beliefs.

AGENCY AND DECISION-MAKING CAPACITY

For autonomy to have expression, two requirements must be present. The first of these is "agency." The patient must be able to establish his or her own values and goals and be able to make appropriate decisions based on those values. The principle of agency has its expression in the clinical realm under the term "decision-making capacity." Decision-making capacity is often confused with the legal term "competence." Capacity is the physician's *clinical* determination of the patient's ability to understand his or her situation and make appropriate decisions for treatment, whereas competence is the *legal* determination that an individual has the right to make life-affecting decisions. A judge's or court's assessment of competence, however, is based in significant part on the clinical assessment of decision-making capacity. In clinical practice, the lack of decisional capacity should be proved and not presumed. Clinical evidence of confusion, disorientation, and psychosis resulting from organic diseases, metabolic disturbances, and iatrogenic interference can adversely affect decision-making capacity.

Several clinical standards are used to assess decision-making capacity:

1. The patient can make and communicate a choice
2. The patient understands the medical situation and prognosis, the nature of recommended care, available alternative options, and the risks, benefits, and consequences of each
3. The patient's decisions are stable over time
4. The decision is consistent with the patient's values and goals
5. The decision is not due to delusions

The second major requirement for autonomy is liberty; that is, the patient must be free to influence the course of his or her life and medical treatment. Many recent court decisions, from the Quinlan case in 1976 to the Cruzan decision in 1990, along with strong support from the medical ethics community, have established the right of patients to influence their care. This right is particularly applicable to the right to refuse any form of medical intervention, even if such refusal will lead to the patient's death. It is important, however, to ensure that a patient's decision is based on sufficient, correct information regarding the treatment or treatments that are being refused. This topic is discussed further in the section on informed consent.

ADVANCE DIRECTIVES AND SURROGATE DECISION MAKING

What if the patient lacks decision-making capacity? How can care decisions be made? One way is the use of an advance directive. An advance directive is a document, or verbal instructions, in which a patient who presently possesses decision-making capacity states choices for medical treatment, or designates an individual who should make treatment choices for the patient, should the person lose decision-making capacity. Advance directives can take several forms: 1) the living will, 2) the durable power of attorney for health care, 3) a document appointing a health care surrogate (in jurisdictions that do not formally recognize the durable power of attorney for health care), and 4) the advance medical care directive. Some states are now attempting to combine the living will and durable power of attorney for health care into one all-around advance directive.

Living Will

The living will arose in response to the tragic case of Karen Ann Quinlan in the mid-1970s. The living will requires two threshold requirements before it takes effect: 1) the patient must be deemed terminally ill, and 2) the patient must lack decision-making capacity. The determination of terminal illness varies from jurisdiction to jurisdiction, and therefore it is important for each physician to be familiar with the local statutes regarding advance directives. In general, the designation of terminally ill is applied to patients whose prognosis for survival is 6 months or less. When activated, the living will provides guidance to the caregivers about what treatments the patient does or does not desire. If the patient has an uncertain prognosis, or is clearly not terminal, the living will does not apply, even if the patient lacks decision-making capacity. This is one of the significant limitations of this type of advance directive.

Durable Power of Attorney for Health Care

The durable power of attorney for health care (DPAHC) is a document that designates a surrogate decision maker should the patient lose decision-making capacity. It does not require that the patient be terminally ill and is therefore an advance directive that is generally more applicable across a broad range of clinical circumstances. Within the DPAHC, the patient can make specific directives concerning different types of treatment such as cardiopulmonary resuscitation (CPR), artificial nutrition, and hydration. The major value of this type of advance directive is that it provides an individual who can dynamically interact with a health care team regarding the great breadth of medical decisions that may need to be made.

The Advance Medical Care Directive

In some circumstances, patients have specific desires never to receive certain forms of treatment. For instance, a member of the Jehovah's Witness faith may choose to refuse the administration of blood or blood products in any and all circumstances. Other individuals may choose to categorically refuse dialysis or a ventilator regardless of the circumstances. The advanced medical care directive is a document that states this categorical refusal for a specific treatment. It may take the form of a no-transfusion card or a statement on a Medic-Alert bracelet or necklace.

With all advance directives, it is important to discuss the values and goals of the patient and to know the contents of the advance directive. In 1990, Congress passed the Patient's Self-Determination Act in response to the Cruzan decision. Its goal was to try to ensure that patients were made aware of their right to have advance directives. Unfortunately, significant numbers of patients still desire to limit life-sustaining therapy, such as CPR, but their physicians are unaware of these desires. The SUPPORT study (2) revealed that for 4,301 patients who died at five academic institutions, only 51% of the patients who desired CPR actually had such an order written for them. Roughly half of the physicians of these patients did not know their patients' desire for life-sustaining therapies. Clearly, much work needs to be done to improve communication between patients and their caregivers in this critical area.

A survey of the literature by Layson et al. *(3)* revealed that the vast majority of patients want to speak with their physicians about life-sustaining therapies and their values and goals for medical care. Most believe such discussions should occur early in the relationship with their physician, and optimally will occur while the patient remains in good health and is not faced with an immediate crisis. Contrary to what most physicians would predict, patients actually want to discuss these issues soon after the diagnosis of a malignancy or other serious illness. The majority also believe that it is the responsibility of the physician to initiate these discussions. For the patient who is facing a life-threatening illness, which includes many hematologic disorders, caregivers have at a very minimum the responsibility to invite a careful discussion of the patient's goals, fears, and choices concerning therapy. Although time-consuming, a good discussion early on in the course of treatment can ultimately save an incredible amount of time and anguish down the line and make subsequent decision making much easier.

Nondesignated Surrogates

Who speaks for a patient when there is no advance directive specifically designating a surrogate? The underlying principle is to find the person, or persons, who most likely knows the patient's values and how the patient would most likely choose if he or she could speak for himself or herself. This individual should also be in the position to interact with the health care team. Different jurisdictions may formally create a specific list of rankings for which individuals can serve in the capacity of surrogate, but the following is a practical approach, in descending order of authority: 1) the patient's spouse, 2) an adult child or the majority of adult children, 3) a parent or parents, 4) an adult sibling or the majority of adult siblings, 5) an adult relative who has exhibited special care and concern, and 6) if no relative can be located, a close friend.

Inescapably, situations arise in which a surrogate's instructions conflict with a patient's previously expressed directive or with those of other family members. It is important to remember that the primary responsibility of the physician is to the patient, and the physician should determine what the patient would choose for himself or herself. In these circumstances, it may be helpful to involve an independent third-party arbitrator, such as an ethics consultant or committee, or legal counsel to help work through the issues. This option is useful only if the physician is unable, for whatever reason, to resolve the conflict.

Medical Futility

As discussed, patients clearly have the right to refuse any and all forms of treatment, including life-sustaining therapy. However, does this right to influence treatment by limiting interventions translate into a right to demand therapy as well, even if the caregivers believe the treatment is a waste of time or "futile"? If caregivers are not ethically required to provide all care demanded by patients or their surrogates, then what criteria can be used for determining what care can be denied?

These are some of the more difficult questions facing physicians today. On the one hand, we have a strong professional tradition in medicine of not offering treatments that do not benefit the patient much, if at all. As Hippocrates wrote in his piece, *The Art*, "First I will define what I conceive medicine to be. In general terms, it is to do away with the sufferings of the sick, to lessen the violence of their diseases, and to refuse to treat those who are over-mastered by their disease, realizing that in such cases medicine is powerless." There is also the issue of personal moral integrity that arises when a caregiver is asked to perform an intervention that he or she believes is more likely to cause harm, or little if any good. On the other hand, if a treatment has some chance of sustaining life, albeit small, and the patient is willing to endure the physical side effects of the intervention and will accept the state of life that the intervention might provide, how can we disregard the patient's value system and potentially let him or her die?

An issue that seems to be frequently associated with the concept of medical futility is medical economics. There is a belief that a tremendous amount of resources are wasted in "futile" care. It is very important early on in this discussion to not confuse the concept of futility with rationing. The fact that a treatment is costly does not necessarily make it futile. Embodied in these concerns are two recognitions: 1) that in some interventions the cost, understood in terms of money or the patient's well-being, is disproportionate to the amount of benefit derived, and 2) that the process of treatment—not just its end points—must be taken into consideration. In general, however, the economic arguments for futility have little factual base to support them. Data from the SUPPORT study (2) and an independent investigation by Halevy et al. (4) revealed that very few cases fall under the frequently proposed futility definitions and, consequently, the savings derived from proposed futility policies would be very modest.

Even if eliminating "futile" care could generate more savings in the health care budget, we would still be faced with the very difficult question of whether futility can be defined in a clinically meaningful way. To begin to answer this question, we need to return to the origins of the word itself. "Futility" is derived from the Latin word *futilus*, meaning leaky. According to the Oxford English dictionary, a futile action is "leaky, hence untrustworthy, vain, failing of the desired end through intrinsic effect." Therefore, a futile intervention is one that cannot achieve the goals of the intervention *no matter how often it is repeated*. Failure may be predicted because of the inherent nature of the intervention proposed.

From this definition, it is clear that there are some situations in which an intervention would be futile, and therefore the caregiver is under no obligation to provide it. For instance, if the proposed treatment has no pathophysiologic rationale, it is, by definition, futile. Similarly, if maximal therapy is already being used but is failing, attempting to add other treatments will not improve the situation. Another example is a request to repeat interventions that have already failed in the context of the care of a specific patient.

These examples, however, are very narrow and do not represent most situations in which a futility escape is often sought. Probably the best-known attempt to create a broader clinical definition of futility was by Schneiderman et al. (5). The definition consists of two parts. First, there is a quantitative definition stating, "when a physician concludes that in the last 100 cases medical treatment has been ineffective," it is, therefore, futile. The authors admit that this is an arbitrary level, believing that it is a threshold with which most would be comfortable. Yet, it has not been shown that a 5% threshold or a 0.5% threshold might be more appropriate, and it is doubtful that universal acceptance of any given threshold will be achieved. In the survey by Murphy et al. (6), 10% of studied patients believe that a 1% chance of survival from CPR was still worth pursuing. Even if we could agree on a 1% threshold, what we are stating is that a positive outcome is unlikely rather than futile. It can work, but it is unlikely to do so. That being the case, then only the patient can weigh the odds, the burdens, and the benefits and determine whether it is consistent with his or her goals for life. To claim otherwise is to assert that the patient's values are irrelevant or inferior to the physician's, an act of significant arrogance and unbridled parentalism in its worst form.

The quantitative definition of futility is also problematic because of our limited ability to quantitate the probabilities of outcomes exactly. We need only go to a classic issue in the question of CPR to illustrate this point. One of the supposedly clear cases of futility in CPR has been in patients with metastatic cancer. The well-known meta-analysis by Ebell *(7)* in 1992 showed that overall survival to dismissal for all patients receiving CPR in 14 studies from 1980 to 1991 was 13.5%. The patients were categorized according to diagnosis, and the overall survival to dismissal was 5.8% in those with a malignant disease and 0% in those with metastatic disease. However, in 1991, Vitelli et al. *(8)* reported that 65.7% of 114 patients receiving CPR at Memorial Sloan-Kettering Cancer Center were successfully resuscitated, and 10.5% survived to dismissal. The presence of metastatic disease was not a determining factor. Schwenzer et al. *(9)* reported that 20% of patients with metastatic cancer who received a resuscitation attempt survived to dismissal. Now, it must be stated that at these institutions the percentage of total patients with cancer and metastatic disease who still requested CPR was small. The reality is that most patients in these situations will probably request a DNR status. What remains is the fact that for those who continue to request CPR, the intervention cannot be considered futile. In fact, the study by Schwenzer et al. concluded

> *the outcome from CPR is a matter of probability, not certainty, ... The administration of CPR in previously defined futile situations, i.e., metastatic disease, could be successful, and therefore cannot be judged to be universally futile in such situations. We found no convenient categories of absolute nonsurvival nor absolute futility.*

It is very difficult to assert a moral claim to be able to define futile care when our own outcomes data are by no means clear in this regard.

The second aspect of the definition by Schneiderman et al. *(5)* is a qualitative notion stating, "any treatment that merely preserves permanent unconsciousness or that fails to end total dependence on intensive medical care," even if it has some physiologic effect on some part of the body, may also be called futile. This is the most troublesome aspect of their definition because it is entirely value-laden. It states that, in life, quality is more important than quantity. Although many of us may agree with this position, many do not. Those in disagreement insist that life has value irrespective of its quality and should be preserved. Some groups of Orthodox Judaism, Roman Catholicism, Protestantism, and other value systems maintain this type of "vitalism" in their world view and belief structure. Once again we must ask, where is the futility involved? The outcome may be unacceptable to some, but the interventions maintaining the life are not futile. They are physiologically effective, but they are maintaining the life in a quality that some would find unacceptable. Again, we are left with the question, whose values should predominate in these situations?

It is also clear that if formal futility definitions such as this are used, they will be inappropriately applied. Uhlmann and Pearlman *(10)* and others have shown that physicians often rate patients' quality of life significantly lower than patients do for themselves. A study by Curtis et al. *(11)* revealed that residents had an incorrect understanding of quantitative futility 33% of the time and described interventions affording a 5% to 10% chance of survival as futile. They also failed to discuss quality of life with communicative patients in whom qualitative futility was invoked one-third of the time. Even more alarming was the finding that residents found interventions futile more often if the patient was not white (2.7 times more often).

To me, the great tragedy of the whole futility issue has been that most who have written about it insist on analyzing the problem as a division of power: the power of patient autonomy versus the power of medical knowledge and judgment. This approach fundamentally misses the real source of power in medicine. The power is in the relationship, the coming together of the afflicted and the healer, blending needs and goals with knowledge and skill to come to as good an outcome as possible. There can be no true healing without this relationship. The futility versus autonomy dichotomy pits caregiver against patient. But healing and caring are not games in which one side plays a trump card against the other to win. To resort to the futility card is to admit that the healing relationship has died or at least is severely impaired.

The best approach to these difficult situations is one of "due process." Here, all efforts are used to negotiate a plan of care that is acceptable to all the involved parties. It is important to recognize and respect moral integrity and values of the patient, surrogates, and caregivers. This approach was first articulated in 1994 by the Christian Medical and Dental Society *(12)*. A similar, more elaborate approach was delineated in *JAMA* in 1996 and has become known as the "Houston Protocol," because it was the joint effort of most of the major hospitals in Houston *(13)*. The Houston Protocol was formally endorsed by the Council on Ethical and Judicial Affairs of the American Medical Association in December 1996.

Briefly, the procedure proposed involves multiple steps. The first involves a careful discussion between the responsible physician and the patient or surrogates concerning the diagnosis, prognosis, reasons why the debated intervention is undesirable or inappropriate, and what alternatives may be available. It is important to emphasize that appropriate medical care and humane care will always be provided to promote comfort, dignity, and emotional and spiritual support. These discussions are also important because many patients have an unrealistic expectation of medical care in their outcomes. Appropriately educating patients can many times resolve these dilemmas. A study by Murphy et al. *(6)* showed that when patients learned the actual outcome statistics for CPR, the number still desiring resuscitation was almost halved.

If these discussions fail to produce agreement, then the responsible physician should offer the patient transfer to the care of another physician or another institution. It may be helpful at this time to request consultation by an independent physician concerning the medical inappropriateness of the intervention in question. Also at this level, institutional resources such as nursing, patient care representatives, chaplaincy, social services, or, perhaps, ethics consultation should be engaged to help resolve the disagreement.

If all these efforts still fail to resolve the dispute, a consultant or end-of-life decisions committee charged with recommending the final course of action should be engaged. The physician should notify the patient or surrogate that this process has been invoked and allow that individual(s) opportunity to meet with the consultant or committee. If the process agrees with the patient and the physician remains unpersuaded, interinstitutional transfer to another physician may be arranged. If the process agrees with the physician and the patient or surrogate remains unpersuaded, intrainstitutional transfer may be sought and should be supported by the institution. If transfer is not possible, the intervention need not be offered, on the grounds of its "futility."

We are left with one final question, and that is how the final committee should make its decision regarding medical appropriateness or inappropriateness. Pellegrino and Thomasma *(14)* have identified three major areas that need to be considered: 1) the likelihood of benefit of the proposed intervention, 2) a proportional weighing of the benefits and burdens incurred to pursue the treatment in question, and 3) the issue of benefit. Benefit is a complex concept involving several considerations. We immediately think of biological or medical benefit, and this is indeed one aspect of the larger concept. However, other forms of benefit must be considered, including psychological or emotional benefit and benefit in terms of the patient's belief system or world view, including spiritual benefit. As such we need to consider whether the patient considers it a spiritual duty to maintain life at all costs. Bringing all of these pieces of information to bear on the question should help make it clear whether a requested intervention should be provided or not.

INFORMED CONSENT

A derivative principle of autonomy, informed consent has two preconditions on the part of the patient: 1) decision-making capacity, and 2) voluntariness, essentially the same as the agency and liberty associated with the principle of autonomy. Beyond these preconditions are the informational requirements of informed consent. The patient should receive accurate, truthful information sufficient to make a reasoned decision. The amount of information shared with the patient should not be guided by only what the physician believes is adequate, but that which the average, prudent person would need to have in order to make an appropriate decision (the reasonable persons standard). Included within this information is a discussion of available alternatives to the proposed treatment. For instance, a patient with Hodgkin's disease amenable to radiation therapy or chemotherapy should receive a thorough discussion of each of the options and their potential complications and side effects, even if the physician may be biased toward one of the treatments. In many hematologic illnesses in which intensive therapy could certainly be used, but may not be curative, or may be associated with significant life-threatening toxicity, the option of supportive, palliative care should also be discussed with the patient. It is the duty of the physician to set aside personal bias and provide detailed information of each treatment course to allow the patient to make a well-informed personal decision. The patient can then take the information and assess it within the context of his or her life goals and quality of life considerations.

After a discussion of available alternatives, the physician should present the patient with a single recommendation that the patient can accept or reject. Patients come to their physicians expecting the caregivers to use their knowledge and experience in providing them with a recommendation. Simply laying out a series of choices before the patient may lead to confusion or the perception by the patient that the physician is unconcerned with his or her welfare. If the patient refuses the recommended treatment and chooses one of the alternatives, the physician should respect the patient's choice.

In certain circumstances a patient may require more information than what the average reasonable person might desire. For instance, some religious belief systems may specifically preclude certain forms of medical intervention that might not trouble another individual in the least. It is important to ensure that patients receive sufficient information within the context of their beliefs to help them make an appropriate choice.

In certain circumstances, informed consent may not be obtainable, specifically in emergency situations in which physicians are compelled to provide medically necessary therapy, without which harm would result. The principle of *implied consent* clarifies that there is a duty to assist a person in urgent need of care. The principle has been legally accepted and it provides the physician a legal defense against battery, although not negligence.

Truth Telling and Sharing Bad News

Truth telling on the part of the physician is an integral part of autonomy. To make the principle of autonomy function, the physician must provide decisionally capable patients with adequate and truthful information on which to base decisions. Without the receipt of sufficient truthful information, patients cannot make truly autonomous decisions about their life plans. Occasionally, however, the physician may withhold part or all of the truth if it is believed that telling the truth is likely to cause significant injury. This is the principle of *therapeutic privilege*. For example, if it can be well ascertained that a patient will attempt harm of himself or herself or others if certain information is received, such as the diagnosis of a malignant illness, then the information may be withheld. However, there is a heavy burden of proof on the withholding physician to establish the likelihood of injury, and the decision for intentional nondisclosure must be fully and carefully recorded in the medical record.

There may be significant differences between patients and cultures as to what may be assimilated from a discussion and as to what the patient expects in regard to the amount of information disclosed by the physician. The news of the diagnosis of malignant disease, while acceptable as a painful truth for one patient, may be devastating and carry profound social and religious implications for another. It is important to be sensitive to these issues, yet willing to give patients as much information as they want or need. We can do so by giving them the permission to ask questions and providing them with the information they want. One must never prejudge the extent to which information will be shared based on a patient's particular ethnic or religious background. Individuals in every tradition may want more information and honest disclosures than their cultural tradition might otherwise imply. Thus, it is extremely important that patients be given the freedom to ask questions and to some extent guide the discussions.

Although sufficient, truthful disclosure is important, it is not always necessary to beat patients with the truth, either. By this I mean it is not mandatory to walk into each examination room clearly stating the exact name of the malignancy, rattling off some survival statistics, listing the treatment options with all the potential side effects, and then leaving. Such brutal honesty would be unacceptable to some patients and will not be assimilated or retained by most. We can temper our discussions and communicate necessary information gradually and sensitively. What cannot be condoned, however, is overtly lying to a patient. If the patient specifically asks, "Is this a cancer?" then we must tell the truth. To lie is to betray the trust placed in us as caregivers. A lie, even for beneficent ends, ultimately undermines any future trust that the patient will place in us.

Having said this, it is also important to acknowledge that telling a patient bad news is one of the hardest things a physician does. Creagan *(15)* offered the following suggestions in the art of delivering bad news. 1. Be sensitive to the physical setting of the discussion. Sit down with the patient, maintaining good, level eye contact. Remove intervening barriers. 2. Preserve patient confidentiality. Know who is with the patient, their relationship to the patient, and whether the patient wants them to be there. 3. Make no assumptions about what the patient knows. It is not necessary to talk down to the patient, but it is necessary to engage in dialogue. Learn what the patient knows and understands and periodically ask, "Does this make sense?" or "Do you have any questions at this point?" 4. Give the patient permission to ask what is important to him or her. 5. Acknowledge the patient's reactions. Emotions are real and they are legitimate. Don't ignore a patient's tears. A moment of silence or a gentle touch allows the patient to be himself or herself and feel accepted. 6. Arrange follow-through, another chance to ask questions or clarify points of information or misunderstanding. Give the patient access to you. Let the patient know that you recognize that all the information you are going to provide during that conversation may not be assimilated. Take the burden off the patient by telling him or her to contact you with additional questions and concerns.

Beneficence and Nonmaleficence

Beneficence is acting to benefit patients by preserving life, restoring health, relieving suffering, and restoring or maintaining function. Beneficence is beautifully illustrated in the statement by Dr. William Mayo, "The best interest of the patient is the only interest to be considered." The physician is obligated to help patients attain the interests and goals as determined by the patient, not the physician. Nonmaleficence is a corollary principle that requires that one should not do evil or harm. The two principles of beneficence and nonmaleficence were classically articulated together in Hippocrates' work *The Epidemics*, "As to diseases, make a habit of two things—to help, or at least do no harm."

THE PRINCIPLE OF DOUBLE EFFECT (BENEFICENCE VERSUS NONMALEFICENCE)

In the medical management of patients, sometimes the pursuit of a beneficent outcome risks the potential for serious injury or harm. Consequently, the moral obligations for beneficence and nonmaleficence conflict. This situation is frequently encountered in the patient with hematologic illness when consideration is given to use of aggressive intervention such as high-dose chemotherapy or bone marrow transplantation. The principle of double effect is a means of trying to analyze the conflict between beneficence and nonmaleficence and to determine whether a proposed intervention is morally acceptable despite the risks. The principle states that an act is acceptable if 1) the act itself is good or morally neutral, 2) the agent intends only the good effect, 3) the bad effect must not be a means to the good effect (e.g., death is the only way to achieve the desired outcome), and 4) the good effect must outweigh the bad effect. A frequent example in the care of patients with malignant disease is the conflict that can develop in the use of analgesia that is adequate to control the patient's suffering but may lead to respiratory depression or failure. By reasoning of double effect, and the higher requirement of beneficence to address the suffering of patients, adequate analgesia for the relief of suffering should always be given even if death is hastened. The analgesics are to be given, however, in such a way as to relieve the pain and not specifically hasten the death of the patient, even in terminally ill patients.

PHYSICIAN-ASSISTED SUICIDE AND EUTHANASIA

This issue leads to another important question facing the profession of medicine and our patients at this time, that of physician-assisted death (assisted suicide or euthanasia). For the past several decades, the percentage of Americans favoring some form of assisted death has approximately doubled; recent surveys indicate that 50% to 80% of the American public believes they should have access to assisted suicide or euthanasia. Recently the populous of the state of Oregon reapproved a law permitting physician-assisted suicide. In 1997 the Supreme Court of the United States voted that laws against assisted suicide were not necessarily unconstitutional, but did allow states such as Oregon to pass laws permitting assisted death. In several recent surveys, as many as 50% of the physicians responding indicated that they also favored some form of legalization of physician-assisted suicide. In some of these, 7% indicated that they had already assisted in a patient's suicide.

What has brought about this significant change in the attitudes of the public and the medical profession? I believe the underlying concerns can be summed up in what may be described as the "Five Fears": 1) the fear of pain, 2) the fear of loss of control over one's life and bodily functions, 3) the fear of being a burden to family members, 4) the fear of technology, and 5) the fear of abandonment, especially from the caregivers. As mentioned, the SUPPORT study *(2)* showed that many patients are receiving treatments and technological interventions that they do not desire. Patients are being maintained in states that are unacceptable to them. Other data from the SUPPORT study also indicate that physicians have not been aggressive enough in the use of narcotics and other analgesics to control pain. However, is access to assisted suicide the best solution to these concerns?

It is beyond the scope of this chapter to engage in a full analysis of the arguments for and against this critical issue. However, the following is a brief summation of the major arguments. The arguments for physician-assisted death are:

> The *autonomy argument:* This is the statement that patients should have the right to determine the time and circumstances of their deaths, including ending their lives overtly through assisted suicide or euthanasia.
>
> The *equivalence argument*: This is the statement that there is no difference between a patient's right to refuse life-sustaining therapy, which may lead to an earlier demise, and a choice to more directly end life via suicide or euthanasia.
>
> The *mercy argument*: This argument states that physicians, out of compassion, should be willing or able to end the suffering of patients via assisted death.
>
> The *best interests argument*: This is the privacy argument, stating that if the patient and physician choose assisted suicide in the privacy of their own relationship, it is their business alone and no one else's.
>
> The *Golden Rule argument*: This states that physicians who would not want to be left in intractable pain themselves and might use their own access to drugs to end their own lives should not deny this ability to their patients. "Do unto others as you would have them do unto you."

The arguments against physician-assisted death are:

> The *sanctity of life argument*: This argument, which dates back to one of the commandments from the Bible, "Thou shalt not kill," and other religious traditions, states that life is intrinsically valuable and something that no one has the wisdom or the right to end deliberately.
>
> The *slippery slope argument*: This complex argument states in essence that if a line is crossed and a current prohibition is eroded, albeit for good reasons, there will logically and inexorably be subsequent steps that cannot be prevented and will lead to occurrences that no one would have wanted in the first place. In the context of this discussion, the slippery slope argument states that even if we try to regulate assisted death carefully by specific criteria, abuses will occur and patients who did not necessarily request assisted death will be euthanized.
>
> The *professional integrity argument*: This argument goes back to the Hippocratic Oath and the fundamental tradition of medicine that physicians do not kill. It states that if physicians now may take a patient's life explicitly, significant trust in the physician-patient relationship will be eroded.
>
> The *finality argument*: This argument states that one should not burn one's bridges and that once the patient has been killed there is no going back for another intervention or because the patient changed his or her mind.

One could engage in arguments from both sides. What would be most helpful would be some clear information or data that demonstrate the validity, or lack thereof, of these arguments. Fortunately, we do have some information that has tremendous bearing on the issue of physician-assisted death for the United States. For several decades, the Netherlands has permitted euthanasia and physician-assisted suicide under specific regulations. Although these practices remain against the law according to the formal statutes, physicians who comply with several specific requirements may directly assist death without prosecution. The Dutch system is very similar to the Oregon Death With Dignity Act and as such the experience in the Netherlands may give us some clues as to what we might expect if these practices are sanctioned in the United States. Comparing the United States with the Netherlands is a fairly valid comparison in that both cultures are strongly dedicated to individual rights and both societies have a history of liberal social ideals. The differences between the societies actually tend to show that the problems that have developed in the Netherlands are more likely to occur in the United States. The socialized medicine in Holland reduces a lot of the financial concerns that may drive many Americans to desire assisted death. The Dutch have always been a very law-abiding people with a careful commitment to social order, in contrast to the shoot from the hip and ask questions later mentality of the United States.

The Dutch program requires that the patient have severe, intractable physical suffering. A second consultation should be performed by an independent physician concerning the competence and informed consent of the patient, and the diagnosis, for example. The Dutch require that the patient be acting voluntarily and that there be a considered request for death. Either euthanasia or assisted suicide may be performed. (In Oregon, the patient must be terminally ill, and only assisted suicide is permitted.) The assisted death must be recorded in the medical record as such and not reported as a natural death. The physician must then notify the local prosecutor and inform him or her of the assisted death. If these regulations are complied with, then no prosecution occurs. (The only other major difference between the Netherlands program and the Oregon program is that the Oregon program mandates a 15-day waiting period from the initial request before a lethal prescription can be given to the patient.)

The most substantial information regarding the Dutch experience has been known as the Remmelink Report, commissioned and first published by the Dutch government in 1991, updated in 1996. According to the data, approximately 2.4% of all deaths in the Netherlands result from euthanasia and 0.4% from assisted suicide. In the 1991 report, 1,000 patients were described who were killed without their request. After these data were challenged, a subsequent publication in 1993 described so-called Life-Terminating Acts Without Explicit Request (LAWER). These apparently accounted for 0.8% of all deaths. In other words, 1 in every 125 deaths was due to a physician overtly taking the patient's life without any prior request from the patient. This was in clear violation of the requirements that the patient be competent and acting voluntarily. In 41% of the cases in which LAWER occurred, there was no knowledge of the patient's wishes about the issue, in 30% of cases no consultation took place with other colleagues, in 83% the decision was discussed with a family member (which means that in 17% of cases the act occurred strictly on the decision and action of the physician alone), and in 36% of cases LAWER occurred in patients possessing decision-making capacity.

The story does not end here, unfortunately. Several recent judicial decisions in the Netherlands have greatly broadened the number of individuals who can be euthanized. In 1993, a three-judge court in the city of Assen ruled that nonterminally ill patients suffering from depression could request physician-assisted death. What was once an exclusionary criterion has now become another reason to end a patient's life. In 1995, a district court in the city of Akmaar refused to convict Dr. Hank Prins for killing a 3-day-old girl who had spina bifida. The patient was in pain and the parents persistently requested euthanasia. The trial proved Dr. Prins guilty of murder, but he was not convicted because the court wanted to establish a precedent for euthanasia candidates unable to request death. Consequently, the court has moved to formally sanction the acts of LAWER. Also in 1995 a Groning court dismissed murder charges against Dr. Gerthardus Kadijik for killing a 3-week-old girl with trisomy 13 (Patau's syndrome). This is a severely disabling congenital syndrome with an extremely poor prognosis. What was particularly trouble-some with the court's decision, however, was the statement from the presiding judge that the physician "had no choice than to kill the child since treatment was futile." The Dutch have therefore moved from a law that allowed competent individuals to voluntarily request euthanasia and assisted suicide to a situation in which physicians have no choice but to kill their patients.

The Dutch experience conclusively demonstrates the great potential for abuse if physician-assisted death is formally sanctioned. It demonstrates in a very concrete fash-ion that slippery slope arguments are not hypothetical but that a slide is indeed quite probable. Let us consider two factors to show how this will happen or is already happen-ing in Oregon. First, we need to examine the prohibition against euthanasia while physician-assisted suicide is permitted. All it takes is one quadriplegic patient, or some-one who is incapable of taking pills alone, to sue the State of Oregon under the Americans With Disabilities Act, claiming that the prohibition against euthanasia is discriminating against his or her right to self-determination. Soon euthanasia will necessarily be permit-ted as well. There is already evidence that the criteria will not be strictly regulated either. In the fall of 1997 an Oregon physician specifically euthanized a patient without the patient's request. The State of Oregon has chosen not to prosecute the physician, and the suspension of his license by the Department of Professional Regulation in that state has been revoked. Physician-assisted suicide and euthanasia will be abused.

What is particularly problematic, however, is that assisted death is really only a cover for the true underlying problems. Our response should be to better address the underlying concerns rather than to paper over the issue by killing the patient. Physicians must commit to better pain control and palliative care. We must personally improve our understanding as practicing physicians in these areas but also make concerted efforts to incorporate these concerns in undergraduate, postgraduate, and continuing medical education. We must also do a better job of recognizing and treating depression. We must encourage and enhance communication between patients and their caregivers about the patient's values and desires for life-sustaining and other forms of treatment. We must do a better job at utilizing and respecting advance directives.

NONABANDONMENT

We must work hard not only as a profession but as a society to make sure that no one feels abandoned. One of the fundamental implications of beneficence and nonmaleficence is the promise of fidelity to the patient even in difficult circumstances. Particularly for patients with neoplastic and potentially terminal diseases, it is critical that physicians see themselves as healers rather than technicians. It is critical that we understand that relation-ship is key and an important part of our overall therapy. One of the most distressing things that can happen to a patient is coming to the point when the physicians no longer have further treatments that hold any reasonable hope of producing a response and then sensing the caregivers pulling away. The tendency is for us to back away from the patient at that point, thinking, if I can't give you any more chemotherapy, there is nothing more I can do for you. However, if relationship is the focal point, then it is critical that we continue to comfort, support, and counsel our patients in this final part of their journey. It is in so doing that we recognize their intrinsic worth and dignity. It is at this point that we become the treatment.

A young medical student *(16)* a few years ago described her struggle with squamous cell carcinoma of the tongue. She went through multiple surgical procedures, radiation, and multiple rounds of chemotherapy, including some experimental treatments. Ultimately she died of her disease, but before her death she wrote:

> *Reflecting on the course of my disease and its treatment, I have often considered the medical profession's power to affect people's lives. Their caring attitudes sustained me through the most daunting procedures. Clearly, I could not have reached this far without the encouragement of physicians, nurses, secretaries, and technicians who have given me their love and concern.*

> *These professionals entered into a relationship with me, their patient, a relationship that plays a powerful role in the healing partnership. Amidst the pain, agonizing decisions, and changing self-image, the one constancy I had was the bond tying healer and afflicted together . . . .*

> *Beyond what machines and medicines and procedures can do for the patient, the act of caring remains a powerful weapon in the fight against disease. It is the one thing that medical technology can never replace. When everything is done that can be done, compassion is the only thing that remains. It is the only thing that brings beauty and meaning to our lives. It is the irreplaceable gift.*

ACKNOWLEDGMENT

Portions of this chapter were previously published in Prakash UBS (editor-in-chief). *Mayo Internal Medicine Board Review 1998-99.* Lippincott-Raven Publishers, Philadelphia, 1998. By permission of Mayo Foundation for Medical Education and Research.

REFERENCES

1. Beauchamp TL, Childress JF. *Principles of Biomedical Ethics*, 4th ed. Oxford University Press, New York, 1994.
2. The SUPPORT Principal Investigators. A controlled trial to improve care for seriously ill hospitalized patients. The Study to Understand Prognoses and Preferences for Outcomes and Risks of Treatments (SUPPORT). *JAMA* 1995; 274: 1591-1598.
3. Layson RT, Adelman HM, Wallach PM, Pfeifer MP, Johnston S, McNutt RA, and the End of Life Study Group. Discussions about the use of life-sustaining treatments: a literature review of physicians' and patients' attitudes and practices. *J Clin Ethics* 1994; 5: 195-203.
4. Halevy A, Neal RC, Brody BA. The low frequency of futility in an adult intensive care unit setting. *Arch Intern Med* 1996; 156: 100-104.
5. Schneiderman LJ, Jecker NS, Jonsen AR. Medical futility: its meaning and ethical implications. *Ann Intern Med* 1990; 112: 949-954.
6. Murphy DJ, Burrows D, Santilli S, Kemp AW, Tenner S, Kreling B, Teno J. The influence of the probability of survival on patients' preferences regarding cardiopulmonary resuscitation. *N Engl J Med* 1994; 330: 545-549.
7. Ebell MH. Prearrest predictors of survival following in-hospital cardiopulmonary resuscitation: a meta-analysis. *J Fam Pract* 1992; 34: 551-558.

8. Vitelli CE, Cooper K, Rogatko A, Brennan MF. Cardiopulmonary resuscitation and the patient with cancer. *J Clin Oncol* 1991; 9: 111-115.
9. Schwenzer KJ, Smith WT, Durbin CG Jr. Selective application of cardiopulmonary resuscitation improves survival rates. *Anesth Analg* 1993; 76: 478-484.
10. Uhlmann RF, Pearlman RA. Perceived quality of life and preferences for life-sustaining treatment in older adults. *Arch Intern Med* 1991; 151: 495-497.
11. Curtis JR, Park DR, Krone MR, Pearlman RA. Use of the medical futility rationale in do-not-attempt-resuscitation orders. *JAMA* 1995; 273: 124-128.
12. Christian Medical & Dental Society. CMDS ethical statement--medical futility. http://www.cmds.org/Ethics/2_2.htm.
13. Halevy A, Brody BA. A multi-institution collaborative policy on medical futility. *JAMA* 1996; 276: 571-574.
14. Pellegrino ED, Thomasma DC. *For the Patient's Good: The Restoration of Beneficence in Health Care.* Oxford University Press, New York, 1988.
15. Creagan ET. How to break bad news—and not devastate the patient. *Mayo Clin Proc* 1994; 69: 1015-1017.
16. Theisen A. The irreplaceable gift. *JAMA* 1991; 266: 1283.

SUGGESTED READING

General Principles of Medical Ethics

Hook CC, Prakash UBS, Dunn WF. Medical ethics, in *Mayo Internal Medicine Board Review 1998-99* (Prakash UBS, editor-in-chief). Lippincott-Raven Publishers, Philadelphia, 1998, pp. 581-591.
Jonsen AR, Siegler M, Winslade WJ. *Clinical Ethics: A Practical Approach to Ethical Decisions in Clinical Medicine*, 4th ed. McGraw-Hill, New York, 1998.

Medical Futility

Emanuel EJ, Emanuel LL. The economics of dying. The illusion of cost savings at the end of life. *N Engl J Med* 1994; 330: 540-544.
Fins JJ. Futility in clinical practice: report on a Congress of Clinical Societies. *J Am Geriatr Soc* 1994; 42: 861-865.
Hook C. Medical futility, in *Dignity and Dying: A Christian Appraisal* (Kilner DF, Miller AB, Pellegrino ED, eds). William B. Erdmans Publishing Company, Grand Rapids, MI, 1996, pp. 84-95.
Teno JM, Murphy D, Lynn J, Tosteson A, Desbiens N, Connors AF Jr, Hamel MB, Wu A, Phillips R, Wenger N, Harrell F Jr, Knaus WA, for the SUPPORT investigators. Prognosis-based futility guidelines: does anyone win? *J Am Geriatr Soc* 1994; 42: 1202-1207.

How to Break Bad News

Buckman R. *How to Break Bad News: A Guide for Health Care Professionals.* The Johns Hopkins University Press, Baltimore, 1992.

Physician-Assisted Death

Canady CT. *Physician-Assisted Suicide and Euthanasia in the Netherlands: A Report of Chairman Charles T. Canady to the Subcommittee on the Constitution of the Committee on the Judiciary, House of Representatives, 104th Congress, Second Session.* United States Government Printing Office, 1996.
Fins JJ, Bacchetta MD. The physician-assisted suicide and euthanasia debate: an annotated bibliography of representative articles. *J Clin Ethics* 1994; 5: 329-340.
Hendin H. *Seduced by Death: Doctors, Patients, and the Dutch Cure.* W.W. Norton & Company, New York, 1997.
New York State Task Force on Life and the Law. *When Death Is Sought: Assisted Suicide and Euthanasia in the Medical Context.* New York State Task Force on Life and the Law, New York, 1994.
Pellegrino ED. Doctors must not kill. *J Clin Ethics* 1992; 3: 95-102.
Pijnenborg L, van der Maas PJ, van Delden JJ, Looman CW. Life-terminating acts without explicit request of patient. *Lancet* 1993; 341: 1196-1199.
Sachs GA, Ahronheim JC, Rhymes JA, Volicer L, Lynn J. Good care of dying patients: the alternative to physician-assisted suicide and euthanasia. *J Am Geriatr Soc* 1995; 43: 553-562.
van der Maas PJ, Van Delden JJ, Pijnenborg L, Looman CW. Euthanasia and other medical decisions concerning the end of life. *Lancet* 1991; 338: 669-674.

van der Maas PJ, van der Wal G, Haverkate I, de Graaff CL, Kester JG, Onwuteaka-Philipsen BD, van der Heide A, Bosma JM, Willems DL. Euthanasia, physician-assisted suicide, and other medical practices involving the end of life in the Netherlands, 1990-1995. *N Engl J Med* 1996; 335: 1699-1705.

Weir RF. The morality of physician-assisted suicide. *Law Med Health Care* 1992; 20: 116-126.

30 Statistical Methods Frequently Used in Hematology Research

Georgene Schroeder, MS

Contents

INTRODUCTION

The use of statistical methods is central to any research endeavor, and the number of textbooks written on this topic could easily fill a small library. Therefore, one chapter cannot begin to cover all the topics and methods necessary to perform and understand detailed statistical analyses. This chapter is not intended to be a reference for investigators who want to perform their own statistical analysis. Instead, the goals are to discuss the role of the statistician in hematology research and to introduce some basic study designs, statistical terms, and statistical methods that are frequently used. For additional information, specific references are provided for each topic.

THE ROLE OF THE STATISTICIAN

The primary role of the statistician in clinical research is to aid the investigator in the design, analysis, and reporting of the research study. Initially, on the basis of the specific research question(s), the statistician helps the investigator choose the best study design. A good study design minimizes the burden on patients while providing the maximal amount of information. An experienced statistician is able to identify unforeseen problems and provide creative solutions. During the patient-entry phase, the statistician often handles routine monitoring of patient compliance, adverse events, questions relating to

From: *Primary Hematology*
Edited by: A. Tefferi © Mayo Foundation for Medical Education and Research, Rochester, MN

bias, and interim toxicity and efficacy reporting. During the analysis phase, the data are checked for accuracy and analyzed. Some statistical designs provide straightforward answers to primary research questions; other designs require more complicated techniques. Regardless, the statistician's job is to analyze the data objectively and assist in the interpretation of the results. The final, and often the most difficult, challenge is reporting the results as clearly as possible in a manner appropriate for the intended audience.

STUDY DESIGNS

Research studies are divided into two major categories: retrospective and prospective. The study design and the context in which the data are collected define the two categories. In a retrospective study design, existing patient records or databases are reviewed to provide insight into a particular question. One advantage of a retrospective study is that it typically can be performed quickly. Major disadvantages of retrospective studies include the method of patient selection (nonrandomized) and the quality and quantity of data available for analysis (the available data are limited to those recorded in the medical record). For these reasons, inherent biases frequently exist with retrospective studies, making interpretation of the results difficult.

One common type of retrospective study is the case-control study. In a case-control study, data abstracted from the records of patients with a particular disease (cases) are compared with data from patients who are free of the disease (controls). Demographic information and other factors that may be associated with the disease are gathered retrospectively from patient records. The goal of the study is to determine whether certain factors exist more frequently in those who have the disease. A case-control study design is especially effective for studying rare diseases because data can be abstracted and retained until an appropriate number of cases are identified. This type of design is also effective when there are many possible unknown origins of the disease. A limitation of the case-control design is potential bias in identifying cases or selecting controls. For more detailed information regarding case-control studies, see Schlesselman (1).

In a prospective study, patients (or research subjects) are identified and enrolled to answer a specific research question. Data pertinent to the research question are collected over time while the patients are actively followed. The major advantage of the prospective study is that study subjects are identified up front and all data are subsequently collected. If the question involves the comparison of two or more treatments, randomization and blinding of the investigators and subjects can be used to eliminate potential bias. Even in a study involving a single treatment group (sometimes referred to as a one-sample study), careful initial planning can aid in minimizing bias.

Examples of commonly used prospective study designs are phase I, phase II, and phase III clinical trials. Phase I and phase II trials typically include a single treatment regimen. The primary goal of a phase I clinical trial is determination of an acceptable drug dosage. The acceptable drug dosage, or maximum tolerated dose, is the highest drug dosage that can be given without causing unacceptable side effects. A typical phase I trial uses a dose-escalation scheme and includes approximately 30 patients. Once toxicity patterns are determined and a maximum tolerated dose is realized, the next step in studying a drug is a phase II clinical trial. A phase II clinical trial is a relatively small, monitored investigation into a drug's efficacy and toxicity. Typical phase II clinical trials require 25 to 50 patients. Frequently, phase II trials are used to select the most efficacious and least toxic

Table 1
Prevalence of Anemia Among Residents of Olmsted County,
Minnesota, Who Received Medical Attention at Mayo Clinic

| Sex | Olmsted County residents | | | |
	Observed number of existing cases	Total number at risk for anemia	Rate[a]	95% CI
Male	1,580	32,470	6.6	6.3–6.9
Female	4,851	36,959	12.4	12.1–12.8
Total[b]	6,431	69,429	9.3	9.1–9.5

[a]Prevalence per 100 persons directly age-adjusted to the structure of the 1990 U.S. white population.
[b]Age- and sex-adjusted.
Abbreviation: CI, confidence interval.
Modified from Ania et al. *(3)*. By permission of Mayo Foundation for Medical Education and Research.

from a large group of possible drugs. Drugs found to be promising in phase II studies need to be compared with the current standard treatment to determine whether a new standard of care is warranted. This comparison occurs in a phase III clinical trial, in which the drug or treatment is evaluated in a large-scale randomized study. Depending on the disease and the research question, phase III trials can include hundreds to thousands of patients. For more information on the conduct of clinical trials, see Pocock *(2)*.

Whether the chosen study design is retrospective or prospective, an understanding of the following commonly used terms is essential to the analysis phase.

COMMONLY USED TERMS

In describing patterns of a disease in a population, "prevalence" and "incidence" are two commonly used terms.

> **Definition**
>
> Prevalence of a disease is the *frequency of existing cases* of a disease in a specific study population during a specific time period. It is defined by the *number of existing cases* of a disease in a specific time period divided by the *total number of people in the study population who are at risk for the disease during the time period*.

Example: To illustrate how prevalence is used, consider the data from Ania et al. *(3)*, who studied the frequency of anemia among residents of Olmsted County, Minnesota, who received care at Mayo Clinic. The data in Table 1 summarize the existing cases of anemia from 1985 to 1989.

In this example, the unadjusted (crude) prevalence rate of anemia among male subjects is 4.9% (1,580/32,470). To facilitate meaningful comparisons between rates calculated from different geographic regions, prevalence rates are often age- and sex-adjusted to a standard reference population. In this example, prevalence was age- and sex-adjusted to the 1990 U.S. white population. The age- and sex-adjusted prevalence rates reported in Table 1 cannot be calculated directly from the data presented. The age-adjusted prevalence rates were 6.6 per 100 persons for male subjects and 12.4 per 100 persons for female subjects; the age- and sex-adjusted prevalence rate is 9.3 per 100 persons, with a 95% confidence interval of 9.1 to 9.5. Confidence intervals are discussed in more detail in the next section.

Definition

Incidence of a disease is the rate at which *new cases* of a disease develop in a specific population during a specific time period. It is defined by the number of *new cases* of a disease in a specific time period divided by the *number of people at risk of getting the disease at the beginning of the time period.*

Prevalence and incidence rates are often calculated by age and sex groupings to assess potential age or sex differences. They also frequently are calculated and compared over time to study the historical trends of a particular disease. Whether a prevalence or incidence rate is appropriate depends on the research question. If the research question concerns the number of *existing cases* of a disease, a prevalence rate is appropriate, whereas if the research question concerns the rate of *new cases* of a disease, an incidence rate is appropriate. For more detailed information regarding the calculation of prevalence and incidence, see Rimm et al. *(4).*

Two additional terms frequently used in medical research are "sensitivity" and "specificity." Sensitivity and specificity are most frequently used to compare new diagnostic tools and screening tests with existing methods.

Definition

Sensitivity is the probability that a test will show a positive result for a disease in a person who truly has the disease.

Definition

Specificity is the probability that a test will show a negative result for a disease in a person who truly does not have the disease.

Example: As an illustration of sensitivity and specificity, consider data from Lozano et al. *(5),* who compared the polymerase chain reaction (PCR) method of detecting clonal immunoglobulin heavy-chain (IgH) gene rearrangements with the traditional Southern blot hybridization (SBH) analysis. Frozen tissue from 147 cases of hematolymphoid proliferations was used to compare the semi-nested IgH-PCR method with the standard SBH method of determining clonality. The results are given in Table 2.

In this example, SBH is considered the true measure, or standard, with which the PCR method was compared. According to the information in Table 2, the sensitivity of PCR is calculated to be 0.715 (60/84), or 71.5%. This can be interpreted by stating that the result of the PCR method was clonal in 71.5% of cases in which the "true" result was clonal (as determined by SBH). Therefore, in 28.5% (that is, 100% – 71.5%) of the cases, the PCR method failed to accurately detect a "true" clonal result. The *false negative rate* is defined as 1 – sensitivity; therefore, the false negative rate for the PCR method is estimated to be 28.5%. Similarly, from Table 2, the specificity of PCR is calculated to be 0.92 (58/63), or 92%, meaning that the PCR result was nonclonal in 92% of cases in which the SBH result was actually nonclonal. A specificity of 92% implies a *false positive rate* of 8%.

Another definition of interest is the *overall concordance rate*, or the percentage of time the two tests produce the same result. For this example, the overall concordance rate was 0.802 (118/147), or 80.2%. For more information regarding sensitivity and specificity, see Rimm et al. *(4).*

Table 2
Comparison of SBH and Semi-Nested PCR
Regardless of the Type of Lymphoid Proliferation[a]

| SBH | Semi-nested IgH-PCR | | | | Total no. |
| | Clonal | | Nonclonal | | |
	No.	%	No.	%	
Clonal[b]	60	71.5	24	28.5	84
Nonclonal[c]	5	8.0	58	92.0	63
Total	65		82		147

[a]Among the total 147 cases, there was overall concordance in 118 cases (80.2%).
[b]IgH rearrangements.
[c]PCRβ rearrangements only or germline configuration.
Abbreviations: IgH, immunoglobulin heavy-chain; PCR, polymerase chain reaction; SBH, Southern blot hybridization.
From Lozano et al. *(5).* © Copyright 1996 American Cancer Society. Reprinted by permission of Wiley-Liss, Inc., a subsidiary of John Wiley & Sons, Inc.

HYPOTHESIS TESTING

In many studies the goal is to answer a specific research question. In such situations, a hypothesis test is often used. A hypothesis test consists of comparing a null hypothesis (H_0) with an alternative hypothesis (H_a). The null hypothesis is the state of nature the investigator is trying to find evidence against, while the alternative hypothesis is the state of nature the investigator suspects to be true. A hypothesis test is based on a test statistic calculated from the data which assesses whether there is evidence against the null hypothesis. One of two decisions results from a hypothesis test: 1) the null hypothesis is rejected, or 2) the null hypothesis is not rejected. In a hypothesis-testing situation, the underlying truth is never known. However, there are conceptually four possible outcomes, as shown in Table 3.

If H_0 is rejected when it is truly *false*, no error occurs. Likewise, if H_0 is not rejected when it is in fact *true*, no error occurs. The remaining two scenarios, however, both result in erroneous outcomes, which are referred to as type I and type II errors.

Definition

A type I error occurs if H_0 is rejected when it is in fact *true*.
The probability of a type I error is commonly referred to as alpha (α), or the size of the hypothesis test.

Definition

A type II error occurs if H_0 is not rejected when it is in fact *false*.
The probability of a type II error is commonly referred to as beta (β).

For example, in a group of patients with multiple myeloma who are anemic, it may be of interest to determine whether the mean pretreatment reticulocyte count in patients who have responded to treatment (μ_1) is different from the mean pretreatment reticulocyte count in nonresponding patients (μ_2). In this example, the null hypothesis is that the two means are equal (H_0: $\mu_1 = \mu_2$); the alternative hypothesis is that a difference exists (H_a: $\mu_1 \neq \mu_2$). Each hypothesis test is designed with a specific size and power, as defined below.

Table 3
Four Possible Outcomes of a Hypothesis Test

Possible result of the hypothesis test	Truth	Outcome
H_0 is rejected	H_0 is false	No error
H_0 is not rejected	H_0 is true	No error
H_0 is rejected	H_0 is true	Type I error exists
H_0 is not rejected	H_0 is false	Type II error exists

Abbreviation: H_0, null hypothesis.

Definition

Power is defined as the probability that H_0 is rejected if H_a is in fact true. Power is equivalent to 1 minus the probability of a type II error $(1 - \beta)$.

From a statistical standpoint, a favorable study design has a small probability of both type I (α) and type II (β) errors. Commonly, the probability of a type I error is specified (convention is to use $\alpha = 0.05$), and then an appropriate sample size is determined to achieve the desired power.

Hypothesis tests can be either one-sided or two-sided. The difference between one-sided and two-sided tests is evident by the way the formal hypothesis is stated:

Two-sided test
$H_0: \mu_1 = \mu_2$
vs.
$H_a: \mu_1 \neq \mu_2$

One-sided test
$H_0: \mu_1 \leq \mu_2$ $H_0: \mu_1 \leq \mu_2$
vs.   or   vs.
$H_a: \mu_1 > \mu_2$ $H_a: \mu_1 < \mu_2$

In a two-sided hypothesis test, any difference between groups is of interest, regardless of direction. In a one-sided hypothesis test, only differences in one direction are considered relevant. In most cases, a two-sided test is used, even if the direction of a suspected difference is known.

A **p-value** for a hypothesis test is the probability of obtaining a result as extreme as that obtained from the study data, given that H_0 is true. A **p-value** ≤ 0.05 is often used to denote statistical significance. However, the context of the problem could always be considered. For more information regarding these topics, see Rosner *(6)*.

COMMONLY USED STATISTICAL METHODS

Many statistical techniques are based on the theory of hypothesis testing. The appropriate technique is specific to each problem. The terms "parametric" and "nonparametric" define two categories of statistical methods. Parametric tests are used when the distribution of the data can be assumed to approximate one of several commonly used probability distributions (such as normal, Poisson, binomial). Nonparametric tests make fewer assumptions about the nature of the data and are used when it is questionable whether the data satisfy the distributional assumptions required for a parametric analysis. Guidelines for using a parametric or a nonparametric test are given for each of the hypothesis tests reviewed here.

Tests for Continuous Variables

Often in hematology research, the end point of interest is a continuous variable. Continuous variables are used for data measured in a scale of equal units, such as age in years, weight in kilograms, or hematocrit in grams per liter. When data are summarized, continuous variables are typically given with the mean and standard deviation (mean ± SD) and sometimes also with the median and range.

TWO-SAMPLE PROBLEMS

Frequently, the answer to a research question involves the comparison of two groups. For randomized prospective studies the groups being compared are typically treatment groups. For nonrandomized studies (prospective or retrospective), the groups are frequently defined by a specific patient or outcome characteristic (such as males vs. females, responders vs. nonresponders). When the end point of interest is a continuous variable, the two-sample *t*-test (parametric) or Wilcoxon rank sum test (nonparametric) is commonly used.

Two-Sample Tests

The following are guidelines for using two-sample tests:

1. Used specifically for comparing the means (two-sample *t*) or medians (Wilcoxon rank sum) of two samples.
2. Used when data are continuous.
3. The data are assumed to be independent. Data are assumed to be **independent** if the value of each data point in no way alters or depends on the value of any other data point.
4a. If both sample populations are assumed to be approximately normally distributed, with equal variances, use a two-sample *t*-test.
4b. If assumption 4a is inappropriate, use the Wilcoxon rank sum test.

The specific hypothesis being tested varies slightly between the two-sample *t*-test and the Wilcoxon rank sum test. The two-sample *t*-test tests the equality of the means of two samples. The rank sum test analyzes the ranks of the individual data points, rather than the actual values. By using the ranks, the test compares the medians of the groups rather than the means.

For more information regarding the calculation of these two-sample tests, see Rosner *(6)*.

Example: Two-Sample *t*-Test: To demonstrate the use of the two-sample *t*-test, consider data from Garton et al. *(7)*, in which 20 patients with the anemia of multiple myeloma and a hematocrit value less than 30 g/L were studied in a randomized, placebo-controlled, double-blind clinical trial. Twenty patients were randomized to receive either epoetin alfa ($n = 10$) or placebo ($n = 10$). Hematocrit levels were determined for each patient at baseline and at 12 weeks. To assess the efficacy of epoetin alfa, the mean change in the hematocrit level from baseline to week 12 (delta) for each individual was compared between the two groups (epoetin alfa and placebo). The following hypothesis test was used:

$$H_0: \text{mean change}_{(\text{epoetin alfa group})} = \text{mean change}_{(\text{placebo group})}$$

vs.

$$H_a: \text{mean change}_{(\text{epoetin alfa group})} \neq \text{mean change}_{(\text{placebo group})}$$

The mean ± SD change in hematocrit level was 2.7 ± 2.2 g/L for the epoetin alfa group and 0.63 ± 1.6 g/L for the placebo group (Table 4).

Table 4
Summary of Change in Hematocrit Level
from Baseline to 12 Weeks in Patients
Receiving Epoetin Alfa or Placebo

Stem	Placebo (n = 10)	Epoetin alfa (n = 10)
−1		6
−1	2	
−0	8	
−0	5 3 1	
0	2	
0	5	
1		0 4 4
1		
2	4	
2	5	5
3		
3	5	
4		0 2
4		5 7
5		3

In this example, the goal is the comparison of two groups, the variable of interest is continuous, and the data are considered independent. Guideline 4a on page 437 states that to use the two-sample *t*-test, the data should be approximately normally distributed, with equal variances. The stem and leaf plots in Table 4 show the data for the change in hematocrit level for each group. From inspection of these plots, there is no evidence of outliers (atypical data points) or other severe departures from what would be expected if the data were from a normal distribution. Furthermore, there is no reason to suspect that the variance in hematocrit level should differ between groups. Therefore, it is reasonable to assume that these data satisfy the assumptions for the two-sample *t*-test. The p-value associated with the two-sample *t*-test for these data is 0.02, indicating a statistically significant difference between groups. Therefore, from these data there is evidence that in patients with multiple myeloma who are anemic and have a hematocrit value less than 30 g/L, the use of epoetin alfa increases the hematocrit level from baseline to week 12 significantly more than does a placebo.

Example: Wilcoxon Rank Sum Test: To illustrate the Wilcoxon rank sum test, consider the data from Billadeau et al. *(8)*, who studied plasma cell proliferative disorders in 43 patients with monoclonal gammopathies. The 43 patients included 8 with smoldering multiple myeloma (SMM) and 15 with multiple myeloma (MM). One comparison made was the percentage of clonal cells detected by allele-specific oligonucleotide-polymerase chain reaction (ASO-PCR) in the two groups of patients. The following hypothesis test compares the difference of the medians between the two samples.

$$H_0: \text{median}_{\text{(SMM group)}} = \text{median}_{\text{(MM group)}}$$

vs.

$$H_a: \text{median}_{\text{(SMM group)}} \neq \text{median}_{\text{(MM group)}}$$

In this example, the goal is the comparison of two groups with respect to a continuous variable. The stem and leaf plots in Table 5 show the data for the percentage of clonal cells

Table 5
Percentage of Clonal Cells Detected in
Smoldering Multiple Myeloma (SMM) and
Multiple Myeloma (MM) With ASO-PCR

Stem	SMM (n = 8)	MM (n = 15)
0	0 0 0 0 0 0 1	0 0 0 0 1 1 2 2 3 4
0		6 7 8
1		
1		
2		
2		
3		
3		
4		
4		
5		
5		
6		0
6		
7		0
7		
8		
8		
9		
9		
10	0	

Abbreviation: ASO-PCR, allele-specific oligonucleo-
tides-polymerase chain reaction.

detected for each group. From evaluation of these plots, outliers are apparent (6.0, 7.0, and 10.0). When outliers such as these are detected, the first response should be to verify that the data are correct and not the result of an error in data recording or entry. In this case, it can be assumed that the data have been verified to be accurate. The presence of outliers makes it unrealistic to assume the data are approximately normally distributed. Therefore, the rank sum test is appropriate. The p-value associated with the rank sum test for these data ($p = 0.06$) showed a borderline significant difference between the two groups in median percentage of clonal cells detected. Therefore, from these data there was some evidence to suggest that patients with active MM had a higher percentage of clonal cells detected than those with SMM.

If the goal of the study is to compare more than two groups with a parametric approach, a one-way analysis of variance (**ANOVA**) is the appropriate statistical method. When more than two groups are to be compared with a nonparametric approach, the **Kruskal-Wallis test** is the appropriate statistical method. For more information regarding these topics, see Rosner *(6)*.

ONE-SAMPLE PROBLEM

In the previous two examples, the goal was to compare two independent distributions. The following two examples are of one-sample problems. In the one-sample problem, the goal is to make an inference based on a single distribution. The test statistic is based on comparing the mean or median of the distribution with a constant using the one-sample *t*-test (parametric) or signed rank test (nonparametric) as appropriate. A **paired comparison** is a special case of the one-sample problem, in which each data point from one sample can be matched to a unique data point from the other sample. This matching implies that the two samples are not independent; therefore, such data should not be analyzed with a two-sample technique. Instead, the matching is taken into account by calculating the difference between each matched pair, resulting in a sample of paired differences that can be analyzed with a one-sample technique. The paired *t*-test often referred to in the literature is actually a one-sample *t*-test comparing the mean of the distribution of paired differences with zero.

One-Sample Tests

The following are guidelines for using one-sample tests:

1. Used specifically to compare the mean of a distribution against a constant, or in the case of a paired test to compare the mean (paired *t*-test) or median (signed rank test) paired difference against zero.
2. Used when data are continuous.
3a. The data are assumed to be normally distributed. In the case of the paired *t*-test, it is the distribution of paired differences which is assumed to be normally distributed.
3b. If assumption 3a is inappropriate, use the signed rank test.

The specific hypothesis being tested varies slightly between the paired *t*-test and the signed rank test. The paired *t*-test compares the mean paired difference with zero. Similar to the rank sum test, the signed rank test uses the ranks of the data rather than the actual values. By using the ranks, the signed rank test compares the median of the distribution against zero.

For more information regarding the calculation of these one-sample tests, see Rosner *(6)*.

Example: Paired *t*-Test: To demonstrate the use of the paired *t*-test, consider again the data from Garton et al. *(7)* used in the example on page 437. The 10 patients who received placebo in the double-blind phase of the study were followed for 12 weeks. It was of interest to study the change in hematocrit level from baseline to 12 weeks in this group of patients. The data in Table 6 show two measurements for each patient, one at baseline (1) and one at 12 weeks (2). Next, for each patient, the difference between (1) and (2) was calculated.

The following is the hypothesis test that was used for these data:

$$H_0: \text{mean difference } \{(1) - (2)\} = 0$$
$$\text{vs.}$$
$$H_a: \text{mean difference } \{(1) - (2)\} \neq 0$$

To perform this test, a paired *t*-test using the above-stated hypothesis was conducted. The mean difference in hematocrit level from baseline to 12 weeks is 1.26 g/L. The p-value for this paired *t*-test is 0.24, indicating that for these data there was no evidence of a significant change in hematocrit from baseline to 12 weeks in patients randomized to receive placebo.

Example: Wilcoxon Signed Rank Test: To summarize the use of the signed rank test, consider the data from Adair et al. *(9)*, in which the effect of food on the bioavailability of chlorambucil in patients with hematologic malignancies was studied. Pharmacokinetic studies were performed on 10 patients during days 1 and 2 of chemotherapy; the question of interest was whether food could affect the time to peak plasma concentration.

Table 6
Change From Baseline to 12 Weeks
in the Placebo Group

Case	Baseline (1)	12 Weeks (2)	Difference: (1) – (2)
1	22.7	22.1	0.60
2	28.0	28.9	–0.90
3	27.6	26.7	0.90
4	24.0	29.0	–5.00
5	26.0	25.9	0.10
6	27.7	28.1	–0.40
7	27.6	25.3	2.30
8	24.5	22.9	1.60
9	26.3	31.1	–4.80
10	26.5	33.5	–7.00

The patients were randomly assigned to fasting on either day 1 or day 2 of treatment. Each patient had paired data consisting of fasting and nonfasting measures of six different pharmacokinetic factors. One of the factors, time to peak plasma concentration (minutes), will be considered for this example (Table 7).

Because there are paired data, a one-sample approach should be used. The distribution of the paired differences is known to be highly skewed for variables such as time to peak plasma concentration; therefore, the use of the paired t-test is not appropriate and the Wilcoxon signed rank test should be used. In this case, the p-value associated with the Wilcoxon signed rank test comparing the median difference (nonfasting minus fasting) with zero gives a p-value < 0.01, indicating that there is a statistically significant difference in time to peak plasma concentration between fasting and nonfasting patients.

Tests for Categorical Variables

Sometimes in hematology research the end point of interest is defined with a **categorical** variable. Unlike a continuous variable, the measurement scale for a categorical variable consists of a set of possible categories or groups. For example, a categorical variable defines response to treatment as complete response, partial response, stable disease, or progression of disease. When two categorical variables are compared, a contingency table is often constructed. Table 8 is a 2×2 contingency table comparing sex and response to treatment.

If the two variables are independent (not associated), the **expected number of events** in each cell can be calculated by multiplying the total number of events in the cell's row by the total number of events in the cell's column and dividing this product by the total number of observations. For the data presented in Table 8, if there is no association between response to treatment and sex, the expected number of males who would have responded to treatment is $(9 \times 12)/20$, or 5.4. The chi-squared test is a statistical method used to test the independence of two categorical variables. The chi-squared test is appropriate when the expected number of events in every cell of the contingency table is 5 or more. Fisher's exact test is very similar to the chi-squared test; however, fewer distributional assumptions are made. When the expected number of events in any cell of a contingency table is less than 5, Fisher's exact test is appropriate.

Table 7
Summary of Time to Peak Plasma Concentration
After Administration of Oral Chlorambucil

Case	*Time to peak plasma concentration, min*		
	Fasting	*Nonfasting*	*Difference*
1	36	38	2
2	70	70	0
3	35	118	83
4	125	230	105
5	35	72	37
6	33	245	212
7	30	118	88
8	29	42	13
9	28	57	29
10	15	29	14

Modified from Adair et al. *(9)*. By permission of
Springer-Verlag GmbH & Company KG.

Table 8
Example of a 2 × 2 Contingency Table

Sex	*Response to treatment, no.*		
	Yes	*No*	*Total*
Male	7	5	12
Female	2	6	8
Total	9	11	20

TESTS FOR INDEPENDENCE OF CATEGORICAL VARIABLES

The following are guidelines for comparing categorical variables:

1. Used to test the hypothesis of independence between two variables.
2. The variables being compared are categorical (can be arranged in an R × C contingency table, where R = number of rows and C = number of columns).
3a. If the sample size is "reasonably" large, use the chi-squared test. The sample size is considered to be reasonably large when the *expected* number of events in *each* of the cells of the contingency table is 5 or more.
3b. If guideline 3a is not met, use Fisher's exact test.

For more details about the chi-squared test and Fisher's exact test, see Rosner *(6)*.

Example: Chi-Squared Test: To demonstrate the chi-squared test, consider data from Pisansky et al. *(10)*, who studied patterns of tumor relapse after mastectomy and adjuvant systemic therapy in patients with axillary lymph node-positive breast cancer. In that study, 564 patients received either cyclophosphamide, 5-fluorouracil, and prednisone (CFP) or CFP and tamoxifen (CFPT). A total of 184 patients achieved a response to treatment. A research question of interest was whether the occurrence of isolated locoregional initial relapses at 3 years differed by treatment among these 184 patients. The following hypothesis test is appropriate for this question:

Table 9
Isolated Locoregional Initial Relapse Distribution by
Treatment Among 184 Patients With Relapse by Year 3

| Treatment | *Initial relapse location* | | | | Total |
| | *Isolated locoregional* | | *Other* | | |
	No.	%	No.	%	
CFP	35	33.3	70	66.7	105
CFPT	33	41.8	46	58.2	79
Total	68	37.0	116	63.0	184

Abbreviations: CFP, cyclophosphamide, 5-fluorouracil, and prednisone; CFPT, CFP and tamoxifen.

H_0: Response to treatment and sex are independent

vs.

H_a: Response to treatment and sex are not independent

The two variables—type of relapse and treatment—are categorical and can be represented in a 3×2 contingency table (Table 9).

In this example, the chi-squared p-value is 0.24, indicating that the null hypothesis should not be rejected because there is not sufficient evidence to suggest, according to the data, that treatment and initial relapse location are associated.

Example: Fisher's Exact Test: Consider the data from Kyle et al. *(11)*, who studied three treatments for primary amyloidosis. Two hundred twenty patients were randomized to receive colchicine alone (C), melphalan and prednisone (MP), or melphalan, prednisone, and colchicine (MPC). The response information for the 134 patients who had an abnormal serum albumin level, by regimen, is summarized in Table 10.

The proportions of patients who had an abnormal serum albumin level at randomization and responded to treatment in the C, MP, and MPC groups were $p_1 = 1/50$ (2.0%), $p_2 = 7/42$ (16.7%), and $p_3 = 6/42$ (14.3%), respectively. In this example, the hypothesis test is testing whether p_1, p_2, and p_3 are equal. Fisher's exact test was the preferred method in this example because guideline 3a on page 442 was not met.

Fisher's exact p-value in this example is < 0.03, indicating that the proportion of patients with an abnormal serum albumin level at randomization who responded to treatment is *not* equal across regimens. One possible interpretation is that in patients who have an abnormal serum albumin level at randomization, those randomized to C have a lower response rate than those randomized to MP or MPC.

Summary

The hypothesis tests described above are those most commonly used in hematology research. The appropriate test depends primarily on the sample size, the type of data being analyzed, and the distributional assumptions required. All of the tests described can be calculated with most standard statistical software. Commonly, a p-value of ≤ 0.05 denotes statistical significance. However, each situation is unique, and therefore the choice of α and the interpretation of a given p-value should be made within the context of the problem. Table 11 summarizes the hypothesis tests and their classification.

Table 10
Response to Treatment Among Patients
With Primary Amyloidosis Who Had an
Abnormal Serum Albumin Level at Randomization[a]

| | Response to treatment | | | | |
| | Yes | | No | | |
Treatment	No.	%	No.	%	Total
C	1	2.0	49	98.0	50
MP	7	16.7	35	83.3	42
MPC	6	14.3	36	85.7	42
Total	14	10.5	120	89.5	134

[a]Not all patients had an abnormal serum albumin level at randomization,
 Abbreviations: C, colchicine; MP, melphalan and prednisone; MPC, MP + C.
 Data from Kyle et al. (11).

Table 11
Summary of Hypothesis Tests

Type of data	Parametric methods	Nonparametric methods	Use
Continuous	Two-sample t-test	Rank sum test	Compare two independent medians
Continuous	One-way analysis of variance	Kruskal-Wallis test	Compare more than two independent medians
Continuous	One-sample t-test or paired t-test	Signed-rank test	Compare one mean against a constant
Categorical	χ^2 test	Fisher's exact test	Study the independence of two variables

Confidence Intervals

The statistical methods considered have been designed to test a hypothesis, that is, to provide a yes-or-no answer to a question. Another important statistical tool is the confidence interval (CI), which is designed to provide information about the precision of one's knowledge about some value. Most statistical methods involve using a sample to estimate some value, such as a rate, a probability, or a mean. Frequently, a CI for these values is calculated. For example, in a clinical trial of 30 patients, if the observed response rate is 60% (18/30) with a 95% confidence interval of 41%-77%, then 60% is the sample-based estimate of the "true" response rate, and 41%-77% is a 95% CI for the "true" response rate. The theory behind a 95% CI is as follows. If the experiment was repeated many times, and each time a 95% CI was calculated, then 95% of the time the CI would contain the "true" response rate. For more information regarding the calculation of CI for various parameters and the connection between hypothesis testing and CI, see Rosner (6).

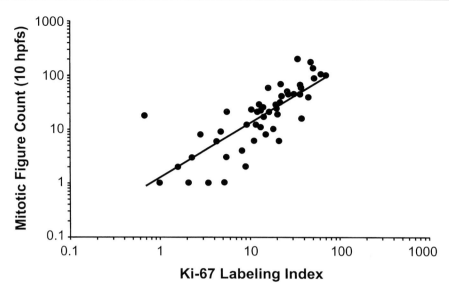

Fig. 1. Scatter diagram of mitotic figure count and Ki-67 labeling index. A log transformation of the data was done to ensure constant measurement variability over the range of measurement. (From Weidner et al. [*12*]. By permission of WB Saunders Company.)

Correlation and Regression

Correlation and regression analyses are statistical methods designed to describe the relationship between two or more continuous variables. Specifically, regression analysis is a method used to predict the value of one variable (the dependent variable) given the value of another variable(s) (the independent variable). For example, in a dose-response study, an investigator varies the dose of a particular drug (independent variable) and studies the effect on patient response (dependent variable).

SCATTER DIAGRAMS

The first step in investigating the relationship between two continuous variables is to plot the data on a scatter diagram. A scatter diagram graphically displays the association between two continuous variables. Each point on the diagram represents the value for one observation in the data set, with the dependent variable represented on the y-axis and the independent variable represented on the x-axis.

Example: Consider the data from Weidner et al. *(12)*, depicted in Figure 1, in which the relationship between two methods of measuring tumor proliferation (mitotic figure count and Ki-67 labeling index) was studied in 50 patients with breast cancer.

Each plotted point on the graph represents an observation for one patient consisting of an x value (Ki-67 labeling index) and a corresponding y value (mitotic figure count). If a regression analysis is intended, the y-axis typically represents the dependent variable and the x-axis represents the independent variable. To assess the statistical significance of the association between the variables, a correlation analysis was performed.

CORRELATION

A correlation analysis is used to study the strength of the relationship between two continuous variables. In general, the **correlation coefficient** (ρ) describes the degree of relationship between two variables. Consistent with statistical methods described previously, there are both parametric and nonparametric approaches to studying correlation. The parametric approach is called the *Pearson product moment correlation* and is used when each of the variables is assumed to follow a normal distribution. The nonparametric approach is called the *Spearman rank correlation* and is appropriate when distributional assumptions are in question. In either case, a sample correlation coefficient (r) is calculated. The correlation coefficient lies between -1 and $+1$ and is interpreted as follows. Two variables having $r > 0$ are defined to be positively correlated, meaning that as one of the variables increases, the other also tends to increase. Two variables having $r < 0$ are defined to be negatively correlated, implying that as x increases, y tends to decrease. The closer r is to $+1$ or -1, the stronger the positive or negative correlation between the two variables. If $r = 0$, the variables are not correlated (not associated). If $|r| = 1$, then the dependent variable can be predicted exactly from the independent variable (and vice versa). The Pearson correlation coefficient for the data shown in Figure 1 is $+0.78$.

Having calculated a sample correlation coefficient of $+0.78$, what conclusions can be drawn about the association between mitotic figure count and Ki-67 labeling index? To make inference on the value of ρ, a hypothesis test that asks the following question is performed: If $\rho = 0$ (no correlation between mitotic figure count and Ki-67 labeling index), what is the chance of obtaining a sample correlation coefficient as extreme as $r = 0.78$? The specific hypothesis test uses the following null and alternative hypotheses.

$$H_0: \rho = 0$$
$$\text{vs.}$$
$$H_a: \rho \neq 0$$

The p-value for this hypothesis test is < 0.0001, indicating that if there were no correlation, a resulting $r = 0.78$ would occur by chance less than 1 time in 10,000. Therefore, the conclusion is that a significant positive correlation exists between the two variables.
Points of caution:

1. The correlation coefficient applies to a linear relationship between two variables. Thus, $r = 0$ does not mean there is no relationship between the two variables, only that a linear relationship does not exist.
2. The observed correlation cannot be extrapolated to points outside the range of the sample data.
3. A strong correlation ($+$ or $-$) between two variables does not imply causation.
   For more information regarding correlation analysis, see Colton *(13)*.

SIMPLE LINEAR REGRESSION

A natural extension of correlation analysis is simple linear regression. Simple linear regression involves fitting a straight line to a scatter of data points such as those in Figure 1. The least complex linear equation that describes the dependence of y on x is of the form $y = a + bx$, where *a* is the *intercept* (the value of y when x is 0) and *b* is the *slope* (the increase in y corresponding to an increase of 1 unit in x).

The simple linear regression model based on the form of the equation $y = a + bx$ is defined as follows:

Definition

Given observed values (x_1, y_1), (x_2, y_2), ... , (x_n, y_n) for an independent (x_i) and a dependent (y_i) variable, the general statistical model for simple linear regression is:

$$y_i = \beta_0 + \beta_1 x_i + \varepsilon_i$$

where i = 1, 2, ... , n. The ε_i are the model residuals and are assumed to be independent and normally distributed, with a mean 0 and a standard deviation σ.

The intercept (β_0) and slope (β_1) are estimated by the **method of least squares** (for more information see Moore and McCabe [14]). In a regression model, β_1 is called the regression coefficient and can be interpreted as the increase in y corresponding to an increase of 1 unit in x. The following hypothesis test can be used to answer the question: "Is x a significant predictor of y?"

$$H_0: \beta_1 = 0$$
$$\text{vs.}$$
$$H_a: \beta_1 \neq 0$$

If the p-value for the hypothesis test is ≤ 0.05, there is significant evidence that $\beta_1 \neq 0$, indicating that x and y are associated and that β_1 is the change in y corresponding to an increase of 1 unit in x.

The definition above can be extended to the fitting of a linear relationship in which there is more than one independent variable. This technique is called *multiple linear regression*. The general statistical model for multiple linear regression is:

$$y_i = \beta_0 + \beta_1 x_{i1} + \beta_2 x_{i2} + \dots + \beta_p x_{ip} + \varepsilon_i,$$

where p is the number of independent variables. The ε_i are the model residuals and are assumed to be independent and normally distributed, with a mean 0 and a standard deviation σ. For more information on multiple regression, see Moore and McCabe *(14)*.

LOGISTIC REGRESSION

The model stated above is for cases in which the dependent variable is continuous. Regression also can be performed when the dependent variable is binary. A **binary** variable is one that takes on one of two possible values (0 or 1, success or failure, yes or no). If the dependent variable is binary, logistic regression is an appropriate statistical method. The goal of logistic regression is the same as that of any regression technique—to find the best model to describe the relationship between a dependent and an independent variable(s). Aside from a different model and set of assumptions, the methods used in logistic regression analysis follow the same general principles used in linear regression. In logistic regression, the association of the independent variable and the binary dependent variable is often expressed using an **odds ratio** (defined in the example below). Multiple logistic regression is appropriate when there is more than one independent variable. For more information on multiple logistic regression and more details on the differences between linear and logistic regression, see Hosmer and Lemeshow *(15)*.

Example: Consider the data from Litzow et al. *(16)*, in which 73 patients who had a bone marrow transplantation between April 1982 and July 1996 were studied. The primary goal was to study the effect of several variables on the severity of veno-occlusive disease. All 73 patients had either severe (*n* = 28) or mild (*n* = 45) disease. The question of interest was the effect of maximal urea value (continuous independent variable) on the severity of veno-occlusive disease (binary dependent variable). The p-value associated with the test of hypothesis for β_1 is 0.001, indicating that there is strong evidence to suggest that the maximum urea value is predictive of the severity of veno-occlusive disease. Specifically, the estimated **odds ratio** for an increase in maximum urea concentration of 50 mg/dL is 4.3. This indicates that for every 50 mg/dL increase in the maximum urea value, the risk of having severe veno-occlusive disease (as opposed to mild) increases 4.3 times.

This summary of regression only begins to introduce a very complex subject. Techniques of nonlinear regression involving more complex mathematical forms are of benefit in other areas of medical research. For a fairly comprehensive coverage of regression, see Draper and Smith *(17)*.

Survival Analysis

When studying many hematologic diseases, the ultimate question often is how long the patients will survive after diagnosis. One way to study this question is to perform a survival analysis. A survival analysis is a summary of patient data in which the time from a well-defined starting point (t_0) to a well-defined end point (such as death) is studied. Although death is the most frequently used end point in survival analysis, others commonly analyzed are relapse, progression of disease, and treatment failure. In a prospective study, t_0 is usually defined as the date of randomization or the beginning of treatment; in a retrospective study, t_0 is often defined as the date of diagnosis. The amount of time from t_0 to the end point of interest is referred to as the *survival time* for a patient.

For most survival studies, patients enter the study at different calendar times and are followed until death or until some point in calendar time that marks the end of the study. At the time of analysis, the actual survival time for many patients will be observed, while some patients will still be alive. If a patient has not reached the end point (died) at the point in calendar time that marks the end of the study, then the survival time for that patient is "censored." For example, if a patient dies exactly 2 years after entering a study, the survival time is 2 years. However, if a patient entered the study exactly 2 years before the analysis was performed and was still alive at the time of the analysis, the patient's survival time would be "censored" at 2 years.

The graphic representation of survival times for a patient cohort is called a *survival curve*. A common statistical problem is to estimate and compare the survival curves of two or more patient cohorts. In many phase III clinical trials, patients are randomized to receive either the standard treatment or the experimental treatment, and the survival curves of the two cohorts are compared. Two methods are commonly used to estimate the survival curve in a patient population: 1) the actuarial, or life-table, method and 2) the Kaplan-Meier method. The Kaplan-Meier method is most commonly used in hematology research.

The survival curve is used to estimate the probability of surviving *t* or more years beyond study entry. When the Kaplan-Meier method is used, the survival curve is calculated taking into account the fact that some patients have "censored" survival times. Because the estimate of the survival curve changes only at the times when an end point is observed, the curve looks like a step function (see the example below). For more information regarding survival analysis and the Kaplan-Meier method, see Collett *(18)*.

LOG RANK TEST

The log rank test is a nonparametric hypothesis test that is used to compare the survival experience between two groups. The null hypothesis is that there is no difference in the survival experience between the two groups; the alternative hypothesis is that there is a difference in survival experience between the two groups. The log rank test statistic is calculated directly from the data and has a corresponding p-value. When the p-value is sufficiently small (usually ≤ 0.05), the null hypothesis of no difference in survival experience is rejected and it can be concluded that the two groups have a difference in survival experience.

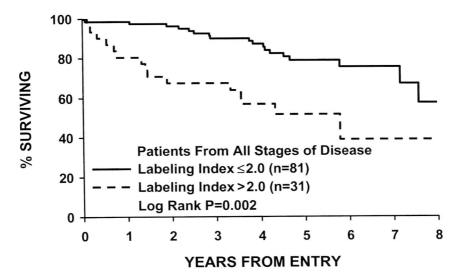

Fig. 2. Overall survival of 112 patients with low-grade non-Hodgkin's lymphomas, according to labeling index ($\leq 2\%$ vs. $> 2\%$).

Example: Consider the study by Witzig et al. *(19)* of 112 patients with low-grade non-Hodgkin's lymphoma, in which a goal of the study was to compare the survival between a group of patients with a bromodeoxyuridine labeling index of 2% or less ($n = 81$) and a group of patients with an index more than 2% ($n = 31$). For each patient, t_0 was defined as date of initial diagnosis. The survival curves for the two patient cohorts, constructed with the Kaplan-Meier method, are shown in Figure 2. The log rank p-value of 0.002 is indicative of a highly significant difference in survival between the two groups.

Another method frequently used for survival analysis is Cox *(20)* proportional hazards regression. When the prognostic significance of several independent variables in predicting time to death is studied, a Cox model may be the appropriate regression model to use. For more information, see Collett *(18)*.

SUMMARY

The statistical aspects of a research project need to be addressed early in the design phase of the study. The type of study design, sample size requirements, and statistical analysis methods are interrelated issues. A thorough understanding of statistics is required to design and carry out a study in a manner that will ensure the research question can be adequately addressed. The aim of this chapter was to introduce some of the frequently used statistical concepts, terms, and methods. Although this chapter is merely an introduction, many of the references provided give detailed descriptions of the statistical methods and their appropriate use. Many software packages are available for performing the statistical methods described. These packages, however, do not guarantee that the appropriate study design was chosen or that the appropriate statistical method is used. There is no substitute for a thorough understanding of the statistical implications inherent in hematology research.

ACKNOWLEDGMENT

The author thanks Daniel J. Sargent, Ph.D., for his thoughtful review of this chapter.

REFERENCES

1. Schlesselman JJ. *Case-Control Studies: Design, Conduct, Analysis*. Oxford University Press, New York, 1982.
2. Pocock SJ. *Clinical Trials: A Practical Approach*. John Wiley & Sons, New York, 1988.
3. Ania BJ, Suman VJ, Fairbanks VF, Melton LJ III. Prevalence of anemia in medical practice: community versus referral patients. *Mayo Clin Proc* 1994; 69: 730-735.
4. Rimm AA, Hartz AJ, Kalbfleisch JH, Anderson AJ, Hoffmann RG. *Basic Biostatistics in Medicine and Epidemiology*. Appleton-Century-Croft, New York, 1980.
5. Lozano MD, Tierens A, Greiner TC, Wickert RS, Weisenburger DD, Chan WC. Clonality analysis of B-lymphoid proliferations using the polymerase chain reaction. *Cancer* 1996; 77: 1349-1355.
6. Rosner BA. *Fundamentals of Biostatistics*, 3rd ed. PWS-Kent, Boston, 1990.
7. Garton JP, Gertz MA, Witzig TE, Greipp PR, Lust JA, Schroeder G, Kyle RA. Epoetin alfa for the treatment of the anemia of multiple myeloma. A prospective, randomized, placebo-controlled, double-blind trial. *Arch Intern Me*d 1995; 155: 2069-2074.
8. Billadeau D, Van Ness B, Kimlinger T, Kyle RA, Therneau TM, Greipp PR, Witzig TE. Clonal circulating cells are common in plasma cell proliferative disorders: a comparison of monoclonal gammopathy of undetermined significance, smoldering multiple myeloma, and active myeloma. *Blood* 1996; 88: 289-296.
9. Adair CG, Bridges JM, Desai ZR. Can food affect the bioavailability of chlorambucil in patients with haematological malignancies? *Cancer Chemother Pharmacol* 1986; 17: 99-102.
10. Pisansky TM, Ingle JN, Schaid DJ, Hass AC, Krook JE, Donohue JH, Witzig TE, Wold LE. Patterns of tumor relapse following mastectomy and adjuvant systemic therapy in patients with axillary lymph node-positive breast cancer. Impact of clinical, histopathologic, and flow cytometric factors. *Cancer* 1993; 72: 1247-1260.
11. Kyle RA, Gertz MA, Greipp PR, Witzig TE, Lust JA, Lacy MQ, Therneau TM. A trial of three regimens for primary amyloidosis: colchicine alone, melphalan and prednisone, and melphalan, prednisone, and colchicine. *N Engl J Med* 1997; 336: 1202-1207.
12. Weidner N, Moore DH II, Vartanian R. Correlation of Ki-67 antigen expression with mitotic figure index and tumor grade in breast carcinomas using the novel "paraffin"-reactive MIB1 antibody. *Hum Pathol* 1994; 25: 337-342.
13. Colton T. *Statistics in Medicine*. Little, Brown and Company, Boston, 1974.
14. Moore DS, McCabe GP. *Introduction to the Practice of Statistics*. WH Freeman and Company, New York, 1989.
15. Hosmer DW Jr, Lemeshow S. *Applied Logistic Regression*. John Wiley & Sons, New York, 1989.
16. Litzow M, Repoussis P, Schroeder G, Schembri-Wismayer D, Batts K, Anderson P, Arndt C, Gastineau D, Gertz M, Inwards D, Lacy M, Tefferi A, Noel P, Solberg L, Letendre L, Hoagland H. Veno-occlusive disease (VOD) of the liver following bone marrow transplantation (MBT): analysis of risk factors and results of therapy with tissue plasminogen activator (tPA) (abstract). *Blood* 1997; 90 Suppl 1: 220a.
17. Draper N, Smith H. *Applied Regression Analysis*, 2nd ed. John Wiley & Sons, New York, 1981.
18. Collett D. *Modelling Survival Data in Medical Research*. Chapman & Hall, London, 1994.
19. Witzig TE, Habermann TM, Kurtin PJ, Schroeder G, Stenson MJ, Greipp PR. S-phase fraction by the labeling index as a predictive factor for progression and survival in low grade non-Hodgkin's lymphoma. *Cancer* 1995; 76: 1059-1064.
20. Cox DR. Regression models and life-tables (with discussion). *J R Stat Soc [Series B]* 1972; 34: 181-220.

INDEX